AF352090

ANNALS OF THE NEW YORK ACADEMY OF SCIENCES

Volume 515

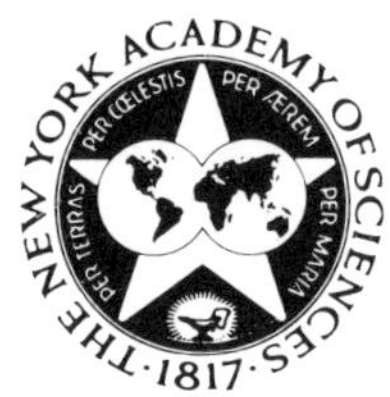

EDITORIAL STAFF

Executive Editor
BILL BOLAND

Managing Editor
JUSTINE CULLINAN

Associate Editor
STEFAN MALMOLI

The New York Academy of Sciences
2 East 63rd Street
New York, New York 10021

CENTRAL DETERMINANTS OF AGE-RELATED DECLINES IN MOTOR FUNCTION

ANNALS OF THE NEW YORK ACADEMY OF SCIENCES
Volume 515

CENTRAL DETERMINANTS OF AGE-RELATED DECLINES IN MOTOR FUNCTION

Edited by James A. Joseph

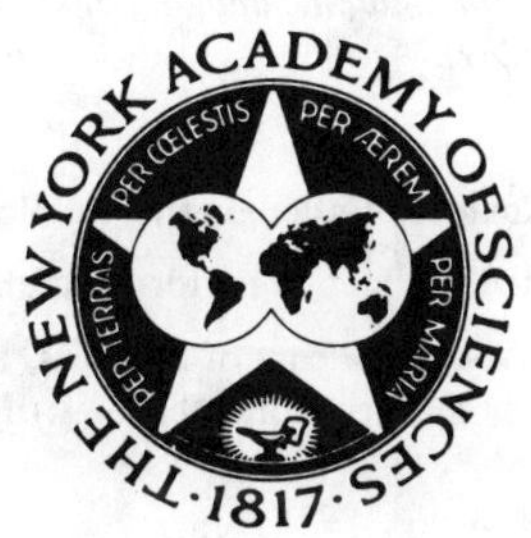

The New York Academy of Sciences
New York, New York
1988

The cover shows positron emission tomographic imaging of striatal dopamine in MPTP-induced parkinsonian monkeys (see page 232).

Library of Congress Cataloging in Publication Data

Central determinants of age-related declines in motor function/edited by James A. Joseph.

p. cm. — (Annals of the New York Academy of Sciences, ISSN 0077–8923; v. 515)
Presented at a conference held by the New York Academy of Sciences on October 1–3, 1986, in Rye Brook, N.Y.
Includes bibliographies and index.
ISBN 0-89766-425-6.   ISBN 0-89766-426-4 (pbk.)
1. Central nervous system — Aging — Congresses.   2. Efferent pathways — Aging — Congresses. 3. Central nervous system — Diseases — Age factors — Congresses.   4. Parkinsonism — Congresses.   I. Joseph, James A.   II. New York Academy of Sciences.   III. Series.   [DNLM: 1. Aging — physiology — congresses.   2. Movement — congresses.   W1 AN626YL v. 515 / WE 103 C397 1986]
Q11.N5 vol. 515
[QP370]
500 s — dc19
[599′.01852] .
DNLM/DLC   87-34319
for Library of Congress   CIP

CCP
Printed in the United States of America
ISBN 0-89766-425-6 (Cloth)
ISBN 0-89766-426-4 (Paper)
ISSN 0077-8923

ANNALS OF THE NEW YORK ACADEMY OF SCIENCES

Volume 515
January 18, 1988

CENTRAL DETERMINANTS OF AGE-RELATED DECLINES IN MOTOR FUNCTION[a]

Editor
JAMES A. JOSEPH

Conference Chairmen
JAMES A. JOSEPH, JAMES MORTIMER, DONALD INGRAM, and WANEEN SPIRDUSO

CONTENTS

[a] The papers in this volume were presented at a conference entitled Central Determinants of Age-Related Declines in Motor Function, which was held by the New York Academy of Sciences on October 1–3, 1986, in Rye Brook, New York.

Part VI. Poster Papers

Financial assistance was received from:
- BAYER AG/MILES
- HOECHST-ROUSSEL PHARMACEUTICALS, INC.
- MATRIX RESEARCH LABORATORIES, INC.—SUBSIDIARY OF PRAXIS PHARMACEUTICALS, INC.
- OFFICE OF NAVAL RESEARCH
- NATIONAL INSTITUTE ON AGING—NIH
- REVLON HEALTH CARE GROUP
- UNITED PARKINSON FOUNDATION
- THE UPJOHN COMPANY

Reaction Time, Speed of Performance, and Age

A. T. WELFORD[a]

Hadsley House
Guernsey, Channel Islands

Ever since the pioneering days of experimental psychology in the second half of the last century, reaction times have been studied in the attempt to discover and measure the mental events that intervene between the receipt of stimuli by the sense organs and the overt responses to them. If it takes longer to react under some conditions than others, then it is a fair question to ask how the difference of time is spent. Today, reaction times are probably the most powerful method that we have of relating so-called mental events to physical measures. They have proved to fit theories of central processing in the brain with astonishing precision in a number of cases and they provide a base on which to build understanding of the timing of movement and of the times taken by complex activities. Reaction times are of obvious importance in the study of aging because one of the most pervasive and striking of the changes that come with age is the slowing of performance.

COMPONENTS OF REACTION TIME

Between the onset of a sensory stimulus and the initiation of a response to it, there are at least six stages:

(1) Conversion of the stimulus by the sense organ into a signal consisting of a series of nerve impulses.
(2) Transmission of these to the brain.
(3) Perceptual identification of the signal.
(4) Choice of the response.
(5) Transmission from the brain to the effector muscles making the response.
(6) Activation of these muscles.

Some methods of measuring reaction time also include the time taken to make the responding movement; however, this is not traditionally included in the definition of reaction time.

The time taken by all these stages increases with age. The increases of transmission time in the second and fifth stages make only a small contribution to the lengthening of the total reaction time (rarely more than about 4 ms per meter of the nerve concerned). However, because the speed of conduction varies with the diameter of nerve fibers, the slowing of conduction in a bundle of mixed diameters will lead to impulses arriving at the far end over a longer period and will thus produce fewer impulses within

[a] Current address: 187A High Street, Aldeburgh, Suffolk, England IP15 5AL.

1

any critical interval for firing the next stage. As regards the first stage, appreciable slowing with age in the eye has been shown using the technique of backward masking: when subjects aged 61–76 were compared with those in their 20s, the interval over which a masking stimulus could negate perception of a previous stimulus was found to be substantially longer, especially if the first stimulus was brief.[1] The stimulus took longer in the older than in the younger subjects to generate a signal to the next stage and thus to avoid interference from a following stimulus.

Slowing is also appreciable at stage 6. For instance, Onishi[2] found that the time from the beginning of EMG recording to muscular contraction was some 18% greater for subjects aged 60–72 than for those in their 20s. Slowing at stage 6 is also implied by the finding of Travis,[3] which states that action tends to be initiated in phase with muscular tremor, and of Tiffin and Westhafer,[4] which states that reaction times are shorter and less variable when stimuli occur at the top and bottom points of a tremor cycle. A slowing of finger tremor from 8–10 cycles per second in the late teens, 20s, and 30s to 6–8 cycles in the 60s and 70s[5] would account for an increase of reaction time of about 16 ms. The increase should presumably not occur with verbal responses, and this is perhaps why Nebes[6] found that the average difference of simple reaction time between mean ages of 18.7 and 67.7 years was 17 ms less for vocal than for manual responses.

The main interest centers in the perception and choice at stages 3 and 4, which take up by far the largest part of the total reaction time. The two stages are difficult to separate, although this has been done in a number of studies (e.g., references 7 and 8). There is also controversy about whether perception has to be completed before choice can begin or whether they can overlap in time. For many purposes, though, the distinction between the two stages is not important and they can be treated together. Some indications of the processes involved in identification and choice are provided by the four experimental findings below.

(i) Reaction time usually increases with the number of possible signals and responses. Many studies have shown the increase to be logarithmic. Hick[9] defined choice reaction time as $a + b \log_2(N + 1)$ and Hyman[10] defined it as $a + b \log_2 N$, where a and b are intercept and slope, respectively, and N is the number of equiprobable signals and responses. In Hick's equation, a represents the delays in the apparatus and should otherwise be zero. In Hyman's equation, a represents the simple reaction time. It has become conventional to use logarithms to base 2 so that $\log N$ for the simple case = 0, for two choices = 1, for four = 2, and for eight = 3. Sometimes Hick's equation and sometimes Hyman's equation will fit the results better for reasons not yet fully understood.[11] Both identification and choice are included in b. When they have been separated, the logarithmic relation with N has been found to apply to both, with the slope somewhat less for identification than for choice.[12] The magnitude of b rises as the relationship between signals and their corresponding responses becomes more complex—for instance, when instead of a row of signal lights corresponding in order to a row of response keys, signals on the right have to be responded to with the left hand and vice versa, or when signals are numbers and responses are made on keys. Presumably, such complications mean that extra processes are required to match responses to signals.

Results of the many studies that have been made of reaction time in relation to age have been collected elsewhere.[13,14] They show that both simple and choice reaction times shorten from childhood to the 20s, lengthen slowly until the 50s, and thereafter change more rapidly. The simple reaction tasks and subjects in different studies have varied to an extent that few are really comparable with one another, but studies in which a simple key press or release was required in response to a light or sound showed rises from the 20s to the 60s of between 0 and 25% and a mean of 14.5%. With choice

TABLE 1. Choice Reaction Times Showing Differences between Age Groups of Intercept a and Slope b according to Hyman's[10] Equation[a]

Author and Task	Range of Choices	Younger				Older			Percent Age Differences	
		Age Range or Mean	a	b		Age Range or Mean	a	b	a	b
Suci *et al.*[15] — Speaking nonsense syllables on the disappearance of one or more of four lights	1,2,3,4	17–38	323	179		60–70	387	302	20	69
Talland & Cairnie[16] — Manual reactions to colored lights.	1,2	20–40	253	80		65–75	309	114	22	43
Griew[17,18] — Responses to lights in semicircle by moving stylus from central disc to corresponding disc in 5-inch radius semicircle. Reaction time was from appearance of light to leaving center disc.	2,4,8	20–28	288	73		48–62	307	94	7	29
Botwinick *et al.*[19] — Card sorting. Movement time included.	2,4,6,8,10	19–35	510	188		65–81	745	242	46	29
Morikiyo *et al.*[20] — Pressing keys under fingers to numbers shown on Nixie tube.	2,4,8	20–29	199	193		50–59	216	234	9	21
Szafran[21] — Pressing microswitches to neon lights.	3,5,8	32.3	272	85		47.7	288	82	6	−4
Same, but with subsidiary task of short-term retention or speaking with delayed auditory feedback.			393	89			447	87	14	−2
Crossman & Szafran[22] — Card sorting. Movement time included.	2,4,8	20–39	584	274		50–80	927	267	59	−3

[a] Reaction time $= a + b \log_2 N$, expressed in milliseconds.

reaction times, increases with age have been found in both the slope b and the intercept a of Hyman's equation, as shown in TABLE 1. Increases have been greater when the relationships between signals and responses have been complex than when they have been straightforward. Examples are given in TABLES 2 and 3.

(ii) If one of the possible signals in a choice reaction task occurs more frequently than others, reaction to it is, on average, faster. The same is true if the signals are equally frequent, but one follows another more often than it would by chance. Dramatic shortening of reaction time has also been found when the subject is told to react as fast as possible to all signals, but to concentrate especially on one. In this case, the shorter times for the signal on which the subject has concentrated are balanced by longer times for other signals, so the overall mean is not changed.[8,27]

(iii) When the signals are vibrations in keys on which the tips of the subject's fingers are poised ready to respond, the slope b has been found to be virtually zero.[11,28,29] Why this is so is not entirely clear, but the finding suggests that the time expressed by b is taken in bridging the gap between the sensory projections and the motor areas in the brain. The gap is substantial when the signals are visual or auditory; however, when they are tactual and the responses are strictly corresponding, the gap is very small because the sensory and motor areas are adjacent. This view is the more plausible because if the signals and responses are not strictly corresponding — as, for instance, when the signals are delivered to the finger of one hand and the responses are made by the corresponding finger of the other — b is substantial. When the responses are by non-corresponding fingers — such as when a stimulus to the right index finger is responded to by the left little finger, and so on — the rise of b has been greater still.[8,11] So far as I am aware, age trends in this type of task are again unknown.

(iv) Average reaction times become shorter in the course of practice. The effect is due almost entirely to a reduction of b, so for various degrees of choice, the shortening is proportional.[30,31] This implies that with sufficient practice (several thousand reactions), b should become zero and that reaction times for different degrees of choice should all be the same. Some evidence that this happens was obtained by Mowbray and Rhoades,[32] who found that, for one subject, two- and four-choice reaction times became equal after 26,000 trials. Presumably, in the course of practice, some kind of

TABLE 2. Two-Choice Reaction Times by Members of Three Generations — Son or Daughter, Parent of Same Sex, and Grandparent of Same Sex[a]

| Mean Age (years) | Responses by Keys on Same Side as Signal | | | Responses by Keys on Opposite Side from Signal | | |
| | Interval between End of Response and Arrival of Next Signal | | | | | |
	2 s	0 s	Percent Difference	2 s	0 s	Percent Difference
19	278	393	41	425	527	24
46	273	398	46	448	545	22
73	340	520	53	602	732	22
Percent Differences						
46–19	−2	+1		+5	+3	
73–19	+22	+32		+43	+39	

[a] The signals were lights and the responses were made by pressing keys under the two index fingers. Times are in milliseconds. Data are from Welford.[23]

TABLE 3. Ten-Choice Reaction Times Showing Effects of Relationships between Signals and Responses[a]

Kay[24,25]	Age Group		Percent Difference
	15–34	65–72	
(A) Keys in corresponding positions close to lights.	0.78 (0)	0.90 (0)	15 (0)
(B) As A, but lights are three feet away from keys.	1.27 (0.16)	1.58 (0.08)	25 (−50)
(C) As B, but lights are turned 180 degrees.	2.71 (0.32)	4.22 (0.27)	56 (−17)
(D) Lights related to keys by number code	2.77 (0.06)	4.24 (0.16)	53 (+248)
(E) The coding of D combined with the transposition of B.	4.91 (0.31)	22.27 (2.40)	452 (+773)
Birren *et al.*[26]	18–33	60–80	Percent Difference
(A) Randomly numbered lights and keys in corresponding positions.	0.62	0.77	24
(B) Lights numbered in random order. Keys numbered serially.	1.04	1.58	52
(C) As B, but with letters instead of numbers.	1.05	1.59	51

[a] Signals were lights. Responses were made by pressing keys. Times are in seconds. Errors per correct response are shown in parentheses. The apparatus used by Birren *et al.* was modeled on and closely resembled that used by Kay.

connections between particular signals and their corresponding responses became established in the brain — "built in" — so that the processes previously taking place during the time represented by b were no longer required and the responses were approximated to reflexes. Similar indications are given by the finding that if signals are digits or letters of the alphabet that are presented visually and responses are speaking their names, b is again virtually zero. Thus, again, reaction times are nearly the same for different numbers of possible signals (e.g., reference 33). Connections between the seen and spoken letters will have been built up in the course of many repetitions during the years of childhood. With an unfamiliar alphabet, b would be appreciable.

Age trends in the effects of practice on reaction times have in some cases been proportional. Therefore, although older subjects are slower initially, they improve in an absolute sense more rapidly than younger subjects, and age differences gradually diminish. In some cases, indeed, older subjects have improved at a rate that is more than proportional, thereby suggesting perhaps that they are slowed initially by some difficulty in comprehending the task rather than by an inability to perform it once it is understood. In neither case, however, have older groups of subjects been found to reach equality with younger: some increase of the intercept a with age remains (see reference 31).

THEORETICAL MODELS

A number of mathematical models have been formulated to account for the logarithmic relationship between reaction time and the degree of choice, N. Almost all of these, however, have failed to account for some important evidence. So far, no model proposed is without difficulties, but one seems promising. It is conceived on two levels: one that may be termed "microbehavioral", which conceives choice reaction time as involving a series of subdecisions to identify the signal and choose the response, while the other level is conceived in quasi-neurological terms.

The microbehavioral version is a modification of a model put forward with some hesitation by Hick.[9] A subject confronted by a multichoice task is conceived as dividing the total possibilities into two or three groups. These are inspected serially until the one containing the signal and the corresponding response is found. This group is then subdivided and the subdivisions are again inspected serially, and so on, until the signal and response required are identified. The exact procedure seems to depend on the type and layout of the display, but the formulation has been found to fit several sets of choice reaction data with remarkable precision (in some cases to well within 1%).[8,27,34] Each inspection is assumed to take an equal amount of time, so a dichotomizing decision such as in a two-choice task will sometimes require one inspection and sometimes two (an average of 1.5 when the frequencies of the signals are equal). Inspection time has been found to be about 100 ms for young subjects (calculated by Hyman's equation from two-, four-, and eight-choice reaction times when the signals were lights in a row and responses were made by corresponding keys under the subject's fingers).[27] Confirmation was obtained in a two-choice task when subjects were instructed to concentrate on one of the signals, which could thereby be reckoned to have always been reached in one inspection, while the other signal was reached in two. The difference of reaction time between the two signals was again about 100 ms. The inspection time thus defined is, of course, two-thirds of b in Hyman's equation and rises with age. The model explains the shorter reaction times to more frequent or more predictable signals by assuming that these tend to be inspected before others.

The figure of 100 ms found for inspection time among young adults makes it tempting to suggest a connection with EEG alpha rhythm, which Surwillo[35,36] and Woodruff[37] have suggested on other grounds as a "modulus" for choice reaction time (see also reference 38). However, the question arises of how to account for cases in which b is much greater than or less than 150 ms, as it is with indirect or specially direct relations between signals and responses. Is it that the figure was a chance coincidence for light-key tasks, or is it that complications in the relationships between signals and responses increase the number of inspections needed and extreme simplifications reduce them? At present, evidence on which to decide is lacking, but it is perhaps significant that in an eight-choice task in which pairs of light-key relationships were reversed, the mean reaction time was almost exactly two inspection times longer than when relationships were straightforward.[27]

At the quasi-neurological level, studies of discrimination have pointed to the idea that for a decision to be made, there must be an accumulation of input data and a buildup of excitation resulting from it until some critical level is reached at which a response is triggered. It is becoming generally recognized that incoming sense data have to be discriminated from a background containing an appreciable amount of moment-to-moment random variation and that this can cause errors. Part of the variation is in the stimulus itself—in audition, this appears as noise; in vision, the variation has been termed "visual noise". For our present purpose, however, the important point is that randomness occurs also in the sense organs, pathways, and brain (so-called "neural noise") and affects not only the reception of incoming stimuli, but the signalling from one part of the brain to another. Neural noise can be regarded as being averaged out as the sample of incoming data is increased, and the buildup required to trigger a response represents the attainment of a critical signal-to-noise ratio sufficient to ensure that errors are kept to an acceptable minimum. The principle is the familiar one underlying tests of statistical significance. Signal-to-noise ratios tend to be lower in older people, partly because of well-known changes in the sense organs and nervous system that reduce signal strength and partly because of an increase in neural noise.[22,39-41]

In studies of the time required to discriminate between two lines of different lengths, Vickers *et al.*[42] were able to measure neural noise and also what they termed "inspection time". The latter, which interestingly turned out to be approximately 100 ms for young adults, was the minimum exposure time required to discriminate accurately between two lines that differed in a ratio of three to two. This inspection time shortens with the increase of mental age from childhood to young adulthood and lengthens progressively beyond the age of about 50.[43]

Vickers *et al.*[42] calculated noise from errors made when lines of closely similar length were exposed for one inspection time. The authors argued that the effect of the noise was to produce moment-to-moment variability in the perceived lines so that when the difference between them was small, the shorter line would sometimes appear the longer, and vice versa. They were thus able to measure noise in terms of visual angle. They applied their concepts to aging by reanalyzing data by Botwinick *et al.*,[44] who had exposed pairs of lines to subjects aged 65–79 and 18–35 for either 0.15 s or 2 s. The time taken by both groups to discriminate rose as the difference between the lines fell from 5% to 1%. With the short exposures, the times of the older subjects were longer than those of the younger ones by a constant amount at all percentage differences, but the older subjects became progressively less accurate as the differences decreased. With the two-second exposures, the older subjects were as accurate as the younger, but they took progressively longer as the differences betweeen the lines decreased. With the short exposures, Vickers *et al.*[42] calculated from the errors made that the standard deviation of the random variation in apparent line length was 0.21° of visual angle for the older subjects and 0.14° for the younger. With the long exposures, it was 0.1° for both groups. With the longer exposures, the older subjects appeared to be able, by accumulating data over a longer time, to build up their signal-to-noise ratio to equality with that of the younger.

The decisions involved in choice reactions, both overall and in component inspections, can be regarded as decision processes in discriminating signals and responses corresponding to signals. A model formulated by Smith[11,29] in these terms envisages that the signal is progressively focused down onto the brain area of the response and builds up activation in it until it reaches a critical level. His model involves three quantities: the signal-to-noise ratio (E), the critical level of this ratio (C), and the rate of transfer from signal to response (K) in a revision of Hick's equation. Smith proposes that

$$\text{Reaction Time} = K\log(NC/E + 1).$$

Normally, E is accumulated until it becomes equal to C, in which case the equation is identical to Hick's. If the equation is rewritten,

$$\text{Reaction Time} = K[\log(C/E) + \log(N + E/C)],$$

then it can be seen that when E is less than C, there will be a constant addition to reaction time for all values of N. This might especially happen with brief exposures of stimuli and among older subjects. In fact, it is also a possible explanation for the results obtained by Crossman and Szafran[22] and by Szafran[21] shown in TABLE 1, where there was a rise in a, but none in b with age. An increase of K would lead to a rise in both a and b and could account for the other results shown in TABLE 1. Any additions to the mediating processes required to relate signals to responses are likely to increase K and could thus account for longer reaction times when there are complex relationships between signals and responses. If K also tends to increase with age, the effects of age and complication would be multiplicative, as they appear to be in TABLES 2 and 3.

Activation of the motor area to produce a particular response appears to spread to adjacent areas and the critical buildup can be conceived as that required to differentiate the appropriate area from its neighbors. Evidence for this is that with straightforward light-key tasks, most errors are made by pressing a key adjacent to the correct one. Errors in this case imply that the buildup has been insufficient; it is consistent with this that error reaction times tend to be shorter than correct ones. With straightforward relationships between signals and responses, older subjects tend to be more accurate than younger, and their longer reaction times may, at least in part, be attributed to this—in other words, they have higher values of C. However, reciprocity between speed and accuracy tends to break down as relationships between signals and responses become complicated, so older subjects tend to become less accurate than younger ones, as is shown by the error figures in TABLE 3. The increased errors with age are presumably due to the confusion in making the complex-mediating manipulations required.

SERIAL EFFECTS

As mentioned earlier, the shortening of choice reaction times to signals that predictably follow others is an example of how reaction times are affected by previous signals in a series. Three other examples have attracted research in relation to age.

Maintaining Optimum Speed and Accuracy

Rabbitt[45,46] found that over a series of choice reactions, times gradually became shorter until an error was made, whereupon the next reaction time was much longer. Over the next few reactions, times again became shorter until another error was made, and so on. Rabbitt suggested that subjects try to keep their speed within a narrow band just below that at which errors are liable to occur. He found that the error reaction times of older subjects were no longer than those of younger ones, although their correct reaction times were longer and also more variable. Because of this variability, he concluded that older subjects need a greater "margin of safety" (higher value of C) to avoid errors and that this is part of the reason for their generally longer reaction times. If so, the result can be regarded as an interesting example of a conscious or unconscious strategy aimed at overcoming a handicap. Brewer and Smith,[47] who found similar, although more pronounced results when comparing young retarded adults with normal, suggested that the lack of fine adjustment could be due either to low signal-to-noise ratio, which would impair ability to observe the speed of response accurately, or to failure to take account of enough previous responses to distinguish between slow drifts and occasional larger deviations to which subjects might overreact. Both are plausible explanations of age effects. Signal-to-noise ratio has already been noted as tending to fall with age, and studies of serial performance have shown that older subjects do indeed take account of fewer previous items, presumably due to some deficiency of running short-term memory.[48,49]

Effects of Repetition

Reaction times within a series have been found to differ according to whether the signals and responses are the same as, or different from, those immediately preceding. These "repetition" and "alternation" effects are not fully understood, but Kirby[50] (on the basis of a thorough survey) concluded that a part explanation must be that some facilitating effect of a signal and response enables a similar reaction to be made more quickly during the following second or so. Because neural aftereffects tend to last longer in older people, it seemed reasonable to suppose that the facilitatory effect would be greater for them.[51] However, direct tests of this hypothesis produced the diametrically opposite result: the reactions of older subjects to repeated signals were, on average, slower than to alternative ones.[23] The results resembled those previously found with intervals between trials that were too long for neural aftereffects to have operated.[52] Even when repetition effects have been found, they have been less for older than for younger subjects.[53] Repetition and alternation effects are affected not only by immediately preceding signals and responses, but by those that are two, three, and four steps back (see reference 50). Age differences in these more remote effects are not known, but the evidence noted above, that older people tend to take account of fewer previous items in a series, suggests that such differences should be less.

Single-Channel Effects

When a stimulus arrives during the reaction time to a previous stimulus, response to the second stimulus is typically delayed. The length of the delay is such as to suggest that the second stimulus has to wait until the response to the previous stimulus has begun. The extensive and somewhat controversial evidence in this area has been surveyed elsewhere.[54,55] The late K. J. W. Craik[56] pointed to the indication that the brain can handle only one decision connecting signal to response at a time, and that once a process of decision has begun, it is protected from interference by subsequent signals until it has been completed. Such "single-channel" operation in the brain occurs even though the decisions do not lead to overt responses. Thus, for example, if a signal for action is preceded by a warning, this will delay reaction to the signal if the interval between it and the warning is very short. Insofar as decision processes become slower with age, the interval has to be longer for older people if delays due to warnings are to be avoided.[57]

Apparent exceptions do not breach the general principle:

(i) When two signals arrive within a period of up to about 100 ms, reaction time to both is longer than would be expected to either singly. They appear to be treated together and to lead to a coordinated response to both. A common example is when a pianist reads a musical phrase from a score and then produces a coordinated playing by both hands.

(ii) A signal to intensify the response to a previous signal may take effect without being delayed. In this case, no new decision has to be made.

(iii) While normally it is impossible to do two things at once unless they are coordinated,[58] they can sometimes be done independently if one of the tasks is relatively simple and thoroughly "built-in" as a result of extensive practice so that little moment-to-moment decision is needed. Thus, a woman can knit a simple pattern while talking. The talking ceases, however, if the pattern is complex or when points are reached, such as the end of a row, where more complex action has to be taken.

(iv) There has been a long-standing controversy, when two tasks are being performed simultaneously, about whether attention (or, more correctly, "capacity for decision") is divided between them or is applied fully to each in rapid alternation [see references 55 and 59 (p. 708–712)]. The answer appears to depend on the time scale on which the performance is considered. On a scale of minutes, the former view is obviously correct, but on a scale of fractions of a second, present evidence points clearly to the latter. Most everyday tasks do not require continuous attention, so another task can be dealt with during spare time left by the main task. The amount of spare time can be assessed from the extent to which the performance of the two tasks together is poorer than when they are performed separately: for example, the demands of car driving under various traffic conditions have been studied by measuring the extent of interference with mental arithmetic carried out while driving. The longer reaction times shown in TABLE 3 that were found by Szafran[21] when an additional task was added to the choice reaction are attributable to similar interference. It is interesting to note that the effects were, as would be expected from single-channel delays, entirely upon the intercept a and not on the slope b in Hyman's equation.

Delays have also been observed when a second signal arrives during or shortly after the response to a previous signal. Apparently, capacity for decision is engaged (to the exclusion of dealing with new signals) by the monitoring of "high points" of the response. A new signal arriving shortly after the beginning of a response is delayed by such monitoring until about 150–200 ms after the response has begun; similarly, a new signal arriving shortly after the end of a response has to wait until about 150–200 ms after the time of ending. Delays due to monitoring seem not to occur when a new signal is waiting. Thus, they do not occur if the new signal arrives before the response to a previous signal has begun. Furthermore, if the new signal arrives during the response to the previous signal, there is no delay due to monitoring the end of the response. Monitoring seems to be important for conscious awareness of what one is doing, and in experiments where it has been arranged that there is always a new signal waiting when the response to the previous one begins, subjects tend to have a curious feeling that their actions are not under voluntary control.[60] Much the same feeling occurs after long practice at some industrial repetition tasks in which action becomes "automatic".

There is little evidence about single-channel effects in older subjects, but it has been found that dual-task performance is adequately accounted for in both older and younger subjects in terms of performance at each task separately; that is, no extra time is taken by either older or younger in switching back and forth between the two. However, insofar as older subjects perform more slowly, interference between tasks is greater for them when time is limited.[61] Older subjects, though, have been found to monitor more than younger, perhaps because lower signal-to-noise ratios make them more liable to error unless they take extra care, and such additional monitoring is a cause of slower performance.[23,38] Failure to suppress the monitoring of the end of the previous response was probably the reason why the reaction times shown in TABLE 2 were higher when there was no gap before the next signal appeared than when two seconds elapsed. The effects can be seen to have been greater for older subjects when relationships between signals and responses were straightforward, but not when they were reversed. Perhaps, this was because the complexity of the latter condition made both groups more likely to monitor their responses.

The concept of single-channel operation has two interesting corollaries. First, once a decision is under way, it cannot be immediately cancelled if the situation suddenly changes: we all know of occasions on which we have committed ourselves to an action that we suddenly realize will be wrong, but are powerless to prevent.

The second corollary is that when an error is made, the time taken to correct it seems to depend upon the stage between input and output where it occurs. Rapid correction can be taken to imply that the central mechanisms have signalled the correct response, but the motor mechanisms have carried it out wrongly. A somewhat slower correction suggests that the signal has been correctly perceived, but an incorrect response has been chosen. An even slower correction would result from incorrect perception of the signal. In short, the time taken to correct an error is an indicator of how much the "work" of reacting has had to be done again.

The longer reaction times and increased monitoring among older people means that the time between committing themselves to an action and being able to modify it is longer for them than for those younger. Also, while errors early in the chain from input to output are likely to take longer for older people to correct, they are able to correct errors later in the chain relatively quickly.

MOVEMENT TIME AND CONTINUOUS PERFORMANCE

The single-channel concept has opened the way to a new understanding of the timing of continuous performance. When the muscular effort required is only light, the speed of performance appears to be limited by the times required for making decisions and for monitoring movements. The movements themselves are "tailored" to fit those times and could easily be made much faster if they were not dependent upon them. For example, the times merely to press the row of ten keys used by Birren et al.[26] (whose results are shown in TABLE 3) were about half of those for their most straightforward reaction time task. Again, the time taken to make movements has been found to be, within limits, independent of the force required: movement time is governed by the times required by decisions to start and stop (see reference 54, p. 144). Movement times, like reaction times, are affected by the context of other movement times; for example, when in a complex task, one component movement has to be made slowly and deliberately, other movements in the cycle tend to be slower than they would otherwise be [see references 54 (p. 152–155) and 62 (p. 105)]. The effect appears to lessen with age, perhaps indicating some loss of integration of performance into higher units.

Several experiments in which decision times and movement times have been measured separately have shown increases in the former associated with age to be much greater than increases in the latter (see references 13 and 62). On the other hand, the time taken to make movements requiring substantial muscular force has been found to increase substantially (and to do so than simple reaction times) with age. For example, Pierson and Montoye,[63] whose subjects had to make a thrust with the whole arm in response to a light, found an increase of 89% in movement time, but only 31% in reaction time between 20s and 60s. Again, Onishi,[2] whose subjects responded to a signal by jumping with the whole body, found increases between the same ages of 18% in the time from the signal to the first EMG activity and 17% from this to the beginning of muscular contraction, but 33% for the muscular contraction itself.

Graded movements aimed to land on a target have been found in several experiments to consist of a series of impulses where each lasts about 100 ms. The first covers about half the distance from the starting point to the target area, the second covers half the remaining distance, and so on until the movement can terminate within the target limits.[64] In young people, these impulses tend to run into each other to make a fairly smooth progression. In older people, they show more definite decelerations and accelerations marking the transition from each impulse to the next.[65] The figure of 100 ms lines up with the finding that repetitive tapping movements are made at a maximum rate of about 10 per second. The series of impulses implies a logarithmic relationship between movement time, amplitude of movement (A), and the accuracy of landing indicated by the scatter of shots on the target (W). The scatter seems to have two additive causes: randomness in the central control of movement, and tremor (t). The results of experiments in which subjects have made movements to-and-fro between targets of various widths and distances apart have been fitted by the equation:

$$\text{Movement Time: } K \log (A + W/2)/(W - t).$$

The equation suggests that the subject controls movement so as, in effect, to choose a landing point within the width of the scatter out of the total distance from the starting point to the far edge of the scatter. Age effects have shown up as small rises of K and t, and as small shifts in the balance between speed and accuracy (towards speed from the 20s to the 40s, and towards accuracy from the 50s to the 70s).[13,66]

The relationships between reaction times and movement times emphasize the important concept of performance depending on several capacities—sensory, central, and motor—of which one may be fully loaded and thus limit performance, while the demands of the task are well within the limits of other capacities involved. This means that in assessing changes associated with age in any performance, it cannot be assumed that all the capacities involved are important. Overall performance cannot, therefore, be reliably predicted from measurements of each capacity separately.

SEX DIFFERENCES

Several studies have found girls and women to have, on average, longer reaction times than boys and men (see reference 14). The most comprehensive results are probably those of Noble *et al.*[67] shown in TABLE 4. Females are slower in every age group except 10–14 and 70–87. The fast reaction times of girls in the former group, if not due to an accident of sampling, may perhaps reflect a tendency for girls to mature earlier than boys. The finding of faster reaction times for women in the 70–87 group is supported by results obtained by Botwinick and Brinley;[68] however, the results are suspect because their women were, on average, about eight years younger than their men. The results were not supported by those of Botwinick and Thompson,[69] which showed older women to be slower. The conflict of evidence suggests the need for care in sampling above the age of about 70. Speed of performance tends to decline rapidly during the few months before death. This fact, together with the tendency for women to live longer than men, could mean that in any institutional or strictly representative sample, the older women would be, on average, fitter than the men and, for that reason, would be likely to show shorter reaction times. At the same time, in a sample recruited on the basis of willingness to be tested, men and women would probably be equally fit because only those reasonably fit would volunteer. The oldest subjects studied by Noble *et al.*[67] appear to have come from a rest home for the elderly. For all other studies,

TABLE 4. Four-Choice Reaction Times Showing Differences between Males and Females[a]

Age Group	Males	Females	Percent Difference
6–9	467	507	+ 8.6
10–14	386	374	− 3.2
15–19	252	277	+ 9.9
20–29	245	287	+ 17.1
30–39	268	316	+ 17.9
40–49	296	346	+ 16.9
50–59	345	388	+ 12.5
60–69	430	467	+ 8.6
70–87	582	538	− 8.2

[a] Times are in milliseconds. Data are from Noble *et al.*[67]

subjects appear to have been volunteers and the women were slower, except in that of Botwinick and Brinley, which has already been noted as suspect.

Why females should tend, on average, to have longer reaction times than males is not clear. It could perhaps be due to females tending to be more cautious, and thus more accurate, but this is not at present known. Apart from such a possibility, it is hard to resist the conclusion that the trend is due to some fundamental biological factor as yet to be identified.

FOR THE FUTURE

Although the study of reaction times came early in the development of experimental psychology and included ingenious attempts to separate times for identification of signal and choice of response,[70] clear understanding of reaction times and models to account for them began to develop only with the publication of Hick's classical paper[9] on the logarithmic relationship between reaction time and degree of choice. Progress since then has been rapid and reaction time has come to be used as a measure (or potential measure) in many other areas such as cognition (e.g., Posner[71]), memory (McNicol and Stewart[72]), personality (Brebner[73]), intelligence (e.g., Jensen,[74] Nettelbeck[43]), and various mental disorders (Nettelbeck[75]). Yet, the more that is done, the more that opens up as needing to be done. For example, we do not yet fully understand the processes involved in translating from signals to responses, and when and why different apparent strategies for doing so are used. We do not know why age effects differ in the ways they do, and why changes with age in choice reaction times should be in one and sometimes another parameter. Finally, we do not know, for certain, under what conditions monitoring of responses can be avoided, or just what happens when performance becomes "automatic".

Along another perspective, changes of reaction time and speed of performance with age have been shown to resemble in many ways those associated with brain damage, cardiovascular disease, and various physiological changes (see references 76 and 77). These resemblances offer stimulating and potentially valuable leads to understanding the causes and processes of change association with age; however, if they are to be established as more than superficial, the mechanisms linking the physical and physiological findings to behavior and performance need to be spelled out.

A special challenge seems to lie in the ubiquitous figure of 100 ms that appears not only in alpha rhythm and tremor, but as an apparent modulus in discrimination, choice, and the control of graded movement. Are the moduli fundamentally the same for all these functions? If the moduli differ between individuals and within individuals under different conditions of stress, drugs, and other factors, do they all do so equally? How far are the effects of age due to the moduli lengthening, and how far are they due to older people requiring more moduli to achieve decisions? An attempt to answer these questions would involve a prodigious research effort in which all these functions would be measured and compared in detail in the same individuals. The laboriousness would be daunting, but the answers obtained would provide a major contribution to the understanding of the mechanisms controlling performance.

REFERENCES

1. KLINE, D. W. & J. SZAFRAN. 1975. Age differences in backward monoptic visual noise masking. J. Gerontol. **30:** 307–311.
2. ONISHI, N. 1966. Changes of the jumping reaction time in relation to age. J. Sci. Labour **42:** 5–16.
3. TRAVIS, L. E. 1929. The relation of voluntary movement to tremors. J. Exp. Psychol. **12:** 515–524.
4. TIFFIN, J. & F. L. WESTHAFER. 1940. The relation between reaction time and temporal location of the stimulus on the tremor cycle. J. Exp. Psychol. **27:** 318–324.
5. BIRREN, J. E. 1965. Age changes in speed of behavior: its central nature and physiological correlates. *In* Behavior, Aging and the Nervous System. A. T. Welford & J. E. Birren, Eds.: 191–216. Thomas. Springfield, Illinois.
6. NEBES, R. D. 1978. Vocal versus manual response as a determinant of age difference in simple reaction time. J. Gerontol. **33:** 884–889.
7. STERNBERG, S. 1969. The discovery of processing stages: extension of Donders' method. Acta Psychol. **30:** 276–315.
8. WELFORD, A. T. 1980. Choice reaction time: basic concepts. *In* Reaction Times. A. T. Welford, Ed.: 73–128. Academic Press. London.
9. HICK, W. E. 1952. On the rate of gain of information. Q. J. Exp. Psychol. **4:** 11–26.
10. HYMAN, R. 1953.. Stimulus information as a determinant of reaction time. J. Exp. Psychol. **45:** 188–196.
11. SMITH, G. A. 1980. Models of choice reaction time. *In* Reaction Times. A. T. Welford, Ed.: 173–214. Academic Press. London.
12. HILGENDORF, L. 1966. Information input and response time. Ergonomics **9:** 31–37.
13. WELFORD, A. T. 1977. Motor performance. *In* Handbook of the Psychology of Aging. J. E. Birren & K. W. Schaie, Eds.: 450–496. Van Nostrand–Reinhold. Princeton, New Jersey.
14. WELFORD, A. T. 1980. Relationships between reaction time and fatigue, stress, age and sex. *In* Reaction Times. A. T. Welford, Ed.: 321–354. Academic Press. London.
15. SUCI, G. J., M. D. DAVIDOFF & W. W. SURWILLO. 1960. Reaction time as a function of stimulus information and age. J. Exp. Psychol. **60:** 242–244.
16. TALLAND, G. A. & J. CAIRNIE. 1961. Aging effects on simple, disjunctive, and alerted finger reaction time. J. Gerontol. **16:** 370–374.
17. GRIEW, S. 1959. Complexity of response and time of initiating responses in relation to age. Am. J. Psychol. **72:** 83–88.
18. GRIEW, S. 1964. Age, information transmission and the positional relationship between signals and responses in the performance of a choice task. Ergonomics **7:** 267–277.
19. BOTWINICK, J., J. S. ROBBIN & J. F. BRINLEY. 1960. Age differences in card-sorting performance in relation to task difficulty, task set, and practice. J. Exp. Psychol. **59:** 10–18.
20. MORIKIYO, Y., H. IIDA & A. NISHIOKA. 1967. Age and choice reaction time. J. Sci. Labour **43:** 636–642.
21. SZAFRAN, J. 1966. Age differences in the rate of gain of information, signal detection strategy and cardiovascular status among pilots. Gerontologia **12:** 6–17.

22. CROSSMAN, E. R. F. W. & J. SZAFRAN. 1956. Changes with age in the speed of information intake and discrimination. Experientia Suppl. **4:** 128–135.
23. WELFORD, A. T. 1977. Serial reaction times, continuity of task, single-channel effects and age. *In* Attention and Performance VI. S. Dornic, Ed.: 79–97. Erlbaum. Hillsdale, New Jersey.
24. KAY, H. 1954. The effects of position in a display upon problem solving. Q. J. Exp. Psychol. **6:** 155–169.
25. KAY, H. 1955. Some experiments on adult learning. *In* Old Age in the Modern World. Report of the 3rd Congress of the International Association of Gerontology, London, 1954, p. 259–267. Livingstone. Edinburgh.
26. BIRREN, J. E., K. F. RIEGEL & D. F. MORRISON. 1962. Age differences in response speed as a function of controlled variations of stimulus conditions: evidence of a general speed factor. Gerontologia **6:** 1–18.
27. WELFORD, A. T. 1971. What is the basis of choice reaction time? Ergonomics **14:** 679–693.
28. LEONARD, J. A. 1959. Tactual choice reactions: I. Q. J. Exp. Psychol. **11:** 76–83.
29. SMITH, G. A. 1977. Studies of compatability and a new model of choice reaction time. *In* Attention and Performance VI. S. Dornic, Ed.: 27–48. Erlbaum. Hillsdale, New Jersey.
30. TEICHNER, W. H. & M. J. KREBS. 1974. Laws of visual choice reaction time. Psychol. Rev. **81:** 75–98.
31. WELFORD, A. T. 1985. Practice effects in relation to age: a review and a theory. Dev. Neuropsychol. **1:** 173–190; 1986. Note on the effects of practice on reaction times. J. Mot. Behav. **18:** 343–345.
32. MOWBRAY, G. H. & M. V. RHOADES. 1959. On the redution of choice reaction times with practice. Q. J. Exp. Psychol. **11:** 16–23.
33. BRAINARD, R. W., T. S. IRBY, P. M. FITTS & E. A. ALLUISI. 1962. Some variables influencing the rate of gain of information. J. Exp. Psychol. **63:** 105–110.
34. WELFORD, A. T. 1975. Display layout, strategy and reaction time: tests of a model. *In* Attention and Performance V. P. M. A. Rabbitt & S. Dornic, Eds.: 470–484. Academic Press. London.
35. SURWILLO, W. W. 1963. The relation of simple response time to brain-wave frequency and the effects of age. Electroencephalogr. Clin. Neurophysiol. **15:** 105–114.
36. SURWILLO, W. W. 1964. The relation of decision time to brain wave frequency and to age. Electroencephalogr. Clin. Neurophysiol. **16:** 510–514.
37. WOODRUFF, D. S. 1975. Relationships among EEG, alpha frequency, reaction time and age: a biofeedback study. Psychophysiology **12:** 673–681.
38. WELFORD, A. T. 1984. Between bodily changes and performance: some possible reasons for slowing with age. Exp. Aging Res. **10:** 73–88.
39. GREGORY, R. L. 1959. Increase in "neurological noise" as a factor in ageing. Proceedings of the 4th Congress of the International Association of Gerontology, Merano, 1957, Vol. 1, p. 314–324.
40. GREGORY, R. L. 1974. Concepts and Mechanisms of Perception. Scribner's. New York.
41. WENGER, L. E. 1977. Estimation of "inspection time" and "noise" in the visual system and age. Paper presented to the 13th Annual Conference of the Australian Association of Gerontology.
42. VIKERS, D., T. NETTELBECK & R. J. WILLSON. 1972. Perceptual indices of performance: the measurement of "inspection time" and "noise" in the visual system. Perception **1:** 263–295.
43. NETTELBECK, T. 1986. Inspection time and intelligence. *In* Speed of Information Processing and Intelligence. P. A. Vernon, Ed. Ablex. Norwood, New Jersey.
44. BOTWINICK, J., J. F. BRINLEY & J. S. ROBBIN. 1958. The interaction effects of perceptual difficulty and stimulus exposure time on age differences in speed and accuracy of response. Gerontologia **2:** 1–10.
45. RABBITT, P. M. A. 1979. How old and young subjects monitor and control responses for accuracy and speed. Br. J. Psychol. **70:** 305–311.
46. RABBITT, P. M. A. 1981. Sequential reactions. *In* Human Skills. D. H. Holding, Ed.: 153–175. Wiley. Chicester, England.
47. BREWER, N. & G. A. SMITH. 1984. How normal and retarded individuals monitor and regulate

speed and accuracy of responding in serial choice tasks. J. Exp. Psychol. Gen. **113:** 71–93.

48. MAULE, A. J. & A. J. SANFORD. 1980. Adult age differences in multi-source selection behaviour with partially predictable signals. Br. J. Psychol. **71:** 69–81.

49. POON, L. W. & J. L. FOZARD. 1980. Age and word frequency effects in continuous recognition memory. J. Gerontol. **35:** 77–86.

50. KIRBY, N. 1980. Sequential effects in choice reaction time. *In* Reaction Times. A. T. Welford, Ed.: 129–172. Academic Press. London.

51. WELFORD, A. T. 1965. Performance, biological mechanisms and age: a theoretical sketch. *In* Behavior, Aging and the Nervous System. A. T. Welford & J. E. Birren, Eds.: 3–20. Thomas. Springfield, Illinois.

52. WAUGH, N. C., J. L. FOZARD, G. A. TALLAND & D. E. ERWIN. 1973. Effects of age and stimulus repetition and two-choice reaction time. J. Gerontol. **28:** 466–470.

53. JORDAN, T. C. & P. M. A. RABBITT. 1977. Response times to stimuli of increasing complexity as a function of ageing. Br. J. Psychol. **68:** 189–201.

54. WELFORD, A. T. 1968. Fundamentals of Skill. Methuen. London.

55. WELFORD, A. T. 1980. The single-channel hypothesis. *In* Reaction Times. A. T. Welford, Ed.: 215–252. Academic Press. London.

56. CRAIK, K. J. W. 1948. Theory of the human operator in control system II. Man as an element in a control system. Br. J. Psychol. **38:** 142–148.

57. TALLAND, G. A. 1964. The effect of warning signals on reaction time in youth and old age. J. Gerontol. **19:** 31–38.

58. KLAPP, S. T. 1979. Doing two things at once: the role of temporal compatibility. Mem. Cognit. **7:** 375–381.

59. WOODWORTH, R. S. 1938. Experimental Psychology. Holt. New York.

60. LEONARD, J. A. 1953. Advance information in sensori-motor skills. Q. J. Exp. Psychol. **5:** 141–149.

61. TALLAND, G. A. 1962. The effect of age on speed of simple manual skill. J. Genetic Psychol. **100:** 69–76.

62. WELFORD, A. T. 1958. Ageing and Human Skill. Oxford University Press for the Nuffield Foundation. London. (Reprinted 1973 by: Greenwood Press. Westport, Connecticut.)

63. PIERSON, W. R. & H. J. MONTOYE. 1958. Movement time, reaction time, and age. J. Gerontol. **13:** 418–421.

64. CROSSMAN, E. R. F. W. & P. J. GOODEVE. 1963. Feedback control of hand-movement and Fitts' Law. Paper to the Experimental Psychology Society, Oxford, July 1963; 1983. Q. J. Exp. Psychol. **35A:** 251–278.

65. MURRELL, K. F. H. & D. G. ENTWISLE. 1960. Age differences in movement pattern. Nature **185:** 948.

66. WELFORD, A. T., A. H. NORRIS & N. W. SHOCK. 1969. Speed and accuracy of movement and their changes with age. Acta Psychol. **30:** 3–15.

67. NOBLE, C. E., B. L. BAKER & T. A. JONES. 1964. Age and sex parameters in psychomotor learning. Percept. Mot. Skills **19:** 935–945.

68. BOTWINICK, J. & J. F. BRINLEY. 1962. Aspects of RT set during brief intervals in relation to age and sex. J. Gerontol. **17:** 295–301.

69. BOTWINICK, J. & L. W. THOMPSON. 1966. Components of reaction time in relation to age and sex. J. Genet. Psychol. **108:** 175–183.

70. DONDERS, F. C. 1868. Over de snelheid van psychische processen. Onderzoekingengedaan in het Physiologisch Laboratorium der Utrechtsche Hoogeschool. 1868–1869, Tweede reeks. **II:** 92–120. (Translated by: Koster, W. G. 1969. On the speed of mental processes. Acta Psychol. **30:** 412–431.)

71. POSNER, M. I. 1978. Chronometric Explorations of Mind. Erlbaum. Hillsdale, New Jersey.

72. MCNICOL, D. & G. W. STEWART. 1980. Reaction time and the study of memory. *In* Reaction Times. A. T. Welford, Ed.: 253–307. Academic Press. London.

73. BREBNER, J. M. T. 1980. Reaction time and personality theory. *In* Reaction Times. A. T. Welford, Ed.: 309–320. Academic Press. London.

74. JENSEN, A. R. 1982. Reaction time and psychometric *g*. *In* A Model for Intelligence. H. J. Eysenck, Ed.: 51–116. Springer-Verlag. New York.

75. NETTELBECK, T. 1980. Factors affecting reaction time: mental retardation, brain damage,

and other psychopathologies. *In* Reaction Times. A. T. Welford, Ed.: 355–401. Academic Press. London.

76. WELFORD, A. T. & J. E. BIRREN, Eds. 1965. Behavior, Aging and the Nervous System. Thomas. Springfield, Illinois.

77. HICKS, L. H. & J. E. BIRREN. 1970. Aging, brain damage, and psychomotor slowing. Psychol. Bull. **74:** 377–396.

DISCUSSION OF THE PAPER

J. MORTIMER (*Veterans Administration Medical Center, Minneapolis, MN*): Are the delays you mentioned unique to the visual modality? Could you talk about other stimulant modalities where at times this aging process also occurs?

A. T. WELFORD (*Aldeburgh, Suffolk, England*): One or two studies, not in relation to the age, of auditory tracking have been carried out and they find the same phenomena as the visual studies. This is true even to the extent that the difficult points in the track are where people start blinking. However, if a second signal occurs within about a tenth of a second of the first signal, it does not get delayed; instead, both signals get delayed and then they are reacted to together. The thing, though, that I wonder so much about is why we have this ubiquitous tenth of a second or hundred milliseconds? Are the cases all linked together? Moreover, how does it relate to alpha rhythm and tremor? Have we got some sort of fundamental modulus there?

M. WOOLLACOTT (*University of Oregon, Eugene, OR*): My question concerns your concept of noise increasing with age and causing increases in reaction time. Could you speculate on what that increase of noise really is in the nervous system and what might contribute to the increase in noise?

WELFORD: I would prefer if a neurologist would answer your question. One idea, though, is tempting and that is that you get a lot more fuzzy activity in EEG recordings. I consulted a colleague about this, but he said that was not the cause of the noise. Instead, he reckoned that if there was a slight mistiming of impulses converging on cells to trigger their firing, then this would have an effect of introducing randomness into the operation of the system.

Characteristic Patterns of Gait in the Healthy Old

DOUGLAS D. LARISH, PHILIP E. MARTIN,
AND MICHAEL MUNGIOLE

Exercise and Sport Research Institute
Arizona State University
Tempe, Arizona 85287

INTRODUCTION

Although impaired gait has been frequently associated with advancing chronological age,[1-5] we are now just beginning to appreciate the degree to which this impaired function compromises the ability of the aged to maintain an active, independent lifestyle.[6-8] For example, in the absence of specific disease, disturbances in gait produce disability in approximately 13% of older adults. Moreover, Teresi *et al.*[9] have recently shown that there is a close relationship between the degree of mobility and functional independence. Because impairments in gait cause serious functional problems, their prevention, delay, and remediation have become principal concerns of geriatricians and others charged with the care of the aged.[10,11] However, appropriate evaluation, training, and rehabilitation programs can only be achieved with a principled understanding of how aging and disease-related processes affect gait. This includes not only identifying age-related and disease-related changes in the gait pattern, but also discovering underlying alterations in musculoskeletal and neuromuscular functions that precipitate these changes.

CRITICISMS OF EXISTING GAIT LITERATURE IN GERONTOLOGY

At present, knowledge about the influence of aging and disease processes on gait is limited. Numerous studies have attempted to describe age-related differences and impairments in the gait pattern. They have failed, however, to identify the nature and extent of the differences or impairments in gait that should be expected as a normal concomitant of the aging process and that result because of pathological conditions affecting the aging motor system. Moreover, few of these research efforts have focused on the causes of impaired gait in the aged.

The majority of existing studies can be characterized as attempts to describe age-related differences in temporal/kinematic parameters of walking, such as velocity, stride length, stride frequency, stance time, swing time, double support time, and stance width.[12-19] The most consistent age-related difference in gait is a decrease in the preferred or freely chosen speed of walking (e.g., references 13, 16, and 18). A shorter stride length has also been shown to be characteristic of gait in the aged, as well as an increased stride frequency, stance width, and double support time, and a decreased ratio of swing to stance time.

Despite the similarity in results from many of these studies, several factors limit the usefulness of the existing data base. Most studies suffer from a significant methodological confounding in that subjects have been instructed to walk at their preferred (freely chosen) speed. Because most temporal/kinematic parameters of gait are speed-dependent, the difference in freely chosen speed between old and young adults will affect comparisons of these gait descriptors. For example, at all but very rapid walking speeds, increased speed is generally accompanied by longer strides.[17] Similarly, the ankle, knee, and hip joints move through a greater range of motion at fast walking speeds than at slow walking speeds.[20] The significance of this speed dependency is that valid conclusions about age-related differences in gait are difficult to form when old and young adults walk at different speeds.

Given the lack of an extensive data base, the descriptive emphasis of the existing research is both understandable and defensible. Such information provides the framework for establishing baseline descriptions essential in evaluating and rehabilitating abnormalities of gait.[21-23] The focus, however, should not be restricted only to mere description, nor to the temporal/kinematic type of analysis. Temporal/kinematic descriptions provide little information about the mechanisms controlling or mediating gait and, in isolation, they offer little insight into the causes of movement and impairments thereof. In our view, a meaningful assessment of gait in the aged must also provide the opportunity to determine the causes of impaired gait, and to do so would require a multidisciplinary tack that combines several types of analyses.

OTHER APPROACHES TO STUDYING GAIT IN THE AGED

Another type of analysis that has been proven useful in gait research, but has received little attention in gerontology, deals with the economy of walking. Economy is operationally defined as the amount of oxygen consumed (per kilogram of body mass) to walk a given distance. Research from the literature on locomotion has resulted in a well-established relationship between the speed of walking and metabolic economy. Simply stated, there is a speed of walking, generally ranging between 1.1 and 1.3 m/s (2.4–3.0 miles per hour), that is most economical (see FIGURE 1). Deviations below or above this range result in higher energy costs to walk the same distance (e.g., reference 17). Moreover, there is evidence to suggest that individuals naturally seek walking speeds that are most economical (e.g., reference 24). For example, the freely chosen walking speed is generally a good approximation of an individual's most economical speed. Inman *et al.*[17] and Sparrow[25] have even proposed that this relationship is a fundamental principle that governs locomotion. There is also evidence that this maximum economy principle extends beyond human locomotion. Hoyt and Taylor,[26] for example, have shown that horses exhibit the typical speed-economy relationship for both walking and trotting.

Alexander[27] and Zarrugh *et al.*[28] have also argued that one's basic pattern of gait is highly related to economy; not only do we tend to select an economical speed of walking, but we also tend to select movement patterns that contribute to economical gait. For example, at any given speed of locomotion, there is a stride length that is most economical.[29,30] Seemingly spontaneous changes in the mode of locomotion have also been attributed in part to the maximum economy principle.[26,27] More specifically, if the metabolic cost of sustaining a given speed becomes too great using one mode of locomotion (e.g., walk), the individual (or animal) will switch to a different mode of locomotion (e.g., jog or run; trot or gallop) that more economically maintains the desired speed. The empirical evidence and examples from the foregoing discussion

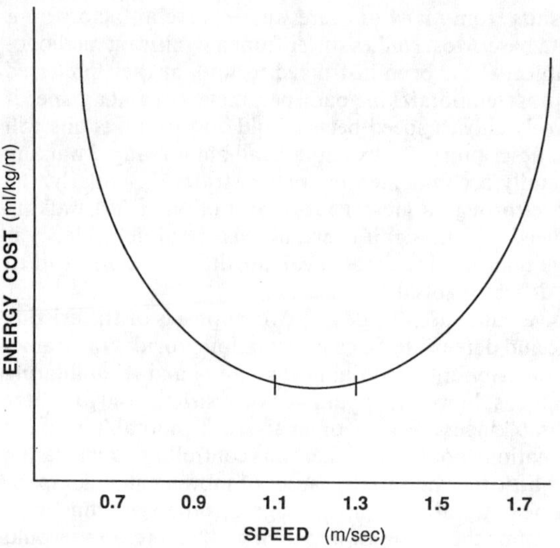

FIGURE 1. Schematic representation of the speed-economy curve.

demonstrate that there can be important interactions between various metabolic and temporal/kinematic factors that govern how we locomote.

An additionally useful, but again rarely used method of studying gait differences between young and old utilizes a kinetic approach in which forces that initiate and alter the motions of the body and body segments are studied directly. It is generally recognized in the biomechanics research literature that kinetic analyses hold more promise in advancing our understanding of human motion because they focus on the causes of movement; thereby they reflect how movements are being controlled and coordinated. Both forces external to the body (e.g., the ground reaction force) and those internal to the body (e.g., muscle forces and contact forces between the bones) are of interest in studying gait. Because the expenditure of energy is associated with muscular activity, knowledge of the muscular force generation patterns would be especially insightful in studying the economy of locomotion. Unfortunately, obtaining valid measures of individual muscle forces remains a challenging task plagued by many methodological problems. Consequently, the researcher is forced to seek alternative kinetic parameters that might be associated with economy of motion. One such measure on a more global level is the ground reaction force because it generally reflects the integrated actions of the musculature that propel the body forward with each step.

With the foregoing discussion in mind, we will shift the focus of this paper to a series of experiments that demonstrate the value of using several types of analyses to study the influence of advancing age on gait. In the initial study, economy of walking was examined in old and young adults. The second study examined walking in the aged by combining temporal/kinematic and kinetic analyses.

ECONOMY OF WALKING IN THE AGED

The maximum economy principle is interesting and potentially important from a gerontological perspective because of the reliable age-related decline in the self-selected

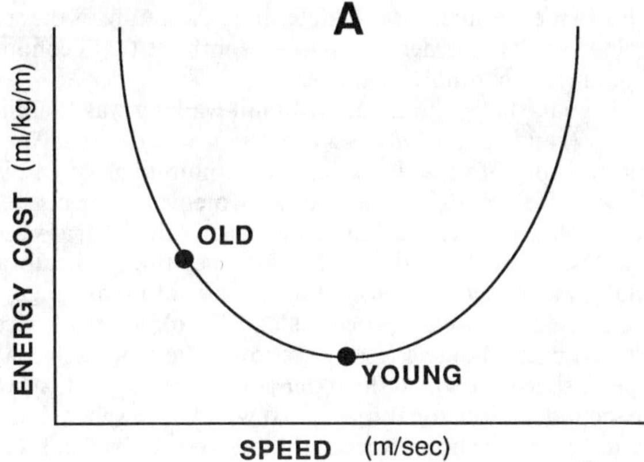

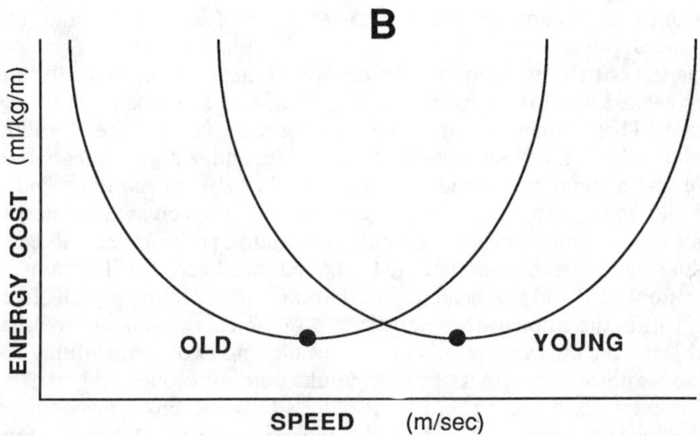

FIGURE 2. Proposed speed-economy relationships between old and young (see text for explanation).

speed of walking. Based in part on the speed-economy relationship, this decline has led some (e.g., reference 4) to conclude that older adults pay a greater metabolic cost per distance walked than do their younger counterparts. This assertion is based on the premise that a single speed-economy curve governs both old and young and that the old simply fall on a less economical portion of this curve (see FIGURE 2A). A second, equally plausible alternative is that the slower freely chosen speed adopted by older adults is most economical and represents an adaptation to age-related changes in musculoskeletal and neuromuscular functions. In this latter instance, the shape of the speed-economy curves may be similar for old and young. It is speculated, however, that the curve for the old would be offset from that of the young (see FIGURE 2B). To our knowledge, neither of these explanations have been addressed empirically. Consequently, the purpose of this first experiment was to determine the nature of the speed-economy relationship in older adults in order to test the hypothesis that economy of walking decreases with advancing chronological age.

To achieve this goal, the economy of treadmill walking was examined in old (M = 70.5 years, n = 17) and young (M = 25.6 years, n = 11) adults. None of the older subjects had a past history of musculoskeletal, neuromuscular, or cardiovascular disease that could have affected walking economy. Moreover, subjects were engaged in a regular regimen of physical exercise that included activities such as walking, jogging, bicycling, aerobic dance, and strength training. This healthy, physically active population of older adults was purposely selected to avoid confounding age-related differences with those caused by disease processes and hypokinesis (physical inactivity).

Each subject participated in two testing sessions. The first session was used to determine the range of speeds at which the older adults were capable of walking on the treadmill. In the second session, the subjects first walked at a speed that they perceived to be their preferred or freely chosen speed and then they walked at six predetermined speeds in ascending order: 0.54, 0.81, 1.07, 1.34, 1.61, and 1.88 m/s. (Younger subjects did not walk at the slowest of these speeds; consequently, no age comparisons were made for this particular speed.) Subjects walked at each speed for approximately five minutes so that an aerobic steady state was achieved. Expired air was collected and analyzed for the last two minutes in order to compute a measure of economy (mL/kg/m) for each speed.

Five aspects of the economy results are worth mentioning. First, the energy cost per meter walked was lowest for the 1.07- and 1.34-m/s speeds for both age groups (see TABLE 1). These values are consistent with the economical range of walking speeds already established in the locomotion literature. Second, a regression analysis showed that there was a significant quadratic relationship between economy and speed for both old and young subjects. As the speed of walking decreased or increased from the two most economical speeds, oxygen consumption per distance walked increased. This finding clearly establishes that the U-shaped speed-economy relationship is characteristic of both old and young alike. Third, it was further found that the freely chosen speed fell within the empirically determined economical range in approximately 82% of the subjects; the only exceptions were three old and two young adults. Fourth, despite the above noted similarities, the older adults were less economical than the younger adults. The energy cost was higher for the older adults at each of the common walking speeds. Finally, and somewhat unexpectedly, the results showed that the preferred (freely chosen) speed of walking on the treadmill was equivalent for old and young adults (1.21 and 1.19 m/s, respectively).

The findings obtained here fail to substantiate either of the two propositions forwarded earlier. There is no support for the notion that older adults are less economical because their freely chosen walking speed falls outside the economical range. In addi-

TABLE 1. Means and Standard Deviations for Economy (mL/kg/m) as a Function of Walking Speed (m/s) and Age

Age		Walking Speed				
		0.81	1.07	1.34	1.61	1.88
Old	M	0.235	0.206	0.202	0.220	0.251
	SD	0.026	0.022	0.022	0.025	0.018
Young	M	0.185	0.162	0.162	0.173	0.187
	SD	0.015	0.011	0.010	0.015	0.018

tion, the results do not support the notion that the economical range is altered by advancing age. The estimated freely chosen speed and economical range of speeds were equivalent for both old and young.

Although there is an age-related difference in walking economy, it appears that age has little influence on the shape of the speed-economy curve and the most economical range of walking speeds. Moreover, the current findings suggest that a decrease in the freely chosen speed of walking may not be as robust an aging phenomenon as currently thought, but may rather be linked to the physical activity patterns of the aged. This further indicates the importance of carefully monitoring and controlling for the physical activity status of subjects studied in aging research.

One of the principal intents of this experiment was to determine whether biological aging processes have an effect on the speed-economy relationship for walking. To minimize the potential for confounding pathological and other age-related conditions [particularly hypokinesis (physical inactivity)], healthy, physically active older adults were specifically selected for this experiment. It may be possible to completely isolate the influence of biological aging processes in human behavioral research, but we and others[31-33] believe that an acceptable approximation can be obtained from older adults who maintain a regular regimen of physical exercise. Therefore, we contend that the diminished economy of the older adults tested here is most likely the result of biological aging processes and not age-related pathological conditions.

The results from this preliminary study answer the question about whether there is an age-related difference in economy of walking. At the same time, they raise another perhaps more important question: Why is there an age-related decrease in economy? One possibility is that the older adults are less economical because of alterations or, perhaps, adaptations in the pattern of gait, which are probably precipitated by morphological and physiological changes in musculoskeletal and neuromuscular functions. The second experiment was designed to consider this issue.

TEMPORAL/KINEMATIC AND KINETIC ANALYSES OF GAIT IN THE AGED

As noted earlier, numerous studies have reported age-related differences in the gait pattern. These findings, however, fail to provide any direct information about why the aged are less economical because of the confounding between age and freely chosen walking speed. As a consequence, the motivation underlying the second experiment was to determine whether there are age-related differences in selected temporal/kinematic and kinetic parameters of gait when speed of walking is controlled, and whether differences in these parameters might explain, at least in part, the age-related decline in economy. More specifically, the intent of this second study was twofold. One purpose was to determine how stride length–stride frequency combinations are affected when old and young adults are required to walk at the same speeds. In addition to decreases in freely chosen walking speed with old age, it has been frequently concluded that there is an age-related decrease in stride length. As noted above, however, this latter conclusion is tenuous because of the speed dependency of stride length and stride frequency. A second purpose was to determine if age-related differences exist in ground reaction force characteristics and whether such differences may help explain the diminished economy of walking in older adults. The ground reaction force was chosen because it represents the net effect of all muscle and intersegmental forces acting within the body and it has been implicated as a parameter that can affect economy of walking.[34,35]

Subjects for the experiment included 13 old ($M = 73.5$ years) and 15 young ($M = 27.5$ years) adults. All older subjects were healthy and free of orthopedic conditions that could have affected the gait pattern. As a group, though, they were less physically active than those older adults in the previous experiment. Each subject completed ten overground walking trials across a force platform under each of three speed conditions: freely chosen, 0.81 m/s, and 1.34 m/s. A timing system consisting of two photocells (one placed on either side of the force plate) and a digital clock was used to monitor and control walking speed. For the two experimenter-determined speeds, subjects were required to maintain an average velocity within 3% of the target speeds. Trials outside this range were repeated. A WATSMART motion analysis system was used to quantify stride length at a sampling frequency of 50 Hz. Infrared markers were placed on the toe and heel of the right foot. Stride length was determined from two successive heel contacts, starting with heel contact on the force platform. The force platform quantifies the vertical, anterior-posterior, and medial-lateral components of the ground reaction force. Only the first two of these, however, were studied in this experiment. The vertical component represents the force exerted downward against the ground and is the principal contributor to the resultant ground reaction force during

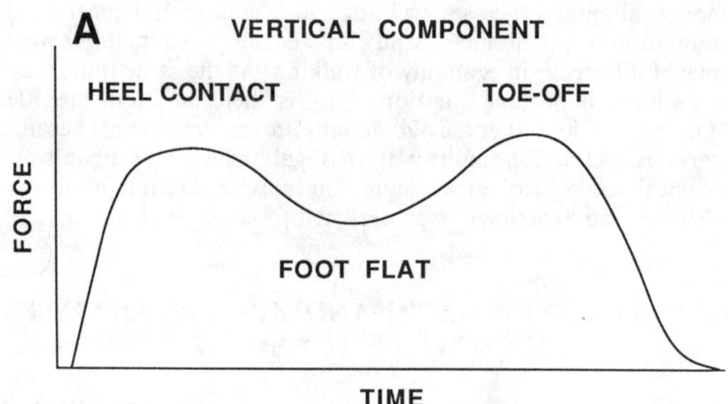

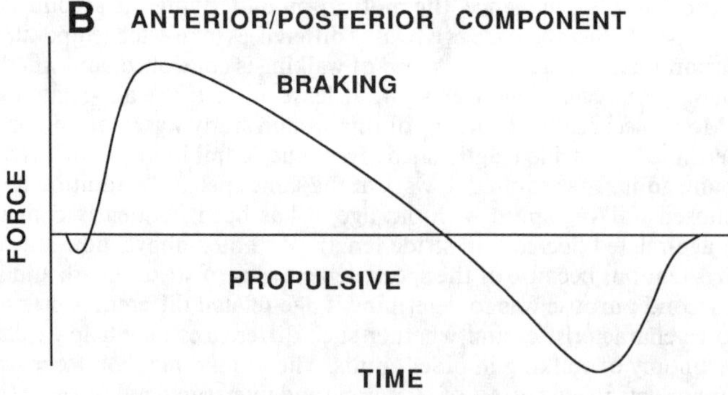

FIGURE 3. Typical patterns for vertical (panel A) and anterior-posterior (panel B) ground reaction forces.

walking. It is characterized by two major peaks that are generally slightly greater in magnitude than body weight (see FIGURE 3A). The first occurs when the leg is receiving the weight of the body shortly after foot contact, whereas the second peak occurs near the end of the contact phase. These two peaks are separated by a valley that is slightly lower in magnitude than body weight, which occurs during midstance.

The anterior-posterior component provides information about the forward-backward application of force to the ground (see FIGURE 3B), and reflects breaking (decelerating the forward motion) and propulsive (accelerating) phases of the contact period. The peak forces associated with each of these phases during walking are approximately 15% of body weight in magnitude and nearly coincide temporally with the two peaks in the vertical ground reaction force component.

Velocity and Stride Length Findings

Analysis of the velocity data showed that for both old and young subjects, the walking velocities in the 0.81- and 1.34-m/s conditions were very close to the desired target times. This finding was, of course, essential to ensure the validity of further age comparisons involving other temporal/kinematic (and kinetic) gait parameters.

Analysis of the stride lengths for the 0.81- and 1.34-m/s conditions showed that longer strides were taken at the faster of these two speeds (see TABLE 2). An interaction was also found between age and speed of walking; there was an age-related decrease in stride length for the 1.34-m/s condition, but not for the 0.81-m/s condition. Other analyses showed that the freely chosen speed was slower for older subjects than it was for younger subjects (1.21 and 1.41 m/s, respectively). In addition, the stride of older adults was shorter than that of the younger adults for the freely chosen condition, which would be expected given the slower freely chosen speed of the older group.

Two important findings emerged from the velocity and stride length analyses. First, it appears that age-related differences in stride length depend on the velocity at which this parameter is measured; this is consistent with data reported by Crowninshield *et al.*[23] In general, stride length differences between old and young are accentuated as the speed of walking is increased. Second, the strategy by which older adults obtain fast speeds of walking appears to differ from the strategy used by younger adults. Increased walking speed can be achieved via increases in stride length, stride frequency, or combinations thereof. As a result of a shorter stride length at the 1.34-m/s speed, older adults had to compensate by increasing stride frequency to a greater degree than younger adults. Thus, old and young subjects used different combinations of stride length and stride frequency to achieve this fast speed of walking. A possible contributor to the decreased stride length may be a reduction in joint flexibility, particularly

TABLE 2. Means and Standard Deviations for Stride Length[a] as a Function of Walking Speed (m/s) and Age

Age		Walking Speed		
		0.81	1.34	Freely Chosen
Old	M	1.31	1.56	1.53
	SD	0.15	0.15	0.18
Young	M	1.35	1.66	1.70
	SD	0.09	0.09	0.10

[a] Normalized to leg length.

at the hip. The interrelationship between flexibility and gait characteristics, though, has not been tested. Additional implications of the stride length–stride frequency difference on economy will be discussed later.

Ground Reaction Force Findings

For the vertical component, the two peak forces for the 0.81-m/s condition were lower than the peak forces for the 1.34-m/s condition (see TABLE 3). Further analysis showed that peak vertical force at heel contact in the older adults was lower than in their younger counterparts for both walking speeds. At toe-off, there was no age-related difference in peak vertical force for the slower walking speed; however, for the faster walking speed, the peak force produced by the older adults was lower than that of the younger adults. The magnitude of the peak vertical force during midstance was equivalent for both age groups and for both experimenter-defined walking speeds. For the anterior-posterior component, the absolute peak forces during the deceleration (braking) and acceleration (propulsion) phases were larger in the 1.34-m/s condition than in the 0.81-m/s condition (see TABLE 4). During the deceleration phase, peak force in the older adults was lower than in the younger adults for both walking speeds. An interaction between age and walking speed was found in the acceleration phase. For the slower speed, there was no difference between the peak forces produced by old and young adults. In contrast, there was an age-related decline in this peak force at the faster speed of walking.

The ground reaction force data obtained here show that the peak forces at heel contact experienced by the older adults are lower than those experienced by the younger adults at both experimenter-defined speeds of walking. In contrast, age-related differences in peak force during toe-off depended on walking speed. The peak forces of old and young adults were equivalent at the slower speed, but were lower in the older adults at the faster speed of walking. (This latter result parallels the interaction between age and speed reported earlier for stride length.) This interaction suggests that the aging motor system attempts to reduce the forces that must be absorbed during the braking phase of stance, even at slow speeds of walking. The speed-dependent nature of the ground reaction force during the propulsive phase of stance suggests that the aging motor system may be unable to produce levels of force comparable to those of younger adults at fast speeds. Another possibility is that this finding reflects an attempt to prevent the musculoskeletal system from experiencing levels of force that are potentially dangerous.

TABLE 3. Means and Standard Deviations for Vertical Ground Reaction Force[a] as a Function of Walking Speed (m/s) and Age

		Walking Speed					
		0.81			1.34		
Age		Heel Contact	Foot Flat	Toe-off	Heel Contact	Foot Flat	Toe-off
Old	M	1.00	0.92	1.02	1.14	0.75	1.06
	SD	0.03	0.02	0.02	0.08	0.05	0.04
Young	M	1.03	0.92	1.03	1.18	0.73	1.12
	SD	0.02	0.02	0.02	0.05	0.04	0.05

[a] Normalized to body weight.

TABLE 4. Means and Standard Deviations for Anterior-Posterior Ground Reaction Force[a] as a Function of Walking Speed (m/s) and Age

		Walking Speed			
		0.81		1.34	
Age		Braking	Propulsion	Braking	Propulsion
Old	M	0.10	0.12	0.17	0.18
	SD	0.02	0.02	0.03	0.03
Young	M	0.12	0.13	0.20	0.22
	SD	0.02	0.02	0.02	0.03

[a] Normalized to body weight.

For the vertical component, the algebraic difference between the peak force at mid-stance and the peak forces at heel contact and toe-off further suggests that there may be an age-related decrease in vertical oscillations of the center of gravity, which results in a lower vertical acceleration in the center of gravity for the older adults. It is possible that this latter finding represents an attempt by older adults to improve economy by minimizing vertical displacements in the center of gravity and by reducing the muscular forces that are required to slow down and speed up the body during walking. Finally, the fact that peak forces were largest for the fastest speed of walking substantiates the speed-dependent nature of the ground reaction force.

GENERAL DISCUSSION

Two criticisms of the existing gait literature in gerontology have been raised here. The most significant of these criticisms pertains to the confounding between manipulations of age and walking speed in a vast majority of studies investigating this problem. Both stride length and ground reaction force data from the present study substantiate the validity of this criticism. Consequently, it is necessary to reevaluate the current status of our knowledge of age-related differences in gait. An in-depth reevaluation of all gait parameters that have been studied is beyond the scope of this paper, but a number of comments are warranted. As noted earlier, a frequent age-related difference has been a decrease in the freely chosen speed of walking. Based on the results from the present study, even this finding can be questioned. For overground walking, the freely chosen speed of older adults was slower than that of younger adults. With treadmill walking, however, the freely chosen speed was equivalent for old and young adults.

One possible explanation for this discrepancy is that treadmill walking may reflect small differences in the pattern of gait from overground walking. This issue has been debated in the locomotion literature, but no consensus has yet been achieved.[36-38] A more likely possibility is that the difference in the level of physical activity maintained by the older subjects of the two experiments influenced the freely chosen speed. Subjects tested in the economy experiment (treadmill walking) maintained a regular regimen of physical exercise. This cannot be said for the majority of subjects tested in the overground walking study. Although the influence of physical activity was not tested in these experiments, the results imply that regular physical activity may help to inhibit deterioration of the gait pattern in the aged.

Using a regression analysis, Crowninshield *et al.*[23] demonstrated that age-related differences in stride length depended upon the speed of walking. This finding was con-firmed here via direct comparisons at two set speeds of walking. These combined results indicate that the currently-held view about age-related decreases in stride length must be qualified. A more accurate conclusion is that age-related decreases in stride length appear only at fast speeds of walking. Another way to conceptualize such a finding is to state that certain age-related differences in gait will surface only when the func-tional capacity of older adults becomes stressed. This idea is further supported by the interaction of age and speed for the ground reaction force during the toe-off period of stance. This interaction has important implications for the study of gait in the aged. The full impact of aging processes on gait may only be realized when gerontologists begin to examine gait patterns across a variety of walking speeds.

The existing research was also criticized because the analysis of gait patterns in the aged has been restricted to temporal/kinematic parameters. It was argued that meta-bolic and kinetic analyses could also further our understanding of the influence that aging and disease processes have on gait. Although the two experiments reported here focused on selected issues, the results overwhelmingly demonstrate the significance of these two additional types of analyses. The metabolic data show that older adults are less economical than younger adults, irrespective of walking speed (at least for ranges of speeds between 0.81 and 1.88 m/s). The ground reaction force data demon-strate that there are age-related differences in at least some kinetic parameters. Crownin-shield *et al.*[23] have also shown that peak joint moments and contact forces at the hip are less in older adults than in younger adults. One of the important challenges con-fronting future work will be to determine the reasons for these differences, as well as their behavioral significance.

An interesting finding from the overground walking study was the different way in which old and young subjects manipulated combinations of stride length and stride frequency to achieve the fastest speed of walking. The question that remains to be answered is why do older subjects have a shorter stride length—and hence a greater stride frequency—than do younger adults at fast speeds of walking? Perhaps, the older adults are forced to take shorter strides because of physical limitations imposed by tissue changes in the musculoskeletal system (e.g., decreased range of motion and muscle strength). One result of the shortened stride may be a corresponding decrease in economy. As noted earlier, not only is economy tied to speed of walking, but, for a given speed, there is also a most economical stride length. An alternative explanation is that the difference in strategy represents an attempt by older adults to minimize the energy cost of walking. Because of changes in the aging motor system, this may be a neces-sary adaptation in the gait pattern to maintain economy. To empirically substantiate either of these possibilities, additional experiments must examine both speed and stride length manipulations on economy.

Although we have proposed that the maximum economy principle may govern the way in which old adults walk, it must be recognized that there are many measures of cost that one might choose to economize and that the chosen variable will probably be determined by the goal that one wishes to achieve.[39] Based on the known changes in musculoskeletal and neuromuscular functions, it is quite reasonable to suppose that the aging motor system opts to economize on other variables; one likely candidate is the minimization of force.

Aging processes produce changes in the structure of bone (e.g., osteoporosis) and joint (e.g., osteoarthritis) that make the musculoskeletal system more susceptible to injury, particularly those caused by undue stresses. As walking speed increases, forces on the musculoskeletal system increase, and fast speeds of walking may create levels of force that place the older adult at risk of injury. The likelihood of an injury caused by large forces could be reduced by modifying the gait pattern or slowing the walking speed. The use of these strategies might also depend on the older adult's level of physical activity. (Deterioration in musculoskeletal function is less in physically active older adults than in sedentary older adults.) As noted earlier, the need to limit forces experienced by the musculoskeletal system may be reflected in some aspects of the ground reaction force data reported here. The stride length findings suggest one way that the aging motor system might achieve this goal is by limiting the length of stride at fast speeds. The need to lessen forces may also be one reason why overground walking studies have found an age-related slowing in the freely chosen speed. Although this alternative view cannot be evaluated without a more detailed analysis of internal stresses on the musculoskeletal system during walking, it raises an important issue about how economy is studied in the aged. Rather than searching for a single variable on which economy is based, a more meaningful approach may be to determine the criteria for selecting one variable over another.

SUMMARY

If the influences of aging processes on gait are to be understood, gerontologists must become better versed in experimental methodology appropriate to locomotion research. They must also begin to conduct experiments that move beyond mere description. Systematic research efforts that are interdisciplinary in nature and that incorporate several types of gait analyses will be needed to discover the causes of adaptations and impairments of gait in the aged. Certainly, this will not be easy to accomplish; however, we hope that the work reported here demonstrates this approach is possible and worthwhile.

ACKNOWLEDGMENTS

We thank Doug Penno, Peter Chase, and Marc Louis for their assistance in collecting the data reported here.

REFERENCES

1. BARRON, R. E. 1967. Disorders of gait related to the aging nervous system. Geriatrics **22:** 113–120.
2. KOLLER, W. C., S. L. GLATT & J. H. FOX. 1985. Senile gait: A distinct neurologic entity. Clin. Geriatr. Med. **1:** 661–669.
3. SABIN, T. D. 1982. Biologic aspects of falls and mobility limitations in the elderly. J. Am. Geriatr. Soc. **30:** 51–58.
4. STEINBERG, F. U. 1966. Gait disorders in old age. Geriatrics **21:** 134–143.
5. SUDARSKY, L. & M. RONTHAL. 1983. Gait disorders among elderly patients. Arch. Neurol. **40:** 740–743.
6. HADLEY, E., T. S. RADEBAUGH & R. SUZMAN. 1985. Falls and gait disorders among the elderly: A challenge for research. Clin. Geriatr. Med. **1:** 497–500.
7. SHEPARD, R. J. & K. H. SIDNEY. 1979. Exercise and aging. Exercise Sports Sci. Rev. **7:** 1–57.
8. SMITH, E. L. & C. GILLIGAN. 1983. Physical activity prescription for the older adult. Physician Sportsmed. **11:** 91–101.
9. TERESI, J. A., R. R. GOLDEN & B. J. GURLAND. 1984. Concurrent and predictive validity

of indicator scales developed for the comprehensive assessment and referral evaluation interview scale. J. Gerontol. **39:** 158–165.

10. HORNSTEIN, S. 1974. Managing gait disorders. Geriatrics **29:** 86–94.
11. PAYTON, O. D. & J. L. POLAND. 1983. Ageing process: Implications for clinical practice. Phys. Ther. **63:** 41–48.
12. AZAR, G. J. & A. H. LAWTON. 1964. Gait and stepping as factors in the frequent falls of elderly women. Gerontologist **4:** 83–84.
13. FINLEY, F. R., K. A. CODY & R. V. FINIZIE. 1969. Locomotion patterns in elderly women. Arch. Phys. Med. Rehabil. **50:** 140–146.
14. GABELL, A. & U. S. L. NAYAK. 1984. The effect of age on variability in gait. J. Gerontol. **39:** 662–666.
15. IMMS, F. J. & O. G. EDHOLM. 1979. The assessment of gait and mobility in the elderly. Age Ageing **8:** 261–267.
16. IMMS, F. J. & O. G. EDHOLM. 1981. Studies of gait and mobility in the elderly. Age Ageing **10:** 147–156.
17. INMAN, V. T., H. J. RALSTON & F. TODD. 1981. Human Walking. Williams & Wilkins. Baltimore.
18. MURRAY, M. P., R. C. KORY & B. H. CLARKSON. 1969. Walking patterns in healthy old men. J. Gerontol. **24:** 169–178.
19. WOLFSON, L. I., R. WHIPPLE, P. AMERMAN, J. KAPLAN & A. KLEINBERG. 1985. Gait and balance in the elderly: Two functional capacities that link sensory and motor ability to falls. Clin. Geriatr. Med. **1:** 649–660.
20. WINTER, D. A. 1983. Biomechanical motor patterns in normal walking. J. Mot. Behav. **15:** 302–330.
21. ANDRIACCHI, T. P., J. A. OGLE & J. O. GALANTE. 1977. Walking speed as a basis for normal and abnormal gait measurements. J. Biomech. **10:** 261–268.
22. CHAO, E. Y., R. K. LAUGHMAN, E. SCHNEIDER & R. N. STAUFFER. 1983. Normative data of knee joint motion and ground reaction forces in adult level walking. J. Biomech. **16:** 219–233.
23. CROWNINSHIELD, R. D., R. A. BRAND & R. C. JOHNSTON. 1978. The effects of walking velocity and age on hip kinematics and kinetics. Clin. Orthop. **132:** 140–144.
24. RALSTON, J. H. 1958. Energy-speed relation and optimal speed during level walking. Int. Z. Angew. Physiol. Einschl. Arbeitsphysiol. **17:** 277–283.
25. SPARROW, W. A. 1983. The efficiency of skilled performance. J. Mot. Behav. **15:** 237–261.
26. HOYT D. F. & C. R. TAYLOR. 1981. Gait and the energetics of locomotion in horses. Nature **292:** 239–240.
27. ALEXANDER, R. M. 1984. Walking and running. Am. Sci. **72:** 348–354.
28. ZARRUGH, M. Y., F. N. TODD & H. J. RALSTON. 1974. Optimization of energy expenditure during level walking. Eur. J. Appl. Physiol. **33:** 293–306.
29. CAVANAGH, P. R. & K. R. WILLIAMS. 1982. The effect of stride length variation on oxygen uptake during distance running. Med. Sci. Sports Exercise **14:** 30–35.
30. HOGBERG, P. 1952. How do stride length and stride frequency influence the energy-output during running? Arbeitsphysiologie **14:** 437–441.
31. SEALS, D. R., J. M. HAGBERG, W. K. ALLEN, B. F. HURLEY, G. P. DALSKY, A. A. EHSANI & J. O. HOLLOSZY. 1984. Glucose tolerance in young and older athletes and sedentary men. J. Appl. Physiol.: Respir. Environ. Exercise Physiol. **56:** 1521–1525.
32. SPIRDUSO, W. W. 1975. Reaction and movement time as a function of age and physical activity level. J. Gerontol. **30:** 435–440.
33. SPIRDUSO, W. W. & P. CLIFFORD. 1978. Neuromuscular speed and consistency of performance as a function of age, physical activity level, and type of physical activity. J. Gerontol. **33:** 26–30.
34. FREDERICK, E. C. 1985. Synthesis, experimentation, and the biomechanics of economical movement. Med. Sci. Sports Exercise **17:** 44–47.
35. HOF, A. L., B. A. GEELEN & JW. VAN DEN BERG. 1983. Calf muscle moment, work, and efficiency in level walking; role of series elasticity. J. Biomech. **16:** 523–537.
36. ELLIOTT, B. C. & B. A. BLANKSBY. 1976. A cinematographic analysis of overground and treadmill running by males and females. Med. Sci. Sports **8:** 84–87.

37. NELSON, R. C., C. J. DILLMAN, P. LAGASSE & P. BICKETT. 1972. Biomechanics of over-
       ground versus treadmill running. Med. Sci. Sports **4:** 233–240.
38. VAN INGEN SCHENAU, G. J. 1980. Some fundamental aspects of the biomechanics of over-
       ground versus treadmill locomotion. Med. Sci. Sports Exercise **12:** 257–261.
39. NELSON, W. L. 1983. Physical principles for economies of skilled movements. Biol. Cybern.
       46: 135–147.

DISCUSSION OF THE PAPER

M. WOOLLACOTT (*University of Oregon, Eugene, OR*): Did you leave out perhaps one other possibility? Specifically, that the subjects have lost the ability to control balance in old age and maybe they do not want to put that foot out quite so far and with quite so much force in front of them because they might lose balance if they did. Could you comment?

D. LARISH (*Arizona State University, Tempe, AZ*): Yes, that could very well be an explanation. However, it is not what we have been looking at and it is not the whole story. In fact, the evidence shows that when older people walk (particularly in those with gait disorders), there is an increase in body sway. Therefore, it has been suggested that the increase in stance width (which is the distance between the two feet as you walk) is a strategy to compensate for the increased sway. Thus, our view is that there are a multitude of factors that could come together to modify the gait pattern as one gets older.

We are looking at the pattern or the component that is of most interest to us because, primarily, that is where our expertise lies. However, what I think your point raises is the need to study movement behaviors in older people from a multidisciplinary perspective. It is a mistake if we just focus on one little corner of the world because there are so many changes in the neuromuscular and muscular skeletal systems that could affect the movements that we are able to produce. Hence, if we just focus on one element, we could miss out on the interaction of other elements.

J. TOBIN (*NIA, Bethesda, MD*): Can you say anything about the level of fitness in relationship to this economy curve?

LARISH: That is a very interesting question and one that we are very much concerned with. In the metabolic economy study that we did, we purposely selected very physically active older adults because we were interested in trying to get our best estimates of what biological aging was doing to the speed economy relationship. For example, one of the individuals in this group was 73 years old and ran four to eight miles, three to four times a week. Another individual client had recently returned from climbing Mount Kilimanjaro. We even had a 88-year-old woman who walked one to two miles a day. The second population of subjects that we tested, though, was not in quite the same category from a physical activity standpoint. I would not classify them as sedentary, but I would put them some place in the middle.

One of our plans now is to bring in a population of sedentary older individuals and to map out the speed economy relationship for them. We need to do this because it may very well be that the curve is going to shift over to the slower end or it may shift up again. However, at this point, we do not know of any data. In fact, speed economy data and the kinematic data are some of the only data that are around in older people.

M. SERBY (*New York University Medical Center, New York, NY*): Was there anything unique about the three subjects who did not demonstrate their optimal economy in the 2.4 miles per hour value?

LARISH: No; in fact, two of them were the younger subjects and they both walked faster. Actually, though, all three of them walked faster than the most economical range. Two of the younger subjects walked at around 3.6 miles per hour, and it also turned out that the 88-year-old woman was the other person that fell outside the range; however, she fell out on the high side rather than the slow side.

Cognitive Aspects of Motor Functioning

TIMOTHY A. SALTHOUSE

School of Psychology
Georgia Institute of Technology
Atlanta, Georgia 30332

The focus of this article is on two sets of phenomena in which cognitive factors have been found to influence motor functioning and that have also been found to have important implications for the interpretation of the effects of aging on motor performance. The approach in each case will be to first discuss the general phenomenon and then to describe the effects of age on that phenomenon, together with an indication of the significance of those effects for research on aging.

It is important to begin by indicating the very restricted sense in which the term motor functioning will be used in this article. Because the phenomena to be discussed involve simple keypress responses, motor functioning will refer to the speed of executing finger depressions of response keys — or what is commonly known as manual reaction time. This is clearly an extremely limited form of motor functioning, but it has had a long history of investigation in psychology. In part, this is because many researchers have felt that an individual's reaction time somehow reflects the integrity of his or her central nervous system. Some theorists have even speculated that reaction time measures might be used to provide a culture-fair index of intelligence; indeed, a number of studies have reported statistically significant correlations between certain reaction time measures and scores on assorted intellectual tests. However, the concern in this article is not with manual reaction time as a measure of cognitive performance, but rather, as the title suggests, on how cognitive factors can influence this very simple type of motor functioning.

SPEED-ACCURACY TRADE-OFF

The first phenomenon to be discussed is what is known as the speed-accuracy trade-off. This is a rather esoteric term for what everyone has experienced in a great variety of activities, such as handwriting, typing, or automobile driving, in which one has control of the speed at which he or she performs, and where it is possible to evaluate the quality or accuracy of that performance. In situations such as these, there is often a point where the quality or accuracy of the performance begins to suffer if one attempts to perform faster. Because, from that point on, speed can be increased only at the cost of reduced accuracy, this phenomenon is referred to as the speed-accuracy trade-off.

The speed-accuracy trade-off phenomenon has been studied in the laboratory with a choice reaction time procedure in which the subject's task is to press one of several keys as rapidly as possible when the appropriate signal occurs. Typical instructions in this type of task are inherently ambiguous because the research subject is usually requested to respond as rapidly and accurately as possible; yet, these are actually contradictory goals when speed and accuracy are reciprocally related. It is therefore quite possible that the instructions are interpreted differently by different people — some individuals emphasize speed more than accuracy, while others emphasize accuracy more than speed.

Recognition of this possibility has led some researchers to advocate measurement of complete speed-accuracy trade-off functions, or what have been referred to as speed-accuracy operating characteristics. Two basic procedures have been employed to generate speed-accuracy operating characteristics, but, in both, the intention is to obtain paired values of speed and accuracy over a range of accuracy from near chance to near perfect levels. One procedure for generating speed-accuracy operating characteristics involves manipulations such as payoffs or instructions to induce people to respond at different levels of speed and accuracy in different sets of trials, and then to use the average speed and accuracy in each set of trials as data points comprising the speed-accuracy operating characteristic.

Another technique that has proven to be more efficient in generating speed-accuracy operating characteristics consists of inducing subjects to perform at many different levels of accuracy within a single set of trials (perhaps by specifying a new goal or criterion time before each trial). The resulting distribution of reaction times is then grouped into discrete time intervals, with the mean speed and accuracy for the trials in each interval used as the data points for the speed-accuracy operating characteristic.

Regardless of the procedure used, the resulting speed-accuracy operating characteristics generally look like the function illustrated in FIGURE 1. It is not yet known whether the function is best characterized by a linear, exponential, or some other form of equation, but it is clear that the optimum reaction time, which is what most researchers employing reaction time procedures are attempting to measure, corresponds to a very narrow region in the function. Moreover, while it is often possible to determine when reaction time is faster than the optimum point because accuracy is less than the maximum, it is much more difficult to determine whether reaction times at the maximum level of accuracy are truly at the optimum because accuracy asymptotes at the optimum point. It is for these reasons that some researchers have argued that reaction times by themselves are uninterpretable and that they must be placed in the context of a speed-accuracy operating characteristic in order to be meaningful.

The preceding argument concerning the importance of speed-accuracy operating characteristics has been generally accepted. However, it has just as generally been ignored because of the greater time and effort required to generate complete speed-accuracy operating characteristics when compared to that required to obtain a single average reaction time. The additional effort, though, may be particularly worthwhile in studies of aging because several interesting questions arise in connection with the effects of age on the speed-accuracy trade-offs. Two of the most important are: (1) do people of different ages perform at different speeds because they have distinct speed-accuracy operating characteristics, or are they simply operating at noncomparable positions along the same function?; (2) do people of different ages differ in the slopes of the speed-accuracy function such that there are differential rates of information acquisition across age groups?

Two studies have recently been reported in which age differences in speed-accuracy operating characteristics have been examined — one[1] employs the procedure with different instructions or incentives for speed as opposed to accuracy in different sets of trials, and the other[2] employs the procedure in which the reaction times within a single set of trials are partitioned into discrete intervals. The results from both studies were similar in suggesting that adults of different ages have distinct speed-accuracy operating characteristics, but that the slopes of the functions were relatively invariant between 20 and 70 years of age; that is, with increased age, the functions appear to shift uniformly

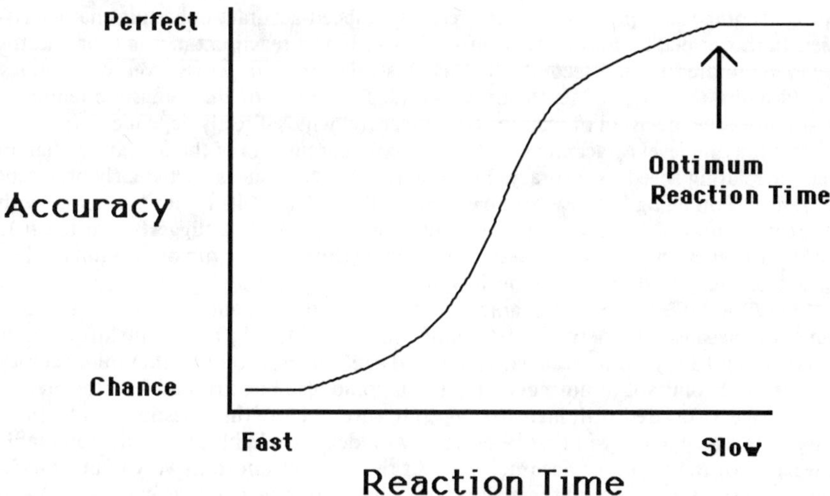

FIGURE 1. Idealized illustration of a speed-accuracy operating characteristic and the position of the optimum reaction time.

to the right such that reaction time is slowed by nearly a constant amount at each level of accuracy. These results thus suggest that age differences in speed do exist independent of the individual's particular emphasis on speed or accuracy, but that there is invariance across age in the rate at which accuracy increases per unit time. However, this latter conclusion should be considered quite tentative because the precision with which the slopes of the speed-accuracy operating characteristics have been assessed has not been great and, consequently, the power of the available comparisons is not known.

Another finding in some studies (e.g., references 1 and 3) is that older adults normally tend to operate with a higher accuracy bias than young adults. Many earlier investigators have made similar observations, but it was only with the advent of speed-accuracy operating characteristics that it became possible to establish that this effect was clearly distinct from the age differences in capacity for speeded responding. Therefore, as age increases, it appears that not only does the speed-accuracy operating characteristic shift to the right, but the region along the function at which one prefers to operate also moves from left to right.

The existence of the speed-accuracy trade-off phenomenon is an example of a cognitive influence on motor functioning because an individual's cognitive emphasis on speed or accuracy clearly affects the rate and quality of his or her motor performance. This particular cognitive aspect of motor functioning is important in research on aging for two reasons—one is methodological and the other is theoretical.

The methodological importance of the speed-accuracy trade-off phenomenon is derived from the realization that if speed and accuracy are reciprocally related, then it may be impossible to derive meaningful interpretations of results from adults of different ages based on only one of the measures. At the very least, ignoring accuracy when attempting to analyze time will greatly reduce the precision of measurement because there is no way of knowing whether or not individuals of different ages are operating at comparable positions in their respective speed-accuracy operating characteristics. In this respect, it may be very misleading to report reaction times in thousandths or even hundredths of a second when the possible variation across levels of accuracy could be on the order of tenths of a second. Regardless of the ostensible temporal resolution, the precision of reaction time measurement is directly dependent upon the accompanying level of accuracy and the specific parameters of the operating characteristic relating speed to accuracy. This methodological issue is particularly pertinent in research on aging because of the evidence that older adults typically operate with a greater emphasis on accuracy than young adults. This thus suggests that the true speeds of older adults may be underestimated relative to those of young adults unless speed-accuracy trade-offs are considered.

Speed-accuracy operating characteristics are also of substantive interest in research on aging because of a desire to determine the reasons for the apparent shift towards accuracy and away from speed with increased age. One possibility is that this accuracy bias is a concomitant of normal aging, but it could also be attributable to the greater experience associated with increased age. However, before this question can be thoroughly investigated, it will first be necessary to identify reliable and easily obtainable measures of the degree of accuracy bias. At the present time, only very indirect techniques have been employed for making this observation (e.g., references 1 and 3) and thus it has been difficult to subject it to systematic investigation.

ANTICIPATORY PROCESSING

The second example of a cognitive influence on motor functioning to be discussed concerns a phenomenon that can be termed anticipatory processing. In many motor tasks, there are severe limits on the rate of performance if one were to rely on strict serial processing in which all of the activity at one postulated stage or level must be completed before any activity can begin at a later stage or level. To illustrate, some estimates suggest that it requires about 100 milliseconds to register and detect a visual stimulus, 50 to 100 milliseconds to interpret the stimulus and decide which response to make, and about 50 milliseconds to execute the response. These estimates sum to a total of about 200 to 250 milliseconds for a choice reaction time, which is close to the value of average choice reaction time for practiced subjects at very high levels of accuracy. However, this figure implies that the maximum rate of repetitive responses should only be about 4 per second, which in the domain of typing would correspond to a rate of approximately 48 words per minute. Because many professional typists are considerably faster than this, it is interesting to ask how these apparently fundamental constraints on processing are circumvented to allow levels of typing performance much faster than that predicted on the basis of the analyses of choice reaction time.

Considerable research has revealed that a major factor contributing to the rapid performance of skilled typists is anticipatory processing; this means that the typists look beyond the immediate to-be-typed character and are often processing characters that are several in advance of the one for which the key is currently being pressed. The strongest support for this inference is derived from research in which the typing rate is measured when the number of characters simultaneously visible to the typist is systematically varied. The typing rate of nearly everyone slows down dramatically as the number of visible characters decreases. This culminates in the average interkey interval when only a single character is visible being virtually identical to that of choice reaction time. FIGURE 2 illustrates typical results with this manipulation.

In a number of recent studies (e.g., references 4–8), I have used this technique of

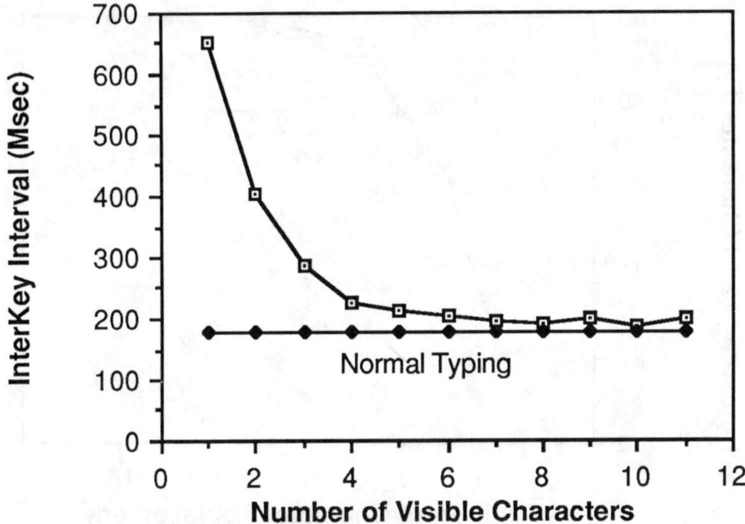

FIGURE 2. Median interkey interval as a function of the number of simultaneously visible characters.

varying the number of visible characters to determine the largest number at which typists exhibit substantial slowing of their typing relative to their rate with no restrictions on the number of visible characters. Because typists are impaired with this number of characters, it can be concluded that they rely upon more than this number in their normal typing. I have referred to this measure as the eye-hand span because it indicates the number of characters intervening between the focus of the eyes and the action of the hand. Across several studies involving slightly different procedures, typists averaging about 60 words per minute have been found to have average eye-hand spans ranging from about 3.4 to 4.9 characters.

The eye-hand span indicates when the typist begins processing a character in advance of the keystroke. Another technique that I have employed provides an estimate of when the typist finishes processing the character and becomes committed to the typing of that particular character. This commitment span is measured by requesting typists to type exactly what appears on a computer monitor and then intermittently changing one of the to-be-typed characters at various positions prior to the relevant keystroke. As FIGURE 3 illustrates, the probability of typing the replaced or second character decreases dramatically as the replacement occurs closer to the keystroke for that character. These results suggest that the typist becomes committed to a keystroke for the original character because he or she can no longer abort that preparation and execute the keystroke corresponding to the replaced character. An individual typist's commitment span can be identified by determining the number of characters in advance of the keystroke corresponding to a 0.5 probability of typing the replaced character. Results from several studies indicate that typists averaging about 60 words per minute have commitment spans ranging from about 2.8 to 3.0 characters.

FIGURE 4 summarizes the results from these two procedures. This manner of representing the results clearly suggests that skilled typists do not rely on strict serial

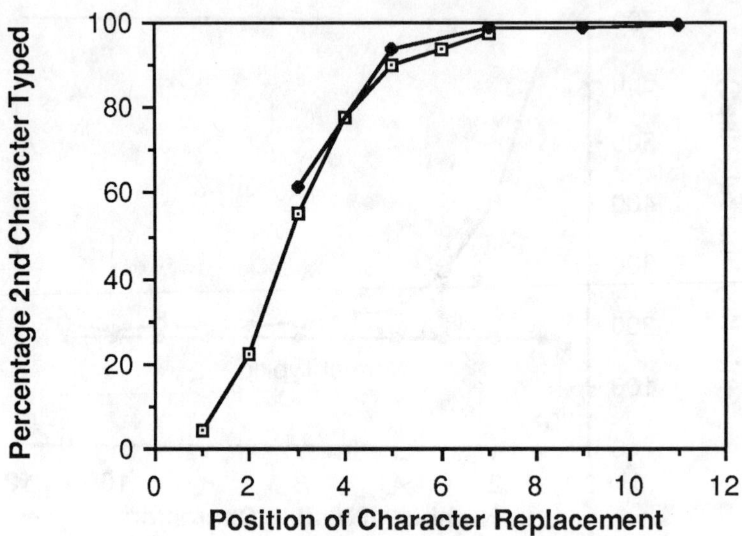

FIGURE 3. Probability of typing the replaced character as a function of the position of the replacement.

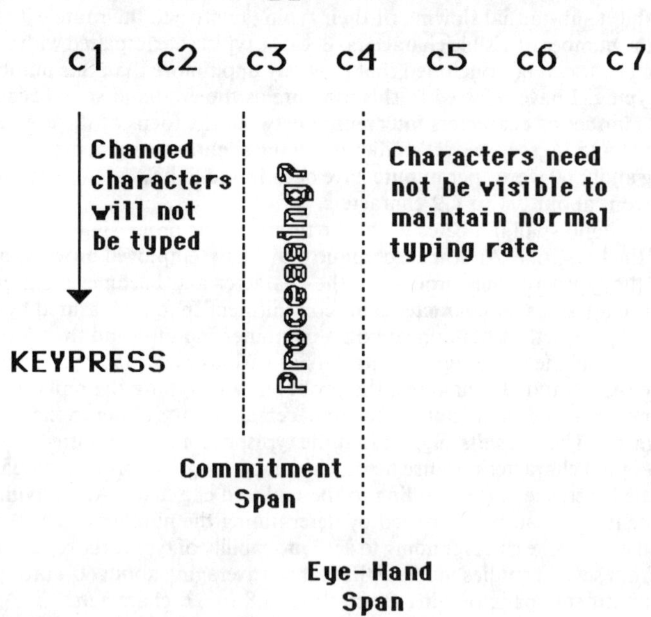

FIGURE 4. Summary illustration of the eye-hand span and commitment span measures of anticipatory processing in typing.

processing, but are instead beginning to process characters two to three in advance while executing the keystroke for a given character. Because these early phases of processing reflect an intricate coordination of perceptual and cognitive information, this anticipatory processing phenomenon is another instance in which cognitive factors influence motor functioning.

I have also examined the effects of age on these measures of anticipatory processing, but only in samples for which there was no correlation between age and average typing speed. Despite this equivalence in overall typing performance, the older typists were considerably slower than the younger typists in the speed of such basic motor processes as repetitive finger tapping and choice reaction time. Because these measures tend to be correlated with speed of typing in the general population, the older individuals would have been expected to be rather slow typists on the basis of their performance on these tasks. However, it was discovered that there were statistically significant positive correlations between age and both eye-hand span and commitment span, thus suggesting that the older typists may have compensated for their slower perceptual-motor processing capacity by expanding the extent of their anticipatory processing. In other words, the older typists apparently began and completed the initial phase of their processing of a character earlier than younger typists and were thus presumably not handicapped by their generally slower rate of perceptual-motor processing.

As with the speed-accuracy trade-off phenomenon, this anticipatory processing phenomenon has two implications for research on aging. The first is methodological and concerns the importance of ensuring that any groups to be compared are equivalent in amount of experience or level of skill. In my typing studies, it was found that the experienced typists, many of whom were older, seemed to employ larger degrees of anticipatory processing than the less experienced, and often younger, typists. Because of this difference in the manner in which the task is performed, levels of basic capacities may not impose the same type of constraints on performance among individuals with different amounts of experience. It is therefore very important that studies of the effects of age on motor functioning involve groups with comparable amounts of experience in the activities that are to be compared.

The second important implication of the anticipatory processing phenomenon is that it indicates that researchers should be very careful in attempting to extrapolate from performance on simple laboratory tasks to prediction of real-world competence. In many instances, performance on a laboratory-type task may have little relevance to functioning in naturally occurring activities, despite the apparent face validity of the tasks. To illustrate, choice reaction time is a valid predictor of typing skill and thus one would have expected the older individuals in the studies described to be poor typists because they tended to have slow reaction times. However, the older individuals had considerable experience as typists and they performed much better than predicted, apparently because they were relying upon cognitive factors (such as expanded anticipatory processing) as effective compensatory mechanisms. Therefore, if one is interested in evaluating the competence of experienced individuals in a reasonably complex motor activity, the performance observations should derive from that activity and not solely from simpler tasks that do not allow the operation of experientially mediated compensatory mechanisms.

To summarize, I have discussed two instances in which cognitive factors influence the level of motor function—one's cognitive emphasis on speed versus accuracy and one's degree of perceptual-cognitive anticipation in sequential activities like transcription typing. Both of these are potentially important to researchers interested in motor functioning because very misleading interpretations of motoric capacity could result if researchers fail to consider their impact. The evidence suggests that this is particularly true in comparisons involving individuals of different ages.

REFERENCES

1. STRAYER, D. L., C. D. WICKENS & R. BRAUNE. Adult age differences in the speed and capacity of information processing: II. An electrophysiological approach. Psychol. Aging. In press.
2. SALTHOUSE, T. A. & B. L. SOMBERG. 1982. Time-accuracy relationships in young and old adults. J. Gerontol. 37: 349–353.
3. SALTHOUSE, T. A. 1979. Adult age and the speed-accuracy tradeoff. Ergonomics 22: 811–821.
4. SALTHOUSE, T. A. 1984. Effects of age and skill in typing. J. Exp. Psychol. Gen. 113: 345–371.
5. SALTHOUSE, T. A. 1984. The skill of typing. Sci. Am. 250: 128–135.
6. SALTHOUSE, T. A. 1985. Anticipatory processing in transcription typing. J. Appl. Psychol. 70: 264–271.
7. SALTHOUSE, T. A. 1986. Perceptual, cognitive, and motoric aspects of transcription typing. Psychol. Bull. 99: 303–319.
8. SALTHOUSE, T. A. & J. S. SAULTS. Multiple spans in transcription typing. J. Appl. Psychol. In press.

DISCUSSION OF THE PAPER

UNIDENTIFIED DISCUSSANT: Have you looked at using nonsense types of words and, if you have, would this show some difference in terms of aging? I am wondering about whether or not the older subjects who are using lots of anticipatory processing are essentially chunking possibly more than the younger typists?

T. SALTHOUSE (*Georgia Institute of Technology, Atlanta, GA*): Yes, there are two ways that we looked at nonsense material. To begin with, we have to take into account the compensation that older typists might employ due to their greater familiarity with the English language, particularly, the sequential dependencies of different letters in the English language. Thus, we looked at both nonsense typing independent of this window manipulation and nonsense typing in the context of it. Our first way of doing this was by taking the same kinds of sentences and simply turning them around, which is very easy to do on the computer (you just start from the end of the array in memory and then go backwards; therefore, the people start with the period that ends the sentence and they end with the capital letter that normally begins the sentence). The advantage of this particular kind of nonsense typing is that it has the same letters, frequencies, spaces, and so forth, but it is completely devoid of meaning.

Another way, though, is to take randomly generated letters so that equal frequency is taken out as well. In both of those cases, the eye-hand spans are greatly reduced; they are shrunken, but you still get this same kind of phenomenon in that the typing rate slows down as you reduce the number of visible characters.

However, the problem is that we do not really know if that shrinking of the range is the cause for the age correlations to go down (which, in fact, they do). Thus, I am answering your question: the correlations between age and these eye-hand spans or anticipatory phenomena are about 0.5 with normal words, whereas they go down to about 0.2 or 0.3 with this nonsense material.

Moreover, though, we do not know whether the attenuation and the correlation are due to the eye-hand span shrinking for everybody. Therefore, the age effects may not be as noticeable, or people may just not be as sensitive to the frequencies differentially with age.

G. LOVELACE: Could you get around that by making the task easier, that is, not having a typing task just have a few buttons?

SALTHOUSE: That is not easier; typing is highly skilled. We did try to do that with number keys and having numbers up on the screen. Then, instead of working with the typewriter keypad, they work with a telephone keypad. However, after 20 sessions of this, the best of our subjects were not even approaching the novice levels of typing. Therefore, it would take an inordinate number of hours to do this.

LOVELACE: You talked about the number of items or characters producing smooth functions when it moves away from normal typing; it breaks off at about five or six items in advance. Now, to me, there is the magic number seven, plus or minus two, which again is a chunk kind of thing. I also wonder if talking in terms of items or characters is to ignore the psychological reality of lexical items; is it five or six because that is the average word length? Remember, they are working a word in advance.

SALTHOUSE: Yes. That is a possibility, but I think that there are a number of factors to argue against it. One is that we still do get these eye-hand spans with nonsense material. They are shrunken, but we still get maybe three to five characters instead of four to six (perhaps a little bit less than that with nonsense material).

The other factor is that when we use very constrained material (such as a study where we just use four-letter randomly arranged words with no semantic meaning because they are just randomly scrambled together) we still get eye-hand spans of about the same length. This argues against the average length of five due to semantic factors because we are still getting eye-hand spans in this same category. I also think that there is a little bit of contribution from the familiarity of meaningful units of words and the fact that they are picking those up in a glance. However, we still get the eye-hand spans with both nonsense material and with words constrained in length of shorter than average length.

A. T. WELFORD (*Aldeburgh, Suffolk, England*): In rapid repetitive movements, usually the dominant hand is a little bit faster than the nondominant hand. Have you separated in terms of your analysis as to which hand is being used and is there a difference in this situation?

SALTHOUSE: In typing, they are obviously using both hands. In the tapping that I used as one of the controls to see what the basic perceptual motor processes were, they either used one hand repetitively (which I balanced across left and right) or they used both hands in alternation. Exactly which one did you want to partial out?

WELFORD: My question is more in relation to those letters that are typed with the right hand and those letters that are typed with the left hand. Can one break up the anticipatory processing time and is it the same?

SALTHOUSE: Typing is very dependent upon hand alternation. Keystrokes are much, much faster if they were preceded by a keystroke on the opposite hand, presumably because there is more actual physical preparation for that next keystroke. Because of factors like this one, I did not try to partial it out.

WELFORD: Presumably, then, alternating fingers are quicker than one finger used repetitively.

SALTHOUSE: That is also true, but that varies with skill levels, as does this alternation effect.

Response Preparation and Posture Control

Neuromuscular Changes in the Older Adult[a]

MARJORIE WOOLLACOTT, BARBARA INGLIN,
AND DIANE MANCHESTER

*College of Human Development and Performance
and Institute of Neuroscience
Esslinger Hall
University of Oregon
Eugene, Oregon 97403*

Two different types of motor abilities are critical for motor coordination at any stage in life. These can be considered under the categories of voluntary movement control (e.g., abilities like eye-hand coordination) and automatic balance control or postural adjustments. Until recently, most of the motor control research on aging has focused on voluntary control skills. However, it is important to realize that the efficient execution of a voluntary movement requires either the prior or simultaneous activation of an appropriate postural set, which is the foundation for accurate movement control.[1,2] Many studies on the control of movements in mammals have presented evidence to indicate that voluntary movements and postural adjustments are activated by the same central command system.[3] In addition, studies on gait disorders in older adults conclude that deterioration of mechanisms underlying balance control is a primary contributor to gait dysfunction.[4-6] Recent work on humans has also shown that the absence of advance (feed-forward) activation of postural muscles before making a voluntary movement is a problem seen in some varieties of neurological disorders.[7,8] It thus might be predicted that deterioration of the postural control system with aging would influence the speed and accuracy of execution of voluntary movement as well.

The following discussion will focus on age-related changes in motor performance in two areas: (1) characteristics of motor control in the postural system itself and (2) characteristics of the interactions between the postural and voluntary control systems during the execution of voluntary movements. We will give evidence to indicate that postural muscle response latencies are significantly longer in the aging adult (compared to the young one) when these responses are activated by external threats to balance. We will also discuss the contribution of visual, proprioceptive, and vestibular system deterioration to changes in balance control with age. In addition, we will show that the feed-forward activation of postural responses before a voluntary movement slows with age. However, this slowing in the activation of postural muscles is smaller than the slowing in the subsequent activation of voluntary responses.

[a] This research was supported by PHS Grant No. AGO 5317-02 from the National Institute on Aging.

BALANCE CONTROL

Early behavioral research on age-related changes in postural control has demonstrated significantly larger amplitudes of body sway during quiet stance both in children (6–14 years) and in older adults (60–80 years) when compared to young adults (16–59 years).[9,10] In order to explore changes in the characteristics of neuromuscular responses that might underlie this increased sway in the older adult, recent studies have examined balance control in a laboratory task similar to that of balancing in a moving bus or ship, or walking on a slippery surface. In order to replicate this type of environmental condition, the position of a movable platform on which the person stood was momentarily shifted in either the anterior or posterior direction, or rotationally, about the axis of the ankle joints. The muscle responses that were subsequently activated and that restored the subject's center of gravity to normal were measured with surface electromyograms (EMGs) that had been rectified and filtered. The characteristics of timing, amplitude, and organization of responses of muscles in the upper and lower legs [gastrocnemius (G), tibialis anterior (TA), hamstrings (H), and quadriceps (Q)] were compared in healthy older (62–78 years) and younger (19–38 years) adults.[11–13]

In order to explore the relative contribution of visual, proprioceptive, and vestibular inputs to the control of balance in both older and younger adults, the sensory information available to the subject was also varied. In order to reduce sway-related proprioceptive information available from the ankle joint and foot, the ankle joint was kept at a constant angle of 90° by rotating the platform around the ankle joint axis in direct proportion to body sway. Visual information available to the subject was manipulated by the use of a visual enclosure that also rotated in direct proportion to body sway. Trials under these conditions were compared to those with eyes open and eyes closed. When both sway-related proprioceptive information was eliminated by keeping the ankle at a constant 90° angle and visual feedback was eliminated with eyes closed, vestibular inputs were assumed to be the dominant inputs controlling posture.

In young adults, it has been shown that unexpected anterior or posterior platform movements cause body sway principally at the ankle joint and that the subsequent stretch of the ankle muscles elicits contractions in the leg that return the center of mass to its normal position. These responses are stereotypically organized into muscle response synergies, with the stretched muscles in the lower leg normally showing activation at about 100 ms, which is followed by the activation of responses in the upper leg (10–20 ms later) on the same side of the body.[14–16] For example, in one study (using ten young adults), when the platform moved forward and the subject swayed backward, responses were activated in TA and Q at 97 $\pm$ 13 ms and 118 $\pm$ 17 ms, respectively.[12]

Recent studies on postural response characteristics in older adults show significant differences in certain parameters of these postural responses: (1) a small, but significant increase in the latency of responses in the ankle joint musculature, (2) occasional disruption in the temporal sequencing of the distal and proximal muscles in certain older adults (5 of 12 adults in one study),[12] (3) increased cocontraction of antagonist muscles, and (4) increased variability in contraction amplitude of proximal and distal muscles within a postural response synergy.

When the response latencies of the two age groups were compared for platform movements causing posterior sway, tibialis anterior response latencies were significantly longer ($p < 0.05$) in the older adult group. Latencies were 102 $\pm$ 6 ms and 109 $\pm$ 9 ms, respectively, for the young and older adult groups. However, due to a large intersubject variability in the older adult group, this difference was not observed for the upper leg. When the responses of individual older adults were examined, two clearly distinguishable response patterns were noted for the distal-proximal muscle response synergy. Seven of the 12 older adults who participated in the study showed a normal temporal response pattern, even though the quadriceps muscle was activated very late (154 ± 15 ms). However, 5 of the older adults showed a reversal of the distal-proximal muscle response sequencing in 10 of the 20 trials, with the proximal quadriceps muscle activated at 101 ± 9 ms, which is in advance of the tibialis anterior (109 ± 9 ms).

In young adults, the absolute amplitude of contraction of muscles varies from trial to trial. However, within a synergic grouping, the proximal and distal muscle response amplitudes remain relatively constant with respect to each other.[15,17] In order to determine if any change occurred in this synergistic amplitude coupling in older adults, the correlations between the amplitudes of tibialis and quadriceps muscle responses (evoked by platform translations causing posterior sway) were calculated and compared for the two age groups. Significant differences ($p < 0.001$) were observed between correlations in the two groups: correlations between 0.82 and 1.0 were seen in all the young adults tested, whereas the older adults showed correlations ranging from a low of 0.12 to a high of 0.86. The amplitude correlation of only one of the older subjects fell within the range for the young adults.[12]

In order to explore the possibility that aging causes changes in the relative contributions of visual, vestibular, and somatosensory inputs and in the ability to rapidly adapt the relative weighting of these inputs to changing environmental conditions, experiments were performed that measured body sway during 10 seconds of stance under the following sensory conditions: (1) somatosensory ankle joint inputs and visual inputs normal (SnVn), (2) somatosensory ankle joint inputs normal and eyes closed (SnVc), (3) relevant ankle joint inputs minimized by rotating the platform in direct relationship to body sway, but vision normal (SsVn), (4) somatosensory ankle joint inputs normal, but relevant visual inputs minimized by rotating a visual enclosure surrounding the subject in direct relationship to body sway (SnVs), (5) both relevant ankle joint and visual inputs minimized by rotating both platform and visual enclosure in direct relation to body sway (SsVs), and (6) relevant ankle joint inputs minimized by platform rotation and eyes closed (SsVc).

In response to the first four conditions, the sway of the older adults was slightly, but nonsignificantly increased in comparison to the younger adults, and sway was well within the limits of stability. This observation is in accordance with the minimal increase in latency of somatosensory-mediated postural adjustments mentioned above. However, the sway of the older adult group deteriorated proportionately more than the younger adults when both the support surface and the visual enclosure were rotated to eliminate relevant ankle and visual inputs or when ankle joint inputs were eliminated with eyes closed. Two of the 12 older adults became unstable and lost their balance under SsVs conditions, while 6 of the 12 older adults lost balance under SsVc conditions. However, on subsequent trials, only one older adult continued to exceed the limits of stability. All others adapted the initial responses sufficiently to maintain balance. No individual in the younger adult group lost balance under any of the conditions tested.[12]

There is physiological evidence to suggest that primary vestibular functions are impaired in the older adult.[18,19] The inability of 6 of the 12 older adults to stand using primarily vestibular orientation inputs (i.e., with eyes closed and the platform rotated to keep the ankle at 90°) may be indicative of impaired peripheral vestibular function or central integrative processes in the aging adult.

VISION AND POSTURE CONTROL

Previous research on the effects of aging on the visual system show that neural circuits activated by stimuli in the peripheral visual field lose sensitivity with age.[19,20] Peripheral vision is also hypothesized to be important in balance control and locomo-

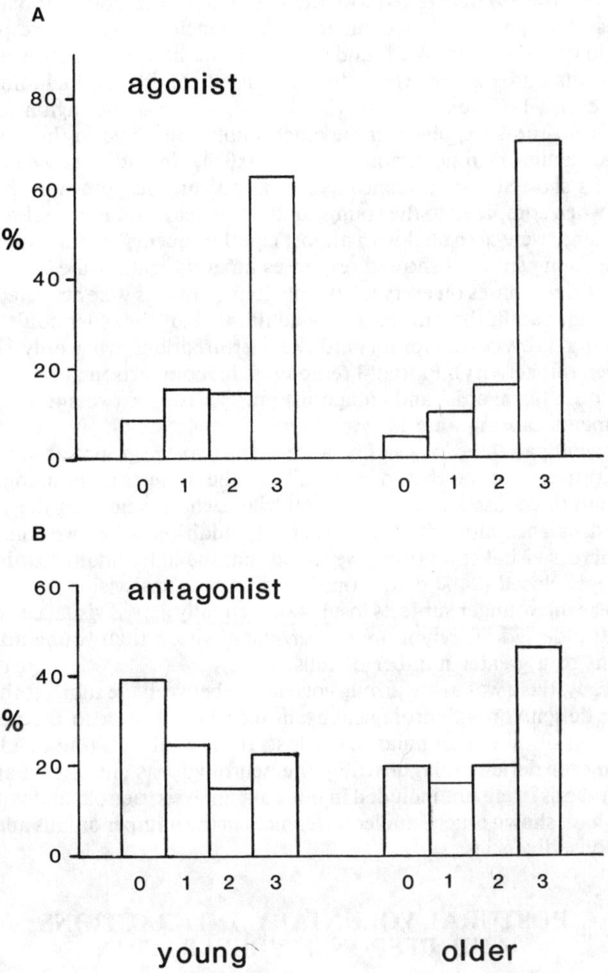

FIGURE 1. Comparison of the frequency of occurrence of postural muscle responses in young (Y) versus older (O) adults for platform movements causing anterior sway. The numbers 0–3 represent the number of trials in which a response was activated out of a total of three trials. Part A shows the frequency of response occurrence in the agonist muscles for the two age groups. Part B shows the frequency of response occurrence in the antagonist muscles.

tion.[20] In order to determine whether there are differential effects of aging on different parts of the visual system controlling posture, a second study was performed in which available visual inputs to the subjects were manipulated by the use of special goggles that limited vision to either (1) central vision only, (2) peripheral vision only, or (3) visual feedback unrelated to body sway (translucent goggles were worn). Trials under these conditions were compared to those with eyes open (with full visual information) and eyes closed. Young adults (mean age of 24 years; $n = 13$) and older adults (mean age of 69 years; $n = 13$) were tested with the same anterior or posterior platform movements as described above. When comparing the latencies of postural responses of the leg muscles in the two groups, we found no significant differences between the younger and older adults under any of the individual visual conditions, including peripheral vision. However, when we combined visual conditions, we once again found significantly longer postural responses in the older adults compared to the younger adults for the tibialis anterior in posterior sway ($p < 0.024$). In addition, we noted that the aging subjects showed a significant increase in postural responses in the antagonist leg muscles when compared to the young adults. Whereas agonist muscles in a postural response synergy were activated with almost equal frequency in old and young adults (62% of the young subjects showed responses on every trial, while 70% of the older subjects showed responses on every trial), antagonist muscles were activated much more often in the older adult than in the young adult (46% of the older adults showed antagonist activity on every trial for forward sway perturbations, while only 22% of young adults showed this activity). FIGURE 1 represents this comparison of the activation frequencies of both the agonist and antagonist muscles for the two age groups for platform movements causing anterior sway.

When we compared the losses of balance of the two age groups under the different visual conditions, we found that, overall, 15% of the subjects in the aging adult group had more than three losses of balance in 60 trials, whereas none of the younger subjects had lost balance more than three times. In addition, when we compared losses of balance across visual conditions, we found that the older adults lost balance most often with eyes closed (24% of the time) and with central vision only (38% of the time), whereas the younger subjects lost balance equally across visual conditions. This suggests that older adults rely more on peripheral vision than young adults, and its absence leads to a greater number of falls.

In this study, there was also a strong correlation between the subjects that presented the stronger deficits on a neurological exam (conducted prior to the postural tests) and the number of times that balance was lost. If the 2 subjects (out of 13) with slight sensory or motor deficits (diagnosed by the neurologist as clumsiness and slight residual hemiparesis) were not included in our data analysis, our old and young populations would have shown much smaller differences in the number of falls and in postural muscle response latencies.

POSTURAL-VOLUNTARY INTERACTIONS
AND RESPONSE PREPARATION

Studies of voluntary reaction time show a slowing of fast reaction time movements with age.[21] Because postural stability has also been shown to deteriorate, and because these systems have been shown to be linked together via a common command pathway,[3] it could be hypothesized that slowing of reaction times in the standing adult for voluntary responses and postural responses are correlated, and that both are linked to underlying changes in the ability of the older adult to adequately prepare postural control systems for movement. In order to determine if the postural control system deterioration is linked to a slowing in voluntary response time, the following experiments were performed. Two groups of subjects—a young adult group (mean age = 26 ± 3; n = 15) and an older adult group (mean age = 71 ±4; n = 15)—were asked to make reaction time arm movements consisting of a push or a pull on a handle placed in front of them at chest height, while they stood on a platform. Surface EMG responses were recorded from the biceps (B) and triceps (Tr) muscles of the arm, in addition to the muscles of the leg (G, TA, H, and Q). Two light-emitting diodes (LEDs) were located on the wall in front of the subject. The illumination of the upper LED indicated a handle push would be required, while the illumination of the lower LED indicated that a handle pull would be required. The trials were triggered with a warning signal that consisted of the illumination (200 ms) of either the upper or lower LED [simple reaction time (SRT) task] or the simultaneous illumination of both LEDs [complex reaction time (CRT) task], which instructed (or did not instruct) the subject in advance about the direction of the arm movement to be performed. The warning signal started a preparatory period of 600 ms. At the end of the preparation period, illumination of one of the LEDs (200 ms), as a response signal, triggered the movement in the corresponding direction (push: upper LED; pull: lower LED). In a series of 20 trials, there were 5 randomly distributed trials for each of the four conditions: push SRT, pull SRT, push CRT, and pull CRT.

Earlier studies on young adults[22] have indicated that the gastrocnemius muscle in the leg is activated consistently before the biceps muscle in the arm when a subject is asked to pull on a handle while standing. Likewise, the tibialis anterior of the leg is activated consistently before the triceps of the arm when a subject is asked to push on a handle while standing. The activation of the gastrocnemius muscle serves to compensate in advance for the change in the center of gravity caused by the handle pull. Response latencies of G and B show means of 190 ± 45 ms and 260 ± 97 ms, respectively, in young adults making simple reaction time arm movements consisting of a handle pull. Those of TA and Tr show latencies of 161 ± 35 ms and 248 ± 90 ms, respectively, for movements consisting of a handle push. When we compared the response of old and young adults for these two movements, we found an increase in the onset latency of postural muscles for the older adult group (G: 217 ± 63 ms for pull; TA: 234 ± 76 ms for push). Thus, there were increases in postural response latencies in older adults of 27 ms for G (nonsignificant) and 73 ms for TA (significant: $p < 0.047$) for simple reaction time tasks. These data show an interesting bias in aging effects on the flexor (TA) versus the extensor (G) muscles of the ankle for these postural adjustments associated with arm movements. This is similar to the aging effect that we noticed for postural responses to external threats to balance, in which TA also shows greater response latency increases than G. We also found large increases in the latencies of the older group for activation of the prime mover muscles of the arm (B: 378 ± 133 ms; Tr: 372 ± 135 ms) (see FIGURES 2 and 3). The concomitant increases in latencies for the prime mover muscles in the older adults for the respective push and pull tasks were 118 ms for B (significant: $p < 0.001$) and 124 ms for Tr (significant: $p < 0.001$).

When we compared the differences in onset times between the postural and voluntary (prime mover) muscles of the young and older adults, we noticed an additional increase in voluntary response slowing in the older adult that was beyond what was due to slowing of the activation of postural responses. Thus, for young adults, differences between B and G onset latencies were 70 ms, while for older adults, they were 161 ms, for pull trials. For push trials, Tr—TA latency differences were 87 ms for the young and 138 ms for the older adult groups, respectively.

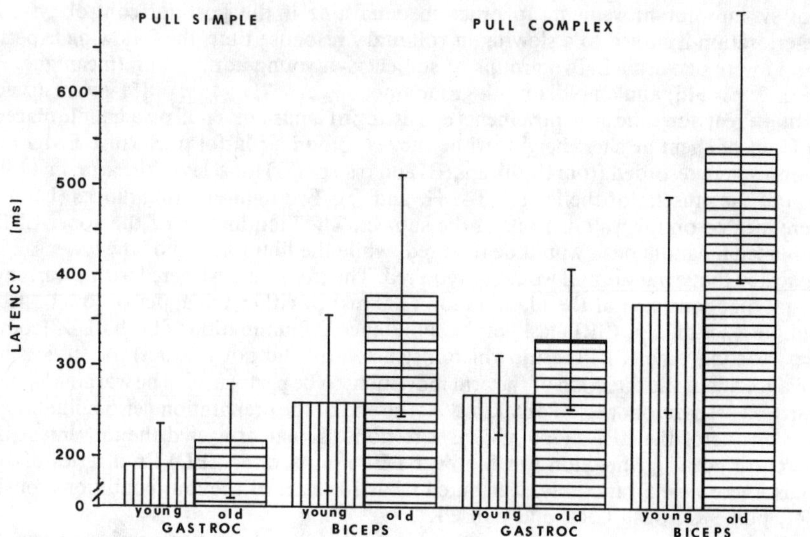

FIGURE 2. Comparison of the onset latencies of postural and voluntary muscle responses in young versus older standing adults for simple and complex reaction time movements consisting of a handle pull.

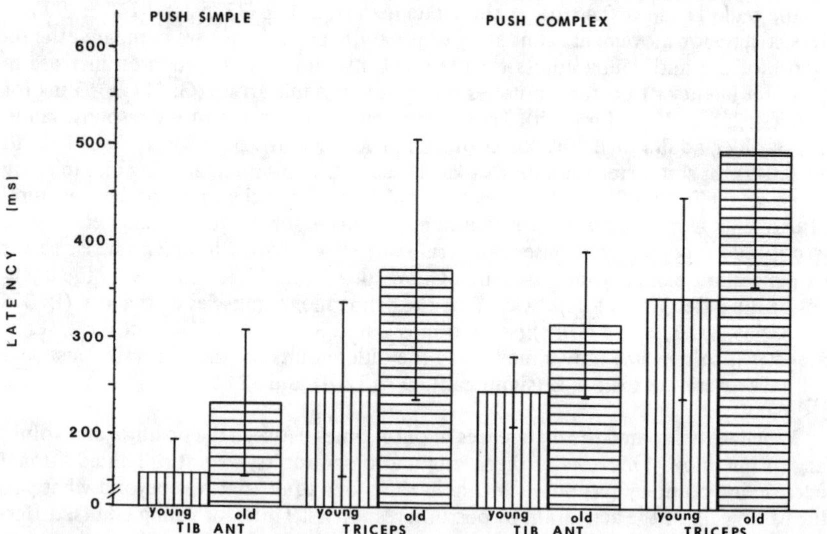

FIGURE 3. Comparison of the onset latencies of postural and voluntary muscle responses in young versus older standing adults for simple and complex reaction time movements consisting of a handle push.

For the complex reaction time task, we noticed additional increases in the onset latencies of both postural and voluntary muscles in the older versus younger adults (see FIGURES 2 and 3). For pull trials, the young adults showed latencies of 269 ± 44 ms for G and 371 ± 119 ms for B, while the older adults showed latencies of 331 ± 78 ms and 543 ± 148 ms for G and B, respectively. For push CRT trials, the younger group showed latencies of 246 ± 36 ms for TA and 344 ± 104 ms for Tr, while the older adults showed latencies of 316 ± 76 ms and 497 ± 141 ms for TA and Tr, respectively. Latency differences for the young versus old groups were highly significant for both postural (G: $p < 0.005$; TA; $p < 0.021$) and voluntary (B: $p < 0.001$; Tr: $p < 0.0001$) muscles. However, as in the SRT task, the onset latencies of the voluntary muscles were slowed to a greater degree than those of the postural muscles.

This suggests that the voluntary control system may be affected to a slightly greater degree than the postural control system during aging. It also implies that deterioration of the speed of activation of the postural control system is not the only factor that limits the speed of voluntary movement onset. It is possible that deterioration of independent preparatory processes within the voluntary control system are an additional cause of slowing in reaction time movements. These results are somewhat different than those that were found by Mankovskii *et al.*[23] when they studied postural preparation for voluntary movements in both young (10–29 years), old (60–69 years), and extremely old (90–99 years) adults. They used a paradigm in which they asked the subjects to voluntarily raise one leg as quickly as possible, by flexion at the knee, in response to the illumination of a lamp. They recorded EMGs from muscles in both the postural (support) leg (Q) and the raised leg (H) (the prime mover). They found a slowing in the postural and voluntary response latencies when comparing their young and old adult groups. In the extremely old adult group, subjects were unable to activate postural muscles sufficiently in advance of the prime mover to keep from losing balance in many of the trials. Instead of showing feed-forward activation of postural muscles, the postural and voluntary muscles were activated almost simultaneously when the extremely old subjects were asked to move as quickly as possible. The differences in the results of our studies and those of Mankovskii and his colleagues may lie either in the experimental paradigm or in the age of the subjects involved in the study. It is possible that the link between the postural control system and the prime movers is different for responses originating totally within the lower limbs than for responses that consist of interactions between the upper and lower limbs.

Alternatively, it is possible that the extent of neurological dysfunction present in the old versus the very old would be significant if it were to be quantified. Mankovskii and his colleagues do not indicate results of neurological examinations of his two older age groups, so it is unclear to what extent each of the groups may have been affected by subclinical sensory or motor problems.

SUMMARY AND CONCLUSIONS

Experiments comparing the characteristics of neuromuscular responses underlying balance control in young and old adults have shown a number of differences between the two populations. Postural muscle response latencies of the ankle musculature activated by external threats to balance are slightly, but significantly, longer in the latter population. In addition, some aging subjects show a temporal reversal of proximal and distal muscle response onset in some trials. There is also a breakdown of the correlation of the amplitude of the muscle responses within a synergy in some of the older subjects tested. Older adults also exhibited cocontraction of agonist and antagonist muscles within a response synergy to a greater extent than young adults. This stiffening of the joints by antagonist cocontraction could be a compensation for the lack of the ability to fine-tune the postural responses to the same degree as the young adults.

Analysis of sensory integration abilities showed an impairment in balance control under conditions of reduced or conflicting sensory information. When they were given inappropriate visual and somatosensory inputs, half of the older adults lost balance on the first trial. In most instances, however, the older adults were able to maintain balance during a second trial consisting of the same sensory stimuli.

When visual cues were reduced by restricting the visual field to either central or peripheral visual cues, we found no difference in postural muscle response latencies. However, the aging adult group showed more losses of balance than the younger group with peripheral vision removed or with eyes closed. In addition, there was a strong correlation between the subjects that showed stronger deficits on an initial neurological exam and the number of times that balance was lost.

Studies on changes in the linkage between postural and voluntary muscle interactions during voluntary arm movements in older adults indicate an increase in the latency of feed-forward activation of postural muscles. However, voluntary muscle response onset latencies show greater increases in the old compared to the young. This suggests that deterioration of the speed of activation of the postural control system is not the only factor that limits the speed of voluntary movement onset. Measurements have not yet been made on the amplitude regulation of feed-forward responses of postural muscles during a voluntary task. It may be that the regulation of the speed of activation of the two systems is less important than the fine tuning of the correlation of appropriate response amplitudes between the two systems. We are currently in the process of analyzing the correlation between the amplitudes of postural and voluntary muscle responses during this task.

REFERENCES

1. BELENKII, V. E., V. S. GURFINKEL & R. I. PALTSEV. 1967. On the elements of voluntary control. Biofizika **12:** 135–141.
2. BOUISSET, S. & M. ZATTARA. 1981. A sequence of postural movements precedes voluntary movement. Neurosci. Lett. **22:** 263–270.
3. MASSION, J. 1984. Postural changes accompanying voluntary movements: normal and pathological aspects. Hum. Neurobiol. **2:** 261–267.
4. MURRAY, M. P., R. C. KORY & B. T. CLARKSON. 1969. Walking patterns in healthy old men. J. Gerontol. **24:** 169–178.
5. GUIMARAES, R. M. & B. ISAACS. 1980. Characteristics of the gait in old people who fall. Int. Rehab. Med. **2:** 177–180.
6. WOOLLACOTT, M. H. 1986. Gait and postural control in the aging adult. *In* Disorders of Posture and Gait. W. Bles & T. Brandt, Eds. Elsevier. Amsterdam.
7. PALTSEV, Y. I. & A. M. ELNER. 1967. Preparatory and compensatory period during voluntary movement in patients with involvement of the brain of different localization. Biofizika **12:** 161–168.
8. TRAUB, M. M., J. C. ROTHWELL & C. D. MARSDEN. 1980. Anticipatory postural reflexes in Parkinson's disease and other akinetic-rigid syndromes and in cerebellar ataxia. Brain **103:** 393–412.
9. SHELDON, J. C. 1963. The effect of age on the control of sway. Gerontol. Clin. **5:** 129–138.
10. HASSELKUS, B. R. & G. M. SHAMBES. 1975. Aging and postural sway in women. J. Gerontol. **30:** 661–667.
11. WOOLLACOTT, M., A. T. SHUMWAY-COOK & L. M. NASHNER. 1982. Postural reflexes and aging. *In* The Aging Motor System. J. A. Mortimer, Ed. Praeger. New York.
12. WOOLLACOTT, M. H., A. SHUMWAY-COOK & L. M. NASHNER. 1986. Aging and posture

control: changes in sensory organization and muscular coordination. Int. J. Aging Hum. Dev. **23:** 97–114.

13. MANCHESTER, D. L., M. H. WOOLLACOTT & N. ZEDERBAUER-HYLTON. 1986. Effects of aging and vision on postural muscle response synergies. Proceedings. NASPSPA Meetings. Scottsdale, Arizona.

14. NASHNER, L. M. 1976. Adapting reflexes controlling human posture. Exp. Brain Res. **26:** 69–72.

15. NASHNER, L. M. 1977. Fixed patterns of rapid postural responses among leg muscles during stance. Exp. Brain Res. **30:** 13–24.

16. NASHNER, L. M. & M. WOOLLACOTT. 1979. The organization of rapid postural adjustments of standing humans: an experimental conceptual model. *In* Posture and Movement. R. E. Talbot & D. R. Humphrey, Eds. Raven Press. New York.

17. NASHNER, L. M., M. WOOLLACOTT & G. TUMA. 1979. Organization of rapid responses to postural and locomotor-like perturbations in standing man. Exp. Brain Res. **36:** 463–476.

18. ROSENHALL, U. & W. RUBIN. 1975. Degenerative changes in the human vestibular sensory epithelia. Acta Oto-Laryngol. **79:** 67–81.

19. SEKULER, R., L. P. HUTMAN & C. J. OWSLEY. 1980. Human aging and spatial vision. Science **209:** 1255–1256.

20. LEIBOWITZ, H. W., C. S. RODEMER & J. DICHGANS. 1979. The independence of dynamic spatial orientation from luminance and refractive error. Percept. Psychophys. **25:** 75–79.

21. WELFORD, A. T. 1980. Sensory, perceptual and motor processes in older adults. *In* Handbook on Mental Health and Aging. J. I. Birren, Ed. Prentice-Hall. Englewood Cliffs, New Jersey.

22. CORDO, P. J. & L. M. NASHNER. 1982. Properties of postural adjustments associated with rapid arm movements. J. Neurophysiol. **47:** 287–302.

23. MANKOVSKII, N., Y. A. MINTS & U. P. LYSENYUK. 1980. Regulation of the preparatory period for complex voluntary movement in old and extreme old age. Hum. Physiol. (Moscow) **6:** 46–50.

DISCUSSION OF THE PAPER

UNIDENTIFIED DISCUSSANT: Is there any evidence from the autopsy studies of deterioration in the vestibular system (especially, for example, hair cells in the macula or the canals) with age?

M. WOOLLACOTT (*University of Oregon, Eugene, OR*): Yes, there have been a number of studies where they have found that there is a significant decrease. In fact, it may be up to about 40% in hair cells in autopsy subjects that were in their 70s or 80s.

G. S. ROTH (*NIA, Baltimore, MD*): In addition to the vestibular system, I want to make a connection between the presentations of today and those that are going to come tomorrow because it will be a bit more biochemical. Could you possibly trace this back to a primary cause (or causes) in the nigrostriatal system? Have you thought about it in that way?

WOOLLACOTT: I certainly have not. I do not know anything about vestibular pathways into the nigrostriatal system.

ROTH: How about apart from the vestibular system? Do you think the vestibular system is really the central defect?

WOOLLACOTT: No, I do not. You cannot take away vestibular inputs from humans without putting them into space, so all I know is what happens when only vestibular inputs remain. If we had taken away vestibular and visual inputs and had only somatosensory cues, we still might have seen exactly the same number of falls.

E. HUE (*Mount Sinai Hospital, New York, NY*): Would you say that the ankle joint is the most important proprioceptive receptor in standing and walking?

WOOLLACOTT: That is what a number of studies that have been done in L. Nashner's lab in Portland seem to indicate. Out of all the joints that are involved in postural control, ankle joints appear to be the most important, though this may vary from one subject to another. In fact, Nashner has shown recently that if you take away a wide base of support and give the subjects a very narrow base of support, they begin to start using information more from their hip joint. Thus, they actually start shifting their weight at the hip instead of at the ankle.

HUE: There are two things that I would like to point out as a clinician. First, there are a substantial number of older people who are bilateral amputees (usually the ones who are going to be walkers are below the knee) and they have been very successful in learning to walk with bilateral prostheses. Of course, they would have absolutely no proprioceptive information from anything below the knee.

The other thing is that there was a study done at Mount Sinai Hospital about 15 years ago by Dujong where they anesthetized cervical spine and found that younger volunteers became ataxic. Thus, I do not know if the ankle is the most important joint because people do walk without ankle joints and without any information from them.

WOOLLACOTT: You are very right. A person can adapt very quickly to losses of information from one area versus another and I have read articles about amputees being able to balance. Therefore, they can shift with experience to using another sensory system; of course, they always have vision and vestibular input relevant and available to them, so people use those when they need to.

One further thing that I would like to mention is that we did have a neurologist, Oscar Marin, look at all of our aging subjects before we did the exams on them. Interestingly, he noticed that 2 out of our 13 subjects had problems that were somewhat greater than the others. One had an inordinate amount of clumsiness in motor coordination, while the second one had slight residual hemiparesis from an accident that occurred long ago. Now, those were the subjects that showed the most significant differences from our young adults. If we had taken those subjects out of our population, we would have found that the older and the young adults would not have been significantly different. Therefore, when doing studies on aging, we should have a neurologist examine the subjects because that can tell us much more about the problems that are contributing to the loss of movement coordination.

A. CAID (*Mount Sinai Hospital, New York, NY*): You seem to have corroborated Lee and Lishman's work back in the 70s that vestibular input is much less important than proprioceptive and visual input in the control of postural sway. They certainly did not have as much sophisticated equipment as you had. However, did you look at anticipatory motor activity in the lower extremities and how that might facilitate or inhibit motor activity after the perturbation?

WOOLLACOTT: Would you clarify that question? What do you mean by anticipatory activity? Do you mean that they knew in advance that there was going to be a perturbation?

CAID: Even if they did not know that there was going to be a perturbation, I still want to know their standing in the instrumentation and what activity might be present at baseline and in the old versus the young. Furthermore, I want to know how that might facilitate or inhibit the future activity of the muscle.

WOOLLACOTT: That is a good point. We did give them certain trials where they had the same platform perturbation over and over again and we did not find that there was a specific increase in tonic background activity level of one particular muscle group. Therefore, it did not appear to be that they were somehow learning and adapting background activity levels in advance. However, I do not know if that was specifically what you meant by responding in advance. They did not know when the platform was going to actually move, so all they could do was increase background activity levels in all muscles to compensate.

CAID: There have been some studies where the individuals have been instructed that there will be a perturbation and then the anticipatory movements (and how they facilitate) were observed. Is that same type of activity present even without knowledge of the timing of the perturbation?

WOOLLACOTT: I have done one study with young adults where we gave them a tone in advance of the postural perturbation (high tone meaning move one way, low tone meaning move another way). We found that they were able to shorten their posture responses by up to about ten milliseconds, but no more than that when they knew in advance which direction it was moving.

Human Motor Behavior and Aging

JAMES A. MORTIMER

*Geriatric Research
Education and Clinical Center
Veterans Administration Medical Center
Minneapolis, Minnesota 55417
and
Department of Neurology
University of Minnesota Medical School
Minneapolis, Minnesota 55455*

An actor playing an aged person relies extensively upon the stereotypic changes in motor function that are usually considered to accompany aging. Foremost among these is the slowness and hesitancy of movement that characterizes the motor behavior of very elderly individuals. Other features that are often included are a stooped posture, shuffling gait, tremor, and diminution of associated movements and facial expression. The similarities between this stereotype of motor function in the elderly and Parkinson's disease have encouraged the view that Parkinson's disease may represent a form of premature or accelerated brain aging.[1,2]

Despite common acceptance of the stereotype of motor impairment in the aged, systematic studies of motor function in the elderly have been few, and the degree to which positive extrapyramidal motor signs (such as rigidity) occur is not well documented. In this paper, the similarities and differences between motor signs in Parkinson's disease and normal aging are explored. In addition, the role of levodopa therapy in slowing the progression of Parkinson's disease is considered in relation to degenerative processes that occur in the dopaminergic system during normal aging.

PATHOLOGICAL AND NEUROCHEMICAL SIMILARITIES BETWEEN PARKINSON'S DISEASE AND NORMAL BRAIN AGING

Although several different brain lesions have been identified in Parkinson's disease, it is widely believed that the major pathological lesion responsible for the characteristic motor signs in this disease is damage to or loss of cells in the *substantia nigra, pars compacta*.[2-4] This nucleus, located in the mesencephalon and caudal diencephalon, is the source of the ascending dopaminergic pathway to the striatum. A strong correlation between loss of cells in the *substantia nigra* and decreased concentration of dopamine in the striatum has been demonstrated.[3] However, the severity of individual motor signs is not well correlated with dopamine levels in the striatum, with the exception of akinesia, which is associated with lower levels of dopamine in both the caudate and putamen.[3]

Morphological[2,4] and biochemical[2,5,6] studies of brains from persons without neurologic disease demonstrate a progressive decline in the dopaminergic system with increasing age. For example, from birth through age 75, the number of cells in the *sub-*

stantia nigra, pars compacta declines from about 400,000 to less than 200,000.[2] However, the degree of cell loss is not as severe as in Parkinson's disease, where cell counts may range from 60,000 to 120,000.[4] Extrapolation of the regression line for normal, age-related cell loss in the *substantia nigra* suggests that the degree of neuronal loss required for manifestation of the clinical syndrome of parkinsonism would not be reached until well over age 100.

Biochemical studies demonstrate an age-related reduction in the caudate and putamen of the activity of tyrosine hydroxylase (the rate-limiting enzyme for synthesis of dopamine),[2] as well as a reduction of dopamine in the caudate nucleus[5] and in the putamen.[6] In each of these cases, the decline follows an exponential pattern, with the greatest reduction occurring at younger ages. Comparisons of dopamine loss in normal controls and in Parkinson patients have demonstrated a higher rate of loss in patients than in normal subjects. Whereas dopamine in the caudate nucleus was found to decline at an average rate of 12.9% per decade in controls, the rate of loss in Parkinson patients varied from 23.3% to 46.55% per decade.[5]

Studies of D2 dopaminergic receptors using positron emission tomography in healthy living subjects have demonstrated a decline in labeled methylspiperone binding with age.[7] These findings are consistent with the age-related declines in D2 receptors documented previously in autopsy material from both animals and humans.[8-10]

The fact that both neurologically normal controls and Parkinson patients show progressive degeneration of the dopaminergic system with increasing age points to a quantitative (rather than a qualitative) difference between Parkinson's disease and normal brain aging. If the motor signs of Parkinson's disease were related solely to the decline in dopaminergic function, one might expect to see a higher rate of occurrence of extrapyramidal motor signs with increased age.

EXTRAPYRAMIDAL MOTOR SIGNS IN NORMAL AGING

Systematic studies of motor signs in normal aging have been few. Based on his clinical experience, Critchley[11] suggested that extrapyramidal motor signs (including flexed posture, muscular rigidity, general poverty of movement, loss of associated movements, slowness, masked facial expression, and infrequent blinking) are very common in old age. However, he did not regard tremor as a common feature of this stereotype. Kokman *et al.*[12] examined 51 socially active normal subjects from 61 to 84 years of age and found no increase of abnormal gait, posture, or muscle tone. Such findings were also rare in the study of Greenhouse *et al.*,[13] who examined 64 persons between 60 and 88. Potvin *et al.*[14] utilized a machine-based neurological battery to examine the associations of tremor, movement speed, and age in 61 males between 20 and 80. They found no significant difference in arm or hand resting tremor, but they did document marked declines in movement speed across the six decades of life.

We studied 74 generally healthy persons aged 45 to 85 with a battery of machine-administered tests used to evaluate extrapyramidal motor signs in patients with Parkinson's disease.[15] The measurement techniques have been described in detail in previous publications.[15,16] Briefly, rigidity is measured using a servo-controlled device that rotates the forearm in a horizontal plane through an arc of 100 degrees at a constant speed of 20 degrees per second. While the arm is being rotated, we measure the torque with which the patient resists or assists the motion and integrate it over five flexion-extension cycles to obtain a measure of total work. This measure is our index of the severity of rigidity. Rigidity measurements are obtained for each arm under two conditions—with the patient instructed to relax and let his arm be passively rotated (resting rigidity), and while the patient performs a pursuit tracking task with the opposite arm (activated rigidity). In most normal subjects and in those with mild Parkinson's disease, resting rigidity values are commonly negative (because subjects or patients assist the motion), thus producing negative work.

We quantify tremor in two different ways. Arm tremor is measured by integrating the rectified envelope of alternating torque about the elbow joint during a 100-second period while the patient maintains a fixed arm position. To provide a standard level of activation, patients are asked to count backwards by twos from 100 during this procedure. We also measure finger tremor with a two-dimensional miniature accelerometer attached to the index finger of the right or left hand. This is done under three different conditions: at rest, while maintaining a posture, and during intentional finger-to-nose movement.

Bradykinesia or slowness of movement is assessed with three measures. For the first (pursuit score), the patient holds a photodetector in his outstretched hand and attempts to cover a bright dot that appears on a CRT screen located in front of him. As soon as he covers the dot, it jumps to a new unpredictable location and he must then cover the dot again. We count the number of times that the patient catches the dot in 50 seconds.

A second measure of upper-limb bradykinesia (pronation/supination rate) assesses the average total number of degrees swept out by repetitive pronation-supination movements of the forearm during three consecutive 10-second periods separated by 10-second rests. This measurement is made while the patient grasps a handle attached to an angular displacement transducer. To encourage maximum effort, the patient can monitor his performance on a meter, which reads out a value proportional to the average rate of pronation and supination.

The last measure of bradykinesia is the walk impairment index, which is obtained by multiplying the number of seconds taken to walk 30 feet by the number of steps

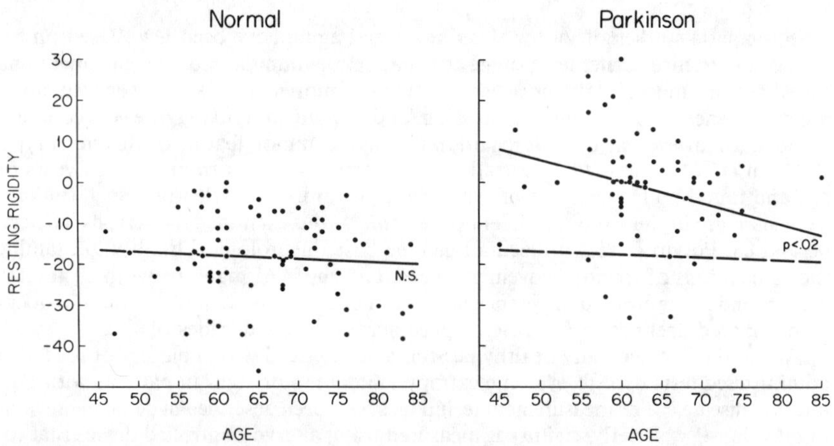

FIGURE 1. Linear regressions of right-sided resting rigidity on age for 74 normal subjects (left panel) and 60 Parkinson patients (right panel). No significant difference was found on any measure between left and right arms. Therefore, in this and all subsequent figures involving measures collected for both arms, data only for the right arm are presented. The dashed line in the right panel corresponds to the regression line for normal subjects in the left panel. (Reprinted with permission from Mortimer and Webster.[15])

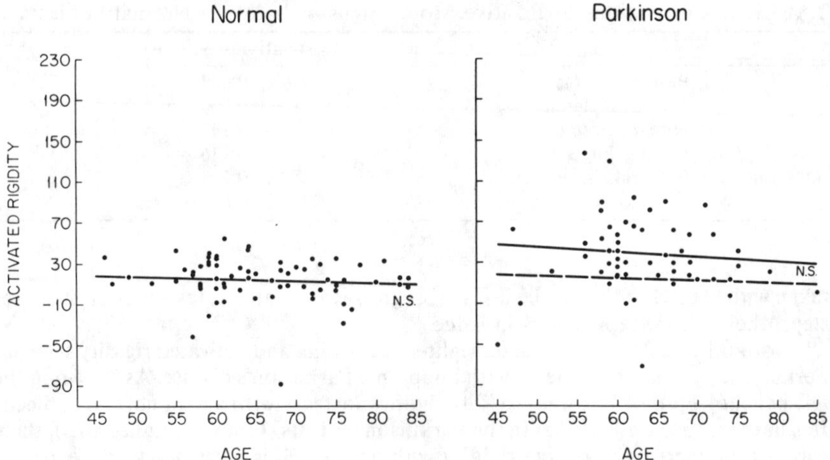

FIGURE 2. Linear regressions of activated rigidity on age for normal subjects and Parkinson patients. Conventions are the same as those in FIGURE 1. (Reprinted with permission from Mortimer and Webster.[15])

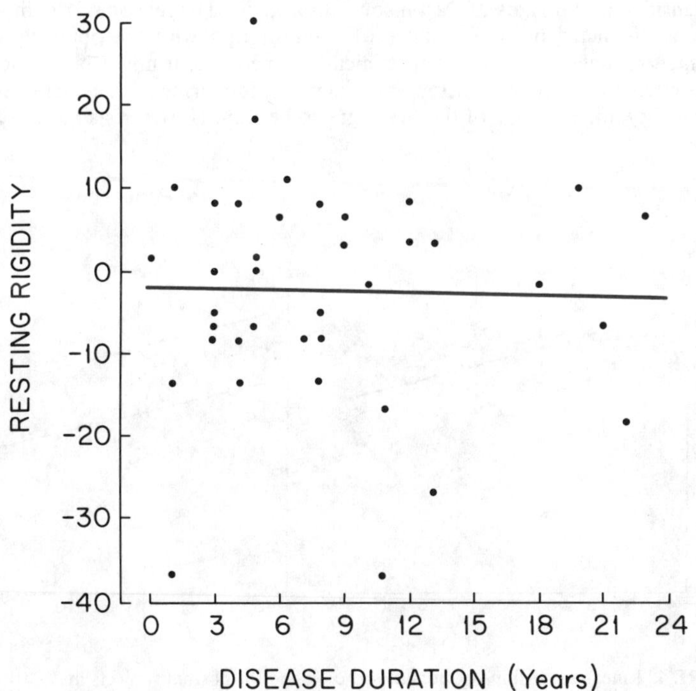

FIGURE 3. Linear regression of resting rigidity on disease duration for the 60 Parkinson patients.

TABLE 1. Correlations of Positive Motor Signs with Age in Normal Subjects

Sign	Correlation Coefficient
Resting rigidity	−0.067
Activated rigidity	−0.090
Forearm tremor	0.197
Resting finger tremor	0.136
Postural finger tremor	0.209
Intention finger tremor	0.099

taken with the right foot. As the disease progresses and patients take shorter or slower steps, the walk index increases in value.

FIGURE 1 and 2 present data on right-sided resting and activated rigidity from 74 normal subjects and 60 patients with idiopathic Parkinson's disease. As shown in the left panel of FIGURE 1, resting rigidity did not increase with age in normal subjects. It is interesting to observe that in the Parkinson patients (FIGURE 1, right panel), there was also no increase in resting rigidity with age, which is what one might expect if this were a motor sign that became more severe as a consequence of age-related changes in the brain. Indeed, what was observed is a decrease in resting rigidity in Parkinson patients with increasing age. This decrease is unlikely to be due to a progressive decrease in rigidity within individual subjects during the disease course. There was, for example, no significant association between rigidity and disease duration (FIGURE 3).

In previous studies, we have found that activated rigidity is one of the earliest and most sensitive motor signs of Parkinson's disease.[17,18] The release of rigidity when a patient is distracted by performance of a motor task with the opposite arm is a phenomenon that is well known to clinicians. Therefore, it might be predicted that if aging were associated with extrapyramidal motor impairment, then increases in activated rigidity might be one of the first signs to be seen. However, as FIGURE 2 shows,

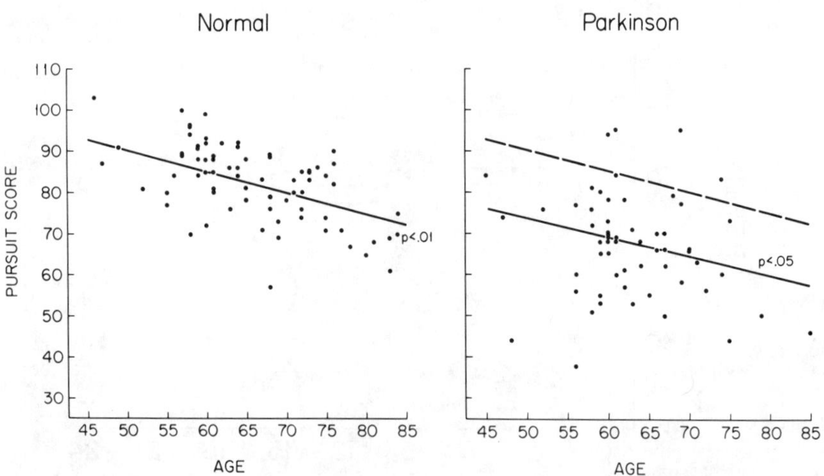

FIGURE 4. Linear regressions of pursuit score on age for normal subjects and Parkinson patients. Conventions are the same as those in FIGURE 1. (Reprinted with permission from Mortimer and Webster.[15])

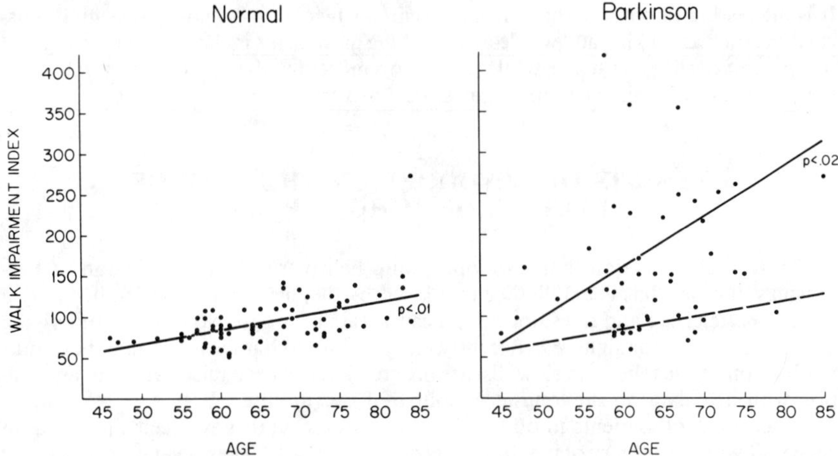

FIGURE 5. Linear regressions of walk impairment index on age for normal subjects and Parkinson patients. Conventions are the same as those in FIGURE 1. (Reprinted with permission from Mortimer and Webster.[15])

there was no age trend in activated rigidity for either normal subjects or for patients with Parkinson's disease.

TABLE 1 summarizes the age correlations within normal subjects for the positive motor signs of Parkinson's disease, namely, rigidity and tremor. There were no significant correlations between age and these positive motor signs.

FIGURE 4 shows the relationship between pursuit score and age when the task was carried out with the right arm. A strong negative correlation between age and maximum motor speed as assessed by this variable is evident. While the scatter of points is greater among Parkinson patients, it is interesting to observe that the slopes of the regression lines for normals and Parkinson patients are virtually identical, thus suggesting that the effects of age and disease may be additive.

The walk impairment index (FIGURE 5) increases linearly in the normal subjects, thus demonstrating progressive slowing of locomotion with increased age. Although there is a significant age trend in the Parkinson patients on this variable, the scatter of points is greater; in addition, there appear to be two groups—a group clustered around the normal control regression line and a group with considerably higher values on the walk index—indicating greater impairment.

TABLE 2 summarizes correlations with age in four motor performance tasks. For all of these tasks, there is a significant decrease in performance with increasing age.

TABLE 2. Correlations of Motor Performance Measures with Age in Normal Subjects

Measure	Correlation Coefficient
Pursuit score	-0.542^a
Pronation-supination rate	-0.423^a
Maximum index-finger tapping rate	-0.236^b
Walk impairment index	0.509^a

[a] $p < 0.01$.
[b] $p < 0.05$.

It is interesting to observe that those movements involving primarily proximal musculature, such as walking and whole-arm reaching movements in the pursuit task, showed the greatest declines with age, while those movements involving more distal musculature, such as index-finger tapping rates, declined less with age.

EFFECTS OF LEVODOPA ON THE RATE OF DECLINE OF MOTOR SPEED

The initial prediction that levodopa would halt or slow the progression of Parkinson's disease[19] has generally been replaced by the view that levodopa has only a symptomatic effect and does not influence the rate of progression of the underlying disease and its motor signs.[20,21] Recently, the possibility that levodopa may both provide symptomatic relief and slow disease progression has been raised again in association with new data on the long-term course of this disease.[22,23]

Since 1962, all patients in our Parkinson's disease clinic have been evaluated on each visit with the battery of machine tests described above. These evaluations provide longitudinal data on the course of Parkinson's disease prior to the availability of levodopa in 1969. Comparable data are available on patients studied since 1969 who were treated with this medication.

TABLE 3 presents data on the mean annual decline in pursuit score for the right and left arms for three groups: the 74 normal controls who were evaluated twice (one year apart), 60 Parkinson patients studied in the 1970s, and 38 Parkinson patients studied in the 1960s before levodopa became available. The normal controls and Parkinson patients studied in the 1970s had approximately the same average rate of annual decline in the pursuit score. On the other hand, patients studied during the 1960s before the advent of levodopa therapy showed about twice the average rate of annual decline as the other two groups. These data suggest that levodopa may have had some type of normalizing or stabilizing effect on the disease process.

An alternative explanation for the difference in the rate of decline of motor speed between Parkinson patients studied in the 1960s and the 1970s is that these groups may have differed in ways other than the types of medications they were receiving. In order to address this issue, we have studied the long-term changes in motor performance in 12 patients whose disease spanned the pre- and post-levodopa era and who were followed for a mean of 6.4 years (3–9 years) before levodopa and for a mean of 10.2 (6–14 years) after this drug was started.

FIGURE 6 shows a 16-year history of the pursuit score in one patient with Parkinson's disease, in whom treatment with levodopa was begun in 1971. Two effects of this medi-

TABLE 3. Mean Annual Rates of Decline of Pursuit Score for Different Groups

	Pursuit Score (% annual decline)	
Group	Right Arm	Left Arm
Normal controls	− 3.55	− 3.51
Parkinson patients with L-dopa	− 2.75	− 4.89
Parkinson patients without L-dopa	− 7.87	− 8.38

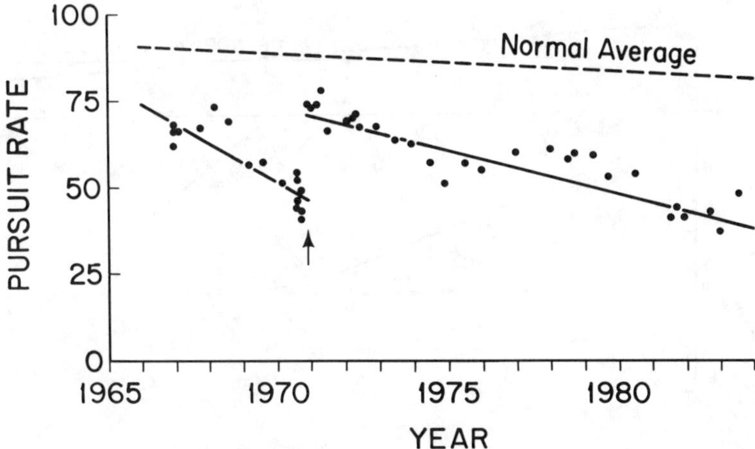

FIGURE 6. Seventeen-year history of pursuit score in a patient with Parkinson's disease. Levodopa therapy was initiated at the time indicated by the arrow. Linear regression lines for pre- and post-levodopa periods are shown. Dots correspond to individual tests or to monthly averages when more than one test was given in a month. Regressions are based on all test scores. Short-term increase in pursuit score and reduction in slope magnitude are both statistically significant ($p < 0.001$). The line labeled "Normal Average" is based on data from the 74 normal control subjects. (Reprinted with permission from Mortimer *et al.*[29])

cation can be observed: a short-term steplike improvement in function soon after the drug was started, and a significant decrease in the absolute value of the slope, thus indicating slowed progression of the bradykinetic deficit. Significant slowing in the progression of bradykinesia was observed in 7 of the 12 patients.

Two other patients had a pattern of response similar to that in FIGURE 7, which consisted of a short-term improvement, followed by a plateau that persisted for two to four years and terminated in an abrupt decline in function. In these patients, the overall effect of the medication was to accelerate the apparent progression of the disease.

Finally, there was a very interesting group of patients who showed little symptomatic relief when levodopa was first given, but in whom there was profound slowing and even reversal in the progression of the bradykinetic deficit. In the particular patient whose data are shown in FIGURE 8, a decline in the pronation-supination rate prior to levodopa was reversed and followed by a period of eight years of slow and gradual improvement.

Data from another patient, who had both a short-term response to levodopa and a long-term progressive increase in function, are shown in FIGURE 9. A very rapid downhill course was halted by levodopa and, over the next 12 years, the patient progressively improved. In fact, nine years after initiation of levodopa therapy, he was performing at a level similar to that of five years before levodopa therapy was begun.

One possible explanation for the slowing or reversal of progression of bradykinesia might be that the dosage of levodopa was increased over time to compensate for disease progression. However, in most of the patients showing long-term slowing or improvement, no major changes in the dosage of levodopa were made over the course of the therapy. For example, in the patient whose data is shown in FIGURE 9, there

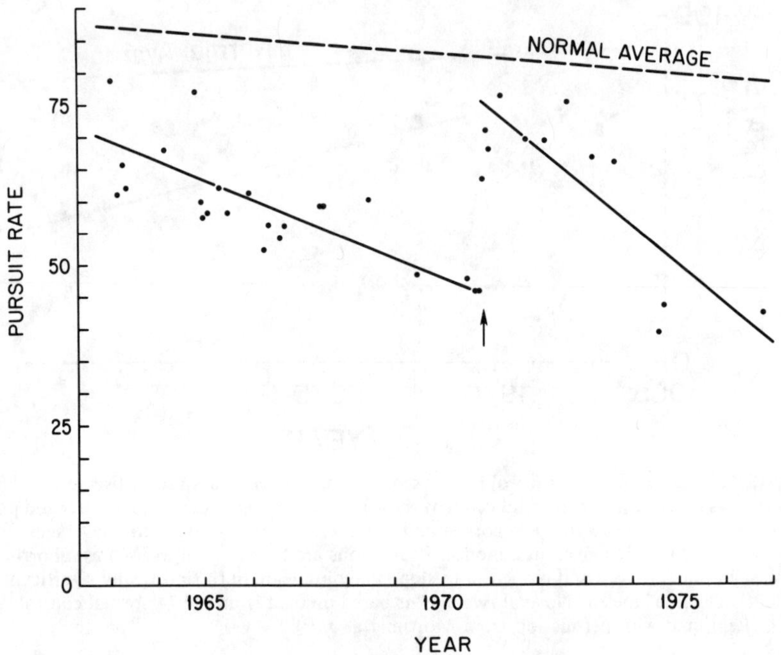

FIGURE 7. Pursuit scores in a patient showing significant short-term response ($p < 0.01$) and a significant increase in slope magnitude ($p < 0.05$) after initiation of levodopa therapy. See the legend of FIGURE 6 for additional details. (Reprinted with permission from Webster *et al.*[23])

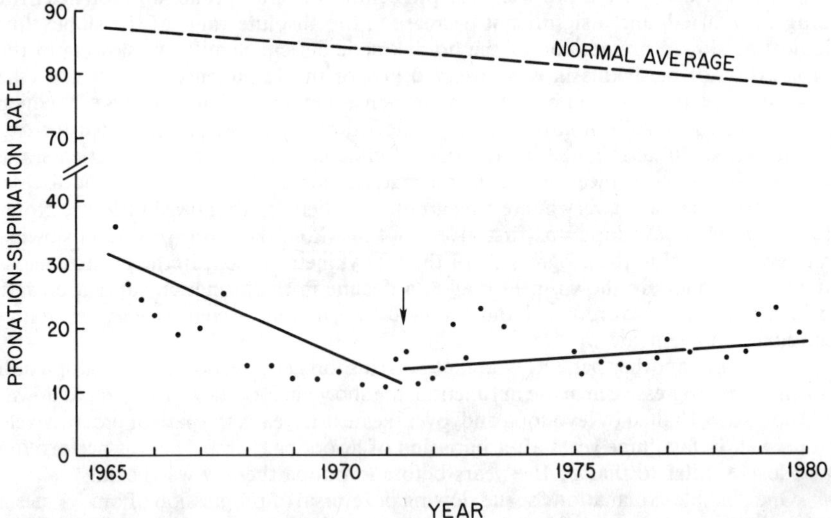

FIGURE 8. Pronation-supination rates in a patient without a significant short-term response to levodopa. Rates are given in hundreds of degrees of total motion. The change in slope is statistically significant ($p < 0.001$). See the legend of FIGURE 6 for additional details. (Reprinted with permission from Webster *et al.*[23])

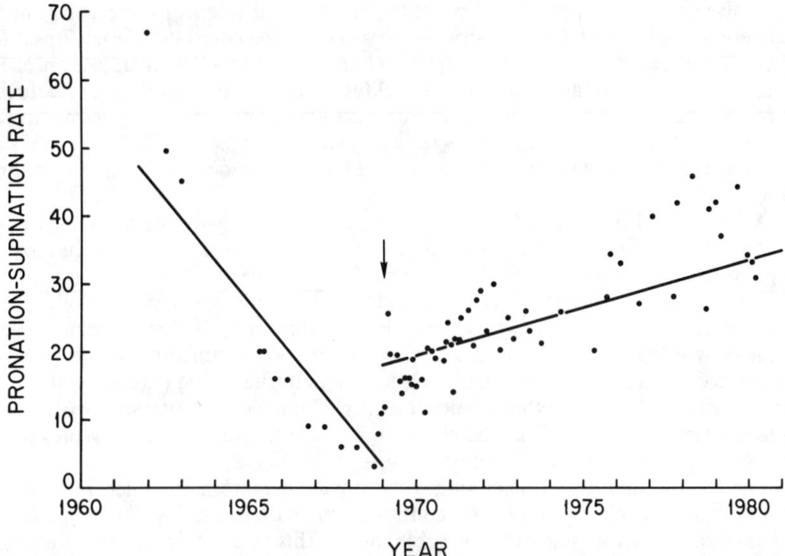

FIGURE 9. Long-term progressive increase in pronation-supination rate ($p < 0.001$) in a patient with a significant ($p < 0.001$) short-term increase in function. See the legends of FIGURES 6 and 8 for additional details. (Reprinted with permission from Webster *et al.*[23])

was no change in the dosage of levodopa from 1969 until 1978, at which time there was slight reduction in dosage. The average daily dose from 1969 to 1978 was 2.5 g.

IMPLICATIONS FOR NORMAL MOTOR AGING

The data presented here generally do not support the view that Parkinson's disease represents premature or accelerated aging of the motor system. Of the signs of Parkinson's disease, only the negative motor signs appear to be expressed during the aging process. Rigidity and rest tremor, which are integral features of Parkinson's disease, are not observed in normal elderly individuals, at least through age 85. In fact, these positive motor signs appear to lessen in severity with increased age in Parkinson's disease. On the other hand, reduced motor speed or bradykinesia is strongly correlated with age in both normal aging and in Parkinson's disease.

Parkinson's disease, when it begins in the 40s or 50s, is usually accompanied by moderate to severe tremor or rigidity (or both). However, when Parkinson's disease begins after age 70, these motor signs are often not as prominent in comparison to the marked slowing in motor behavior. Recent studies of Alzheimer's disease provide important distinctions between an early onset or presenile form of the disease, which involves damage to many different neurotransmitter systems, and a late onset form in which the damage is limited primarily to the cholinergic system.[24-26] Although age-related subtypes of Parkinson's disease have not been as well characterized pathologically and biochemically, the possibility that early onset cases may differ from those beginning later in life is suggested by the clinical differences between early and late onset disease. Other recent data[27] point to important differences in neuropsychological deficits as well — verbal memory impairment being a correlate of early onset Parkinson's disease, and visuospatial impairment being a characteristic of late onset Parkinson's disease. The fact that the major clinical and neuropsychological features of late onset Parkinson's disease (bradykinesia, visuospatial impairment, gait impairment) are also features of normal aging suggests that the late onset form of Parkinson's disease may result largely from the same type of lesions that occur during normal brain aging.

Akinesia and bradykinesia appear to be closely associated with damage to the dopaminergic system; in fact, these are the motor signs in Parkinson's disease that respond best to dopaminergic medications. On the other hand, rigidity and tremor, while they seem to have some relationship to the dopaminergic lesions, likely involve other neurotransmitter systems as well. The fact that the principal change in motor behavior with age is slowing in the maximum rate of movements may be related to circumscribed damage to the dopaminergic system during aging (as has been demonstrated both pathologically and biochemically). Relative preservation of other neurotransmitter systems, such as the cholinergic[28] and noradrenergic, may prevent the appearance of positive extrapyramidal signs in normal aging.

The finding that levodopa cannot only provide symptomatic relief, but can also slow the rate of decline of motor speed that occurs with increasing chronological age in Parkinson's disease, suggests a possible role for this medication in ameliorating the progressive dopaminergic system degeneration that occurs during normal aging.

REFERENCES

1. BARBEAU, A. 1973. Aging and the extrapyramidal system. J. Am. Geriatr. Soc. **21:** 145–149.
2. McGEER, P. L., E. G. McGEER & J. S. SUZUKI. 1977. Aging and extrapyramidal function. Arch. Neurol. **34:** 33–35.
3. BERNHEIMER, H., W. BIRKMAYER, O. HORNYKIEWICZ, K. JELLINGER & F. SEITELBERGER. 1973. Brain dopamine and the syndromes of Parkinson and Huntington. Clinical, morphological and neurochemical correlations. J. Neurol. Sci. **20:** 415–455.
4. McGEER, P. L. & E. G. McGEER. 1978. Aging and neurotransmitter systems. *In* Parkinson's Disease–II. Aging and Neuroendocrine Relationships. C. E. Finch, D. E. Potter & A. D. Kenny, Eds.: 41–57. Plenum. New York.
5. RIEDERER, P. & S. WUKETICH. 1976. Time course of nigrostriatal degeneration in Parkinson's disease. J. Neural Transm. **38:** 277–301.
6. CARLSSON, A. & B. WINBLAD. 1976. Influence of age and time interval between death and autopsy on dopamine and 3-methyoxytyramine levels in human basal ganglia. J. Neural Transm. **38:** 271–276.
7. WONG, D. F., H. N. WAGNER, R. F. DANNALS, J. M. LINKS, J. J. FROST, H. T. RAVERT, A. A. WILSON, A. E. ROSENBAUM, A. GJEDDE, K. H. DOUGLASS, J. D. PETRONIS, M. F. FOLSTEIN, J. K. T. TOUNG, H. D. BURNS & M. J. KUHAR. 1984. Effects of age on dopamine and serotonin receptors measured by positron tomography in the living human brain. Science **226:** 1393–1396.
8. SEVERSON, J. A. & C. E. FINCH. 1980. Reduced dopaminergic binding during aging in the rodent striatum. Brain Res. **192:** 147–162.
9. THAL, L. J., S. G. HOROWITZ, B. DVORKIN & M. H. MAKMAN. 1980. Evidence for loss of brain [^{3}H]spiroperiodol & [^{3}H]ADTN binding sites in rabbit brain with aging. Brain Res. **192:** 185–194.
10. RIEDERER, P. & K. JELLINGER. 1982. Morphological and biochemical changes in the aging brain: pathophysiological and possible therapeutic consequences. Exp. Brain Res. Suppl. **5:** 158–166.
11. CRITCHLEY, M. 1956. Neurologic changes in the aged. J. Chronic Dis. **3:** 459–477.

12. KOKMAN, E., R. W. BOSSEMEYER, J. BARNEY & W. J. WILLIAMS. 1977. Neurological manifestations of aging. J. Gerontol. **32:** 411–419.

13. GREENHOUSE, A. H., H. S. M. UHL, W. MCINNES & C. GOLDEN. 1981. The neurology of normal aging: do changes occur in the neurological examination? Ann. Neurol. **10:** 100.

14. POTVIN, A. R., K. SYNDULKO, W. W. TOURTELLOTTE, J. A. LEMMON & J. H. POTVIN. 1980. Human neurologic function and the aging process. J. Am. Geriatr. Soc. **28:** 1–9.

15. MORTIMER, J. A. & D. D. WEBSTER. 1982. Comparison of extrapyramidal motor function in normal aging and Parkinson's disease. *In* The Aging Motor System. J. A. Mortimer, F. J. Pirozzolo & G. J. Maletta, Eds.: 217–241. Praeger. New York.

16. WEBSTER, D. D. & J. A. MORTIMER. 1977. Failure of L-dopa to relieve activated rigidity in Parkinson's disease. *In* Parkinson's Disease. Neurophysiological, Clinical and Related Aspects. F. S. Messiha & A. D. Kenny, Eds.: 297–313. Plenum. New York.

17. WEBSTER, D. D. 1968. A critical analysis of disability in Parkinson's disease. Mod. Treatment **5:** 257–282.

18. MORTIMER, J. A. & D. D. WEBSTER. 1978. Relationships between quantitative measures of rigidity and tremor and the electromyographic responses to load perturbations in unselected normal subjects and parkinsonian patients. *In* Cerebral Motor Control in Man: Long Loop Mechanisms. J. E. Desmedt, Ed.: 342–360. Karger. Basel, Switzerland.

19. COTZIAS, G. C. 1971. Levodopa in the treatment of parkinsonism. J. Am. Med. Assoc. **218:** 1903–1908.

20. FAHN, S. & S. B. BRESSMAN. 1984. Should levodopa therapy for parkinsonism be started early or late? Evidence against early treatment. Can. J. Neurol. Sci. **11** (suppl.): 200–205.

21. LESSER, R. P., S. FAHN, S. R. SNIDER, L. J. COTE, W. P. ISGREEN & R. E. BARRETT. 1979. Analysis of the clinical problems in parkinsonism and the complications of long-term levodopa therapy. Neurology **29:** 1253–1260.

22. HOEHN, M. M. M. 1985. Result of chronic levodopa therapy and its modification by bromocriptine in parkinson's disease. Acta Neurol. Scand. **71:** 97–106.

23. WEBSTER, D. D., J. A. MORTIMER & M. A. KUSKOWSKI. 1987. Long-term effect of levodopa on progression of Parkinson's disease. *In* Parkinsons's Disease. M. D. Yaur & K. J. Bergmann, Eds.: 473–476. Raven Press. New York.

24. MOUNTJOY, C. Q., M. ROTH, N. J. R. EVANS & H. M. EVANS. 1983. Cortical neuronal counts in normal elderly controls and demented patients. Neurobiol. Aging **4:** 1–11.

25. SELZER, B. & I. SHERWIN. 1983. A comparison of clinical features of early- and late-onset primary degenerative dementia. Arch. Neurol. **40:** 143–146.

26. ROSSOR, M. N., L. L. IVERSON, G. P. REYNOLDS, C. Q. MOUNTJOY & M. ROTH. 1984. Neurochemical characteristics of early and late onset types of Alzheimer's disease. Br. Med. J. **288:** 961–964.

27. MORTIMER, J. A., M. A. KUSKOWSKI, F. J. PIROZZOLO & D. D. WEBSTER. 1985. Prevalence and age distribution of intellectual deficits in Parkinson's disease. J. Clin. Exp. Neuropsychol. **7:** 603.

28. CHUI, H. C., W. BONDAREFF, C. ZAROW & U. SLAGER. 1984. Stability of neuronal number in the human nucleus basalis of Meynert with age. Neurobiol. Aging **5:** 83–88.

29. MORTIMER, J. A., K. HEPBURN & G. J. MALETTA. 1985. Alzheimer's disease: the intersection of diagnosis, research and long-term care. Bull. N.Y. Acad. Med. **61:** 331–342.

DISCUSSION OF THE PAPER

D. MORGAN (*University of Southern California, Los Angeles, CA*): I am very intrigued by the fact that L-dopa seems to retard the rate of progression of Parkinson's disease. One hypothesis for the loss of neurons—a burnout hypothesis—is that the neurons have to work hard; then, if you lose some of them, they have to work harder, thus causing them to degenerate even more rapidly. This is a positive defect system.

However, the L-dopa might tend to prevent this burnout due to the increased hyperactivity to compensate. Do you think your data will be consistent with that hypothesis?

J. MORTIMER (*Veterans Administration Medical Center, Minneapolis, MN*): It would certainly be consistent with that hypothesis, but there is another possible mechanism and that is that dopamine is known to scavenge superoxide. If superoxide radicals are scavenged, damage to dopaminergic neurons might be prevented. The ideal situation is to have dopamine levels in neurons not be too high or too low. Obviously, there are also situations where too much dopamine will cause damage to the nerve cell.

G. BRODY (*Detroit, MI*): What is the measurement index for the pursuit rotor? When you measured the movement speed, did you look at the accuracy as to when they had hit the target? Did you observe whether they missed the target, how far off, and so forth? Also, in regard to the discussion earlier on speed accuracy trade-off, could the Parkinson's patients have moved slower because they were focusing more on accuracy than on motor speed?

MORTIMER: We did not measure accuracy on this task. It is a very simple task and the accuracy is determined obviously by being able to contact the target. In other experiments, we have observed that Parkinson patients tend to be very conservative and favor accuracy over speed. This could be an explanation, at least in part, for the reduced pursuit speed in Parkinson patients.

BRODY: In terms of looking at motor control for pursuit rotor and maybe some other kinds of tasks, a proportion of the movement is devoted to a ballistic stage followed by a honing-in or error-corrective stage. Have you planned to or have you done any looking at acceleration throughout that movement to see whether there is a greater proportion of time spent in one phase versus the other? This would be of interest to people who are just looking at motor performance.

MORTIMER: We have not done that particular experiment. However, we have done some related experiments that look at acceleration in movements that require no accuracy versus those that do require accuracy. The general result from that series of experiments is that Parkinson patients are capable, for the most part, of fairly high acceleration movements when you remove the accuracy criterion. We have seen many patients who were hardly able to walk up a hallway and who had a great deal of difficulty lowering themselves into a chair. However, when we strapped them into our apparatus and had them hit karate bags, their movements were just as fast as age-matched control subjects. When an accuracy requirement was added, they immediately slowed down. Therefore, we do not believe that gross motor speed is very compromised in Parkinson's disease. What does seem to be compromised is this ability to perform accurate movements at high speed.

BRODY: Now that is what I was referring to in terms of error correction. That last part of movement is the error correction.

MORTIMER: Well, whether this is a problem with error correction or the need for visual monitoring in Parkinson's disease is not clear.

GENERAL DISCUSSION OF PART I

D. Ingram (*NIA, Baltimore, MD*): There are often very strong statements made about producing a marked conceptual dichotomy between aging and disease. Now, with the exception of J. Mortimer, who addressed this issue, the rest of the panel treated their data as being representative of aging. However, how would the panel respond to the possible criticism that the responses that they are observing are not what one would call normal aging, but are instead related to a specific disease or yet unspecified disease process?

M. Woollacott (*University of Oregon, Eugene, OR*): When we performed neurological examinations of our subjects, we noticed that our subjects with clinical manifestations were the ones that had the most significant effects on our motor performance tasks. What we, as people working in aging and motor control, have to do in all of our studies is to decide what we define as normal aging. If you look in the literature, you will find articles that include any adult over 65 years of age in the population and call that normal aging. Then, there are other researchers who will actually eliminate anybody with any problem whatsoever. There was one study where they took something like 13 subjects out of 1,100 (and in that case, they found no differences at all with aging), so I think it is very, very critical to define yourself very carefully when you do a particular research study.

J. Mortimer (*Veterans Administration Medical Center, Minneapolis, MN*): I want to say that when we are studying people (say, men over age 80), we are looking at a highly selective survivor population. If the people who died before they were 80 had lived to longer ages, we might have seen much more of a drop-off in terms of function than what is seen in survivors. Thus, we are biased by virtue of the survivorship effect: there is a biasing of the data in the direction of making older people look faster and more efficient.

M. Serby (*New York University Medical Center, New York, NY*): I would like to add that we might have another conference just on the appropriate cognitive and neurological exams needed to quantify normal aging.

M. B. Smith: I want to comment on J. Mortimer's presentation. I was intrigued by the results because we went back and looked at long-term exposure to an L-dopa–supplemented diet. What we found was what appeared to be an apparent slowing of motor decline when we looked at the animals in the longitudinal sample or the cross-sectional sample.

D. B. Calne (*University of British Columbia, Vancouver, British Columbia, Canada*): What about the fluctuations that occur so characteristically in Parkinson's disease? How did you, J. Mortimer, take that into account in obtaining your values in the treated patients.

Mortimer: Some of these treated patients obviously did have fluctuations and we were not able to measure them several times a day in order to capture them at several times. This, of course, increased the variability of the data from the Parkinson patients from time to time. Therefore, it was even somewhat more remarkable that they showed fairly nice regressions on age given the fact that they did have some variability. In addition, as you probably are aware, it was a fairly conservative method of treatment of Parkinson patients and the side effects in this particular sample were reasonably low.

A. T. Welford (*Aldeburgh, Suffolk, England*): I guess another implication of my question is that there might be some interest in those patients who are fluctuating by looking at them at their worst. Maybe we can even get a better indication of the pathological substratum without pharmacological interference.

MORTIMER: That is a very important point. All the patients whose data I have shown were on long-term levodopa. Therefore, I do not think that we are really curing the disease, but certainly the effect of levodopa on the motor activity is changing it.

J. TOBIN (*NIA, Bethesda, MD*): What we have heard so far is not only concerned with normal aging versus disease; in addition, a recurrent theme seems to be adaptability or ways of compensating for things that may be happening—whether it is sway, risk-taking behavior, or speed and accuracy. How then are we able to separate compensations for something that is going wrong?

WOOLLACOTT: Are you asking whether the nervous system has enough plasticity to actually compensate or whether we can shift over to vestibular information accurately if we lose proprioceptive information?

TOBIN: Yes, you are tearing apart the mechanisms by which we maintain our balance. Part of the reasons why we lose balance may be due to disease, but they may also be due to aging changes. This is also true for the speed and accuracy and psychology tests as well.

WOOLLACOTT: One set of experiments that we did was on adaptability to changing environmental conditions. On the first trial, when we took away sensory inputs, half of our subjects fell when they had no visual input (which was their proprioceptive input). Thus, when we took away the proprioceptive input, the older subjects on the first trial tended to fall in 50% of the cases. However, if we gave them five successive trials, they adapted to the changing conditions just like the young adult would and they were giving very, very good responses by the fifth trial. Therefore, they can adapt to changing conditions and their adaptability is very good in that particular task situation.

W. SPIRDUSO (*University of Texas, Austin, TX*): I want to return to a comment that J. Mortimer made about age differences in reaction time depending upon the modality. I would like you to talk about that in terms of the response expression instead of the stimulus modality. I am sure that you are all aware of the three or four papers that show there are no age differences in vocalized reaction time; that is, when the subject has had to express the reaction time by saying yes or no instead of a manual response, there are no age differences. We have recently replicated that and, in addition, set up a situation where we had a manual complexity level and a vocalized complexity level. We found no age interaction with the vocal response whatsoever, but an age interaction was found with the manual response. Thus, is vocalizing reaction time being spared in aging?

WELFORD: The point is that if you look in much greater detail than we normally look at performance in relation to age, you will find that older people are again and again performing, doing the same tasks, possibly even achieving the same performance, but doing it in a different way. I am afraid that modern research has been so streamlined and so hurried that we seldom take the time to look in sufficient detail at these various subtleties and consider what they mean.

Now I can answer W. Spirduso's question. There are two points to be made. First, the verbal responses to auditory stimulation are usually responses that have been very well practiced. The identification of letters, speaking, is an activity where the relationship between the stimulus and the response have been very thoroughly practiced over the years.

The second point is that motor responses were shown in (I think) 1928 and since then to be initiated in phase with tremor. Thus, if you work it out, the effect of a slowing of tremor from about 10–12 to about 7–8 cycles is likely to add a very considerable and appreciable amount to the reaction time of an older person if his or her responses are initiated in phase with tremor.

D. LARISH (*Arizona State University, Tempe, AZ*): There are two other points that I can think of that might explain the potential difference between arm movements, for example, and the speech system. I do not know that much about the anatomical structure of the muscles controlling speech, but, for example, in muscles that move the arm or move the legs, I think it is well established that there is a decrease in the number of type-2 muscle fibers that one can activate as you get older. Now, the type-2 muscle fibers are your fast twitch muscle fibers, which are the muscle fibers responsible for you being able to produce rapid movements. Hence, in many of the reaction time–type tasks, they use arm movements in which those muscles would be used, but I do not know what happens with the speech muscles with age.

The second point from a biomechanical standpoint is that a number of the studies that look at speeded movements with the arms and legs talk about moving a larger mass than with the jaw. Therefore, the ability to move that larger mass with not being able to crank up the type-2 muscle fibers may be part of the explanation.

MORTIMER: Perhaps M. Woollacott wants to answer this question also from the point of view of whether or not there is a postural preparation for speech movements versus those that are carried out by the limbs, where obviously there is a postural preparation. If one could eliminate the postural component, one could probably eliminate a lot of the differences in reaction time.

WOOLLACOTT: All I can say is that we are beginning to look at studies doing that type of thing. We have a subject make a reaction time task in which the whole body is stabilized, except for the specific joint that is moving. Thus, we are attempting to see whether there are very different types of changes in preparation for movement under these conditions versus those under conditions where postural responses are needed.

UNIDENTIFIED DISCUSSANT: What percentage of decrement in the reaction time is accounted for by the postural decrement length?

WOOLLACOTT: In latency? I think I might have given some of those figures. The difference between young and old is 124 milliseconds between tibialis and triceps versus 73 milliseconds, so about 50 milliseconds.

Motor Performance Variability during Aging in Rodents
Assessment of Reliability and Validity of Individual Differences

DONALD K. INGRAM

Molecular Physiology and Genetics Section
Laboratory of Cellular and Molecular Biology
Gerontology Research Center [a]
National Institute on Aging
Francis Scott Key Medical Center
Baltimore, Maryland 21224

Incorporated into the gerontological maxim that motor performance manifests an age-related decline is the hypothetical principle of increased interindividual variability with increased age. From his extensive survey of research in aging and human skill, Welford[1] offered the following observation:

> . . . there is the increasing variability between one individual and another as we go up the age scale, which means that more often than not we find a substantial number of old people performing at a level at least equal to that of the average of a group of younger subjects (p. 283).

This view of human aging as a highly individual process has been supported by the results of large-sample studies incorporating both cross-sectional and longitudinal analyses.[2,3]

The perspective of an age-related increase in motor performance variability is illustrated hypothetically in FIGURE 1. This perspective would be derived from cross-sectional data on a parameter free of ceiling and floor effects that would tend to distort estimates of variability across age. The statistical picture is one of an age-related decrease in mean performance, but with an associated increase in variability. The apparent increase in variability can be expressed in FIGURE 2 with real data that were derived from age comparisons of motor speed taken from a tracing task.[4] This presentation depicts an age-related increase in the standard deviation of the performance variable.

An important assumption derived from FIGURES 1 and 2 (which are based upon cross-sectional data) is that the age-related increase in variability indicates differential trajectories of motor aging across the adult life span. This assumption is illustrated in FIGURE 3A, which is derived from a hypothetical longitudinal analysis of motor performance. The large variance within older age groups measured cross-sectionally presumably results because individuals X, Y, and Z have aged in motor performance at different rates.

---

[a] This institution is fully accredited by the American Association for the Accreditation of Laboratory Animal Care.

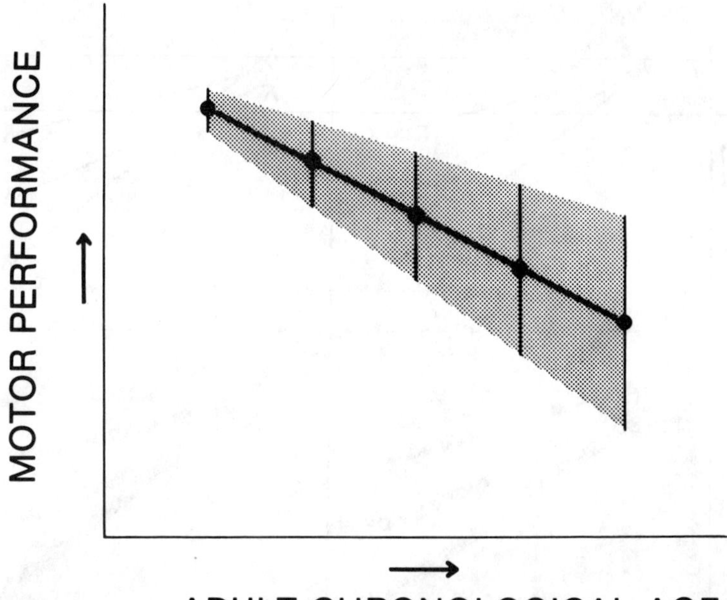

FIGURE 1. Hypothetical function illustrating an age-related decline in motor performance (depicted as means measured cross-sectionally) accompanied by an increase in variability (e.g., standard deviation).

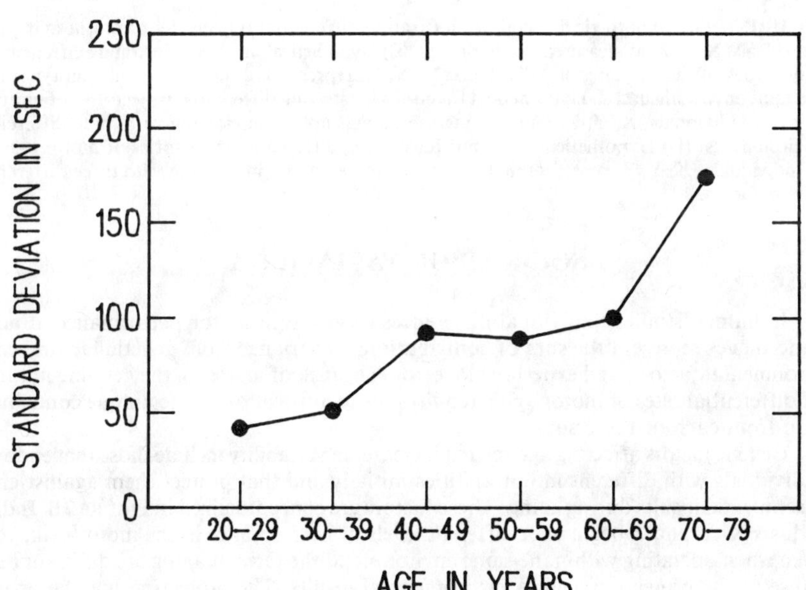

FIGURE 2. Standard deviation of motor speed in a tracing task as a function of age in humans. Data are from Brown,[4] cited in Welford.[1]

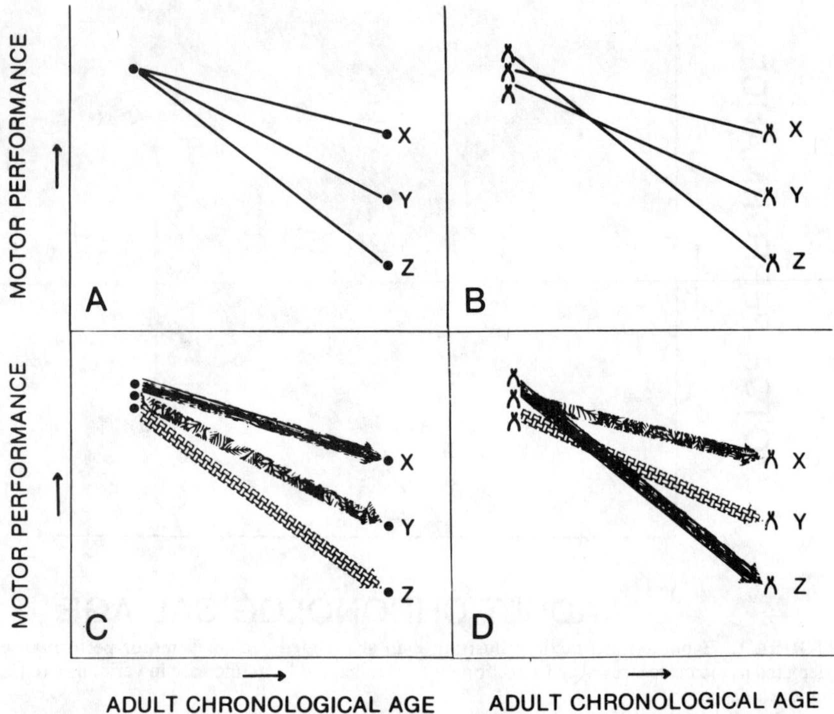

FIGURE 3. (A) Hypothetical functions illustrating differential trajectories of motor aging in individuals, X, Y, Z, as measured longitudinally. (B) Hypothetical functions illustrating differential trajectories of motor aging in individuals, X, Y, Z, representing three different genotypes in the same environment. (C) Hypothetical functions illustrating differential trajectories of motor aging in individuals, X, Y, Z, representing the same genotype interacting with three different environments. (D) Hypothetical functions illustrating differential trajectories of motor aging in individuals, X, Y, Z, representing three different genotypes interacting with three different environments.

SOURCES OF VARIABILITY

In human studies, individual differences observed in motor performance at advanced ages represent the sum of contributions to variance from genetic factors, environmental factors, and experimental error. The task of assessing the genuine nature of differential rates of motor aging requires the identification of the unique contribution from each of these sources.

Genetic factors affecting age-related increases in variability include those that endow individuals with different motor abilities initially and that protect them against environmental insults during aging. These factors are conceptualized in FIGURE 3B. Individuals X, Y, and Z begin with different levels nef performance in the motor task, yet even when operating within the same environment, the rates of aging are different because of the protection against environmental insults. The protection may be operating in a totally different physiological sphere from motor performance, but it is manifested in the reduced negative slope of performance with age.

Environmental factors affecting age-related increases in variability would be those due to differential experiences. These experiences may stem from gross influences that affect the rate of environmental insults to a given genotype or from specific influences (such as those directed by different nutritional experiences or behavioral conditioning) that affect motor performance. The impact of environmental factors on the rate of aging is stylized in FIGURE 3C. Individuals X, Y, and Z, all with identical genetic endowments affecting a motor task, may manifest differential aging in this performance based upon their interactions with different environments.

Error of measurement represents variability that has little inherent scientific interest regarding the issue of differential rates of motor aging. Yet, it is imperative to first identify the degree of variance ascribed to this source before the degree to which individual differences ascribed to genetic and environmental sources can be assessed. Error of measurement may reside in the methods, in the equipment, or within the subject (such as time-of-testing effects or fatigue). It may also be manifested in the form of extraneous variation that confounds the variable of interest, that is, motor performance.

In this light, the influence of disease on the age-related increase in motor performance variability must be addressed. This is a very complex issue for gerontology in general.[5] The separation of "normal aging" from disease has been extremely problematical.[3,6] First, the question of assigning the influence of disease to genetic or environmental factors would depend upon whether the etiology was viewed as intrinsically (genetically) or extrinsically (environmentally) linked. If one were attempting to measure "normal aging" exclusively, then variability due to disease would be viewed as a measurement error that must be eliminated.

Overall, at present, it is very difficult in studies of human aging to identify the various influences of genetic factors, environmental factors, and measurement error (including disease) on the phenomenon of individual differences in motor aging. The complexity of this task is illustrated in FIGURE 3D. Disregarding the issue of measurement error, one sees that variability in motor performance at advanced ages has resulted because different genotypes have interacted with different environments during aging.

The use of laboratory rodents offers an opportunity to identify components of this variability. This is not to say that variability observed among aged rodents is homologous to that observed among aged humans. What the use of laboratory rodents does permit is the testing of hypotheses relating to how particular genetic and environmental factors influence the rate of aging to produce individual differences. Drawing from past investigations from our laboratory,[7-9] this discussion will exemplify how this issue can be addressed. The focus is on the assessment of the reliability and validity of individual differences observed in the motor performance of aged laboratory rodents.

ADVANTAGES OF RODENT MODELS

Many of the problems inherent in analyzing specific factors underlying individual differences in motor performance among aged humans can be alleviated through the study of inbred strains of laboratory rodents. First, there are the practical advantages of analyzing individual differences among experimental subjects that possess only about 3% of the life-span potential of human counterparts. Second, treatments can be used that ethical considerations might prohibit in human research. Third, it is possible to specify conditions of morbidity and pathology. Fourth, and most important to the problem at hand, it is possible to characterize the genetic and environmental conditions of the subjects.

Specifically, the genetic homogeneity provided in inbred rodent strains permits comparisons of motor performance between genotypes reared in similar environments. Similarly, the influence of different environmental treatments on motor performance can be assessed within one genotype. Therefore, it is possible to hold one source of variation constant, while manipulating the other. Such an analysis of genotype-environment interactions can disengage some of the apparent complexity of individual differences manifested in motor aging.

PARAMETRIC PERSPECTIVE OF MOTOR AGING IN RODENTS

Numerous studies have documented the parameters of age-related decline in motor performance in laboratory rodents, including rats,[10] mice,[11] and hamsters.[12] The great majority of such studies focus on mean comparisons between typically two to three age groups from one rodent strain. Results focus on the main effects of aging in the one parameter of interest. The behavioral description of these findings suffice for many studies, whereas others seek to link the behavioral observations to neurobiological mech-

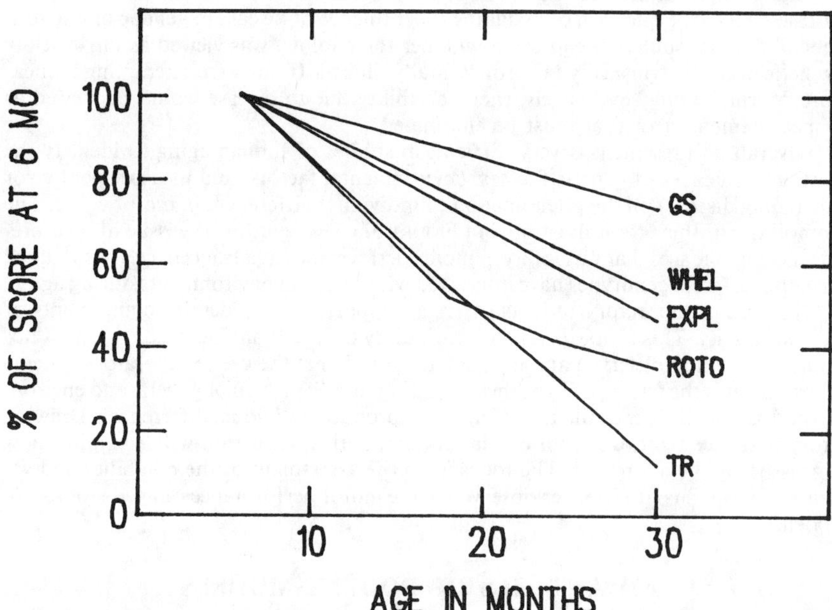

FIGURE 4. Parametric view of age-related decline in psychomotor performance in male C57BL/6J mice. Functions are based on a previous regression analysis[8] with an estimated score at six months set as 100%. (GS) Grip strength score represents the mean pull (in grams) of front paws on a strain gauge over three trials. (TR) Tightrope score represents the mean latency to fall (s) when suspended by the front paws from a taut string over three trials. (ROTO) Rotorod score represents the falls from a plastic rod rotating at 3 rpm during 3-min exposure to the rod. Regression has been based on the reciprocal of falls; thus, this function is not linear. (EXPL) Forced exploration represents the number of quarter-turns in an oval runway during a 10-min trial under darkened illumination. (WHEL) Wheel activity was measured as the mean daily revolutions over a 96-h period.

anisms. Attempts are made to correlate various neuromorphological,[13] neurophysiological,[14] and neurochemical[15] parameters to the behavioral observations. Experimental linkage of psychomotor function to the proposed neurobiological mechanisms is usually made with pharmacological manipulations.[16] This approach has been fruitful in linking motor impairments to specific age-related alterations at neurobiological levels. However, this specific approach has been limited in determining the generalization of the findings. Part of this limitation (which diminishes its relevance to the human condition) stems from the lack of analysis of the genetic and environmental factors that can impinge on the observations of age-related motor performance decline.

At the Gerontology Research Center, we have conducted several studies that provide a parametric perspective of psychomotor aging in laboratory rodents. For example, performance in the inbred mouse strain, C57BL/6J, declines as a linear or near-linear function of age. This parametric view is presented in FIGURE 4 in several psychomotor tasks that have been described in detail previously.[7] "Psychomotor" (instead of "motor") is the preferred terminology to describe this battery because it implies that performance might be influenced by motivational and learning factors. Correlations of the mean performances of different age groups with chronological age for each task yielded Pearson coefficients ranging from 0.78–0.94.

Thus, it is clear that aging impacts markedly upon these measures. However, two questions are posed: (1) Does this parametric perspective apply to other genotypes; and (2) To what extent can environmental factors alter this perspective within a genotype?

GENETIC INFLUENCES ON PSYCHOMOTOR AGING

As shown in FIGURE 5, there is a wide range of variability in life span among inbred mouse strains.[17] This variability is indicative of differential aging rates among strains that might be manifested in differential rates of motor aging.

Although inbred strains of mice vary widely in motor responses, few studies have been conducted that make strain comparisons of age-related decline in motor responses.[18-21] Examples from an earlier study from our laboratory illustrate that aging can differentially affect specific motor performances in inbred mouse strains.[19] We examined three adult life-span representative groups of male A/J and C57BL/6J mice in a psychomotor test battery.

FIGURE 6A provides data on a balance-beam task in which the mouse was placed on a narrow wooden rod and in which the time spent on the rod before falling was recorded and averaged over three trials. The performance of the C57BL/6J strain was generally superior to that of the A/J strain; however, the rate of decline with age was similar for both strains.

In contrast to this pattern of aging are the data in FIGURE 6B, which depict performance in a tightrope task. In this test, the time that the mouse could remain suspended from a taut string by its front paws was recorded and averaged over three trials. Both strains appear equally capable in this task at the youngest age. Although we observed an age-related decline in this ability in the C57BL/6J strain, there was no evidence of a decline in the A/J strain.

What might account for the differential effects of age on these psychomotor performances? Clearly, the principal factors contributing to this differential pattern of aging must be genetic in origin. The mice had been obtained from the same vendor, had been reared in similar cages in the same room with the same husbandry, had eaten the same diet, and had been tested in the same battery. Moreover, it should be noted that the difference was not because the A/J strain was longer-lived. Indeed, estimates

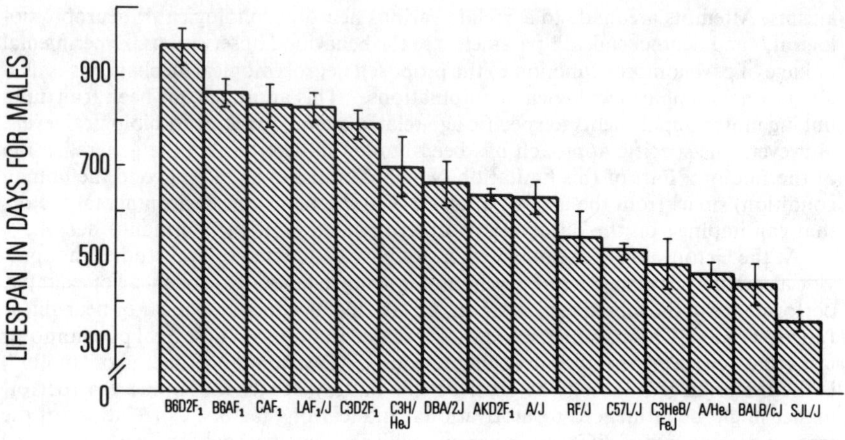

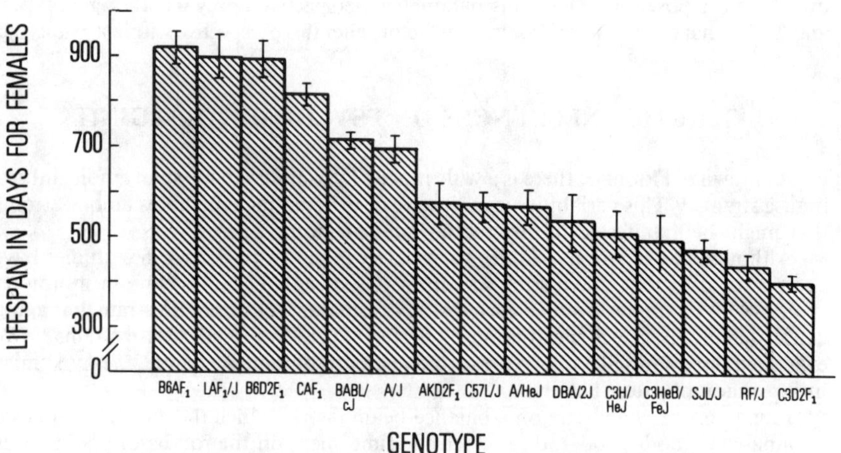

FIGURE 5. Mean life spans of various inbred strains of male and female mice.[17]

from our laboratory indicate that the mean life span of A/J mice is about 22 months, as compared to 26 months for the C57BL/6J strain.[22]

What further use might this strain difference provide beyond this behavioral description? First, the behavioral difference might organize a search for possible neurobiological mechanisms of this differential pattern of aging. Second, further genetic analysis using conventional Mendelian techniques of hybridization and backcrossing or more modern genetic tools (such as recombinant inbred strains or bilineal congenic strains) that shortcut this lengthy process could be used to identify the number and location of genetic loci involved in this strain difference.[23]

As regarding neurobiological correlates of strain differences in psychomotor performance, there has been ample research of this type using young mice from inbred

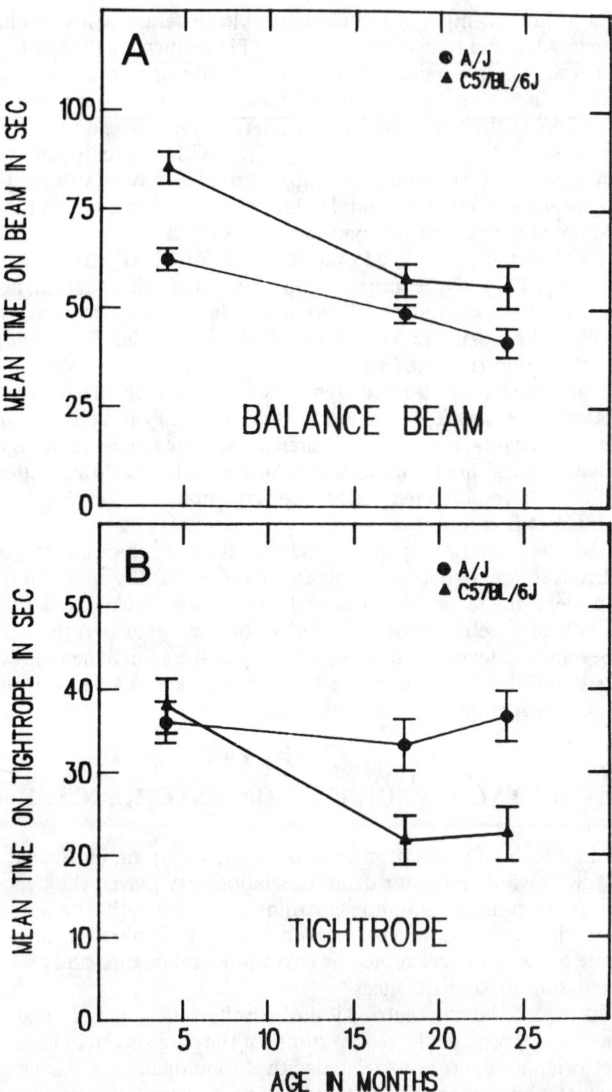

FIGURE 6. Age and strain comparisons (*ns* = 15–29) of male C57BL/6J mice (A) in a balance-beam test and (B) in a tightrope test.[19]

strains.[24] Little investment has been made to compare neurobiological parameters of aged mice from different strains.

In the same two inbred strains in which we studied psychomotor performance, the age and strain differences in neurotransmitter synthetic enzyme activities were also analyzed.[25] FIGURE 7 provides examples of patterns of aging that were observed in the striatum and hippocampus for choline acetyltransferase (ChAT), glutamic acid decarboxylase (GAD), and tyrosine hydroxylase (TH), which are the synthetic enzymes for the cholinergic, GABA-ergic, and adrenergic systems, respectively. With respect to regional ChAT, increases in hippocampal activities with age were observed in both strains (FIGURE 7A). In the striatum, though, ChAT activity increased in the C57BL/6J strain and decreased in the A/J strain (FIGURE 7B). With respect to GAD, age-related increases were again observed in hippocampal activities in both strains (FIGURE 7C); however, an age-related decline in striatal GAD activity was observed in the A/J strain, while an age-related increase of this parameter was observed in the C57BL/6J strain (FIGURE 7D). This pattern paralleled that observed for ChAT activities. The pattern of age differences in TH activities also varied with strain. In the striatum, no age differences were observed in either strain (FIGURE 7F); in the hippocampus, though, TH activity increased with age in the A/J strain, but showed no significant age differences in the C57BL/6J strain (FIGURE 7E).

It should be noted that strain differences have been reported in postsynaptic parameters as well.[26] How differential aging patterns in enzyme activities and receptor concentrations can be linked to strain differences in motor aging remains to be determined. Pharmacological manipulations that probe each neurotransmitter system to affect a specific motor response (e.g., tightrope performance[16] or exploratory activity[21]) may be helpful in this regard.

There is also the potential for taking the search for mechanisms to genetic levels of analysis. Invertebrate models of aging are advanced in this direction of investigation. For example, using recombinant inbred strains, Johnson[27] has identified several loci involved in motor behavior of nematodes and has calculated the heritability of these traits. Several loci involved in the heritability of life span in nematodes have also been identified, and these appear to exert effects that are independent of those loci controlling the motor responses analyzed thus far.

ENVIRONMENTAL INFLUENCES ON PSYCHOMOTOR AGING

Even within an inbred strain of mice in the same vivarium, individuals die across a range of ages. Previous estimates from our laboratory placed the degree of heritability of life span among several mouse strains around 50%.[22] The questions posed are: (1) Do the differences in life span within a cohort of inbred mice reflect differences in the rate of aging as determined by environmental factors; and (2) Can psychomotor tests measure these differences?

FIGURE 4 provided the parametric view of psychomotor aging in male C57BL/6J mice. FIGURES 8 and 9 provide the scatter plots for the data shown in FIGURE 4.[7] When individual performance data are correlated with chronological age, the resulting coefficients are considerably less than those obtained when correlating mean performance for different age groups with chronological age.

There is clearly marked variability in performance. To what degree does this variability reflect individual differences in the rate of psychomotor aging? First, it should be clear that the variability is not genetic in origin. This is an inbred strain. Second, it is assumed that a portion of the variability must be due to experimental error. Thus, the variability that cannot be attributed to experimental error reflects genuine individual differences that must be due to environmental factors.

What could be the possible sources of environmental variation within an inbred strain? Great effort has been made to assure environmental homogeneity. However,

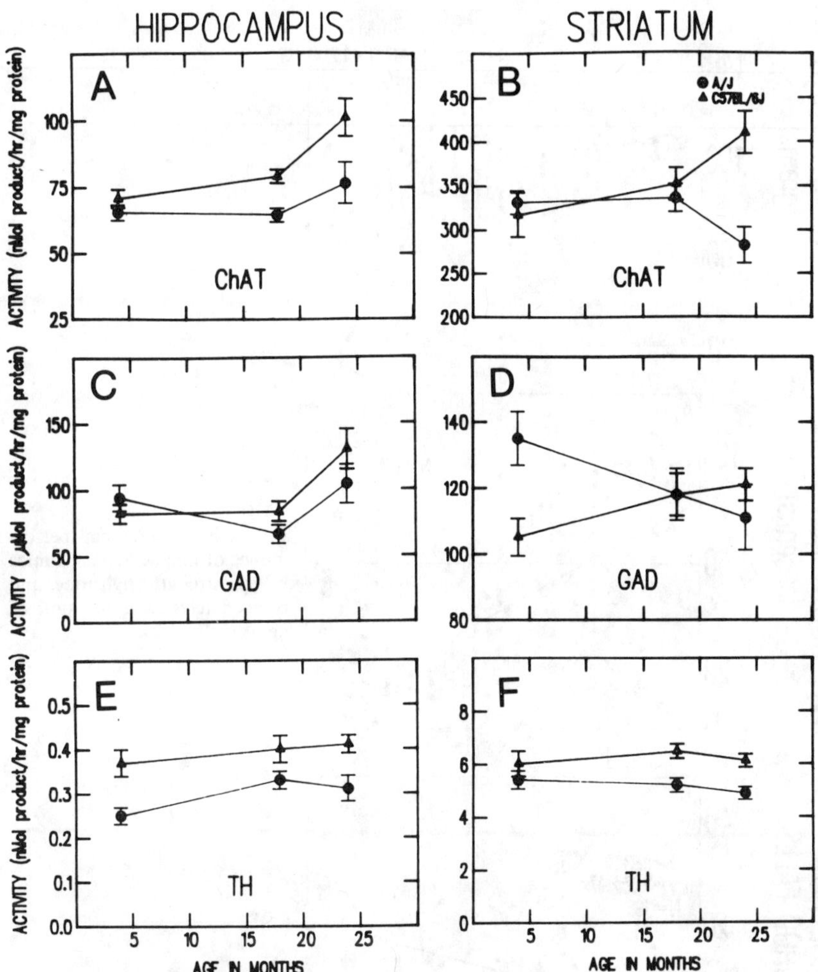

FIGURE 7. Age and strain comparisons (ns = 15–29) of neurotransmitter synthetic enzyme activities of choline acetyltransferase (ChAT), glutamic acid decarboxylase (GAD), and tyrosine hydroxylase (TH) in hippocampus and striatum of C57BL/6J male mice.[25]

it is evident that not all elements of the microenvironment can be controlled. Among possible uncontrolled environmental factors that could produce individual differences are the following: (1) nutritional influences that can begin *in utero* to affect development; (2) social factors that could influence neuroendocrine development; (3) maternal factors that could influence development; (4) specific environmental experiences that permit learning; and (5) specific pathological influences. Thus, the search is for reliable and valid measures of this behavioral phenotype.

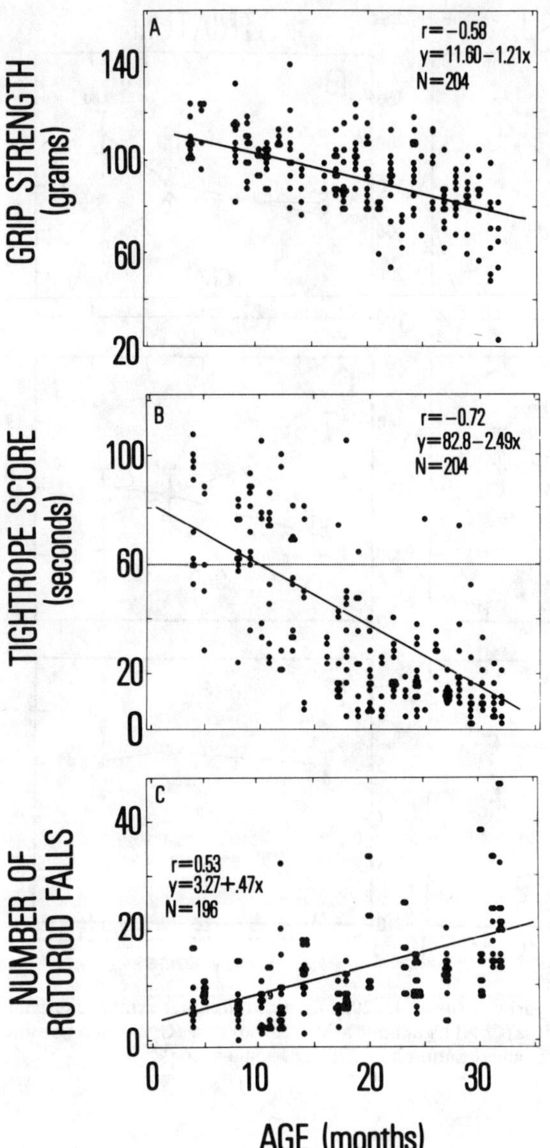

FIGURE 8. Individual performance of male C57BL/6J mice in grip strength, tightrope, and rotorod tests as a function of age.[8]

Reliability

To assess the degree to which variability reflects experimental error, one needs to address the issue of the reliability of the tests. One method of assessing the reliability of a particular measure is to estimate the retest correlation. The question addressed is how stable are the individual differences over a short time interval? Will the individ-

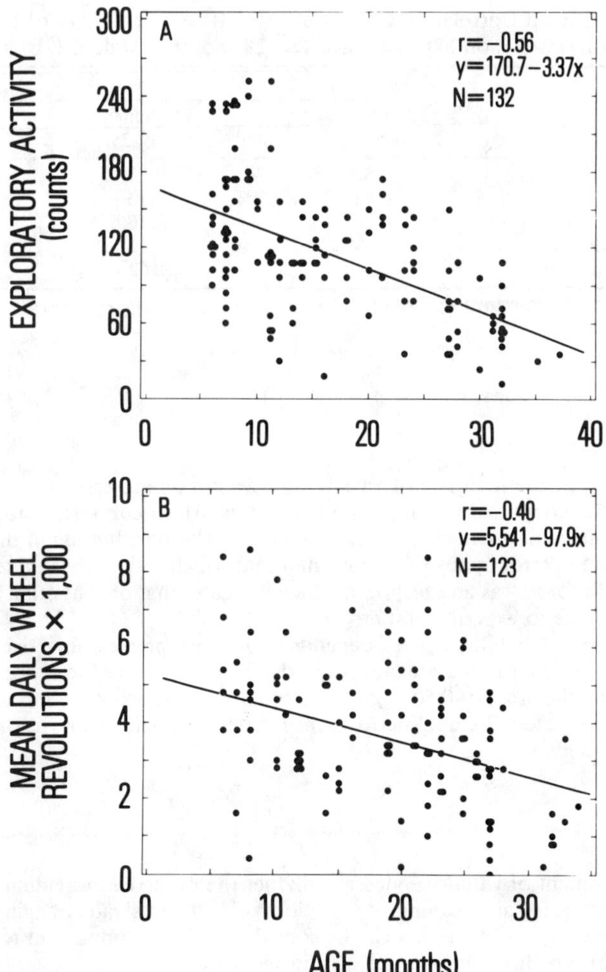

FIGURE 9. Individual performance of male C57BL/6J mice in exploratory activity and run-wheel tests as a function of age.[8]

uals that scored high during the first test session continue to score high, and will those that scored low continue to score low?

TABLE 1 provides data on the retest reliability of the psychomotor tests for the age patterns that were presented in FIGURE 4. Two additional age groups of C57BL/6J mice (young: 6–9 months; aged: 26–28 months) were tested in the psychomotor battery and then retested one week later.[7] For the young group, it is evident that in the tightrope, rotorod, and forced exploration tasks, virtually all the variability was due to experimental error; that is, the individual differences were not stable. Individual scores in the grip strength and wheel activity tests showed some degree of stability,

TABLE 1. Pearson Correlation Coefficients for Retest Reliability of Psychomotor Tests in Young (6–9 months) and Aged (26–28 months) Male C57BL/6J Mice

| | r | | |
| | All | Young | Aged |
Test[a]	$(n \sim 50)$[b]	$(n \sim 25)$	$(n \sim 25)$
Grip strength	0.67^c	0.55^c	0.41^d
Tightrope	0.66^c	0.16	0.43^d
Rotorod	0.86^c	0.10	0.83^c
Forced exploration	0.39^d	0.12	0.44^d
Runwheel activity	0.80^c	0.62^c	0.63^c

[a] Parameters are described in FIGURE 4.
[b] Sample size.
[c] $p < 0.005$.
[d] $p < 0.01$.

but in both tests, the majority of variability was still due to error — over two-thirds in fact (estimate obtained by squaring the coefficient). In contrast, among the aged group, all tests demonstrated significant retest correlations, but again the degree of variability due to error appeared higher than that which reflected genuine individual differences. Rotorod was an exception, which indicates that only about a third of the variance was due to experimental error.

The degree of reliability desired depends upon the expressed objective of the test. If the objective were to separate groups on the basis of test performance, then retest coefficients on the order of 0.50 might be acceptable. On the other hand, if the objective were to evaluate individual performance, retest coefficients on the order of 0.95 would be desired.

Validity

The assessment of validity concerns whether the observed individual differences in psychomotor aging are meaningful reflections of differential rates of aging in general. Several different types of validity can be considered. All are important to the overall assessment of whether a measure is a valid test of aging.

Predictive Validity

Predictive validity refers to the ability to correlate with a criterion measured at some future time. To the extent that correlation of present performance with future performance on a test is an objective, this might be considered a further evaluation of the retest reliability. However, if the interval is sufficiently long, then the inference is that the correlation between performances over this interval will reflect differential rates of psychomotor aging. Such would be the view in FIGURE 10. These data reflect the correlation coefficients obtained for male C57BL/6J mice when comparing performances in various psychomotor tasks at 24 months of age and at later ages in the same tasks.[9] With the exception of the rotorod task, all other tests show some degree of predictive validity, albeit not to a high degree. Most coefficients are less than 0.50, but these are reasonably high estimates when given the moderate retest reliability of

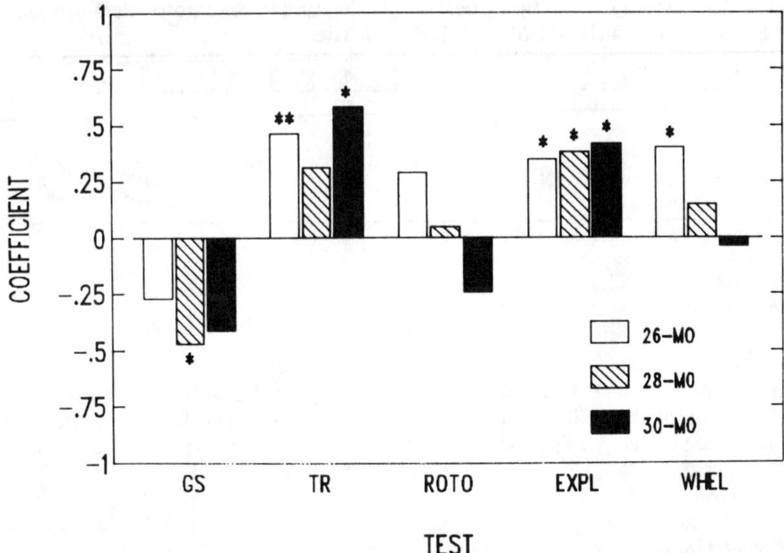

FIGURE 10. Pearson correlation between test scores obtained at 24 months and those obtained at 26, 28, and 30 months in male C57BL/6J mice.[9] The asterisk stands for $p < 0.05$; the double asterisk stands for $p < 0.01$.

the tests. The greatest stability of individual differences appears in the tightrope and exploratory activity tasks.

The correlations for the grip strength test require further explanation. These represent negative correlations between performance at 24 months and future performance; that is, those mice scoring high at 24 months scored relatively lower at older ages. This pattern of correlation indicates confounding by learning, which will be discussed later.

The preceding analysis assessed predictive validity with respect to the correlation between scores obtained at different ages. The criterion for prediction was intrinsically bound within each test. Predictive validity might be further addressed by assessing the correlation with an external criterion. Life span has been proposed as a suitable criterion to assess differential rates of aging.[7,9,28] As with the previous comparisons of strain differences in life spans, the underlying assumption is that variability among individual rates of aging will correlate with individual differences in life spans. Therefore, if individual differences in psychomotor performance reflect differences in the underlying rate of biological aging, then they should be correlated with individual life spans. Past studies of aged humans have shown significant, but modest correlations between life span and psychomotor performance.[29]

TABLE 2 provides data from a previous study in our laboratory to illustrate this possibility.[9] These data reflect the correlations between psychomotor performance scores obtained for male C57BL/6J mice at 24 months of age and subsequent life span. With the exception of the rotorod test, scores in all other tests were significantly correlated with life span; however, again, the relatively low coefficients indicated that most of the variability in life spans was not accounted for by individual test scores.

TABLE 2. Pearson Correlation Coefficients Relating Psychomotor Performance to Life Span in 24-Month-Old Male C57BL/6J Mice

Test[a]	n[b]	r
Grip strength	79	0.38[c]
Tightrope	82	0.32[d]
Rotorod	78	−0.04
Exploratory activity	77	0.41[c]
Runwheel activity	76	0.51[c]

[a] Parameters are described in FIGURE 4.
[b] Sample size.
[c] $p < 0.001$.
[d] $p < 0.005$.

A multiple regression analysis revealed that a linear combination of these test scores could account for about 40% of the variance in life span. Thus, evidence of the predictive validity of the battery was provided. An effort to replicate this validity met with marginal success.[9]

Construct Validity

Evidence of the predictive validity of a particular test would support the construct validity of the test. Construct validity refers to how well the test measures the hypothetical construct of aging. The objective of this process would be to determine how well different tests of psychomotor aging reflect the underlying rate of biological aging. Long-term stability of individual differences and correlation with life span were used to quantify predictive validity as the degree to which individual differences in performance reflected underlying differences in biological aging.

Construct validity can be assessed by an alternative approach that diminishes the need for an identifiable, quantitative criterion and that instead assumes a comparative approach. Specifically, if individual differences in a psychomotor test reflect variability in the rate of biological aging, then the test should be able to discriminate between groups of individuals that have undergone a treatment or experience that presumably has altered the rate of biological aging. Such experimental situations are rare. In the human realm, the population of the Japanese atom bomb victims was thought to provide an opportunity for such an analysis.[30] In the rodent realm, various regimens of dietary restriction have been suggested as a means by which different rates of biological aging can be studied.[31,32]

The typical dietary restriction experiment compares survival and various parameters of biological function between a control group of rodents reared on a conventional *ad libitum* diet and an experimental group reared on a diet in which caloric intake has been restricted 10–50% by various means. The actuarial evidence for differential rates of aging between the groups is based upon different slopes of mortality.[32]

Another view of the actuarial evidence is provided in FIGURE 11. These data from our laboratory represent the survival curves of two groups of male C57BL/6J mice on two dietary regimens.[33] One group was provided an *ad libitum* (AL) diet (4.2 kcal/g), while the other group was provided the same diet, but given every other day (EOD); this resulted in about a 15–20% reduction in food intake over the life span. It is clear that the EOD diet enhanced survival because of the evidence of the increased median and maximum life spans (∼11%) of this group when compared to the AL group. In

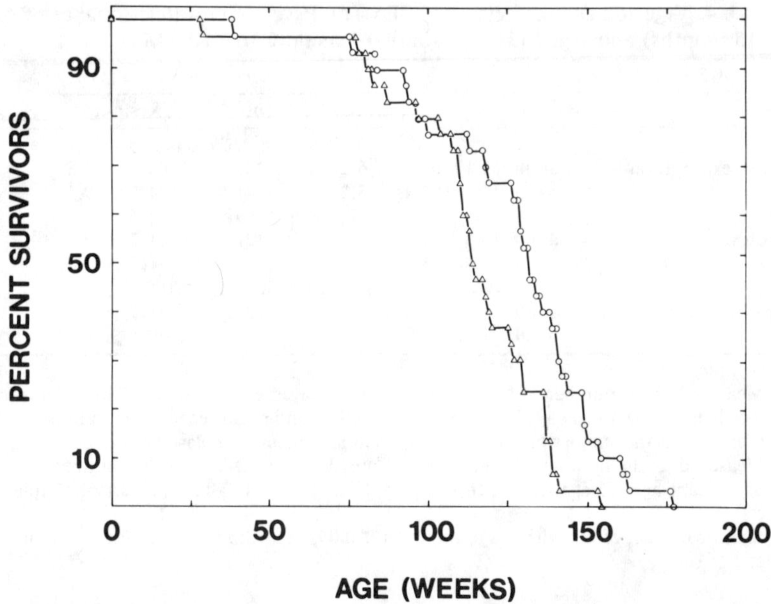

FIGURE 11. Survival distribution of male C57BL/6J mice fed either *ad libitum* (Δ) or every other day (O).[33]

effect, the survival curve of the EOD group was shifted to the right of that of the AL group. If one assumes that these differences in survival indicate that the underlying rate of aging has been altered, then psychomotor tests that purport to reflect individual differences in the rate of aging should be able to discriminate between these different diet groups.

TABLE 3 provides a comparison of scores between two groups of 26-month-old male C57BL/6J mice in the psychomotor battery previously described.[7,8] As noted, the performances of the EOD groups were superior to those of the AL group in every test (except grip strength, in which there were no significant differences). Thus, these data suggest that several of the psychomotor tests were capable of discriminating between individuals (in this case, groups of individuals) that differed in the rate of biological aging.

TABLE 3. Comparison of Means for Psychomotor Performance of Male C57BL/6J Mice Fed either *Ad Libitum* (AL) or Every Other Day (EOD)

Test[a]	AL $(n \sim 15)$[b]	EOD $(n \sim 15)$
Grip strength	79.1	76.4
Tightrope	18.2	33.3[c]
Rotorod	7.8	4.9[c]
Forced exploration	104.4	122.3[c]
Runwheel activity	1620.3	4217.9[c]

[a] Parameters are described in FIGURE 4.
[b] Sample size.
[c] $p < 0.05$, according to two-tailed t test.

TABLE 4. Age and Diet Effects ($\overline{X} \pm$ SEM) on Psychomotor Performance of Adult (11–15 months) and Aged (31–35 months) Female C3B10RF$_1$ Mice

		Diet			
Test	Age	Control	$(n)^a$	Restricted	(n)
		Beam interruptions			
Forced exploration[b]	adult	102.8 ± 6.2	(15)	104.9 ± 5.8	(15)
	aged	103.4 ± 8.2	(14)	104.5 ± 9.5	(13)
		Number of falls			
Rotorod[c]	adult	1.5 ± 0.4	(12)	1.7 ± 0.3	(13)
	aged	6.9 ± 2.2[e]	(15)	1.4 ± 4[f]	(12)
		Wheel revolutions × 1000			
Runwheel activity[d]	adult	35.4 ± 6.0	(12)	51.2 ± 6.2[f]	(12)
	aged	40.0 ± 5.4	(11)	49.5 ± 4.5[f]	(11)

[a] Sample size.

[b] Measured as the number of beam interruptions by a series of four equally spaced infrared photocells in an oval runway during a 10-min period under darkened illumination.

[c] Measured as the number of falls during a 3-min placement on a plastic rod rotating at 3 rpm.

[d] Measured as the number of wheel revolutions during a 72-h access to an activity wheel.

[e] Significant age effect within diet group, $p < 0.05$, according to an F test of simple main effects.

[f] Significant diet effect within age group, $p < 0.05$, according to an F test of simple main effects.

These findings have been confirmed partially in a recent study of another mouse strain — female C3B10RF$_1$.[34] The diet restriction was different and much more restrictive ($\sim$40% reduction in caloric intake). As shown in TABLE 4, among the aged group (31–32 months), restricted mice had higher performances in wheel activity and rotorod, but not in exploratory activity. However, in this case, there was no age difference noted in exploratory or in wheel activity, which is an observation that again indicates strain differences in the pattern of psychomotor aging.

Other environmental manipulations might provide opportunities to examine whether tests of psychomotor aging have construct validity. These include exercise,[35] a breeding regimen,[36] dietary antioxidants,[37] and hypophysectomy.[38] All treatments are purported to affect aging rate, but none are established as well as diet restriction in this capacity.

Extraneous Error

Before accurate conclusions about the validity of psychomotor tests can be drawn, further consideration must be given to possible sources of extraneous error. Several extraneous factors can impinge upon the validity of the measurement.

Body Weight

Individual differences in body weight represent a potential source of extraneous variation. For example, if heavier animals do more poorly in a tightrope task compared to lighter animals, the conclusion regarding individual differences in biological aging might be confounded by this correlation. As shown in TABLE 5, when performance in the psychomotor battery was examined across the life span of male C57BL/6J mice, there were significant correlations between body weight and performance in three

TABLE 5. Pearson Correlation Coefficients and Partial Correlation Coefficients Reflecting the Relationship between Test Scores and Chronological Age (CA) and Body Weight (BW) in Adult Male C57BL/6J Mice

Test[a]	n[b]	rCA	rBW	rCA·BW
Grip strength	204	-0.58^c	0.02	-0.62^c
Tightrope	204	-0.72^c	-0.44^c	-0.68^c
Rotorod	196	0.52^c	0.25^d	0.52^c
Forced exploration	132	-0.56^c	0.04	-0.58^c
Runwheel activity	123	-0.40^c	-0.24^d	-0.43^c

[a] Parameters are described in FIGURE 4.
[b] Sample size.
[c] $p < 0.001$.
[d] $p < 0.01$.

of the five tests—tightrope, rotorod, and wheel activity.[7] However, when this correlation was statistically controlled by a partial correlational technique, the correlation between performance and chronological age was virtually unaffected.[7] This relationship existed despite the correlation between body weight and performance; thus, the experimenter need not be concerned that body weight is an extraneous variable in this analysis.

What about individual differences within the same age group? In TABLE 2, we see that body weight was positively correlated with life span in 24-month-old C57BL/6J mice.[9] This means that heavier mice at that age might be biologically younger, so mice with lower body weight would have a steeper trajectory toward death. Thus, tests in which performance was correlated with body weight might have their correlations with life span confounded by this extraneous relationship. However, after conducting a partial correlational analysis controlling for body weight, the correlations between psychomotor performance and life span were observed to be relatively unaffected.[9]

The assessment of possible confounding by body weight differences is more difficult in regard to performance differences due to dietary restriction. The use of partial correlational techniques are more problematical when the covariant (body weight) is also affected by the treatment (diet). However, regarding the data on the correlation between body weight and performance in TABLE 5, it is possible that body weight differences could confound the comparison of rotorod performance in TABLE 4. Thus, this means that diet-restricted mice might perform better not because they are biologically younger than control mice, but because they are lighter. This did not appear to be the case because an analysis of covariance of the rotorod performance data still revealed the significant interaction between age and dietary treatment.[34]

Motivation

Similar caution must be taken in regard to motivational factors. In comparisons of *ad libitum* and diet-restricted animals, for example, it may be possible that performance differences reflect motivational differences to perform. This might be most acute in a task such as runwheel performance, which is sensitive to the degree of food deprivation. Procedural consideration of this potential source of confounding was provided in producing the data in TABLE 4 with regard to this issue.[34] These had been obtained after a period of several weeks in which the experimental group (diet-restricted) had been fed the control diet, which was in fact below an AL level. Again, investigators interested in maintaining the reliability and validity of their psychomotor measures must be cognizant of such possibilities. Regarding all the tests depicted in FIGURE 4, it is difficult to assess whether age differences existed in the motivational factors required for optimum performance.

Learning

The degree to which the task stresses learning to perform offers us another area to consider as a possible source of confounding in the analysis of psychomotor aging. If the test is more heavily weighted on assessing the acquisition of skills necessary to perform than on assessing skills that already exist or require little learning to perform accurately, then construct validity might be compromised. Again, to emphasize, the term "psychomotor aging" has been used instead of "motor aging" because of the implicit recognition that motivational and cognitive factors may be involved in the performance of the task. However, what should be considered is whether the test is too heavily weighted on learning. This could be to such an extent that the individual differences reflect differences in learning abilities to a greater degree than motor abilities.

One way to assess the influence of this extraneous variation is to perform multiple tests over time on the same individuals. This longitudinal perspective might reflect the extent to which learning factors are involved in age and individual differences. If learning is involved, then performance might improve as a function of experience — in this case, with age. Representative data highlighting this issue are presented in FIGURE 12. These data represent psychomotor performance in male C57BL/6J mice as measured in the test battery every two months beginning at 24 months of age.[9] By assessing the percentage change in performance across age relative to performance at 24 months, it is clear that performance declines in all tasks except in the grip strength test. In this task, mice improved their performance with age, which indicates that learning is possibly confounding performance. This suggestion is further supported in FIGURE 10, which shows the inverse correlation between grip strength at 24 months and at later ages.

Rate of Aging

A longitudinal analysis can also be utilized in a different way to assess further the construct validity of psychomotor tests. If subjects can be measured repeatedly, then it is possible to estimate a linear slope of each individual's performance with age. If psychomotor performance is reflecting the rate of biological aging, then these slopes should be correlated with life span. This is the analysis presented in TABLE 6. For all mice that were tested at least three times from 24 months of age in the battery shown in FIGURE 12, a linear slope was computed and correlated with life span.[9] Grip strength was not included in this analysis for the reasons described above. As observed, the slope of performance in all tests was positively correlated with life span. This should have indicated that those mice with less decline in psychomotor performance lived the longest. However, with a sample of only 29 mice, only the coefficient for the tightrope test was statistically significant, and then the coefficient reflected only about 30% of the variance in life span.

Disease

A final source of extraneous variation that needs to be considered is the influence

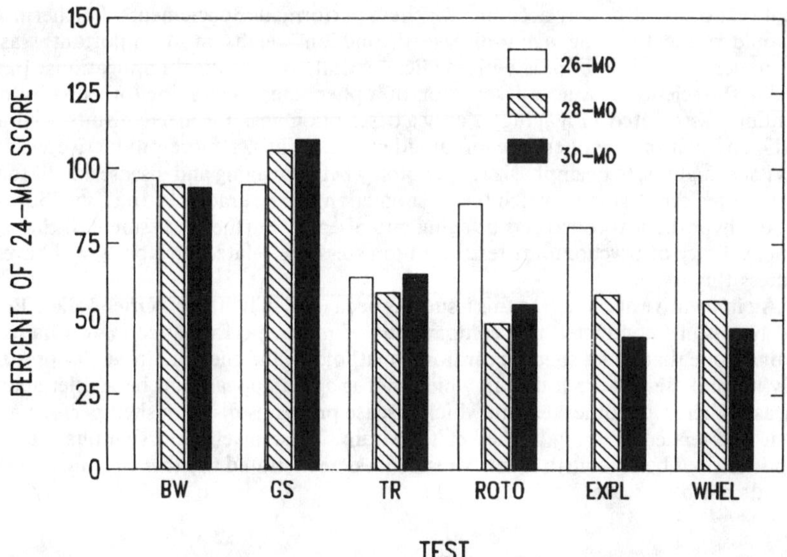

FIGURE 12. Mean test scores of 26-, 28-, and 30-month-old male C57BL/6J mice expressed as the percent of the score obtained at 24 months.[9]

of disease on psychomotor performance. The argument can be made that aging per se has little role in the decline of psychomotor performance observed over the life span in rodents. Instead, disease, which might affect function in musculoskeletal, cardiovascular, and sensorimotor systems, is the principal cause of the impairment. This is a very important point that can be interpreted to have far-reaching consequences to gerontological research and geriatric practice.[3,5,6] To our shortcoming, we have not been able to properly address this issue in our paradigms due to the lack of collaboration with pathologists experienced in the assessment of aged rodents. This should be a very important consideration for all studies in this area.

In defense, I would assert that many of the age-related declines in psychomotor performance that we and others observe begin relatively early after maturity and continue as linear or log-linear functions with age. This then would diminish the argu-

TABLE 6. Pearson Correlation Coefficients Relating Rate of Psychomotor Decline[a] to Life Span in Male C57BL/6J Mice

Test[b]	n^c	r
Tightrope	27	0.55[d]
Rotorod	27	0.28
Forced exploration	27	0.22
Wheel activity	26	0.34

[a] Individual linear slopes across at least three ages measured two months apart beginning at 24 months.
[b] Parameters are described in FIGURE 4.
[c] Sample size.
[d] $p < 0.01$.

ment that overt pathology accounts for these performance decrements. Furthermore, I would argue that the aging-disease distinction weighs most importantly as a phenomenological descriptor with medical, social, and political implications. In regard to the scientific issue, a description of a phenomenon as aging (or as pathology seemingly associated with aging) is only a description until the mechanism(s) that underlie and control the phenomenon are identified. Thus, a more productive view of this issue might be to deemphasize a dichotomy between aging and disease and to focus instead on a dimension in which the phenomenon can be graded by the contributions of both hypothetical constructs of aging and disease.[5] Further assessment of the construct validity of psychomotor tests used to assess age-related variability will have to address this issue.

An innovative approach to this issue has been used in hamsters. Ottenweller, Tapp, and Natelson[12] conducted age comparisons of motor performance in two hamster strains—one that had a specific cardiomyopathology and the other that was presumably normal. Tests were found in which motor aging appeared to be accelerated by disease. There were other tests in which disease processes distinguished performance from that related to aging in the healthy strain. These investigators emphasized the importance of being able to identify tests that demonstrated whether the rate of aging was altered by disease.

DEVELOPING A NEW PSYCHOMOTOR TEST

From the preceding discussion of past results in our laboratory, it should be clear that no test has met all objectives of reliability and validity to a high degree in regard to accuracy in assessing individual differences in psychomotor aging. A strategy for assessing these features has been established, but modification and expansion of the test battery is needed.[7-9].

Over the past several months, we have endeavored to develop a new test that might improve on several features when compared to the tests examined thus far. The new test is intended to be a measure of the maximum running speed in mice. Previous research examined maximum running capacity as a function of age in rats and found an age-related decline.[39] However, that study emphasized endurance because the measurement involved was the time spent running at a high rate (20 m/min) on a treadmill. This current study, though, emphasizes capacity to run at the highest speed and attempts to minimize endurance factors.

The test being developed utilizes a commercially made, automated drum exerciser (DREX, Columbus Instruments, Columbia, Ohio). This apparatus consists of a drum (30 cm in diameter and 9.5 cm wide) that contains a corrugated, rubber running mat on its circumference. Through a microprocessor-controlled motor, the drum can be programmed to rotate at various speeds for various time intervals. The drum is enclosed within a Plexiglas box with a stainless steel grid shelf (15 cm × 9 cm) that is located at one end of the wheel at a height about one-sixth below its diameter. Pulsed footshock (~0.5 mA at 0.5 s) is delivered through the grid floor. Located two cm horizontally above the grid floor are a series of four infrared photocells that can register whether the animal is present on the grid floor. These photocells thereby permit the microprocessor to record the number of visits to the grid floor, the time spent on the grid floor, and the time spent on the drum. All these data can be printed out after each predesignated trial.

The procedure that is currently being applied has the following features. First, mice are given a training session on one day and a test session on the following day. The training session consists of placing the mouse on the rotodrum while the drum is stationary. This 2-min trial permits the mouse to discover that the grid floor is electrified. Then, the rotodrum is activated to turn at a speed of 1 cm/s for one minute. At this slow speed, all mice have little trouble staying on the rotodrum and thus avoid the electrified grid. Following this trial, there is a 1-min rest trial in which the rotodrum is not activated. The remainder of the session involves these 1-min running trials, separated by 1-min rest sessions, with the speed increased in the following increments: 3, 5, 10, 15, 20, 25, 30, 35 cm/s. The upper limit of this range was derived empirically as being near the highest level of capability on the first day of training. If the mouse remains on the electrified grid for 45 seconds during any trial, it is removed from further testing. This criterion appears stringent, but it is somewhat contaminated at present because the mouse's tail can also activate the infrared photocells. However, if this is the case, it is usually because the mouse is at the end of the rotodrum and is striving to run when its tail is activating the photocells. Prior to the trials when this begins to happen, the mouse is running at the top of the rotodrum with its tail far removed from the photocells. During the second session on the following day, the first 1-min trial begins at a speed of 10 cm/s and is incremented 2 cm/s for each additional 1-min trial (following a 1-min rest trial between each increment in rotodrum speed). The criterion for removal on the second day is two consecutive trials in which the photocells have recorded 45 seconds on the grid (which again includes deflection by the tail). The rotodrum is sponged with hot soapy water every day after the last session on both days. Mice are run during diurnal hours 9:00 A.M. – 4:00 P.M.

What are the features of this test that have been improved over those of the tests described previously? First, there is almost no interaction between experimenter and subject. Second, an attempt is made to reduce extraneous variation due to motivational and learning factors. This is accomplished by having shock-avoidance as the motivational manipulation. The experimenter is reasonably assured that the subjects are motivated to perform at their highest ability. Moreover, because the rotodrum velocity is slowly and gradually incremented, the experimenter is assured that the animals have the opportunity to learn the relevant features of performance, that is, to run on the rotodrum at a speed that permits them to avoid the shock grid. Two sessions are given to further offset any learning effects. Pilot studies indicated that maximum performance was not enhanced appreciably (< 2 cm/s) when a third session was given 24 hours after the second one to mice of different age groups. The objective is to measure the mouse's highest ability with respect to this task, that is, its maximum running speed.

FIGURE 13A presents our preliminary results with this test in male C57BL/6J mice. As noted, there was an age-related decline in performance. Between 8 and 25 months, maximum running speed declined about 22%. As observed, there was no age-related increase in variability in this case. Performance also appeared unaffected by individual differences in body weight. The correlation between body weight and performance was positive, $r = 0.27$, but not significant, $p \geqslant 0.05$. Thus, body weight did not appear to be an extraneous performance factor.

An additional factor extraneous to the variable of interest might be fatigue. The initial procedure used to reduce the influence of fatigue was by having short test trials separated by rest trials. To further offset this possibility, a more recent procedure has been introduced that differs in two ways from that described above. First, to reduce the total number of trials required during the second session, the speed on the first trial was changed from 10 to 20 cm/s. Second, beginning at the trial with a rotodrum velocity of 30 cm/s, the length of the rest trial was increased from 1 to 2 min. FIGURE 13B demonstrates the age comparisons of performance resulting from this protocol in male C57BL/6J mice. The results were very similar to those observed in FIGURE

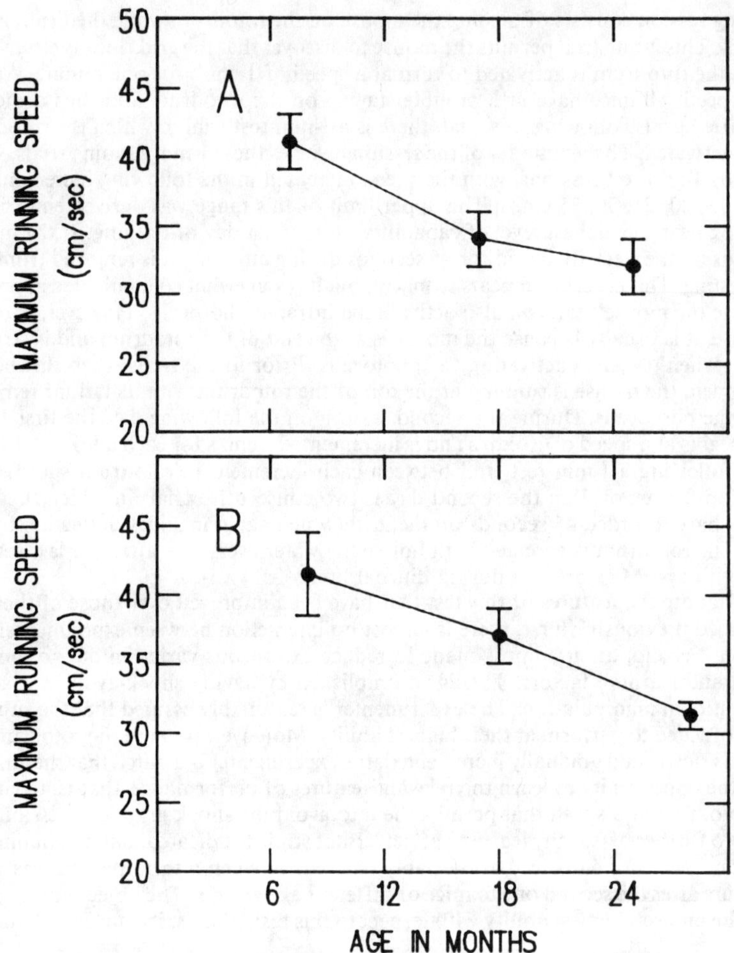

FIGURE 13. Maximum running speed in male C57BL/6J mice as a function of age.

13A. Therefore, fatigue does not appear to be an extraneous factor affecting the age comparisons. Again, there was no age-related increase in variability. If anything, there was a decrease, but the measures of variability here are the standard errors of the mean that were affected by markedly different sample sizes. Again, similar to that found in the first study of this test, there was no correlation between body weight and performance, $r = -0.01$.

Further analysis is planned to examine the reliability and validity of the running speed test. Specifically, we will assess the short-term and long-term stabilities of individual differences and the correlation with life span. In addition, a correlational analysis will be conducted to determine what relationship the rotodrum test has to the previous tests examined. Finally, work is also under way to determine if performance in the rotodrum test is correlated with individual differences in striatal dopamine receptors.

CONCLUSIONS

The objective of this discussion was to document that motor aging may be analyzed from the perspective of individual differences. By comparing inbred rodent strains, investigators can analyze genetic influences on the type and rate of age-related performance decline. Once reliable strain differences are documented, then further analysis can be conducted to determine mechanisms at physiological, cellular, and genetic levels. By analyzing individual differences within inbred strains, investigators can analyze the effects of environmental manipulations (such as nutrition) on the rate of motor aging within a particular genotype. By focusing upon the behavioral phenotype within uniform and different environments, investigators can assess whether parameters of motor aging reflect the underlying rate of biological aging and thereby link common mechanisms. With these research objectives in mind, the task becomes one of developing reliable and valid measures of motor aging.

Emphasis on individual differences has implications for other areas of geropsychology, including assessment of age-related memory dysfunction.[40] An important application is provided in the assessment of therapeutic interventions. For example, Gage, Dunnett, and Björklund[41] first identified a subset of aged rats that were impaired in a learning task before submitting them to a fetal neural grafting procedure that improved the deficit in this experimental group.

In summary, further research interest in assessing individual differences in inbred animal models will likely help to elucidate the rich variability that exists in motor performance during human aging. Thus far, interest in this line of research remains at a threshold.[23]

ACKNOWLEDGMENTS

The author acknowledges the valuable contributions of John Freeman and Edward Spangler for assistance in behavioral testing and animal husbandry, of Richard Hiner, Maurice Zimmerman, and Gunther Baartz for construction of many pieces of equipment, of George Roth and Elaine Bresnahan for critical reviews of the manuscript, of Paul Ciesla for artwork and computer-aided graphics, and of Rita Wolferman for clerical assistance.

REFERENCES

1. WELFORD, A. T. 1958. Ageing and Human Skill. Oxford Univ. Press. London/New York.
2. PALMORE, E., E. W. BUSSE, G. L. MADDOX, J. B. NOWLIN & I. C. SIEGLER, Eds. 1985. Normal Human Aging III: Reports from the Duke Longitudinal Studies (1975–1984). Duke Univ. Press. Durham, North Carolina.
3. SHOCK, N. W., R. C. GRUELICH, R. ANDRES, D. ARENBERG, P. T. COSTA, E. G. LAKATTA & J. D. TOBIN. 1984. Normal Human Aging: The Baltimore Longitudinal Study of Aging. NIH Publ. No. 84-2450. U.S. Govt. Printing Office. Washington, D.C.
4. BROWN, R. A. 1957. Age and paced work. Occup. Psychol. **31:** 11–20.
5. HALL, D. A. 1984. The Biomedical Basis of Gerontology. John Wright. Littleton, Massachusetts.

6. WILLIAMS. T. F. 1986. Geriatrics: The fruition of the clinician reconsidered. Gerontologist **26:** 345–349.
7. INGRAM, D. K. 1983. Toward the behavioral assessment of biological aging in the laboratory mouse: Concepts, terminology, and objectives. Exp. Aging Res. **9:** 225–238.
8. INGRAM, D. K. 1984. Biological age: A strategy for assessment. *In* Geriatrics and Gerontology Yearbook (U.S.S.R.). F. Chebortarev, A. V. Tokar & V. P. Voitenko, Eds.: 30–38. Institute for Gerontology. Kiev.
9. INGRAM, D. K., & M. A. REYNOLDS. 1986. Assessing the predictive validity of psychomotor tests as measures of biological age in mice. Exp. Aging Res. **12:** 155–162.
10. WALLACE, J. E., E. E. KRAUTER & B. A. CAMPBELL. 1980. Motor and reflexive behavior in the aging rat. J. Gerontol. **35:** 364–370.
11. DEAN, R. L., J. SCOZZAFAVA, J. A. GOAS, B. REGAN, B. BEER & R. T. BARTUS. 1981. Age-related differences in behavior across the life span of the C57BL/6J mouse. Exp. Aging Res. **7:** 427–451.
12. OTTENWELLER, J. E., W. N. TAPP & B. H. NATELSON. 1986. Use of motor performance tests to differentiate aging effects from disease effects. Exp. Gerontol. **21:** 13–21.
13. FREDDARI, C. B. & C. GIULI. 1980. A quantitative morphometric study of rat cerebellar glomeruli during aging. Mech. Ageing Dev. **12:** 127–136.
14. ROGERS, J., M. A. SILVER, W. J. SHOEMAKER & F. E. BLOOM. 1980. Senescent changes in a neurobiological model system: Cerebellar Purkinje cell electrophysiology and correlative anatomy. Neurobiol. Aging **1:** 3–11.
15. JOSEPH, J. A., G. S. ROTH & J. R. WHITAKER. 1983. Importance of striatal dopamine receptor changes in senescence. *In* Intervention in the Aging Process, Part B: Basic Research and Preclinical Screening. W. Regelson & F. M. Sinex, Eds.: 187–202. Alan R. Liss. New York.
16. GIBSON, G. E. & C. PETERSON. 1983. Amelioration of age-related deficits in acetylcholine release and behavior with 3,4 diaminopyridine. *In* Aging of the Brain. D. Samuel, S. Algeri, S. Gershon, V. E. Grimm & G. Toffano, Eds.: 337–348. Raven Press. New York.
17. INGRAM, D. K., M. A. REYNOLDS & E. P. LES. 1982. The relationship of genotype, sex, body weight, and growth parameters to lifespan in inbred and hybrid mice. Mech. Ageing Dev. **20:** 253–266.
18. GOODRICK, C. L. 1975. Behavioral differences in young and aged mice: Strain differences for activity measures, operant learning, sensory discrimination, and alcohol preference. Exp. Aging Res. **1:** 191–207.
19. INGRAM, D. K., E. D. LONDON, M. A. REYNOLDS, S. B. WALLER & C. L. GOODRICK. 1981. Differential effects of age on motor performance in two mouse strains. Neurobiol. Aging **2:** 221–227.
20. SPROTT, R. L. & B. E. ELEFTHERIOU. 1974. Open-field behavior in aging inbred mice. Gerontologia **20:** 155–162.
21. REIS, D. J. 1983. Genetic differences in numbers of chemically specified neurons in brain: A possible biological substrate for variations in onset of symptoms of cerebral aging in man. *In* Aging of the Brain. D. Samuel, S. Algeri, S. Gershon, V. E. Grimm & G. Toffano, Eds.: 257–270. Raven Press. New York.
22. GOODRICK, C. L. 1975. Life-span and the inheritance of longevity of inbred mice. J. Gerontol. **30:** 257–263.
23. SPROTT, R. L. 1980. An appraisal of the utility of genetic techniques for the study of neurobiology of aging in mice. *In* Psychobiology of Aging. D. Stein, Ed.: 187–202. Elsevier. New York.
24. INGRAM, D. K. & T. P. CORFMAN. 1980. An overview of neurobiological comparisons in mouse strains. Neurosci. Biobehav. Rev. **4:** 421–435.
25. WALLER, S. B., D. K. INGRAM, M. A. REYNOLDS & E. D. LONDON. 1983. Age and strain comparisons of neurotransmitter synthetic enzyme activities in the mouse. J. Neurochem. **41:** 1421–1428.
26. LONDON, E. D. & S. B. WALLER. 1984. Relations between choline acetyltransferase and muscarinic binding in aging rodent brain and in Alzheimer's disease. *In* Dynamics of Cholinergic Function. I. Hanin, Ed.: 69–83. Plenum. New York.
27. JOHNSON, T. E. 1986. Molecular and genetic analyses of a multivariate system specifying behavior and lifespan. Behav. Genet. **16:** 221–235.

28. BROWN, K. S. & W. F. FORBES. 1976. Concerning the estimation of biological age. Gerontologia **22:** 428–437.

29. BOTWINICK, J., R. WEST & M. STORANDT. 1983. Predicting death from behavioral test performance. J. Gerontol. **33:** 755–762.

30. HOLLINGSWORTH, J. W., A. HASHIZUMA & S. JABLON. 1965. Correlations between tests of aging in Hiroshima subjects—an attempt to define physiologic age. Yale J. Biol. Med. **38:** 11–26.

31. MASORO, E. 1984. Food restriction and the aging process. J. Am. Geriatr. Soc. **32:** 296–300.

32. SACHER, G. A. 1977. Life table modification and life prolongation. *In* The Handbook of the Biology of Aging. C. E. Finch & L. Hayflick, Eds.: 582–638. Van Nostrand–Reinhold. Princeton, New Jersey.

33. TALAN, M. I. & D. K. INGRAM. 1985. Effect of intermittent feeding on thermoregulatory abilities of young and aged C57BL/6J mice. Arch. Gerontol. Geriatr. **4:** 251–259.

34. INGRAM, D. K., R. WEINDRUCH, E. L. SPANGLER, J. R. FREEMAN & R. L. WALFORD. 1987. Dietary restriction benefits learning and motor performance of aged mice. J. Gerontol. **42:** 78–81.

35. SAMORAJSKI, T., D. COURTNEY, L. DURHAM, J. M. ORDY, J. A. JOHNSON & W. P. DUNLAP. 1985. The effect of exercise on longevity, body weight, locomotor performance, and passive-avoidance memory of C57BL/6J mice. Neurobiol. Aging **6:** 17–24.

36. INGRAM, D. K., E. L. SPANGLER & G. P. VINCENT. 1983. Behavioral comparison of aged virgin and retired breeder mice. Exp. Aging Res. **9:** 111–113.

37. MIQUEL, J. & K. LINDSETH. 1983. Determination of biological age in antioxidant-treated *Drosophila* and mice. *In* Intervention in the Aging Process, Part B: Basic Research and Preclinical Screening. W. Regelson & F. M. Sinex, Eds.: 187–202. Alan R. Liss. New York.

38. REGELSON, W. 1983. The evidence for pituitary and thyroid control of aging: Is age reversal a myth or reality? The search for a "death hormone". *In* Intervention in the Aging Process, Part B: Basic Research and Preclinical Screening. W. Regelson & F. M. Sinex, Eds.: 187–202. Alan R. Liss. New York.

39. HOFECKER, G., M. SKALICKY, A. KMENT & H. NIEDERMULLER. 1980. Models of the biological age of the rat. I. A factor model of age parameters. Mech. Ageing Dev. **14:** 345–359.

40. INGRAM, D. K. 1985. Analysis of age-related impairments in learning and memory in rodent models. Ann. N.Y. Acad. Sci. **444:** 312–331.

41. GAGE, F. H., S. B. DUNNETT & A. BJÖRKLUND. 1984. Spatial learning and motor deficits in aged rats. Neurobiol. Aging **5:** 43–48.

DISCUSSION OF THE PAPER

G. LOVELACE: When you showed the plot with the diverging X, Y, Z curves, presumably that was conceptually a plot against chronological age of performances of some sort. If the abscissa had not been chronological age, but functional age, might they have then represented three lines of individuals who were simply biologically aging at different rates?

D. INGRAM (*NIA, Baltimore, MD*): The task in a nutshell is: does the variability observed among individuals of the same chronological age really represent differences in functional age? If one makes the assumption, then one has to provide tests that demonstrate that the individual differences are reliable and that they are meaningful (in the context that you can predict that the individual differences can predict something). Therefore, we need to know the criteria for this. Is it going to be how long the person lives? Is it going to be the age at which he or she develops a chronic disease? So far, the advocates for measures of biomarkers of aging have yet to come up with a suitable criterion with which we can measure those things. We demonstrated that some variability in life span can be predicted by motor performance. What I failed to say is that we do not know how much of that is related to disease because we did not do specific pathology on the animals; however, you will note that the pattern of longitudinal decline starts early, thus implying that decline over that long of a period of time could not be attributed to a specific pathology for most animals.

W. SPIRDUSO (*University of Texas, Austin, TX*): When you establish an animal's performance level at 6 months, 12 months, 24 months of age, etc., do you test that animal for three, four, five, etc., days and take that as some kind of an estimate of the best performance of the animal at each age? Or, on the other hand, are you testing those animals for one shot and then coming back 12 months later and testing them again? Therefore, is the age-related decline the capacity of the animal or the change in variability within the subject consistency of the animal?

INGRAM: All the data I presented today were based on one shot; however, there is a possibility of confounding of learning. I just measured one shot using several trials (three to five trials) depending upon the task (the tightrope task had five trials, while the grip strength task had three trials). It is a very short exposure to the test experience, but that short exposure can have effects two months later; this can be seen in the grip strength test, where the animals learned to perform better in that task.

Thus, the best design is to put the animals up to their capacity. We get the animal up at a young age to a capacity (a high level of capacity) and then assess the aging effects longitudinally. That is the objective, though it is not the current status of the data I presented.

M. BRENNAN (*Revlon Health Care, Tuckahoe, NY*): The strain differences present interesting models to evaluate genetic influence as a source of variance in the effects of age. Therefore, can we make cross-sectional comparisons between strains that have slightly different life spans? What is the significance in observing a difference between the two strains in terms of both behavior and any of the neurochemical or neurobiological markers underlying those differences?

INGRAM: I would defer to my previous comment that we definitely need longitudinal analysis. There are so many factors that can impinge upon that one performance. It could be motivational in nature and, if one repeatedly tested the animals, some acclimation to the test environment might wash out that strain difference altogether. A well-developed battery that has demonstrated reliability and that is conducted in longitudinal fashion is the best.

BRENNAN: My question was more in terms of context of differential survivorship rather than in the same subject population.

INGRAM: Well, on the tightrope task, you will notice that the A/J strain that did not show an age-related decline is actually the shorter-lived strain.

Adaptivity as a Paradigm for Age-dependent Changes Exemplified by Motor Behavior

B. JÄNICKE, H. COPER, AND G. SCHULZE

Institute for Neuropsychopharmacology
Freie University
D-1000 Berlin 19, Federal Republic of Germany

The ability to adapt to one's environment and to appropriately react to changes within it is a prerequisite for the development and preservation of each species. This reciprocal interrelationship between external stimuli and the internal regulation of all functions in the homeostatic system varies in stability, capacity, and reserve. The adaptivity must be subdivided into the acute reactions of an individual (as determined by the current regulation capacity in each phase of life) and the dynamic processes of adaptive mechanisms over a period of time. These processes include not only regeneration and aging, but also acclimatization and training effects.

The stability of the regulatory systems, as characterized by susceptibility to disturbances, can be quantified by the intensity of the stimulus causing the deviation from the norm. The capacity for compensation and its control can be determined by the extent and speed of a response and can be tested by finding the limits to an overtaxation of the system (testing the limits). The reserve of functions can be measured by an improved performance after practice.

The homeostasis is maintained by inherent and learned regulation processes that are multiply ensured, thus allowing partial weaknesses to be covered up and compensated for. These differentiated possibilities of adapting are expressed differently during the course of ontogeny, thereby resulting in characteristic changes. By taking individual and species-specific compensation mechanisms into consideration, the aging process can be demonstrated at different levels—molecular, cellular, endocrinous, at the level of the organs[1-5]—as well as in changes in the functions of the whole organism.

Numerous studies have shown that compensation reactions become delayed, less effective, or nonexistent with increasing age.[6-8] This has especially been demonstrated for reaction to changes in ambient temperature, pressure, and amount of oxygen, or in increased peripheral resistance in the circulation.[9-14]

Deviations in adaptivity due to increasing age can be especially well demonstrated at the level of motoric behavior. Determination of central control is mainly responsible for reduced performance. Limitations in the periphery are only secondary contributors to the etiology of movement deficits and they only work in a modulatory way.[1,15-19] The low stability of unpracticed behavioral reactions, due mainly to missing or incorrectly functioning correctional mechanisms, has been observed in man and animals many times and is, in principle, applicable to all age stages.[20-26] However, with increasing chronological age, it has been observed that adaptivity is especially diminished; in some cases, though, clarification is needed to determine whether reduced performance represents an exhaustion of effective capacity or a defective use of adaptive regulation. A change in the time pattern in which the organization and execution of motor processes take place, in the sense of a prolongation, also leads to a reduction in effectiveness — an example being the synchronization of reaction processes with the demands.

The deviations affect the speed as well as the power components of physiological reaction patterns, especially those of adaptive reactions to endogenous and exogenous stimuli. Subdivisions into mainly speed-dependent and speed-independent abilities are especially important in clinical diagnostics and in the validation of pharmacodynamic effects.[27] In the following, we will proceed with this differentiation despite existing interactions and relationships.

Many studies have confirmed that aging, with respect to the speed component of motoric processes, is rule governed and can be considered a valid and reliable characteristic of the aging process.[16,28,29] Despite great multiplicity, this process tends to be manifested as a slowing down. In contrast, the aging process of the power component is not so clear and must be examined for each individual quality. The verification of reduced abilities is methodically problematic because various adaptation strategies that can compensate for restrictions in partial functions are developed during the course of ontogeny. This compensation is constantly produced by many regulatory elements. Thus, the ensurance of integrative functions is a system property of the organism that guarantees its survival.[30]

A difficulty in determining the aging process of behavior mainly independent of speed is due to the fact that little-used and seldom-taxed abilities are less routinized and thereby more susceptible. Therefore, in determining their efficiency, it is necessary to know how often they have been regularly used and, thus, their availability. This is true to the same degree for the corresponding counterbalancing processes.

The rats used in our experiments were female Wistar rats (Hagemann,

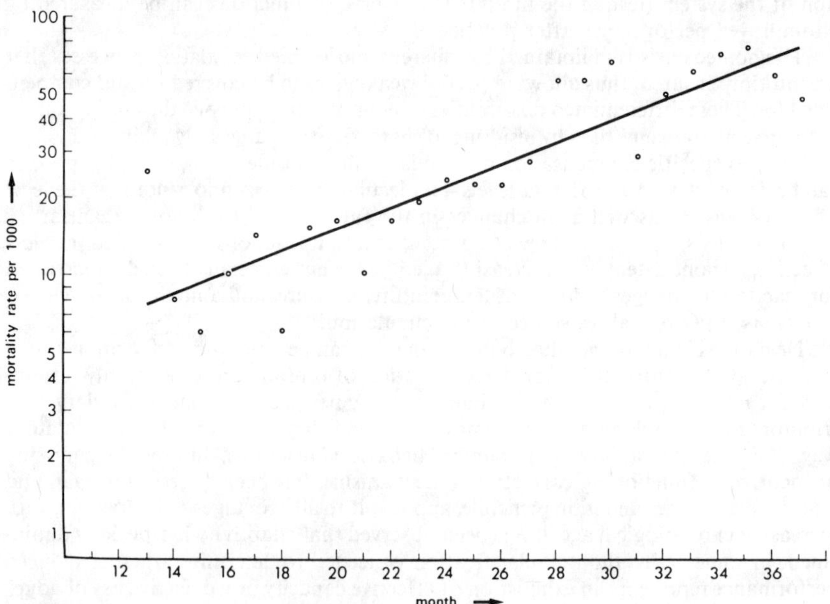

FIGURE 1. Gompertz curve of 280 female Wistar rats (breeder: Hagemann, Bösingfeld) showing the age-specific mortality rate.

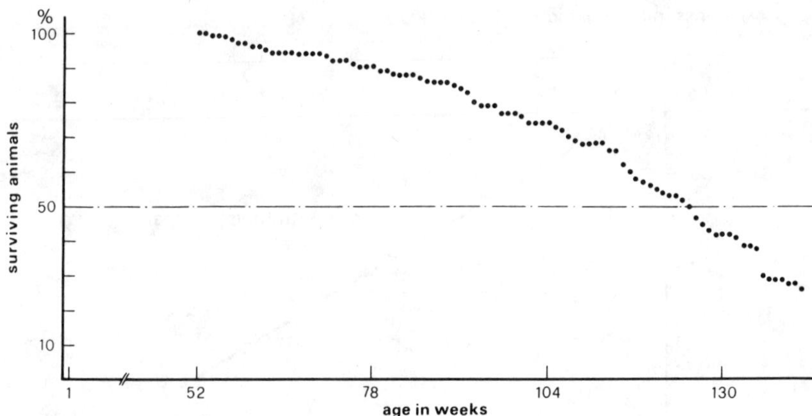

FIGURE 2. Survival curve of 280 female Wistar rats. The 50% survival limit is at 125 weeks.

Lippe/Bösingfeld) whose weights were registered weekly. The Gompertz curve indicates that it was an aging population (FIGURE 1) with the 50% survival limit at 27 months (FIGURE 2). The data are based on an observation period that currently spans three years. It is noteworthy that a closer analysis of the death rates shows characteristic weight processes for long-lived rats (older than 27 months) and animals with an average life span, thus confirming Everitt's[31] findings with male Wistar rats (FIGURE 3).

Motor ability was examined by using a battery of motor tests of graduated complexity in a cross-sectional analysis. Compared to a longitudinal analysis, this only represents a description of the skill profiles of different-aged organisms, but it has the advantage that comparative examinations can be performed in a relatively short time period.

The results showed that vital behavior (which includes spontaneous activity in a familiar and unchanged environment) was quantitatively unchanged in young and old rats (FIGURE 4).[32] There were also no significant differences between the age groups in the swimming test. The positive results of others on this test are probably due to different methods or to specific breed characteristics.[33–36]

Supplementary data on food and fluid intake over several weeks[37–39] underscore that motility is only slightly impaired by age. All tests have in common a high survival value and a lack of an immediate time component which, as mentioned before, is responsible for most age differences.[40,41] In tests measuring the ability to react (passive-avoidance test; Porsolt-Test),[42] passivity does not represent a low level of performance, but a behavior appropriate to the circumstances.[43] In addition, during the course of ontogeny, behavioral stereotypes based either on experience or heredity can develop and cause the behavioral repertoire to appear limited, independent of the time factor. However, the speed component could be of importance in such a case as when Wilcox[44] uses the reactions of a rat suddenly thrown into water as a measure of its fitness. Test situations that are unfamiliar to an animal could cause a strong stress stimulus that, for example, could be marked by increased defecation. This reaction is more pronounced in old rats. On open-field tests, it has been observed that old rats are more strongly emotionally affected by the new situation.[45–48] The emotional response disappears with practice, but older rats require considerably more time than young ones.[49]

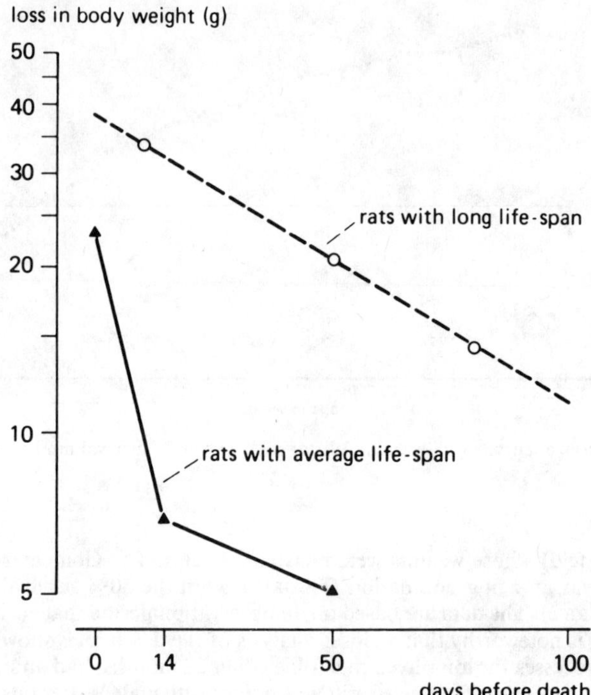

FIGURE 3. Course of weight-loss in female rats during the last 100 days of life. ▲—▲: rats with average life span; O—O: rats with long life span.

Although there is a definite time component in the climbing test and the chimney test (FIGURE 4), our experiments were designed to allow the animals to perform the task without a time constraint. Nevertheless, in both tests, there were considerable differences between the age groups with respect to their reactions to the situation and especially in the manner that the tasks were performed. Old rats climbed more hesitantly, more tensely, and, in a sense, with more errors (as was determined by the course of movements of their extremities). Thus, one can exclude the possibility that the comparatively longer amount of time they required to complete the task was due to cautious movements and increased precision.

The rotorod test with three rotation speeds tested the coordination capacity of motor functions. Not only did the rats need to learn a complex pattern of movements (motoric learning), but after overcoming initial nervousness, they needed to maintain their attention and concentration over a specific period of time. Therefore, in addition to the speed and power components, this test measured other factors such as vigilance.

FIGURE 5 shows the performance on the rotorod test as a function of the number of starts at the lowest rotation speed (10 rpm). The age difference can be clearly seen in the time it took to reach the criterion at two-minutes running time. An analysis of the frequency of starts as a function of the rotation speed revealed that even the oldest rats demonstrated training effects despite an increase from 10 to 40 rpm. This observation led to the conclusion that, in contrast to the climbing test, the power com-

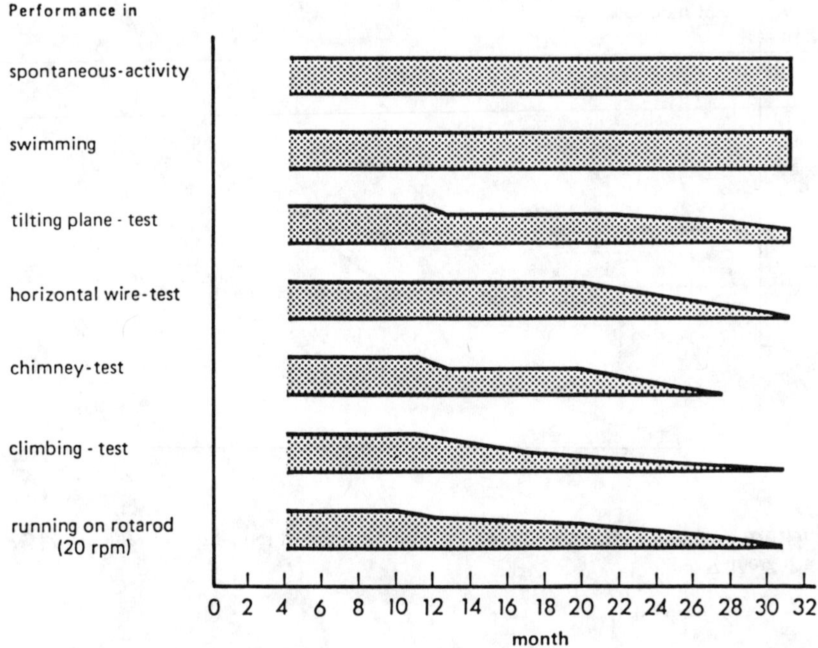

FIGURE 4. Changes in motor performance with increasing age in reference to performance of 4-month-old rats.

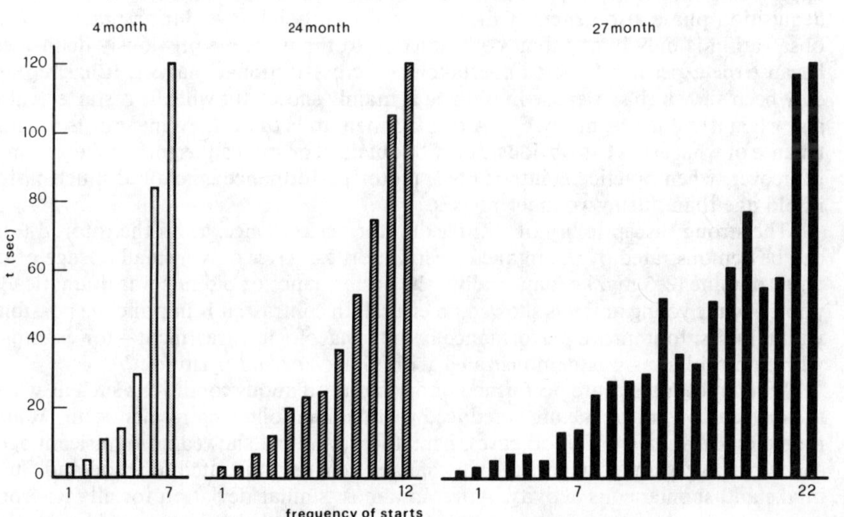

FIGURE 5. Rotorod performance of rats of different age—frequency of starts for a rotation speed of 10 rpm until the chosen criterion was met. (Median values ± SEM; n = 30 each.)

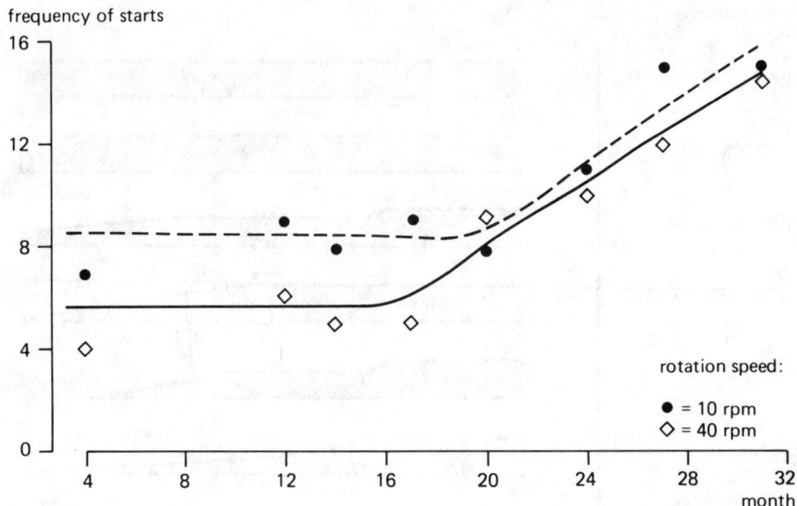

FIGURE 6. Training effect on rotorod test in different aged rats. (Median values; $n = 30$ in each group.)

ponent was of secondary importance to the speed component because the coordinated motoric achievements were determined by speed factors. The effectiveness of training, however, was limited. This was seen when the 27- and 29-month-old rats exhausted their allowed 15 starts without being able to complete the task (FIGURE 6); thus, they approached their limit of performance. Old rats with a low achievement level in the acquisition phase also generally did not significantly improve during practice. This observation is only in apparent contradiction to the principle previously delineated because the experiments were undertaken as a cross-sectional analysis. It has repeatedly been shown that exercise in old age is mainly successful when it is started early and when it is done regularly.[50-53] A displacement to better achievement or the maintenance of what exists can obviously only be obtained by strict adherence to the training. Moreover, when practice is interrupted, motor performance is reduced much faster in old age than during younger phases.

The strong susceptibility of complex motor performance, as on the rotorod test, can be demonstrated by the intake of certain drugs. After only a small dosage of *d*-amphetamine (2–3 mg/kg/day, orally), the performance of old rats was dramatically poorer, while young animals showed no effects. In contrast, it is in principle possible, within limits, to improve performance by pharmacological treatment — for example, with nootropics, as was demonstrated with piracetam and pyritinol.[37,54]

When motor tasks are performed under more strenuous conditions such as when the oxygen content of the air is reduced to 10%, the following results occur. While physiological values for blood gases, hematocrit, and pH showed no significant age-specific changes under hypoxia, such changes were demonstrated for food and fluid intake and spontaneous activity. After an almost similar deviation for all rats from norm values in the sense of attenuation (power component), age groups could be clearly distinguished in the adaptation phase (speed component). In old rats, the time span for recovery was clearly longer and the capacity was measurably reduced (FIGURE 7).[12]

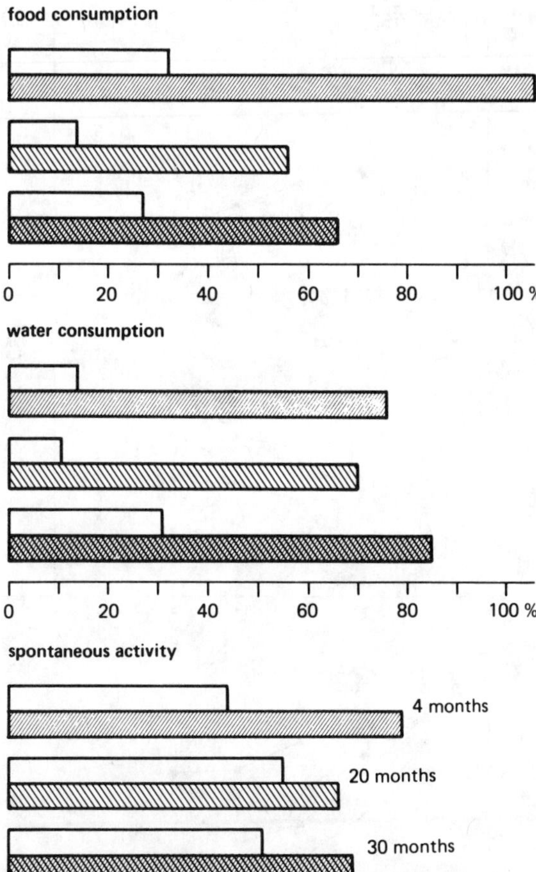

FIGURE 7. Influence of hypoxia (10% O_2) on food and water consumption and spontaneous activity of rats of different ages in percent related to normoxic conditions (20% O_2); ($n = 10$ in each group, blank area = 24-h hypoxia, shaded area = 96-h hypoxia).

Learning the existing spatial setup of a maze, in which motor behavior is important, is a task that has frequently been examined in rats. In our experiments, a closed-pipe system was used. The rats needed to correctly make six right-left decisions in order to reach the goal and be rewarded with food. The movements of the animals were registered by infrared light barriers and the impulses were transferred to a computer for analysis. In addition to more errors (frequency entering cul-de-sacs), the data showed a preferential changing away from "speed reactions". This is expressed as a definitely longer time to complete the task and a longer decision latency at intersections for the 27-month-old rats as compared to the 4-month-old ones.

Initial results with an analogous transparent maze confirmed these results (FIGURE 8). The total running time was a composite parameter that was determined by the number of time-dependent and time-independent factors. Among the time-dependent factors are the length of the nonlocomotor behavior and the resulting overall length of orienting

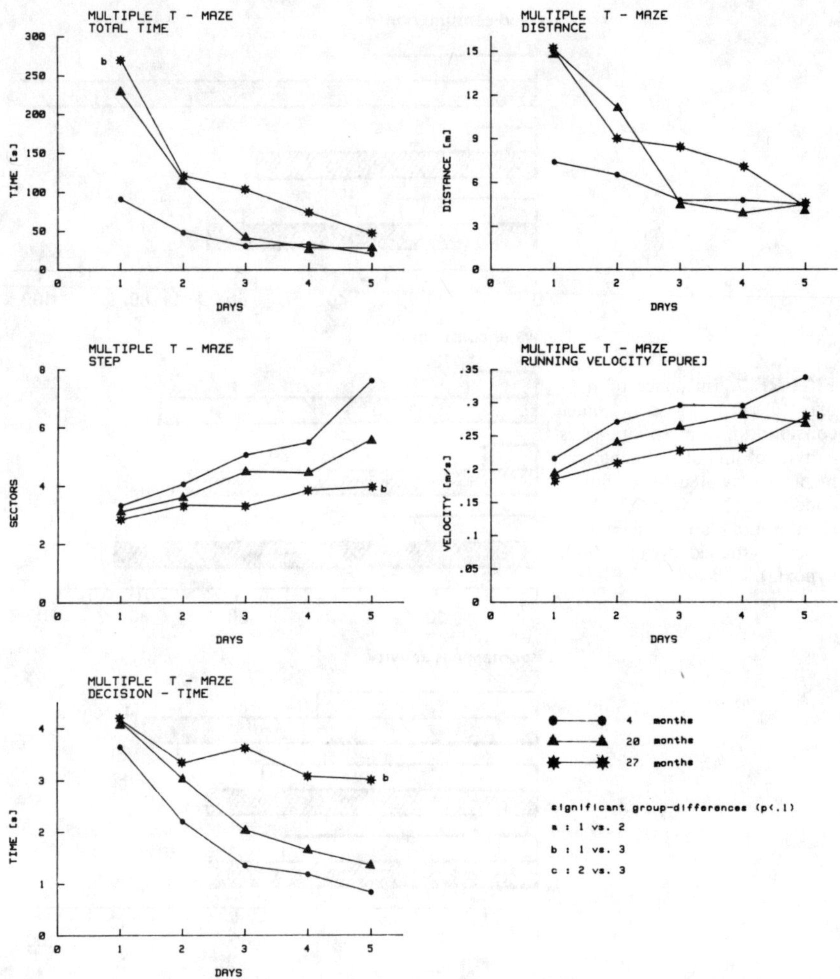

FIGURE 8. Training effects on behavior of different aged rats in a multiple *t*-maze. (Median values; *n* = 30 in each group.)

scenting, which also contains the orienting scenting during decision-making. The running velocity is also a time-dependent factor in the locomotor phases. Time-independent factors are the length of the area covered within the maze (distance). Additionally, the so-called running phase (step) is shown, that is, running activity without interruption. It was evident that differences existed in a number of factors between the various age groups. The age-related deviations still remain with time-dependent factors even if training effects have been obtained. In almost all of the time-independent factors, the age-related factors are nearly eliminated by training.

Chronic treatment with diazepam (2 mg/kg/day, i.p.) led to a significantly shorter running phase in the young rats, whereas the old ones were not affected by the drug. Thus, in this area, the differences between the age groups were diminished. However, the total activity of the old rats was simultaneously much more strongly reduced than that of young rats. The more frequent and longer periods of inactivity caused them to remain in the maze much longer. In analyzing age differences for the entire duration in the maze from start to finish (in addition to other factors such as frequency of errors, length of running phase, decision-making time, etc.), the total activity must also be taken into consideration.

Although the activity within the maze was dependent on many other variables (motivation, vigilance, orientation), it could be concluded, with the inclusion of findings from other researchers, that traversing a maze is also age dependent.[55,56]

In summary, the examples presented demonstrate that differentiated changes occur in motor behavior in old age. These changes are asynchronous and graduated, depending on the complexity and conditions presented (treatment with drugs, exposure to hypoxia). They reveal individual differences, but they also show a common tendency for decline in achievement and adaptivity with increasing age. The variety in which they are manifested can be found in both intra- and inter-individual variability and in the increasingly limited modifiability of decline.

As expected, these changes mainly affect the "speed component" of behavior. In addition, there is a loss of flexibility in the mutual change and the interdependent influence between environment and an organism's ability to integratively process stimuli affecting it from inner and outer milieus, as well as in its ability to maintain its capability for functioning and being vital. This occurs in terms of reduced capacity, diminished stability, and a lack of reserve—all of which affect adaptation. However, the examples also provide possibilities that would allow an old organism to ameliorate performance loss through practice and/or treatment with medication.

REFERENCES

1. SHOCK, N. W. 1977. Systems integration. *In* Handbook of the Biology of Aging. C. E. Finch & L. Hayflick, Eds.: 639–665. Van Nostrand–Reinhold. Princeton, New Jersey.
2. FINCH, C. E. 1975. Aging and the regulation of hormones. Adv. Med. Biol. **61:** 229–238.
3. FINCH, C. E. 1976. The regulation of the physiological changes during mammalian aging. Q. Rev. Biol. **81:** 49–83.
4. ADELMAN, R. C. 1975. Disruptions in enzyme regulation during aging. Basic Life Sci. **6:** 304–311.
5. ROTH, G. S. 1985. Changes in hormone/neurotransmitter action during aging. *In* Aging, Vol. 30, Homeostatic Function and Aging. B. B. Davis & W. G. Wood, Eds.: 41–58. Raven Press. New York.
6. WELFORD, A. T. 1977. Motor performance. *In* Handbook of the Psychology of Aging. J. E. Birren & K. W. Schaie, Eds.: 450–496. Van Nostrand–Reinhold. Princeton, New Jersey.
7. POON, L. W., Ed. 1980. Aging in the 1980s. Amer. Psychol. Assoc. Washington, D.C.
8. CRAIK, F. I. M. & S. TREHUB, Eds. 1982. Aging and Cognitive Process. Plenum. New York.
9. COLLINS, K. J. & A. N. EXTON-SMITH. 1983. Thermal homeostasis in old age. J. Am. Geriatr. Soc. **31:** 519–524.
10. SCHULZE, G. & P. BÜRGEL. 1977. The influence of age and drugs on the thermoregulatory behaviour of rats. Naunyn-Schmiedeberg's Arch. Pharmacol. **283:** 143–147.
11. REYNOLDS, M. A., D. K. INGRAM & M. TALAN. 1985. Relationship of body temperature stability to mortality in aging mice. Mech. Ageing Dev. **30:** 143–152.
12. SCHULZE, G. & B. JÄNICKE. 1986. Effects of chronic hypoxia on behavioral and physiological parameters. Neurobiol. Aging **7:** 199–203.
13. HOFFMANN, W. E., D. PELLIGRINO, D. J. MILETICH & R. F. ALBRECHT. 1984. Cerebrovas-

cular and metabolic response of the aged rat to hypoxia. *In* Monogr. Neural Sci. M. M. Cohen, Ed. **11:** 8–16. Karger. Basel.

14. VERZAR, F. & E. FLÜCKINGER. 1955. Lack of adaptation to low oxygen pressure in aged animals. *In* Old Age and the Modern World. Third International Congress of Gerontology, London, p. 524–532. Livingstone. Edinburgh.

15. SPIRDUSO, W. W. 1982. Physical fitness in relation to motor aging. *In* The Aging Motor System. J. A. Mortimer, F. J. Pirozzolo & G. J. Maletta, Eds.: 120–151. Praeger. New York.

16. WELFORD, A. T. 1982. Motor skills and aging. *In* The Aging Motor System. J. A. Mortimer, F. J. Pirozzolo & G. J. Maletta, Eds.: 152–187. Praeger. New York.

17. GUTMANN, E. & V. HANZLIKOVA. 1972. Basic mechanisms of aging in the neuromuscular system. Mech. Ageing Dev. **1:** 327–349.

18. FROLKIS, V. V., O. A. MARTYNENKO & V. P. ZAMOSTYAN. 1976. Aging of the neuromuscular apparatus. Gerontologia **22:** 244–279.

19. SCHIEBEL, M. E. & A. B. SCHEIBEL. 1977. Differential changes with aging in old and new cortices. Adv. Behav. Biol. **23:** 39–58.

20. SHOCK, N. W. & A. H. NORRIS. 1970. Neuromuscular coordination as a factor in age changes in muscular exercises. *In* Medicine and Sport, Physical Activity and Aging, Vol. 4. E. Jokl & H. Hebbelinck, Eds.: 92–99. Karger. Basel.

21. DE VRIES, H.A. 1970. Physiological effects of an exercise training regimen upon men aged 52 to 88. J. Gerontol. **25:** 325–336.

22. ADAMS, G. M. & H. A. DE VRIES. 1973. Physiological effects of an exercise training regimen upon women aged 52 to 79. J. Gerontol. **28:** 50–55.

23. WALLACE, J. E., E. E. KRAUTER & B. A. CAMPBELL. 1980. Motor and reflexive behavior in the aging rat. J. Gerontol. **35:** 364–370.

24. MARSHALL, J. F. 1982. Sensorimotor disturbances in the aging rodent. J. Gerontol. **37:** 548–554.

25. DAVIS, R. T. 1985. The effects of aging on the behavior of rhesus monkeys. *In* Behavior and Pathology of Aging in Rhesus Monkeys. Vol. 8. R. T. Davis & C. W. Leathers, Eds.: 57–82. Alan R. Liss. New York.

26. MARSHALL, P. H., J. W. ELIAS & J. WRIGHT. 1985. Age related factors in motor error detection and correction. Exp. Aging Res. **11:** 201–206.

27. OSWALD, W. D. & U. M. FLEISCHMANN. 1983. The Nürnberg gerontopsychological inventory—A new assessment in psychometrics. *In* Gerontopsychiatric Diagnostics and Treatment—Multidimensional Approaches. M. Bergener, Ed.: 153–161. Springer Pub. New York.

28. CAMPBELL, B. A., E. E. KRAUTER & J. E. WALLACE. 1980. Animal models of aging: Sensorymotor and cognitive function in the aged rat. *In* Psychobiology of Aging: Problems and Perspectives. G. Stein, Ed.: 201–226. North-Holland/Elsevier. Amsterdam.

29. POTVIN, A. R., K. SYNDULKO, W. W. TURTELLOTTE, J. A. LEMMON & J. H. POTVIN. 1980. Human neurologic function and the aging process. J. Am. Geriatr. Soc. **28:** 1–8.

30. COPER, H., B. JÄNICKE & G. SCHULZE. 1986. Biopsychological research on adaptivity across the life-span of animals. *In* Life-Span Development and Behavior. Vol. 7. P. Baltes, D. L. Featherman & R. M. Lerner, Eds.: 207–232. Erlbaum. Hillsdale, New Jersey.

31. EVERITT, A. V. 1957. The change in food and water consumption and in feces and urine production in aging male rats. Gerontologia **2:** 21–32.

32. JÄNICKE, B., G. SCHULZE & H. COPER. 1983. Motor performance achievements in rats of different ages. Exp. Gerontol. **18:** 393–407.

33. HOFECKER, G., A. KMENT & H. NIEDERMÜLLER. 1978. Die motorische Aktivität als Altersparameter der Ratte. Aktnelle Gerontologie **8:** 271–279.

34. MARSHALL, J. J. & N. BERRIOS. 1979. Movement disorders of aged rats: Reversal by dopamine receptor stimulation. Science **206:** 477–479.

35. YU, B. P., E. J. MASORO & C. A. McMAHAN. 1985. Nutritional influences on aging of Fischer 344 rats: I. Physical, metabolic and longevity characteristics. J. Gerontol. **40:** 657–670.

36. INGRAM, D. K., E. D. LONDON, M. A. REYNOLDS, S. B. WALLER & C. L. GOODRICK. 1981.

Differential effects of age on motor performance in two mouse strains. Neurobiol. Aging **2:** 221–227.

37. JÄNICKE, B. & D. WROBEL. 1984. Changes in motor activity in age and the effects of pharmacological treatment. Exp. Gerontol. **19:** 321–328.

38. MARTIN, J. R., A. FUCHS, R. BENDER & J. HARTING. 1986. Altered light/dark activity differences with aging in two rat strains. J. Gerontol. **41:** 2–7.

39. PENG, M-T., M-J. JING & H-K. HSÜ. 1980. Changes in running wheel activity, eating and drinking and their day/night distribution throughout the life span of the rat. J. Gerontol. **35:** 339–347.

40. WELFORD, A. T., A. H. NORRIS & N. W. SHOCK. 1969. Speed and accuracy of movement and their changes with age. Acta Psychol. **30;** Attention and Performance. Vol. 11. W. G. Koster, Ed.: 3–15. North-Holland. Amsterdam.

41. WELFORD, A. T. 1984. Between bodily changes and performance: some possible reasons for slowing with age. Exp. Aging Res. **10:** 73–88.

42. PORSOLT, R. D. 1977. Behavioral despair in mice: a primary screening test for antidepressants. Arch. Int. Pharmacodyn. **229:** 327–336.

43. LAPSLEY, D. K. & R. D. ENRIGHT. 1983. A cognitive developmental model of rigidity in senescence. Int. J. Aging Hum. Dev. **16:** 81–93.

44. WILCOCK, J. 1972. Water-escape in weanling rats: A link between behavior and biological fitness. Anim. Behav. **20:** 543–547.

45. DOTY, B. & L. A. DOTY. 1967. Effects of handling at various ages on later open field behavior. Can. J. Psychol. **21:** 463–470.

46. GOODRICK, C. L. 1971. Free exploration and adaptation in open field as a function of trials and between-trial-intervals for mature-young, mature-old, and senescent Wistar rats. J. Gerontol. **26:** 58–62.

47. ELIAS, P. K., M. K. ELIAS & B. E. ELEFTHERIOU. 1975. Emotionality, exploratory behavior and locomotion in aging inbred strains of mice. Gerontologia **21:** 46.

48. LUPO-DI-PRISCO, C. & F. D. DESSI-FULGHERI. 1980. Endocrine and behavioral modifications in aging male rats. Horm. Res. **12:** 149–160.

49. BRONSTEIN, P. M. 1972. Repeated trials with the albino rats in open field as a function of age and deprivation. J. Comp. Physiol. Pharmacol. **81:** 84–93.

50. McCAFFERTY, W. B. & D. W. EDINGTON. 1974. Skeletal muscle and organ weights of aged and trained male rats. Gerontologia **20:** 44–50.

51. INGRAM, D. K., M. REYNOLDS & C. GOODRICK. 1982. Relationship of sex, exercise, and growth rate to life span in Wistar rat: a multivariate correlational approach. Gerontology **28:** 23–31.

52. SAMORAJSKI, T., C. DELANEY & L. DURHAM. 1985. Effect of exercise on longevity, body weight, locomotor performance, and passive-avoidance memory of C57BL/6J mice. Neurobiol. Aging **6:** 17–24.

53. McDONALD, R., J. HEGENAUER & P. SALTMAN. 1986. Age-related differences in the bone mineralization pattern of rats following exercise. J. Gerontol. **41:** 445–452.

54. JOSEPH, J. A., R. T. BARTUS, D. CLODY, D. MORGAN, C. FINCH, B. BEER & S. SESACK. 1983. Psychomotor performance in the senescent rodent: reduction of deficits via striatal dopamine receptor up-regulation. Neurobiol. Aging **4:** 313–319.

55. DEAN, R. L., J. SCOZZAFAVA, J. A. GOAS, B. REGAN, B. BEER & R. T. BARTUS. 1981. Age-related differences in behavior across the life-span of the C57BL/6J mouse. Exp. Aging Res. **7:** 427–451.

56. KUBANIS, P. & S. F. ZORNETZER. 1981. Age-related behavioral and neurobiological changes: A review with an emphasis on memory. Behav. Neural Biol. **31:** 115–172.

Aging-dependent Emergence of Sensorimotor Dysfunction in Rats Recovered from Dopamine Depletion Sustained Early in Life[a]

TIMOTHY SCHALLERT

Department of Psychology
and
Institute for Neurological Science
University of Texas at Austin
Austin, Texas 78712

In the study of aging-related motor decline and its central determinants, it is important to consider that older individuals may be subject to sensory impairment or weakness from hypophagia or other events that might influence movement adversely and thus obscure measurements of the integrity of motor function. In addition, previous exposure to neurotoxins, minor cerebral insults, or related perturbations of brain function throughout the life span might affect the operation of motor systems during old age. Two approaches using animal models are considered in this report.

First, an objective, easy to administer, test of somatosensory function will be described, and its value will be illustrated in young versus old rats. This test was developed to assess sensory function, with high resolution, independently from motor, nutritional, or other aging-related events.[1-4] The data indicate that most old rats are generally resistant to somatosensory dysfunction, but many suffer from deficits in movement initiation that can affect the response segment of orienting behavior and thus can affect measures of responsiveness to sensory stimulation.

Second, the effects of aging in rats that had long since recovered from the behavioral signs of unilateral dopamine depletion occurring in adulthood are described. Using a unilateral lesion preparation and neurological tests of sensorimotor asymmetry, selective aging-lesion interactions were isolated. Specifically, unilateral behavioral signs of the earlier brain damage reappear during old age and can be distinguished from noncentral motor dysfunction or other erosive events of the aging process, which, when present, act bilaterally. Because the behavioral effects are asymmetric, nonspecific sensory dysfunction, generalized motor slowing or fatigue, illness, and nutritional factors can be ruled out. The role of aging-related decline in the function of dopaminergic versus nondopaminergic systems will be discussed.

[a] This work was supported by Grant Nos. NS 17274 and NS 23964 to T. Schallert, and Grant No. AA 06761 to W. W. Spirduso and T. Schallert.

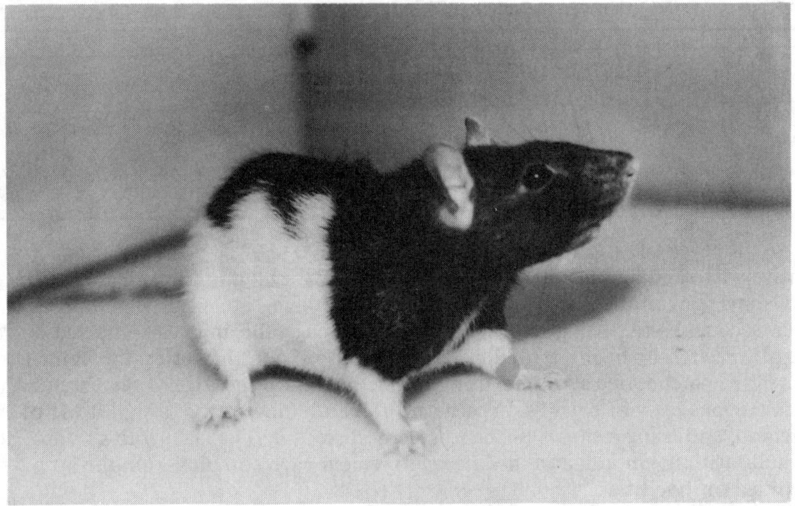

FIGURE 1. A rat with adhesive patches on the radial aspect of each forelimb.

INTACT ANIMALS

Sensorimotor function was determined first in male rats with no brain damage. There were 24 hooded Long-Evans rats — 13 of which were old (28 mo) and 11 of which were young adults (8 mo). There were 10 albino F-344 rats — 5 of which were old (25 mo) and 5 of which were young (4 mo). As in previous work, a palatable diet supplement was used when necessary to offset aging-related nutritional requirements, particularly abnormal weight loss.[5]

The tests were designed to assess sensory asymmetry reliably. All tests were carried out in the home cage, which is relatively free from competing stimuli that otherwise distract the animals and prevent them from orienting toward specific somatosensory stimuli.[1,6,7] In the first test, two small pieces of adhesive-backed paper patches (of equal size: 113.1 mm^2) were used as bilateral tactile stimuli occupying the distal-radial region on the wrist of each forelimb (see FIGURE 1). The animals were removed from their cages briefly so that the patches could be firmly attached. The animals were ex-

TABLE 1. Latency[a] for F-344 Rats to Contact and to Remove Adhesive Patches from Radial Aspect of Forelimb

	Contact	
4 mo	1.8 s	(1.0–2.8)
25 mo	10.5 s	(8.5–88.8)
	Remove	
4 mo	3.6 s	(1.6–11.0)
25 mo	16.3 s	(8.6–120.0)

[a] Median and range of the latency are shown.

TABLE 2. Percentage of F-344 Rats Removing Patch in Less than 40 s versus 15 s

Remove in Less than 40 s	
4 mo	100%
25 mo	80%
Less than 15 s	
4 mo	100%
25 mo	40%

tensively handled in this way before testing so that they did not struggle, vocalize, or show any signs of distress while the patches were being attached, which takes only a few seconds. After being returned to the home cage, the animals contacted one or the other patch by lifting a forelimb to the mouth. Soon thereafter, the animals removed the patches one at a time, using the teeth to grasp the edge of the patch, using simultaneous upward head and downward forelimb movements to pull it off of the forelimb, and using a thrust of the tongue to discard it. The latency to contact each stimulus with the mouth and the latency to remove each stimulus from the limb were recorded on five trials.

TABLE 1 shows the latencies to contact and to remove the adhesive patches for the young versus old F-344 rats. The young rats responded significantly faster than the old rats ($p < 0.05$). All of the young F-344 rats, but only 40% of the old rats, removed an adhesive patch in less than 15 s (TABLE 2). Of the Long-Evans rats, 91% of the young rats, but only 53% of the old rats, removed a patch within 40 s (TABLE 3).

Because these data may reflect sensory impairment rather than movement initiation, an additional type of adhesive-removal test was carried out that estimates the ability to discriminate the relative magnitude of two stimuli that are of slightly different size. In this test, the size of the stimulus on one limb (i.e., intensity, as defined by the limb area occupied by the adhesive patch) was systematically increased while the size of the other stimulus was decreased by increments of 7.0–14.1 mm² each. The widest diameter of a given stimulus was oriented transversely (rather than longitudinally) around the radial aspect of the wrist. When the size of one stimulus is sufficiently larger than the simultaneously applied stimulus on the opposite limb, a response bias occurs (as measured by the order of stimulus contact). Rats usually contact the larger of the two patches first, even if movement initiation (and therefore overall latency) is impaired.[2,6] In other words, the order (rather than the latency) of patch removal is the most important outcome in this measure of somatosensory acuity.

The patch sizes were adjusted until a response bias was detected (i.e., the larger of the two patches was contacted on 80% or more of the trials). Then, 4–5 additional "bias-confirmation" trials were conducted, alternating with 4–5 "nonbias" trials in which the sizes of the two patches were made just similar enough that no bias could be reliably detected (i.e., the larger of the two patches was contacted on 50% or fewer of the trials). For each rat, the median JND (just noticeable difference) was computed in the following way. The size of the larger patch used in the nonbias trials was subtracted from the size of the larger patch used in the bias confirmation trials. This difference was added to the difference between the sizes of the smaller patches used in the nonbias

TABLE 3. Percentage of Long-Evans Rats Removing Patch in Less than 40 s

8 mo ($n = 11$)	91%
28 mo ($n = 13$)	53%

TABLE 4. Somatosensory Acuity Index (JND) in Young versus Old Rats

4 mo	24.2 mm²
25 mo	19.6 mm²

versus the bias confirmation trials. For most animals, this value was simply the mean difference in the size of the left versus right patch found in the "bias confirmation" trials. In cases where a rat initially preferentially contacted the patch on the left or right limb when the patches were of equal size (endogenous asymmetry), the size of the preferred patch was decreased and the size of the nonpreferred patch was increased until the bias was neutralized and again until the bias was reversed. The large patch size in 4–5 reversal trials was subtracted from the large patch size in 4–5 bias neutralization trials, and this value was added to the difference between the small patch sizes in 4–5 bias neutralization versus bias reversal trials to obtain the JND (see TABLE 4).

The above experiments indicate that although old rats are slightly slower than young rats to react to somatosensory stimulation, their somatosensory acuity (as estimated by the capacity to discriminate readily between two stimuli of slightly different size) is comparable to that of young rats. This does not mean that absolute thresholds for detection of sensory stimuli are unaffected by age. In an additional study, patch sizes were reduced to 58, 28, 14, 7, or 3.5 mm² on different trials. The cutoff latency to respond to a patch on any given trial was five minutes. As shown in FIGURE 2, as patch size was reduced, the percentage of rats responding to the patch within the five-minute

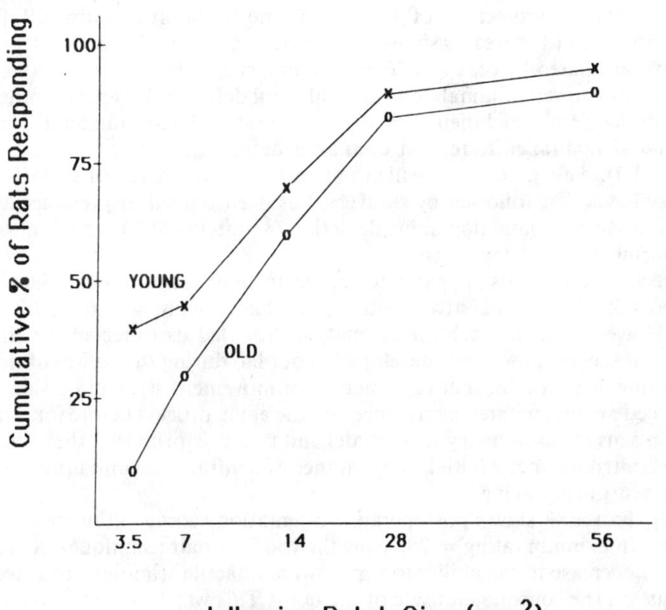

FIGURE 2. Threshold test: Cumulative percentage of old versus young rats responding as adhesive patch size is reduced.

period decreased. Significantly fewer old rats responded to the smallest pa ch size (p < 0.01). However, because the smallest patches yield relatively longer latencies to respond than the larger patches, this effect could be attributed in part to age differences in movement initiation.

UNILATERAL DOPAMINE-DEPLETING LESIONS

Animals that have recovered from brain damage show measurable impairment again during old age. Sensorimotor behavior was examined in 11-month-old rats treated either with the catecholaminergic neurotoxin 6-OHDA or unilateral electrolytic lesions (1 mA for 25 s, anodal) aimed at the far posterolateral hypothalamic area through which mesotelencephalic dopaminergic neurons (and several other systems) project. Sham operations were performed in control groups. The rats were tested for their ability to orient toward somatosensory stimuli (a von Frey hair calibrated to exert 4 g of force) presented at seven regions on each side of the body, and they were rated as in Marshall *et al.*[8-10]

Following surgery, the brain-damaged animals showed deficits in the ability to orient toward tactile stimulation of the contralateral body surface. The animals with electrolytic lesions recovered from this deficit during the first postoperative month and, as the animals became old (about two years), there was a reappearance of contralateral sensorimotor impairment.[5] Twenty-five rats received unilateral microinfusions of 6-OHDA (4–6 µg of free base in 2 µL of artificial CSF, 0.1% ascorbic acid) along the mesotelencephalic dopaminergic projection. All rats were pretreated with a systemic injection of desmethylimipramine (15 mg/kg of free base, i.p., 30 min before 6-OHDA) to provide relative protection of norepinephrine-containing neurons.[11] Five days postoperatively, 17 of these rats showed extensive impairment in contralateral orientation, with contralateral scores = 4.26 ± 1.6 and ipsilateral scores = 27.90 ± 0.4. The remaining rats showed minimal or no contralateral deficits. By three months, 6 of the rats with deficits recovered their ability to localize stimuli (contralateral score = 22.6 ± 2.8) and 11 rats failed to recover even after more than a year (contralateral score = 5.11 ± 1.7). This pattern, in which only a small percentage of 6-OHDA-treated rats showed a deficit followed by recovery, has been typical of previous studies.[8-10] A narrow range of striatal dopamine depletion (about 75–90%) is needed to produce this impairment-recovery pattern.

The recovered animals appeared to redevelop significant impairment as they became aged at 25–27 postoperative months (contralateral score = 11.63 ± 1.8; surviving n = 4). However, further behavioral analyses have led us to reevaluate the results.

Based on sensorimotor tests developed in our lab during the course of this experiment, we now hypothesize that asymmetries of movement style and a slowing of response speed are precipitated or enhanced by the aging process before (or rather than) changes in sensory asymmetry magnitude, and that it is primarily these "motor" effects that contribute to the initial reappearance of contralateral impairment in the von Frey hair test during aging.

Briefly, FIGURE 3 shows postoperative orientation scores in unilateral 6-OHDA-treated rats (maximum rating = 28, using the von Frey hair technique). After surgery, there was a decrease in the ability to turn toward a tactile stimulus presented at multiple points on the contralateral side of the body. This was followed by recovery and, eventually, a reappearance of orienting deficits when the animals became old (about 25 months old). Because this effect is a relatively unilateral one, this indicates that nonspecific behavioral impairment cannot account for the aging-dependent effect.

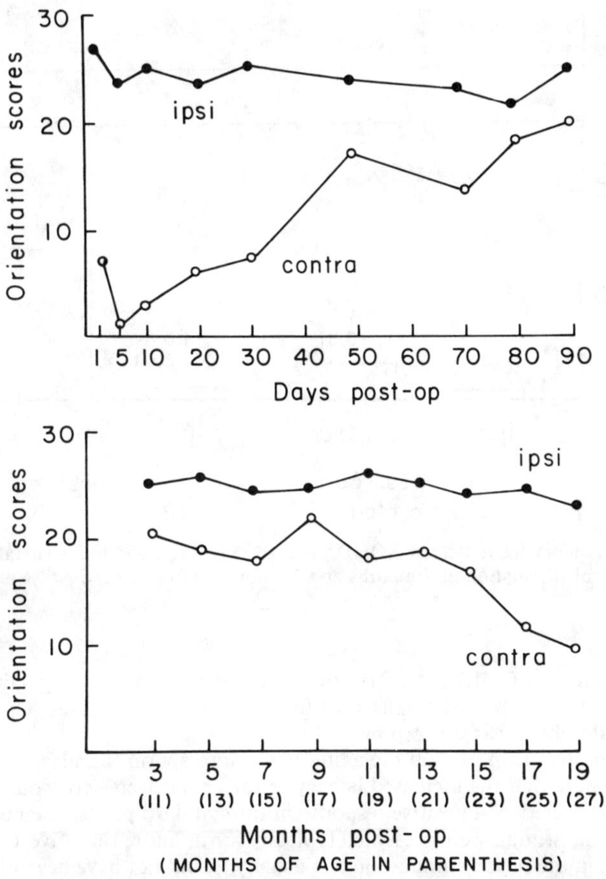

FIGURE 3. Chronic orientation scores as a function of time following unilateral 6-OHDA. Note that reactivity to contralateral stimulation was impaired, but it recovered soon after surgery. During old age, contralateral impairment reappeared.

A further study revealed more about the nature of this effect. Response-completion time seems to be an important factor in the reappearance of dysfunction during aging. As shown in FIGURE 4, relatively "recovered" animals (7 months post-op; 15 months of age) took an average of 3.5 s to turn toward and contact a von Frey hair brushed back and forth tonically at the distal aspect of the contralateral vibrissae (versus 0.3 s to turn toward stimulation of the ipsilateral vibrissae). This latency (3.5 s, with an average range of 2.1–5.3 s) was sufficiently fast that it was not scored as neglect or impaired orienting behavior. The contralateral orienting response was accurate in that the animal contacted the stimulus, but it appeared to be initiated more slowly (the impression gained from videotape observations is that initiation latency, rather than response completion time, is most affected; see also references 12 and 13). As the animals became older (20 months post-op; 28 months of age), they took an average of 13.3

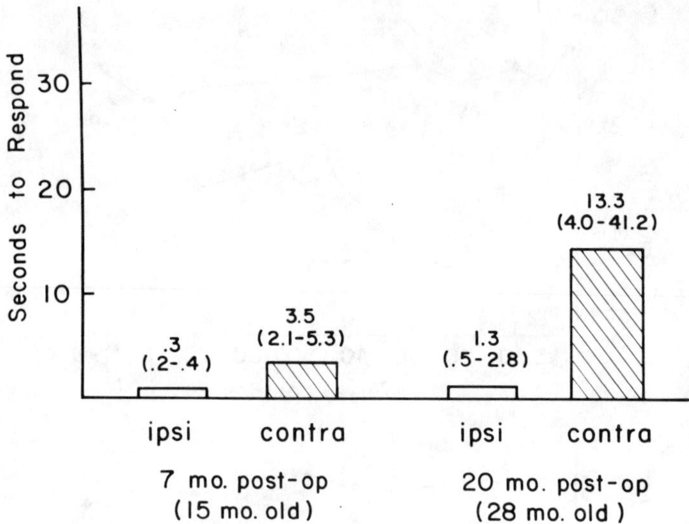

FIGURE 4. Latency for unilateral 6-OHDA-treated rats to respond to ipsilateral versus contralateral perioral stimulation at 7 months and 20 months after surgery.

s (average range = 4.0–41.2 s) to turn toward and contact a von Frey hair presented on the contralateral vibrissae versus 1.3 s for the ipsilateral vibrissae. On some contralateral trials, there was no response.

These data may help explain the aging-lesion interaction found previously.[5] It is important to note that the increased latency to turn contraversively would have been too long to be scored as a positive response in the standard probe-orientation test in which the tactile stimuli were presented typically for no more than five seconds; that is, a response in the probe-stimulation test usually would not have been observed because the experimenter stopped the stimulation from continuing at that particular body point. Thus, one behavioral component responsible for the age-linked changes in orienting capacity (illustrated in FIGURE 3) may be a progressive slowing of movement initiation to tonic tactile stimulation of the contralateral side of the body, and a gradual decrease in the probability of responding in the contralateral direction toward briefly presented tactile stimuli.

Although the mechanisms for the aging-dependent phenomenon undoubtedly are complex, several points seem relevant. It is well documented that alterations appear in a variety of neuronal and supporting activities in the aged brain.[5,14-21] Nigrostriatal dopaminergic levels, cell number, turnover, synthesizing enzymes, axonal transport, and postsynaptic receptor density can decrease with advanced stages of aging (although these effects are not universally observed[14]). These and other potentially important changes often appear to be present in the absence of obvious behavioral symptoms that can be measured by perioral probe-orientation tests. Similarly, compensatory reactions to subtotal brain damage can mediate recovery and maintain function in young rodents and probably in other mammals including man, especially if the damage occurs gradually. In contrast, if the initial brain damage is nearly total (i.e., greater than about 95% in the nigrostriatal system), the compensatory reactions are not sufficient to mediate recovery.[22,23] In humans, it is believed that some neuropathology exists long before parkinsonian symptoms become clinically evident.[24-29] Perhaps it occurs perinatally.[30] Like the animals with subtotal early brain damage in the present study, these people may be at risk for Parkinson's disease because of this vulnerability in the brain. It may be that aging provides the additional dopamine deficiency sufficient to precipitate the overt signs.[5,26,28,31-34]

Recently, Hall and Schallert[35] observed in recovered 6-OHDA-treated rats that the type of response made to contralateral perioral stimulation was abnormal. Therefore, they examined more completely the deficit in movement initiation, its recovery, and its reemergence in old age. Prior to recovery, the typical 6-OHDA-treated rat will respond at first to contralateral stimulation by circling in an ipsiversive direction instead of making a rapid lateral movement of the head as they do both preoperatively and ipsilaterally. If the probe is always quickly removed from the cage by the experimenter before the rat is able to contact it, the rat eventually will learn to inhibit its ipsilateral turns and respond contralaterally without circling. However, the movement the rat makes is an unusual rotatory movement, which involves twisting the head and upper torso such that the teeth engage the probe from underneath. This response can be made quite rapidly (<1 s) so that contralateral and ipsilateral latencies can reach a point (with recovery) where they might not differ by very much. At first, this movement only permits the animal to contact the probe when it is placed a few degrees from the midline. Over several weeks of practice, the rat becomes able to orient to the probe placed more laterally; however, a new movement must be learned. Following the rotatory movement of the head or entire forequarters, the animal makes a ventral tucking movement of the trunk. Together, the rotatory movement, followed immediately by the tucking movement, permits contact with the probe. Other animals use a sequence of small backward and forward movements of the head and forequarters to gradually bring the snout close enough to the mouth so that a positive response can be recorded. Either of these multiple-movement strategies would have been considered to be a recovered response using standard measures. Recovery, though, appears to represent a form of response substitution.[36,37] The rat, unable to initiate its usual response, is forced to discover or develop alternative means of responding to contralateral stimulation.

These data suggest that the aging-lesion interaction may not be caused by aging-related decline in nigrostriatal function (at least not exclusively). An alternative possibility is that the interaction is due to a decline in cortical, cerebellar, or other brain systems[38-41] that might be involved in the mediation of the learned response sequences that ordinarily are not used by the animal in orienting to perioral stimulation. Perhaps, as the animals become old, it is more difficult to rapidly initiate these particular movements toward contralateral perioral stimulation (it may also be that the old animal requires more frequent training to maintain the learned response[42]).

Other data are consistent with this possibility as well. We administered a relatively high dose of 6-OHDA (median striatal dopamine depletion = 93.9%, as measured by HPLC-EC). Using the patch removal test, which does not require lateral head movements,[1,2] we found that there was consistent adhesive-removal bias in every 6-OHDA-treated rat following surgery. As a group, and individually, the latencies to contact and to remove the stimulus located on the ipsilateral radial forelimb were shorter than the latencies to contact and to remove the stimulus on the contralateral radial forelimb.[1,2,43]

These same rats failed to make lateral head turns directed toward von Frey hair (probe) stimulation of the contralateral body surface (median contralateral score = 0). In the probe tests, most rats never recovered. However, in a variation of the patch removal test, there was progressive recovery of function in the so-called nonrecovered animals. Gradations of recovery occurred beginning in the first postoperative month. By adjusting the size of the sensory fields occupied by the contralateral (C) and ipsilateral (I) stimuli (specifically, by increasing the C/I ratio), animals with unilateral nigrostriatal damage can be induced to contact both stimuli with equal frequency.[2,3,6] The minimum C/I ratio that consistently neutralizes the ipsilateral bias may well be a fairly precise reflection of the magnitude of the perceptual asymmetry caused by the brain damage. We used this ratio measure over the period of several months in the rats with severe 6-OHDA depletions that had not yet recovered from their strong ipsilateral adhesive removal or neglect of contralateral perioral stimulation. We found that the minimum ratio that neutralizes the sequence of adhesive removal gradually diminishes in every animal (although at different rates for individual animals). The adhesive-removal test, perhaps because it works relatively independent of postural biases, is able to detect behavioral recovery reflecting early postoperative events (such as compensatory increases in dopaminergic receptor density) in otherwise unrecovered animals. These data are interesting when contrasted with studies showing that behavioral recovery does not occur following chronic-neglect producing dopamine depletion.

The C/I ratio obtained in the patch removal test, which is sensitive to unilateral changes in nigrostriatal function, was used to analyze potential interactions of brain damage and aging. It was surprising to find that there was no aging-lesion interaction using this measure. The animals were examined through 28 months of age, yet no animal showed an increased asymmetry from its recovery level as it became old (median C/I ratio at postoperative day 2 = 2:1; day 7 = 5:1, which was the peak magnitude of asymmetry; day 30 = 3:1; month 18, or 28 months of age = 2.2:1).

In a previous paper,[5] it was argued that unilateral dopamine depletion early in life left the animals asymmetrically vulnerable to aging-related bilateral dopaminergic decline. Although this continues to be a parsimonious explanation for the aging-lesion interaction, it now seems equally likely that the reappearance of slow contralateral responses observed in the probe-stimulation (von Frey hair) test might reflect (at least in part) aging-related problems in the operation of brain functions that are not normally an integral part of the nigrostriatal dopaminergic system. In preliminary work consistent with this view, sedative-hypnotic drugs (which might alter brain function somewhat nonspecifically, as the aging process might do) were given to young adult rats recovered from unilateral nigrostriatal damage and to intact controls. For example, diazepam or ethanol, at doses selected to differentially disrupt complex movement sequences such as those learned by the rat to compensate for the loss of large lateral head movements (2–3 mg/kg diazepam, i.p.; 1–2 g/kg intragastric ethanol; versus vehicle control), reinstated the severe probe-orientation asymmetries in the brain-damaged animals (contralateral, not bilateral, impairment).

It is important to note that the probability of neurological disease may increase during aging for multiple reasons. For example, in related experiments, dopaminergic receptor antagonists reinstated behavioral deficits caused by damage to a non-dopaminergic system in the paramedian pontine reticular formation associated with head nystagmus and equilibrating functions.[45,46] Moreover, damage to striatal or nigrostriatal cells can precipitate a novel behavioral effect if there exists previous damage to neocortical tissue.[35] The behavioral effect was qualitatively different from that occurring after damage to either region alone. Thus, in addition to the aging-lesion interactions noted above and in a previous paper,[5] a decline in striatal function with age conceivably could interact adversely with focal damage to nondopaminergic brain areas, with the latter occurring early in life.

To summarize, generally, somatosensory function does not appear to decline appreciably with age in intact animals. In recovered brain-damaged animals, as well as in neurologically intact animals, behavioral abnormalities may be caused primarily by deficits in the speed of movement initiation. Finally, although acquired deficits in nigrostriatal dopamine function alone clearly can affect response speed, it remains plausible that aging-lesion interactions and the decline in motor function with normal aging can be caused by progressive detrimental changes in nondopaminergic brain systems on a background of dopamine deficiency.

ACKNOWLEDGMENTS

I very much appreciate the efforts of Margaret Upchurch, Timothy Barth, Waneen Spirduso, Stuart Hall, and Theresa Jones.

REFERENCES

1. SCHALLERT, T., M. UPCHURCH, N. LOBAUGH, S. B. FARRAR, W. W. SPIRDUSO, P. GILLIAM, D. VAUGHN & R. E. WILCOX. 1982. Pharmacol. Biochem. Behav. **16:** 455–462.

2. SCHALLERT, T., M. UPCHURCH, R. E. WILCOX & D. M. VAUGHN. 1983. Posture-independent sensorimotor analysis of interhemispheric receptor asymmetries in neostriatum. Pharmacol. Biochem. Behav. **18:** 753–759.

3. SCHALLERT, T., T. D. HERNANDEZ & T. M. BARTH. 1986. Recovery of function after brain damage: Severe and chronic disruption by diazepam. Brain Res. **379:** 104–111.

4. BARTH, T. M. & T. SCHALLERT. 1987. Somatosensory function of the superior colliculus, somatosensory cortex, and lateral hypothalamus in the rat. Exp. Neurol. **95:** 661–678.

5. SCHALLERT, T. 1983. Sensorimotor impairment and recovery of function in brain-damaged rats: Reappearance of symptoms during old age. Behav. Neurosci. **97:** 159–164.

6. SCHALLERT, T. & I. Q. WHISHAW. 1984. Bilateral cutaneous stimulation of the somatosensory system in hemi-decorticate rats. Behav. Neurosci. **98:** 518–540.

7. SCHALLERT, T. & I. Q. WHISHAW. 1985. Neonatal hemidecortication and bilateral cutaneous stimulation in rats. Dev. Psychobiol. **18:** 501–514.

8. MARSHALL, J. F. 1984. Behavioral consequences of neuronal plasticity following injury to nigrostriatal dopaminergic neurons. *In* Aging and Recovery of Function in the Central Nervous System. S. W. Scheff, Ed.: 101–128. Plenum. New York.

9. MARSHALL, J. F., B. H. TURNER & P. TEITELBAUM. 1971. Sensory neglect produced by lateral hypothalamic damage. Science **221:** 389–391.

10. FAIRLEY, P. C. & J. F. MARSHALL. 1986. Dopamine in the lateral caudate-putamen of the rat is essential for somatosensory orientation. Behav. Neurosci. **100:** 652–663.

11. SCHALLERT, T. & R. E. WILCOX. 1985. Neurotransmitter-selective brain lesions. *In* Neuromethods: Neurochemistry, General Techniques. Volume 1. A. A. Boulton & G. B. Baker, Eds.: 343–387. Humana Press. Clifton, New Jersey.

12. EVARTS, E. V., H. TERAVAINEN & D. B. CALNE. 1981. Reaction time in Parkinson's disease. Brain **104:** 167–186.

13. SPIRDUSO, W. W., P. E. GILLIAM, T. SCHALLERT, M. UPCHURCH, D. M. VAUGHN & R. E. WILCOX. 1985. Reactive capacity: a sensitive behavioral marker of movement initiation and nigrostriatal dopamine function. Brain Res. **325:** 49–55.

14. MORGAN, D. G. & C. E. FINCH. 1988. Dopaminergic changes in the basal ganglia: a generalized phenomenon of aging in mammals. *In* Central Determinants of Age-Related Declines in Motor Function. J. A. Joseph, Ed. Ann. N.Y. Acad. Sci. This volume.

15. CARLSSON, A. 1985. Neurotransmitter changes in the aging brain. Dan. Med. Bull. **32** (suppl. 1): 40–43.

16. DEMAREST, K. T., G. D. RIEGLE & K. E. MOORE. 1980. Characteristics of dopaminergic neurons in the aged male rat. Neuroendocrinology **31:** 222–227.

17. CARLSSON, A. & B. WINBLAD. 1976. Influence of age and time interval between age and autopsy on dopamine and 3-methoxytyramine levels in human basal ganglia. J. Neural Transm. **38:** 271–276.

18. McGEER, E. G. 1981. Neurotransmitter systems in aging and senile dementia. Prog. Neuro-Psychopharm. **5:** 435–445.

19. SABEL, B. A. & D. G. STEIN. 1981. Extensive loss of subcortical neurons in the aging rat brain. Exp. Neurol. **73:** 507–516.

20. WILCOX, R. E. 1984. Changes in biogenic amines and their metabolites with aging and alcoholism. *In* Alcoholism and the Elderly. J. T. Hartford & T. Samorajski, Eds.: 85–115. Raven Press. New York.

21. RANDALL, P. K. 1980. Functional aging of the nigrostriatal system. Peptides **1** (suppl. 12): 177–184

22. ZIGMOND, M. J. & E. M. STRICKER. 1977. Behavioral and neurochemical effects of central catecholamine depletion: A possible model for "subclinical" brain damage. *In* Animal Models in Psychiatry and Neurology. I. Hanin & E. Usdin, Eds. Pergamon. New York.

23. LJUNGBERG, T. & U. UNGERSTEDT. 1976. Sensory inattention produced by 6-hydroxy-dopamine-induced degeneration of ascending dopamine neurons in the brain. Exp. Neurol. **53:** 585–600.

24. HORNYKIEWICZ, O. 1973. Metabolism of dopamine and 1-DOPA in human brain. *In* Frontiers of Catecholamine Research. E. Usdin & S. H. Snyder, Eds. Pergamon. New York.

25. LLOYD, K. G. 1977. CNS compensation to dopamine neuron loss in Parkinson's disease. *In* Parkinson's Disease: Neurophysiological, Clinical, and Related Aspects. F. S. Messiha & A. D. Kenny, Eds. Plenum. New York.

26. FINCH, C. E., P. K. RANDALL & J. F. MARSHALL. 1981. Aging and basal ganglia functions. Annu. Rev. Gerontol. Geriatr. **2:** 49–87.

27. MARSDEN, C. D. 1982. Basal ganglia disease. Lancet **ii:** 1141–1146.

28. CALNE, D. B. & J. W. LANGSTON. 1983. On the aetiology of Parkinson's disease. Lancet **2:** 1457–1459.

29. RIEDERER, P. & S. WUKETICH. 1976. Time course of nigrostriatal degeneration in Parkinson's disease. J. Neural. Transm. **38:** 277–301.

30. DE COURTEN, G. M. & T. RABINOWICZ. 1981. Intraventricular hemorrhage in premature infants: Reappraisal and new hypothesis. Dev. Med. Child Neurol. **23:** 389–403.

31. LANGSTON, J. W. & P. A. BALLARD. 1984. Parkinsonism induced by 1-methyl-4-phenyl-1,2,3,6-tetrahydropyridine: implications for treatment and the pathophysiology of Parkinson's disease. Can. J. Neurol. Sci. **11:** 160–165.

32. HORNYKIEWICZ, O. 1982. Brain neurotransmitter changes in Parkinson's disease. *In* Neurology 2: Movement and Disorders. C. D. Marsden & S. Fahn, Eds. 41–58. Butterworths. London.

33. SNYDER, S. H. & R. J. D'AMATO. 1986. MPTP: A neurotoxin relevant to the pathophysiology of Parkinson's disease. Neurology **36:** 250–258.

34. BARBEAU, A. 1984. Etiology of Parkinson's disease: a research strategy. Can. J. Neurol. Sci. **11:** 24–28.

35. HALL, S. H. & T. SCHALLERT. 1987. Unpublished data.

36. GOLDSTEIN, K. 1930. Die restitution bei schadigungen der hirnrunde. *In* Symposium on Restitution of Function after Lesions of the Nervous System (20th Annual Convention of the German Neurological Society). Z. Nervenherk, Ed. **116:** 2–26.

37. FOERSTER, O. 1930. Die restitution bei schadigungen der hirnrunde. *In* Symposium on Restitution of Function after Lesions of the Nervous System (20th Annual Convention of the German Neurological Society). Z. Nervenherk, Ed. **116:** 2–26.

38. ROGERS, J. 1988. Neurobiology of cerebellar senescence. *In* Central Determinants of Age-Related Declines in Motor Function. J. A. Joseph, Ed. Ann. N.Y. Acad. Sci. This volume.

39. RAPOPORT, S. I., R. DUARA, E. D. LONDON, R. A. MARGOLIN, M. SCHWARTZ, N. R. CUTLER, M. PARTANEN & SHINOHARA. 1983. Glucose metabolism of the aging nervous system. *In* Aging of the Brain. D. Samuel, Ed.: 111–121. Raven Press. New York.

40. HOFFER, B. 1988. Age-related changes in cerebellar noradrenergic function. *In* Central Determinants of Age-Related Declines in Motor Function. J. A. Joseph, Ed. Ann. N.Y. Acad. Sci. This volume.

41. GAGE, F. H., P. A. T. KELLY & A. BJÖRKLUND. 1984. Regional changes in brain glucose metabolism reflect cognitive impairments in aged rats. J. Neurosci. **4:** 2856–2865.

42. JÄNICKE, B. 1988. Adaptivity as a paradigm for age-dependent changes exemplified in motor

behavior. *In* Central Determinants of Age-Related Declines in Motor Function. J. A. Joseph, Ed. Ann. N.Y. Acad. Sci. This volume.

43. DUNNETT, S. B., D. M. LANE & P. WINN. 1985. Ibotenic acid lesions of the lateral hypothalamus: comparison with 6-hydroxydopamine-induced sensorimotor deficits. Neuroscience **14:** 509–518.

44. BECK, C. H. M. 1980. Normal aging of the human brain potentiates the neuropathologies of Parkinson's disease, depression, and Alzheimer's disease: Behavioral implications. Can. Counsellor **14:** 110–120.

45. SIRKIN, D. W., T. SCHALLERT & P. TEITELBAUM. 1980. Involvement of the pontine reticular formation in head movements and labyrinthine righting in the rat. Exp. Neurol. **69:** 435–457.

46. SCHALLERT, T. 1985. Unpublished data.

DISCUSSION OF THE PAPER

P. RANDALL (*University of Southern California, Los Angeles, CA*): Do you have data on where mediation of the normal lateral head movement is going downstream from the striatum?

T. SCHALLERT (*University of Texas, Austin, TX*): I do not specifically. However, there are many areas in the brain that, when damaged with neurotoxins of various sorts, give lateral head movement deficits. The nigrostriatal system is not unique.

RANDALL: That is exactly what I am thinking because the nigrostriatal pathway leaves the nigra reticulosis straight to the superior colliculus, which would give you a direct pathway.

SCHALLERT: An interesting thing about unilateral superior colliculus lesions is that despite the head movement deficit, no change is seen in sensory-motor asymmetry as measured by this adhesive removal test; the animal looks exactly the same as it did before surgery. This is not the case following nigrostriatal lesions.

RANDALL: Can lateral head movement be restored pharmacologically in old animals? Do dopamine agonists do that?

SCHALLERT: We have been working on that. Some change is seen in the speed of movement, but the animal gets very, very reactive. My tendency, though, is to say yes. If dopamine is put back in, the animals respond; the lateral head movement actually can come back, but there is a lot of variability.

M. SERBY (*New York University Medical Center, New York, NY*): When you reproduce the deficit with sedatives, does it just seem to be a nonspecific effect? Or can you actually look at some specific pharmacological neurotransmitter?

SCHALLERT: We are looking at the effects of a variety of drugs. A project very active in our lab right now is finding what agents can reinstate this deficit and what agents will not. We started with sedative hypnotics because I thought we should try something that produces impaired cognitive learning function, and we got it. There are a number of other drugs that I want to try; for example, I want to try anticholinergics.

UNIDENTIFIED DISCUSSANT: Have you looked at any unoperated controls at an advanced age and seen any evidence of lateralization of any sensory neglect measurement?

SCHALLERT: We always try to look for lateralization, but endogenous asymmetries are labile. The aging process, though, does not seem to exaggerate an animal's own natural asymmetry if it is there.

UNIDENTIFIED DISCUSSANT: Are these all male rats?

SCHALLERT: Yes.

F. Gage (*University of California, San Diego, CA*): Must these lesions be partial lesions?

Schallert: Yes.

Gage: If you've got the complete lesion unilaterally, will the animals fail to recover?

Schallert: These are subtotal, but if a complete lesion is done (at least as measured by our neurochemistry), you must give the animal more time to respond. You have to be patient with the animal because the animal has a difficult time making that lateral movement. The animal will orient, but the response substitution is difficult. It is going to be delayed. If you look at this adhesive removal test, though, you will always see some gradual recovery. Hence, it really depends on the task.

Gage: However, does the group that you are dealing with show recovery by 90 days after the lesion?

Schallert: Yes, of course.

Gage: Under those conditions, if you measure dopamine at 90 days under a partial lesion condition, what percentage return of dopamine content are you measuring in, say, the ventral lateral quadrant of the caudate, relative to what it was before?

Schallert: About 70%.

Gage: Thus, it is substantial.

Schallert: Yes, plus or minus 20%. It is variable.

Gage: Therefore, the behavioral recovery that you are looking at is most likely related to compensatory or collateral sprouting responses of residual dopaminergic fibers into the ventral lateral quadrant of the caudate. It is not necessarily some substituting system.

Schallert: That is the leading hypothesis and that is the one we have to go on. I suggest, though, that there is a possibility that this is not true for recovery in general. These neurochemical changes may be mediating behavioral recovery only in certain tests. They might not be mediating all forms of recovery. Furthermore, the aging-dependent decline of the behavior might be due not to an inability to sustain these particular compensatory mechanisms, but perhaps due to an erosion of nondopaminergic mechanisms that are acting to facilitate recovery via response substitution. However, the data does not discriminate between the two. I think they raise a hypothesis and maybe we need to look at both.

Age-related Variability

RICHARD L. SPROTT

National Institute on Aging
National Institutes of Health
Bethesda, Maryland 20892

The widespread belief that variance of many, or most, physiological and behavioral variables increases with advancing age is perhaps best summed up in the principle: "The older people become, the less like each other they become."[1] This principle is widely held for several reasons:

(1) It seems intuitively obvious, despite equally widespread age stereotyping. We all know elderly persons who maintain some functional capacities at the apparent level of much younger persons, and others who lose functions at relatively early ages.
(2) Individual differences in genetic dispositions can be magnified by lifetimes of interaction with the environment.[2]
(3) Organisms with identical genotypes (e.g., inbred mice or human identical twins) will show varied responses if raised in different environments.[3]
(4) The incidence of disease and subsequent pathology varies across individuals, thus producing significant differences in experience and morbidity.[4]
(5) Aging processes may differ in various tissues and organs. If the rate of progress of any of these processes varies between individuals, then individual differences will grow larger as a cohort ages.[5,6]

While all of these factors could (and probably do) contribute to increased variance in older individuals, there has been remarkably little empirical research on the magnitude and nature of these changes. If, as most investigators believe, variance increases with advancing age, then the important questions become:

(1) Does variance increase in most or all parameters?
(2) What is the significance of increased variance for gerontological research? For clinical practice? For prediction of life span functional capacity?
(3) Is the observed increased variance due to performance differences, functional capacity differences, or both?

Some indication of the presumed importance of increased variance can be obtained from Shock's discussion of the need for longitudinal studies.[7] Shock argues that few individuals are average (the value obtained from a cross-sectional study); that is, few individuals "follow the pattern of age changes predicted from averages based on measurements made on different subjects." In a discussion of changes in the endocrine system, Minaker argues that physiological changes in endocrine function are substantially modified by disease, medications, alcohol, smoking, diet, exercise, social factors, and experimental conditions: "Failure to consider these variables in study design no doubt contributes to the increased variance in physiologic performance observed in many studies of aging, and the clear variability in performance of patients with age associated disease."[4] While both of these investigators make important references to increased variance with advancing age, neither provides quantification of the variances. A perusal of the literature of the last decade shows that this is most often the case.

The point to this discussion is not that variance does not increase with advancing age (it clearly does for many variables), but rather to suggest that the nature and importance of increases in variance are poorly understood. For example, performance changes in behavior may reflect underlying physiological changes, but they may just as well reflect variance in motivation or experience.[2]

Increased variance can often be inferred from data presented in reports of physiological changes in young and old subjects. What cannot be inferred are the causes or generality of the variance changes. An example of the problems of inferring causation can be found in the observation that human gestation requires a mean of 280 ± 5 days, the onset of menarche requires a mean of 151.8 ± 14.1 months, and the mean age of menopause is 50 ± 8 years.[5] Each of these variables represents a virtually universal developmental event for the human female, and variance clearly increases with advancing age. In addition to the obvious problem of comparing apples and oranges, this example also illustrates the problem of the "floor effect" contained in any developmental variable. The amount of variation seen in the average age of onset of menopause (16 to 18 years) is simply not possible in an early event like gestation, which has a mean of 280 days.

The opportunity to conduct a systematic assessment of variance changes in a mammalian model system is inherent in a major new initiative of the National Institute on Aging (NIA). The major purpose of this initiative, which is expected to be ongoing for the decade 1988 to 1998, is the development of reliable biomarkers of aging. The concept of biomarkers of aging rests on the assumptions that aging is the result of one or many basic biological processes and that interventions in these processes could alter the rate of aging of an organ or an organism. The concept of increased variance with advancing age rests upon the same assumptions. A change in the rate of aging of the organism should be measurable in any nonrenewable cell population of the organism or in the renewal rate of the remaining cell populations. If individuals within a species age at different rates, then "biological age" and "chronological age" are not interchangeable. Increased variance at older ages would then be a measure of variability in rates of aging. Biomarkers of aging are measures that reflect differences in aging rates for tissues, organs, or organisms, and they can be used as better estimates of remaining life span than chronological age. A number of criteria for validity and utility are generally agreed upon. They include:

(1) The rate of change of the biomarker must be measurable and predictable.
(2) The biomarker must be related to basic biological processes, not to disease.
(3) The biomarkers should be reproducible within and across laboratories.
(4) The greater the species generality of the biomarker, the greater its utility.
(5) To be useful for human clinical practice and research or for longitudinal research in any species, the biomarker measurement must be obtainable without altering the underlying biological processes, without altering the later behavior of the organism, and without the use of invasive procedures.
(6) To be experimentally useful, the biomarker should show significant changes in relatively short periods of time.

While the biomarker concept has been a topic of discussion, and even debate, for 15 to 20 years, and was specifically addressed by an NIA conference in 1981,[8] progress has been slow primarily because of variations in animal models, animal husbandry differences, diet differences, and variations in experimental procedures. In order to eliminate as many sources of variation as possible in future biomarker research, the

NIA, in cooperation with the National Center for Toxicological Research (NCTR), is currently creating a major new colony of aged mice and rats at NCTR facilities in Jefferson, Arkansas. Four mouse genotypes (C57BL/6NNia, DBA/2NNia, B6D2F1, B6C3F1) and three rat genotypes (Fischer 344, Brown-Norway, F344 × BNF1) are being placed in a closed, specific pathogen free (SPF) barrier colony. Animals in this colony are fed carefully defined diets either *ad libitum* or under conditions of dietary restriction. These animals will be made available to investigators nationwide for biomarker research grants. Among the conditions required for the awarding of these grants will be the agreement to maintain the animals (once they are received in the investigator's laboratory) in comparable barrier conditions and to feed the animals the same diets, which will be provided by the NCTR. Questions about access to animals from this colony and procedures for appropriate grant applications should be addressed to myself [telephone: (301) 496-4996].

While the purpose of this initiative is biomarker development, it should be obvious that it provides an unparalleled opportunity to obtain empirical evidence of the nature and magnitude of changes in variance with advancing age. The initiative is intended to produce research in all major organ systems and over a broad spectrum of behaviors. As a result, the variance data could be obtained for all of the same systems and behaviors by using common genotypes of animals reared identically. Collection of the appropriate data over the next ten years should provide definitive answers to most, if not all, of the questions raised in this presentation.

REFERENCES

1. ROWE, J. W. & K. L. MINAKER. 1985. Geriatric medicine. *In* Handbook of the Biology of Aging. Second edition. C. E. Finch & E. L. Schneider, Eds.: 932–959. Van Nostrand–Reinhold. Princeton, New Jersey.
2. SPROTT, R. L. 1978. The interaction of genotype and environment in the determination of avoidance behavior of aging inbred mice. *In* Genetic Effects on Aging. National Foundation, vol. XIV. D. E. Harrison, Ed.: 109–120. Alan R. Liss. New York.
3. SPROTT, R. L. & B. E. ELEFTHERIOU. 1974. Open-field behavior in aging inbred mice. Gerontologia **20:** 155–162.
4. MINAKER, K. L., G. S. MENEILLY & J. W. ROWE. 1985. Endocrine systems. *In* Handbook of the Biology of Aging. Second edition. C. E. Finch & E. L. Schneider, Eds.: 433–456. Van Nostrand–Reinhold. Princeton, New Jersey.
5. BAKER, G. T., III, G. McCLEARN & R. L. SPROTT. 1987. Biomarkers of aging. Exp. Gerontol. Special edition. In press.
6. LANDFIELD, P. W. 1982. Measurement of brain age: conceptual issues and neurobiological indices. *In* Endocrine and Neuroendocrine Mechanisms of Aging. R. C. Adelman & G. Roth, Eds.: 183–207. CRC Press. Boca Raton, Florida.
7. SHOCK, N. W. 1985. Longitudinal studies of aging in humans. *In* Handbook of the Biology of Aging. Second edition. C. E. Finch & E. L. Schneider, Eds.: 721–743. Van Nostrand–Reinhold. Princeton, New Jersey.
8. REFF, M. E. & E. L. SCHNEIDER. 1982. Biological markers of aging. NIH Publication No. 82-2221. U.S. Department of Health and Human Services. Bethesda, Maryland.

Quantitative Analysis of Behavioral Pharmacological Data

PATRICK K. RANDALL[a]

Department of Physiology and Biophysics
University of Southern California Medical School
Andrus Gerontology Center
Los Angeles, California 90089

Over the past several years, we have worked on a number of problems on striatal dopaminergic (DA) function that have demanded increased attention to the quantification techniques used for behavioral data.[1-6] Certainly, it is well established that dopaminergic receptors are altered during aging,[6-8] and it is probable that their regulation is compromised to some extent.[1] It is difficult to establish, however, whether these changes have functional consequences and, if they do, whether those consequences are consistent with the type of receptor alterations observed at a biochemical level. On another level, it is critical to determine whether biochemical observations are consistent with motoric difficulties experienced by the elderly, including the increased risk for major motoric side effects from neuroleptic drugs.[9]

It rapidly became apparent from the steadily increasing sophistication in statistical evaluation of binding models available to our biochemically oriented collaborators (e.g., LIGAND,[10] ALLFIT[11]) that the usual techniques for evaluating behavioral data are painfully inadequate. While it is true that mechanistic models of the behavioral action of DA agonists and antagonists are still very distant, we are not totally ignorant of the biochemical and physiological substrates involved. Work on quantitative estimation of drug-receptor parameters in similar, though simpler, pharmacological systems (systems in which the receptor → response function is unknown) began in the latter part of the last century with early formulations of receptor occupation theory[12] and is still under active development.[13,14] Both the general orientation and the specific "null" methods developed in that literature are uniquely suited for the analysis of the complex response variables in behavioral pharmacology. The purpose of this presentation is to show that with methods derived from classical pharmacology and from more modern nonlinear techniques, many current hypotheses on the relationships between receptor alteration and behavioral drug response are expressible and testable in discrete quantitative form.

The common aspect of all the methods to be discussed is the focus on the horizontal behavior of the dose-response curve across the dose axis. In view of the fact that we are unaware of the properties of the function directly relating receptor occupation and response, the direct comparison of response magnitude between two groups differing in receptor properties is nearly meaningless. This orientation was also stressed by Trendelenberg[15] when describing the tendency to compare response magnitude rather than horizontal shifts in early supersensitization experiments as "vertical bias".

[a] Current address: Institute for Neurological Sciences Research, University of Texas, Austin, Texas 78712.

The emphasis on shifts along the *x*-axis rather than differences in response magnitude at different doses is extraordinarily important for behavioral work. Behavioral variables are typically measured on dimensions that are difficult, if not impossible, to relate to fundamental biochemical properties; they have a tendency to be highly variable; and they quite often have a very ambiguous measurement status (e.g., observational rating scales). Assessment of shifts along the *x*-axis has the desirable effect of emphasizing the analysis of an indisputably quantitative scale, that is, dose administered.

DESCRIPTIVE USE OF HORIZONTAL ANALYSIS

The experiment in which we first investigated this type of analysis was an attempt at the seemingly straightforward task of comparing the sensitivity of different mouse strains to dopamine agonists.[4] Because CBA/J and BALB/cJ mice differed in their density of DA receptors[2] (defined by D-2 antagonist binding), it was important to determine whether this difference was of functional consequence. We had originally found that BALB/cJ mice showed higher ratings than CBA/J mice given a standard 2.0 mg/kg dose of apomorphine, and we suggested that this strain had the higher sensitivity to the agonist (as was expected from the higher DA receptor number).[2] Fink and Reis,[16] on the other hand, came to the opposite conclusion. In order to determine the factors responsible for these opposing results, we decided to reevaluate the question from fundamental principles.

Rating Scale Data

Typically, in the intact rodent, the response to DA agonists is evaluated by an observational procedure in which the observer employs a rating scale. The subject is assumed to pass through a sequence of recognizable behavioral states as a function of dose. The states are assigned sequential integer designations such that increasing ratings are associated with response patterns observed at increasing doses. This type of behavioral quantification has a long history in research on the behavioral effects of dopamine agonists — usually referred to as "stereotypic" behavior. Although the resulting data are often used in standard ANOVA analysis,[1,2] it is clear that the technique does not provide a ratio (i.e., a rating of 4 is not necessarily twice as great as a rating of 2) nor an interval (i.e., the interval between 1 and 2 is not necessarily the same as the interval between 3 and 4) measurement scale.

Though much debated, this criticism of rating scales carries much less weight when viewed in light of the fact that even seemingly much better behaved scales (e.g., locomotor activity) have an indeterminant relationship with receptor occupation. While 100 locomotor counts is clearly twice 50 and few would argue the acceptability of parametric statistical tests, it is only locomotor activity that is being analyzed, not drug sensitivity nor receptor occupation. It is clear, however, that if we can determine doses of an agonist that result in equivalent states in two experimental conditions, then we should be able to determine the horizontal behavior of dose-response curves based on rating scale data. In many ways, a reliable rating scale is superior to a univariate, "quantitative" measure because different drug-induced behavioral states are often more easily recognized by direct observation. In this respect, we have found that maintaining the categorical nature of rating scales will preserve a great deal of information that is lost when data are used as if they represented a continuous measurement.

Regardless of the type of measurement done, response magnitude is a dubious measurement on which to base inferences on receptors. The more convincing demonstration would be that CBA/J and BALB/cJ mice show a similar progression of behaviors across doses, but that the BALB/cJ mice traverse this progression at lower doses. The type of data resulting from application of a rating scale is best viewed as the placement of observations into a set of ordered categories.

Ordered Categorical Data

Rating scale data assign observations to ordered categories. The probability of meeting or exceeding the thresholds for the different categories defines a series of quantal dose-response curves; that is, for each category rating, an animal either exceeds the threshold for that category or does not. Inherent in this formulation is that all animals, regardless of rating, contribute to the analysis of every member of the set of quantal curves. For example, an animal receiving a rating of 2 has exceeded the thresholds for 1 and 2, but has not exceeded the thresholds for 3, 4, or 5. This, of course, results from the ordered nature of the categories. This formulation also has the advantage of maintaining an underlying monotonic response function. Counts of individual behaviors are often (in fact nearly always) curvolinear with dose, declining at high doses. This influence of the processes responsible for the subsequent decline on the points to the left of the maxima is usually not considered.

A number of investigators have suggested interpretations of the processes that give rise to quantal dose-response curves,[17,18] and a number of fields from achievement testing[19] to signal detection[20] have also used similar models. All of them have in common the concept of a stimulus along some internal continuum that will produce a response if it exceeds a threshold. Although space precludes a detailed analysis here, reasonable approximations of the distributions of the stimulus (or the threshold) map to a lognormal distribution along the dose-administered axis, which can be compared to a stationary threshold.

More formally, the extension of these quantal models to the ordered categorical response (i.e., rating scales as described above) is straightforward. We consider each of the data points (number in each category at each dose) to be the result of interactions between the underlying curves for probability of a rating being greater than or equal to x, and that of being greater than or equal to $x+1$. Therefore, the ED_{50}'s of the component curves refer to transition doses between categories. The probability of each rating can be expressed as

$$\Pr(R \geq 0) = 1,$$

$$\Pr(R = x) = \Pr(R \geq x) - \Pr(R \geq x + 1),$$

$$\Pr(R \geq n) = 0,$$

where n = number of categories. For example, in the above model, Pr(rating = 2) = Pr(rating $\geq$ 2) − Pr(rating $\geq$ 3). The ED_{50}'s and slopes of the curves for Pr(rating $\geq x$) constitute the parameters of the model.

Logistic Function

In all the work here, we use the logistic function to represent the dose-response curve. It is far more tractable mathematically than is the cumulative normal and it is used extensively for this purpose (i.e., logit or log-logit analysis). In most applications, we use the forms below to represent the two-, three-, and four-parameter curves, respectively:

$$\frac{A^P}{A^P + K^P} \quad \text{or} \quad \frac{1}{1 + e^{P[\ln(K - A)]}},$$

$$\frac{MA^P}{A^P + K^P} \quad \text{or} \quad \frac{M}{1 + e^{P[\ln(K - A)]}},$$

$$D - \frac{M}{1 + \left(\dfrac{A}{K}\right)^P} \quad \text{or} \quad D - \frac{(D - M)}{1 + e^{P[\ln(K - A)]}},$$

where A is the agonist dose, K is the ED_{50}, and P is the logistic slope. The parameter M (maximum response) is added to the second expression and D (minimum response) is added to the last. The form on the right is most often used internally in the fitting routines.

The logistic function has the advantage of being used almost identically in the ordered categorical and continuous variable problems. Also, as expressed here (Waud[21,22] and DeLean *et al.*[11]), it has parameters that are familiar to pharmacologists (e.g., ED_{50}, logistic slope). Nearly all reasonable dose-response curves can be expressed in at most four parameters. With the use of weighted nonlinear least squares or maximum likelihood techniques, the problem of inappropriate weights given the least reliable data points by linearization techniques is circumvented. Finally, by sharing information across curves and by fitting across an entire experiment, the problem of a series of nonindependent fits for individual curves does not exist. This is particularly the case with ordered categorical data where individual data points contribute to all of the curves.

Analysis Technique

Because we can express the probability of an observation falling into each category as a function of the ED_{50}'s and slopes of the logistic curves, we can use standard weighted least-squares algorithms to determine the best-fitting parameters by fitting the actual data, that is, by fitting the number in each category, rather than by a transformation. In this experiment, values are weighted inversely by the expected frequency to provide a minimum χ^2 fit — for example, determination of those parameter values for the logistic curves that minimize the χ^2. Alternatively, we have extended Waud's[21] methodology for quantal dose-response curves to determine maximum-likelihood parameters. Although, as yet, we have not done extensive simulations comparing these two criteria, the resulting parameters in this and several other data sets were nearly identical. Similar to LIGAND,[11] we can also determine the effect of sharing any set of parameters across curves or constraining them to a constant value. For example, a significant increase in the χ^2 resulting from sharing ED_{50}'s across strains relative to a fit where the ED_{50}'s are allowed to vary independently suggests a difference between strains in that parameter. Sharing parameters that are not, in fact, different increases the degrees of freedom for parameter estimation, along with causing a consequent decrease in the error of the estimate.

Strain Analysis

An analysis of this type of the strain experiment described above revealed a differential effect of strain on different behavioral categories. The ED_{50}'s for the two lower ratings that we were able to fit (2 and 3) were similar across strains. The ED_{50}'s for the two higher ratings, however, were much greater for the CBA/J mice than for the BALB/cJ mice (i.e., they eventually showed the more highly rated behaviors, but at much higher doses). In addition, the analysis provided a very compelling explanation for the divergent findings previously reported. The scale employed by Fink and Reis[16] did not employ climbing behavior. The mice were run in smooth-walled enclosures that not only eliminated climbing behavior, but also failed to provide an appropriate stimulus to which gnawing behavior might be directed. Climbing behavior is the most distinguishing feature between a 4 and the lower ratings in our scale. The separation between the ED_{50}'s for a 3 and 4 in the CBA/J mice was much greater than that in the BALB/cJ's. Thus, CBA/J mice continue to show continuous sniffing behavior (the primary indicator of a 3) at doses at which most of the BALB/cJ's would have progressed on to more highly rated behaviors. We noted during the experiment that CBA/J mice often show very vigorous sniffing behavior while they move across the floor of the enclosure. We now view this to be the continuation of 3 behavior, which is relatively uncontaminated by the intrusion of climbing, biting, etc. Sniffing was the predominant behavior of the Fink and Reis scale.

FORMAL NULL METHODS

The formalization of the analysis of shifts in dose-response curves is the general class of null models.[24] They rest on the technique of establishing doses of an agonist that will result in equal effects under two different conditions.

Pharmacological null methods have the following assumptions:

(1) The interaction of an agonist with a receptor gives rise to a stimulus inside the tissue or cell proportional to the receptor occupancy.
(2) The response is an unknown function of the stimulus.
(3) Equal responses imply equal stimuli; that is, the function has an inverse.

Thus, if S and S' are stimuli associated with equivalent agonist responses in two experimental conditions, we can write $S = S'$, which is the null equation of the system. In most cases, these equations are solved for the dose-ratio (DR): the degree of shift to the left or right in the dose-response curve resulting from the experimental manipulation.

Null Method For Competitive Antagonists

Competitive antagonists produce parallel shifts in agonist dose-response curves; that is, the shift in the dose-response curve is not dependent upon agonist concentration. By assessing the shift in the agonist dose-response curve resulting from pretreatment with an antagonist, the dose of antagonist corresponding to its dissociation constant, K_d, can in theory be calculated. This value should be invariant across agonists acting at the same receptor.

The basic assumption of the null model is that equal responses with and without the antagonist correspond to equal tissue stimuli. By simple mass action kinetics, fractional receptor occupancy in the control conditions and in the presence of the antagonist can be represented as

$$\frac{[A]}{[A] + K_A}$$

and

$$\frac{[A]}{[A] + K_A\left(1 + \dfrac{[B]}{K_B}\right)} \, ,$$

respectively, where K_A is the agonist dissociation constant, $[B]$ is the concentration of antagonist, and K_B is the dissociation constant of the antagonist. If $[A]$ and $[A]'$ represent concentrations of the agonist giving equivalent responses without and with the antagonist, respectively, and ε is the efficacy of the agonist, then

$$\frac{\varepsilon[A]}{[A] + K_A} = \frac{\varepsilon[A]'}{[A]' + K_A + \left(1 + \dfrac{[B]}{K_B}\right)} \, ,$$

that is, the null equation. Solving for the dose-ratio, we obtain

$$\frac{[A]'}{[A]} = \frac{[B]}{K_B} + 1.$$

The latter relationship is often expressed as

$$DR - 1 = \log([B]) - \log(K_B),$$

which is the basis of the Schild plot.[25] It is important that the dose-ratio is dependent only upon antagonist characteristics. It is not influenced by agonist distribution as long as the concentration of agonist is a linear function of the dose injected, which is most likely to be the case at peak response.[24] The effective K_B calculated would be weighted only by a route-of-administration constant for the antagonist.

Experimentally, the estimation of K_B is best accomplished by estimating several agonist dose-response curves in the presence of different doses of the antagonist. Although the technique is more time-consuming and costly in animal resources than is the more common determination of an IC_{50} at a single agonist dose, the benefits are substantial. First, determination of an IC_{50} from inhibition under the latter conditions is dependent upon the particular agonist and dose of agonist employed. In well-behaved receptor binding assay systems, a K_d for an unlabeled ligand can be extrapolated from a single IC_{50} against a labeled ligand, provided a good estimate of the K_d of the labeled ligand is available.[26] Theoretically similar calculations are possible for dose-response data, but the resulting expressions are extremely cumbersome, depending upon both the affinity and the efficacy of the agonist employed. In addition, such calculations require that the assumptions of the null model hold directly in the raw values of the dependent measure employed. Construction of several dose-response curves permits tests of both the parallel shift expected between individual doses of the antagonist and the overall unity slope of the Schild plot. Deviations from either of these expectations suggest that additional factors (e.g., agonist or antagonist acting at more than one receptor, or interactions between different behavioral components of the drug response) are operating.

Analysis Methods

The treatment of data from null experiments has changed enormously over the past 15 years. If we use the competitive antagonist model as an example, the original sequence of procedures would be as follows.

First, an estimate of the ED_{50}'s of the dose-response curves under control conditions and with various concentrations of the antagonists would be obtained. This was often done by graphical methods or by linear regression on a transformation of the data (e.g., a log-logit analysis). The dose-ratios would then be estimated; a Schild plot would be constructed (or linear regression would be performed), usually in the form $\log(DR - 1) = \log([B]) - \log(K_B)$; and the intercept would be used as an estimate of the K_B.

Each step has associated error that appears in the final result as a complex combination of several sources in the Schild plot. The problem is further compounded by the use of linearized forms of the dose-response curves in the first step, which will often distort the distribution of doses, thus giving inappropriate weights to data arising from low doses, as well as propagating error in the dose achieved onto both axes. Similar considerations have been exhaustively discussed with respect to Scatchard analysis of binding experiments.[27]

In the late 1960s, iterative nonlinear fitting routines for families of dose-response curves began to appear, primarily as a result of the work of Waud.[21-23] These techniques eliminated the complex weighting problems of linear regressions on transformations by fitting the raw data directly. Also, they permitted sharing of parameters across curves and parameter estimation using all of the available data in the experiment. Increases in the precision of parameter estimation can be striking under these conditions. In addition, this constrained simultaneous curve-fitting approach provided a reasonably discrete test of hypothesized differences between parameters in the various curves. Ratios of residual variance from fits constraining parameters to be shared across curves versus fits in which the parameters are permitted to diverge form an approximate F test with a null hypothesis of equality of parameters. DeLean *et al.*[11] describe the method as testing for differences in parameters by examining the consequences of forcing them to be equal. With this development, the family of dose-response curves (including the control and those at different antagonist doses) could be analyzed across the entire experiment and without linearization techniques. The estimates of ED_{50} ratios can be subjected to a Schild regression.

In addition, these techniques provide an initial test of whether the data are consistent with the underlying null method model: sharing the slope parameter across curves should not significantly degrade the fit, that is, if the curves are parallel as required by the model.

The final development was to combine the Schild analysis into the initial overall fit.[28] This can be accomplished by forming a model equation that could represent any point in the experiment. Because the null model itself is based on shifts away from the control curve, we simply divide the dose of agonist by the dose-ratio before substitution into the logistic equation. The competitive antagonist experiment can then be expressed as

$$R = \frac{MA^P}{A^P + K^P\left(1 + \dfrac{[B]}{K_B}\right)^P},$$

where R is the response, and the parameters of the overall model equation can be determined by least squares methods.

Testing the effect of sharing the K_B across all curves is equivalent to testing the linearity of the Schild plot, and the resulting estimate of K_B will then be based directly on all of the available information in the model. Comparing fits sharing the K_B with those allowing divergent values of the same parameter for different classes of behaviors provides a statistical test for differential sensitivity of behaviors to antagonists known to differ in affinity for different receptor types in binding experiments.

Null Method For Receptor Occlusion

Because maximal tissue response can occur at less than full receptor occupancy, the determination of an ED_{50} in and of itself has little relevance to the K_A, the dissociation constant of an agonist. A number of experimental designs using null methodology have been proposed for assessing the K_A in pharmacological systems;[24] one of which can be readily adapted for the analysis of super- or sub-sensitivity resulting from changes in receptor density.

Estimates of agonist affinity may be made by comparing control dose-response curves with those derived after occlusion of a subset of receptors with an irreversible antagonist. Again, the analysis is done by estimating the doses required to produce equivalent responses in the two conditions. The basic null equation is

$$\frac{\varepsilon[A]}{[A]+K_A} = \frac{\varepsilon[A]'}{[A]'+K_A} \, (1 - y_i),$$

where $[A]$, $[A]'$, and K_A have their usual meanings and y_i is the proportion of receptors removed from the population.

Solving for the dose-ratio yields

$$\frac{[A]'}{[A]} = \frac{1}{(1 - y_i)} + \frac{1}{K_A} \frac{y_i}{(1 - y_i)} \, [A]'.$$

In contrast to the competitive antagonist null equation, the shift in the dose-response curve is dependent upon the concentration of the agonist; therefore, the curves will not, in general, shift in parallel fashion. Also implicit in the formulation is a dependence upon the efficacy of the drug because this parameter will determine the range of receptor occupation over which the biological response will occur. For full agonists, the entire range of tissue response occurs at relatively low fractional receptor occupation. Because the dose shift is a linear function of the agonist dose, then the higher the efficacy, the less the shift, extrapolating to an asymptotic value of $1/(1 - y_i)$; for example, a shift of 1.43 with a 30% receptor occlusion.

The full model for the experiment can be expressed as

$$R = \frac{MA^P}{A^P + K^P\left(\dfrac{1}{(1 - y_i)} + \dfrac{1}{K_A} \dfrac{y_i}{(1 - y_i)} A\right)^P}.$$

Although there are currently no sufficiently specific irreversible antagonists of DA receptors to be used with any confidence behaviorally, this model does have interesting applications to situations with alterations of receptor number (e.g., supersensitivity, strain differences, etc.). The supersensitivity experiment, for example, is equivalent to receptor occlusion by either interchanging the roles of the control and treated groups or by allowing y_i to take on negative values. A similar model was suggested by Seeman[28] in an attempt to explain large changes in apparent drug sensitivity associated with modest elevations in DA receptor number in supersensitization experiments. The model presented there, however, holds only for partial agonists that require full occupancy for maximum response.

Time-Course

One of the most straightforward uses of horizontal analysis is the analysis of the time-course of response. With or without data on the clearance of the drug employed, it is possible to calculate reasonable descriptions of the disappearance of the drug response with time. The added advantage of analyzing time-course is that such analysis allows the use of the entire data set for the estimation of the ED_{50} at maximum response. For example, with apomorphine-induced stereotypic behavior, we commonly sample the behavior every six minutes for a total duration of one hour (ten time periods). With the addition of a single parameter, we gain the use of nine additional data points.

From either a null methodology approach or simply intuitively, it is clear that the dose of the drug should be modified by an expression representing the degree to which the drug has been metabolized or eliminated. At a time when half the drug has been eliminated, the ED_{50} should be twice the estimate of the ED_{50} at maximal response. In the simplest case, this would be a single compartment exponential e^{-kt}. Thus, the model equation would be

$$ R = \frac{MA^P}{A^P + K^P(e^{kt})^P} $$

with substitution into the three-parameter logistic equation. In this case, the uppercase K is the ED_{50} of the dose-response curve at a designated time at, or subsequent to, the time of maximum response. Dose-response curves at later times should be shifted to the right by a degree defined by this exponential. The superiority of this method over the typical comparison of response magnitude and pharmacokinetic data should be restated at this point. We have little idea of the functional relationship between receptor occupation and response. Clearance rate can be over- or under-estimated depending upon the characteristics of the function mapping tissue stimulus and response. In particular, if that function is represented as a logistic curve, then cases where the logistic slope is high would tend to overestimate the rapidity with which the drug clears and low logistic slopes would tend to underestimate this quantity. In addition, as can be inferred from the model equation above, the slope should not be altered. These estimates are on a continuous variate and do not depend on the characteristics of the scale on which response magnitude is measured. However, they do depend upon the degree of precision in matching responses at the two times, and the model at present cannot handle concentration-dependent effects on clearance rate.

USING THE NULL MODEL TO PREDICT AND ANALYZE EXPERIMENTAL RESULTS

Supersensitization

There have been few attempts to explicitly define the expected consequences of the supersensitization experiment in the dopaminergic system, but it has been suggested that physiological and behavioral supersensitivities are greater than that expected from the modest increases in receptor density (usually 20–40%). Using the null model described above, it is possible to predict the manner in which the curve should shift as a result of changes in receptor number given an arbitrary control curve. As is evident above, the degree of shift is dependent both on the dose of agonist administered and the K_A of the agonist. We can express the shift in terms of the ratio of the K_A of the agonist and the ED_{50} of the behavioral response. A large ratio indicates the high efficacy of a full agonist and that the entire dose-response curve occurs at low agonist concentration. Lower ratios define lower efficacies ranging into partial agonists. FIGURE 1 depicts two experimental outcomes — one with a strong full agonist and one with a partial agonist.

As can be seen with a full agonist, the shift resulting from a 30% change in receptor density would be small (approximately 1.4-fold) and indistinguishable from a parallel shift. Under these conditions with simulated data, we have found that ANOVA techniques would only detect a difference between these curves about 15% of the time when the variance is at values common in rotational behavior experiments. The results from a partial agonist are shown in the right panel. It is clear that the modest change in receptor number does result in a substantial increase in response, but the change has a very characteristic form. Responses at low doses of the agonist are altered to a much lesser extent than are those at higher doses, with the shift being a linear function of the agonist dose.

Supersensitization Data

We have used this type of analysis to examine lesion-induced supersensitization in the nigrostriatal DA system.[4] In this experiment, rats first received unilateral lesions

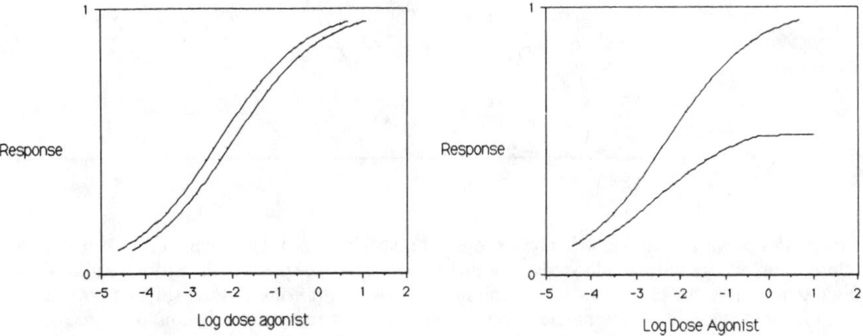

FIGURE 1. Effect of a 30% increase in receptor number on the dose-response curve to a full (left panel) and partial (right panel) agonist.

of the striatonigral pathway. DA agonist-induced rotation in this preparation is thought to result from action in the contralateral, normosensitive striatum.[29] A control dose-response curve for apomorphine-induced rotation was then determined. The same animals then received a 6-OHDA lesion on the side contralateral to the striatonigral lesion and a dose-response curve was again determined. Consistent with other investigators using a similar design with rats,[30,31] we found in this experiment a 30-fold parallel shift to the left in the dose-response curve resulting from the 6-OHDA lesion. This is clearly at odds with the outcome predicted by the null model for the 20–40% increase in receptor number known to result from the lesion.

A second experiment examining the effect of chronic haloperidol-induced supersensitization provided data that were more consistent with theoretical predictions.[3] Here, we observed a 1.52-fold shift in the family of quantal dose-response curves defined by our rating scale. The actual value of the shift and the fact that curves for all ratings shifted to the same extent are quite compatible with both full agonist action of apomorphine and a 30% increase in receptor number resulting from the treatment.

Finally, we have recently performed a more formal experiment[32] in an attempt to resolve the discrepancy between these two systems that have equivalent effects on receptor number, but very different effects on agonist response. It is well known that depletion of nucleus accumbens DA will enhance the locomotor effects of DA agonists and will probably enhance the rotational behavior in the unilateral preparation.[33] It is also possible that the contribution of nucleus accumbens is responsible for the failure of receptor

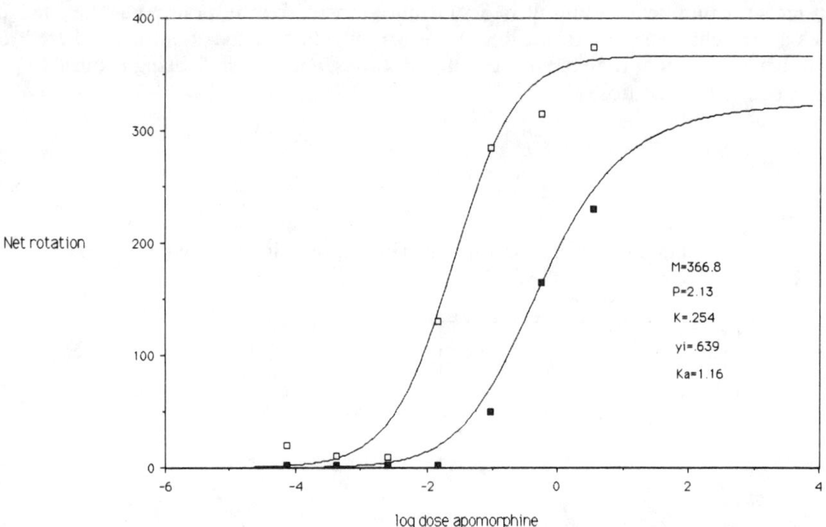

FIGURE 2. Rotational behavior before and after specific striatal DA depletion. Control curve (closed squares) was obtained after striatonigral lesion. Supersensitive curve (open squares) was obtained in the same animals after a depletion of DA on the contralateral side. Curves are derived from the best-fitting parameters of the null model for receptor occlusion. M = maximum response, P = logistic slope of the control curve, K = ED_{50} of the supersensitive curve, y_i = proportion of receptors occluded, and K_A is the dose of agonist corresponding to the agonist K_A. The y_i corresponds to a threefold increase in receptor number. The measured increase in ^{3}H-spiperone binding was 30–35%.

number to account for the supersensitive dose-response curve. In this experiment, the same dual lesion technique was employed (striatonigral followed by 6-OHDA), except that 6-OHDA infusions were directed at different loci to achieve different patterns of DA depletion with respect to striatum and nucleus accumbens. MFB placements depleted both striatal and accumbens DA, while a placement in the tail of the caudate[34] depleted striatal DA without affecting accumbens. Increases in ^{3}H-spiperone binding were 30–35% in both groups.

The animals receiving both striatal and accumbens depletion (data not shown) showed a large shift to the left in the dose-response curve that was comparable to previous experiments and that was much larger than those receiving only striatal depletion. This suggests that at least a portion of the shift normally seen is due to accumbens depletion. We were then interested in whether the effect of striatal depletion alone was consistent with the measured receptor number increase. These data were fit using the null-occlusion model described above and they are shown along with the best-fitting curves in FIGURE 2.

As can be seen, the null equation fits the data relatively well. However, the actual parameter values obtained are very different from the biochemical values. They are most consistent with a greater than threefold (300%) increase in receptor density. As shown previously, the modest alteration in receptor number results in major changes in the dose-response curve when the agonist in question has low efficacy. Even that case does not account for the change described here. The shift in the dose-response curve should be small at low doses and should increase with increases in dose. The shift at low doses in these data is quite substantial. It would seem more likely that the shift here is related to failure of the monotonicity assumption of the null model. At higher doses, competition between behaviors lowers the magnitude of response. If the dose-response curve for rotation is more affected by denervation than that for the competing behaviors, we would expect an artificial elevation in the rotation of the supersensitive group because the effective dose range of the two competing classes of behavior are further apart. Unfortunately, the resolution of the video technique used did not permit quantification of the likely competing behaviors.

Time-Course Data

We have preliminary data using this technique on aging C57BL/6J mice. From the equation above, the ED_{50} at each time point should be related to that at maximum response in the following manner:

$$\log (ED_{50}) = \log (ED_{50(max)}) - kt,$$

where $ED_{50(max)}$ is the ED_{50} at maximal response, k is the exponential constant, and t is the time. Thus, the log of the reciprocal of the ED_{50} should be linearly related to time. Because this experiment utilized rating scale data and an ED_{50} was determined for each rating (see above), we used the geometric mean of the several response ED_{50}'s as the overall ED_{50} indicator. In a more complete analysis, a test would be made to determine that all component ED_{50}'s shifted to the same extent as indicated by the model. The resulting data are shown in FIGURE 3. This figure strongly suggests that the greatest differences among the four different ages of mice are related to drug clearance. In addition, it suggests that the older mice are slightly less, rather than more sensitive to the agonist as would be suggested by an examination of the "total" ratings measures.

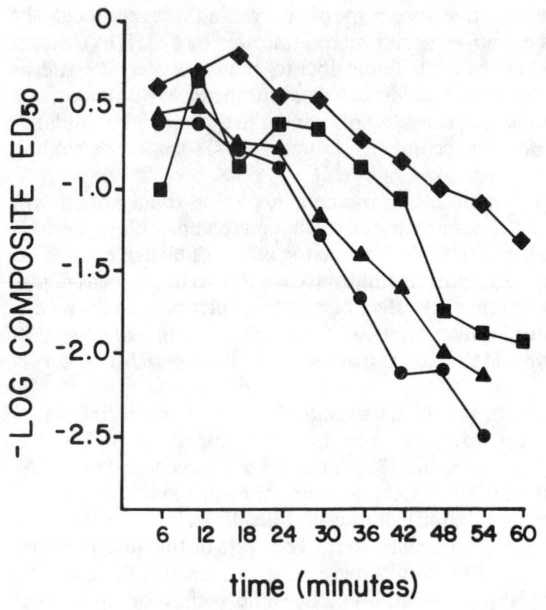

FIGURE 3. Alteration in ED_{50} for apomorphine-induced stereotypic behavior as a function of time in C57BL/6J mice. The negative log of the composite ED_{50} (geometric mean) for different behavioral categories was used as the ED_{50} indicator because it should decline linearly with dose. Diamonds = 4-month-old, squares = 8-month-old, triangles = 18-month-old, and circles = 24-month-old at the start of the experiment. (Composite ED_{50} = mean of ED_{50}'s of component curves.)

PROBLEMS AND FUTURE DEVELOPMENTS

We feel that the approach described has already yielded results of sufficient importance to warrant further development. The first experiment described suggests that a great deal of quantitative information can be obtained using rating scale measurements that allow us to make use of very powerful observational techniques. The experiments on supersensitization are, to our knowledge, the first tests of the DA supersensitivity hypothesis in which behavioral results can be directly related to receptor number. The increase in sensitivity as measured in the rotational model is, in fact, greater than is predicted by the receptor number increase. Whether the behavioral hypothesis or more sophisticated models at a biochemical level (e.g., agonist affinity states) explain this discrepancy remains to be seen. Although the experiments have yet to be done, the methods for dissociating D-1 and D-2 contributions to the effects of nonspecific agonists and antagonists are relatively clear. Finally, the use of horizontal analysis for behavioral time-course, even in the simple form presented here, provides a much more rational interpretation than the simple correlation or comparison of drug levels and response magnitude.

There are several obvious issues that require more work. These will now be listed below.

(1) Alternative models: Most of the similar techniques that have proven successful in receptor binding experiments use residual F tests between alternative models (e.g., one- and two-site fits). Similarly, in the behavioral context, it is relatively easy to determine whether different parameters should be shared by examining residuals of fits where they are forced to be shared versus those in which they are allowed to diverge. For example, in the strain study described above, we found that sharing ED_{50}'s across strains for the curves representing ratings of 2 or greater or 3 or greater made little difference in the resulting χ^2 value. However, sharing the ED_{50}'s for 4 or greater or

5 or greater increased the χ^2 substantially. Similar tests can be used with continuous variates, utilizing residual variance, rather than a χ^2. Alternatively, differences in parameter values may be tested by constructing approximate t tests that utilize the parameter estimates and their standard errors in the dispersion matrix.

In some circumstances, alternative models are relatively easy to determine. Testing whether an antagonist is acting at a single site to influence several behavioral measures can be accomplished by testing a fit where the K_d's for all curves are shared versus one where they are allowed to vary.

The problem, though, can be somewhat more complex. As can be seen in the supersensitization experiment, problems in the relationship between biochemical and behavioral parameters do not necessarily appear as poor fits. One alternative is to fit the null model with y_i being constrained to the constant value determined with the biochemical data. A similar technique is often used in competition experiments using LIGAND in which the K_d of the labeled ligand is constrained to a predetermined value. This fit could then be tested against a fit in which the y_i is allowed to vary (e.g., a single versus multiple site fit). Often, the best alternative may be to test the model fit against a completely unconstrained fit of the empirical curves by using the logistic function.

(2) The residual F tests with nonlinear least squares techniques are approximate.[11] Presumably, they are reasonably well behaved in binding experiments because of limited variance. It remains to be seen whether these tests are reasonably valid with the degree of variance common in behavioral experiments.

(3) The criteria for best fit for the ordered categorical data are not completely clear. Presumably, for the relatively small sample sizes involved, maximum likelihood would be preferred over the minimum χ^2. One reasonable alternative would be to use a modification of log-linear analysis that is now highly developed for hypothesis testing. Even here, Monte Carlo studies on these distributions would be helpful.

(4) The monotonicity assumption is critical for null models. Equal responses must map to equal stimuli. However, as previously mentioned, this assumption is unlikely to be met over the long run with behavioral data. This is often the result of competitive interactions between behaviors arising at different doses of the agonist. Certainly, the locomotor activity effect of amphetamine is constrained by the appearance of stereotypic behavior at higher doses. Diminution of the response by the appearance of competing behaviors not only affects fits of null models, but it can also have drastic effects on estimation of both the maximum response and ED_{50} of the underlying dose-response curve. We are currently investigating two different approaches to this problem—the use of multiple, interacting logistic curves to describe behavioral response, and the use of multivariate response functions.

We first consider a drug response comprising behavior A and B, where B appears at higher doses and is incompatible with A (e.g., ambulation and focused stereotypic activity). We assume that A has an underlying dose-response curve, $L1(a)$, representing the response in the absence of B. Then, the overt behavior, $E(a)$, can be modeled as $E(a) = L1(a) - bL2(a)$, where $L2(a)$ is the dose-response curve for behavior B and where b is a constant. Alterations in dose-response curves similar to our interpretation of the supersensitization experiment might be modeled in this manner. The curve represented by $L1$ then may shift according to the null model even though the actual behavioral output shifts to a greater extent. This analysis, of course, may be extended to several behaviors that have different degrees of compatibility. For example,

$$
\begin{aligned}
E_1(A) &= L_1(A) + a_{1,2}L_2(A) + a_{1,3}L_3(A) + a_{1,4}L_4(A), \\
E_2(A) &= \qquad\qquad\quad L_2(A) + a_{2,3}L_3(A) + a_{2,4}L_4(A), \\
E_3(A) &= \qquad\qquad\qquad\qquad\quad L_3(A) + a_{3,4}L_4(A),
\end{aligned}
$$

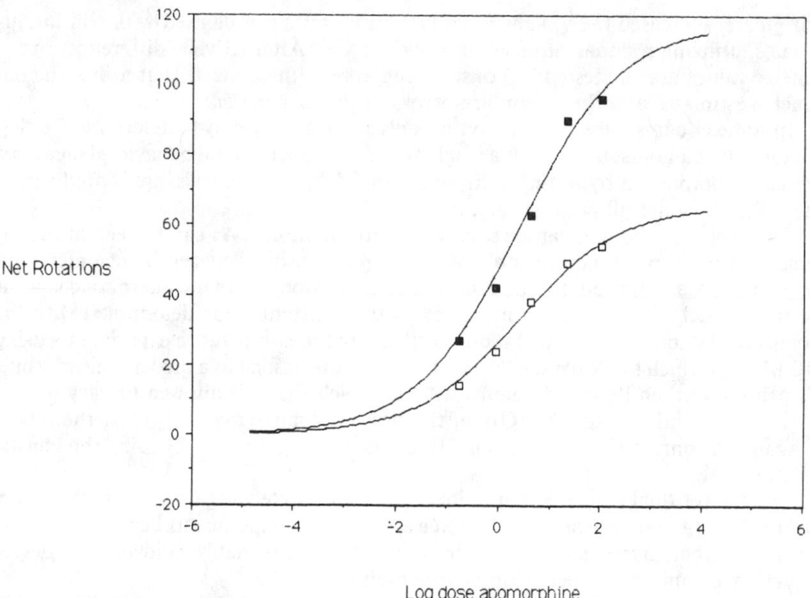

FIGURE 4. Effect of pretreatment with 0.01 mg/kg spiperone on apomorphine-induced rotation in C57BL/6J mice with striatonigral lesions. The best-fitting curves are three-parameter logistic curves calculated with ALLFIT.[11] ED_{50} and slope parameters were not different and were therefore shared in the analysis.

where the E_i represent the different behavioral measures, the L_i represent the corresponding underlying logistic curves, and the $a_{i,j}$ represent the compatibility constants between behaviors. These models would not have to be unidirectional (i.e., behaviors common at lower doses could affect the appearance of higher dose behaviors) nor would anything prevent the compatibility constants from taking positive values (i.e., one behavior could increase another).

Alternatively, the strength of the null models for behavioral work could be easily increased by examining the monotonicity assumption itself. If we deal with a multivariate response, then the assumption is generalized to one of uniqueness. In the simplest case, linear combinations of the response variables define equivalent responses rather than equality on a single univariate response. We have experimented with the construction of dose-response curves with discriminant functions with some success. However, the wide range of available techniques (e.g., canonical correlation, profile analysis) remains to be assessed.

(5) More recent work on null models has focused on physiological or functional interaction. In these experiments, the action of one drug alters the response to a first drug by its actions on a second, distinct receptor. These models provide, if nothing else, a remarkably succinct and precise manner in which to summarize and describe the types of interaction between, for example, D-1 and D-2 agonists or cholinergic and dopaminergic agonists. In the former case, we have found that in mice with discrete striatonigral lesions, pretreatment with 0.01 mg/kg spiperone (see FIGURE 4) nearly doubles the maximum response parameter of the apomorphine-induced rotation dose-response curve. The ED_{50} was not affected. Interestingly, these results have precisely

the same pattern as the cyclic-AMP efflux assay of Stoof and Kebabian,[36] where DA-induced c-AMP efflux was enhanced by coincubation with sulpiride, another D-2 antagonist, but the molar potency was not altered.

REFERENCES

1. RANDALL, P. K., J. A. SEVERSON & C. E. FINCH. 1981. J. Pharmacol. Exp. Ther. **219:** 695–700.
2. SEVERSON, J. A., P. K. RANDALL & C. E. FINCH. 1981. Brain Res. **210:** 210–215.
3. MANDEL, R. J. & P. K. RANDALL. 1985. Brain Res. **330:** 358–363.
4. RANDALL, P. K. & J. S. RANDALL. 1986. Behav. Neurosci. **100:** 85–92.
5. RANDALL, P. K. 1985. Life Sci. **37:** 1419–1423.
6. RANDALL, P. K., J. A. SEVERSON, S. HURD & W. O. McCLURE. 1985. Brain Res. **333:** 85–95.
7. SEVERSON, J. A. & C. E. FINCH. 1985. Brain Res. **192:** 147–162.
8. SEVERSON, J. A. & P. K. RANDALL. 1985. J. Pharmacol. Exp. Ther. **233:** 361–368.
9. THAL, L. J., S. G. HOROWITZ, B. DVORKIN & M. H. MAKMAN. 1980. Brain Res. **192:** 185–194.
10. MUNSON, P. J. & D. RODBARD. 1980. Anal. Biochem. **107:** 220–239.
11. DeLEAN, A., P. J. MUNSON & D. RODBARD. 1978. Am. J. Physiol. **235:** E97–E102.
12. EHRLICH, P. 1960. *In* The Collected Papers of Paul Ehrlich. Vol. III: Chemotherapy. F. Himmelweit, Ed. Pergamon. London.
13. MACKAY, D. 1981. Br. J. Pharmacol. **73:** 127–134.
14. EMMERSON, J. & D. MACKAY. 1981. Br. J. Pharmacol. **73:** 135–141.
15. TRENDELENBERG, U. 1963. Pharmacol. Rev. **15:** 225–276.
16. FINK, J. S. & D. J. REIS. 1981. Brain Res. **222:** 335–349.
17. HEWLETT, P. S. & R. L. PLACKETT. 1956. Biometrics, p. 72–85.
18. HEWLETT, P. S. & R. L. PLACKETT. 1979. The Interpretation of Quantal Responses in Biology. University Park Press. Baltimore.
19. ANDRICH, D. 1979. Biometrics **35:** 403–415.
20. SWETS, J. A. 1961. Science **134:** 168–177.
21. WAUD, D. R. 1972. J. Pharmacol. Exp. Ther. **183:** 577–607.
22. WAUD, D. R. & R. B. PARKER. 1971. J. Pharmacol. Exp. Ther. **177:** 13–24.
23. PARKER, R. B. & D. R. WAUD. 1971. J. Pharmacol. Exp. Ther. **177:** 1–12.
24. TALLARIDA, R. J. & L. S. JACOB. 1979. The Dose Response Relation in Pharmacology. Springer-Verlag. New York/Berlin.
25. GADDUM, J. H., K. A. HAMEED, D. E. HATHWAY & F. F. STEPHENS. 1955. Q. J. Exp. Physiol. Cog. Med. Sci. **40:** 49–74.
26. CHENG, Y. C. & W. H. PRUSOFF. 1973. Biochem. Pharmacol. **22:** 3099–3108.
27. KLOTZ, I. M. 1983. Trends Pharmacol. Sci. **4:** 253–255.
28. WAUD, D. R. 1981. Trends Pharmacol. Sci. **2:** 52–55.
29. SEEMAN, P. 1981. Pharmacol. Rev. **32:** 229–313.
30. MARSHALL, J. F. & U. UNGERSTEDT. 1977. Eur. J. Pharmacol. **41:** 361–367.
31. NEVE, K. A., M. R. KOZLOWSKI & J. F. MARSHALL. 1982. Brain Res. **244:** 33–44.
32. HARTGRAVES, S. L., R. J. MANDEL, J. A. SEVERSON, J. J. WOODWARD, R. E. WILCOX & P. K. RANDALL. 1985. Soc. Neurosci. Abstr. **11:** 686.
33. PYCOCK, C. J. & C. D. MARSDEN. 1978. Eur. J. Pharmacol. **47:** 167–175.
34. JACKSON, E. A., J. L. NEUMEYER & P. H. KELLY. 1983. Brain Res. **87:** 15–23.
35. MANDEL, R. J. & P. K. RANDALL. 1986. Soc. Neurosci. Abstr. **12:** 1188.
36. STOOF, J. C. & J. W. KEBABIAN. 1981. Nature **294:** 366–368.

DISCUSSION OF THE PAPER

G. S. ROTH (*NIA, Baltimore, MD*): Have you considered the possibility that these particular motor responses that we have available to us are simply too complicated to establish a rigorous stoichiometric relationship between receptor occupancy?

P. RANDALL (*University of Southern California, Los Angeles, CA*): No, I have never considered that.

ROTH: If somebody wanted to establish a relationship between dopamine receptor occupancy and response, they would be much better off trying to do it with something like adenylate cyclase because you could get away from possibly other neurotransmitter systems that might be involved.

RANDALL: However, you do not know the nature of the functional output. The kinds of questions I am interested are concerned with the physiological output. At a certain level, the cyclase is maybe involved, but we do not know yet. Therefore, it is not that I consider that less worthwhile, but it is that I am more interested in that other question.

One question that *is* complicated is one that comes up all the time. You have to look very carefully at the assumptions of what I am calling horizontal analysis. The major assumption is that we can recognize animals in similar behavioral states. That is the only real assumption for talking about the spread of dose-response curves. By looking at horizontal shifts, we no longer worry about magnitude at all (there can be 150 cascade amplifiers in the middle, but they do not make any difference). We are looking at shifts across the *x*-axis. If we can equate and match the responses of these two groups, then we can pull it off. The real problem, though, is the monotonicity assumption: that equal responses imply equal occupancy. This is the assumption that has to be true. In the long run, it is not going to be true with a univariate measure of behavior; almost any particular single thing that we measure is eventually nonmonotonic and the response curves eventually come back down.

Almost any behavioral variate is going to end up being nonmonotonic. What we can do in that case (and this is where our next phase is going) is extrapolate from a univariate model into a multivariate model. Because all we are doing is trying to match responses, we can measure that response on any number of different dimensions. Moreover, we can match responses in terms of a number of different criteria whether it is least squares or whatever else one wants to use. For instance, we can use profile analysis; we also have tried using discriminate functions to construct dose-response curves. The key, though, is the matching of behaviors and we can do that anyway we want. The main question is can we tell when two animals are in the same state. In terms of the apomorphine stereotypic behavior example, I think that we are pretty close.

D. MORGAN (*University of Southern California, Los Angeles, CA*): In the rightmost curve of the data that you showed, the animals never quite achieved the same maximal response that it did in the leftmost curve. I was also struck by the correlation with the partial agonist curves that you were showing. Are you restricting yourself to looking at apomorphine as a full agonist or as a partial agonist?

RANDALL: No, we were uncommitted on that. However, it is quite obvious that it is more valuable to have a partial agonist than a full agonist. There is more that you can do with it.

UNIDENTIFIED DISCUSSANT: If you had a response that was affected by two receptor systems, is it possible to add a second receptor site to this and do a two-site analysis similar to what you can do with the receptor system?

RANDALL: Yes.

UNIDENTIFIED: How many data points would one need to do that adequately with behavioral data? Are there enough animals?

RANDALL: You would not want to take the equivalent of an agonist binding curve and try to do it. We always wondered why we saw so little evidence of discontinuities in dose-response data when we used to use analysis of variance on it; that is, why they behaved so well. We have dose-response curves that explain at least 98% of the between-group variance. Why did it behave so well? It behaved so well because there are six of these little transitions that are equivalent to six sites. If you look at binding, those K_d's have to be really far apart before you can distinguish them. However, you can deal with multiple sites if you deal with, say, a nonspecific agonist and a specific antagonist. Then you can either share or let K_d values diverge for different behaviors. Hopefully, the best circumstance would be if different receptor types were related to different behavioral measures rather than to the same one.

GENERAL DISCUSSION OF PART II

D. MORGAN (*University of Southern California, Los Angeles, CA*): In looking at the data that D. Ingram showed, I noticed that the variance was not increasing in the older animals within a strain. Do you think that this was simply because of the fact that you controlled environment and genetics so well that there was no longer an increase in variance with age?

D. INGRAM (*NIA, Baltimore, MD*): It depends on what one uses as a measure of variability. In fact, we use the coefficient variation because the means are going down with age. Thus, if you looked at variability as a function of the mean value, you would get a decrease in variability. However, the whole mathematical issue of how one assesses the hypothetical age-related increase in variability is one that has yet to be addressed fully.

INGRAM: What value, if any, is there in the animal literature right now as far as modeling any aspect of motor aging? Are there possibilities of observing parallel processes in an animal model and humans?

B. HOFFER (*University of Colorado Health Science Center, Denver, CO*): A very important aspect is that we really cannot do very invasive things in man. In animals, when we set the mode of behavior, we can also report on the different parts of the brain. There are very profound regional differences on how motor behavior is regulated — histologically, chemically, etc. — and so far we cannot make the same kinds of necessary invasive measurements in man. Therefore, I think that animal research has a very important aspect to it in terms of aging and in terms of any other problems associated with changes in motor control.

P. RANDALL (*University of Southern California, Los Angeles, CA*): Would you argue that the particular animals you are using are good in the sense of being likely host representatives of what happens in human systems? Is it good for particular species or across strains?

INGRAM: Much is known about the biology of the laboratory rodent. There are pros and cons as to their use. They do not mimic aging in every aspect observed in humans; for example, their cardiovascular parameters are not particularly what one associates with cardiovascular aging in humans. They are not perfect models, but we can do invasive kinds of analyses to determine the mechanisms of phenomena that we are observing. Then, if it appears to have some relevance to the human condition, then one has a clinical trial possibility.

RANDALL: There is something different about the human that makes him respond differently to, say, a chronic neuroleptic when he is older. Why do old rats not show tardive dyskinesia? It may have something to do with the oral musculature or tongue, which is controlled centrally, and that may provide a clue for us as to where to look in the human.

INGRAM: The animal model for aging that is used is an animal that has been hanging around a cage for a couple years of his life and has not been interacting with his environment outside of that cage very much. Therefore, we have not even addressed that issue of whether we are seeing aging or disuse. W. Spirduso's presentation will have some comments in that regard, but we have to take into consideration the validity of the environment in affecting the life span as well.

J. A. JOSEPH (*Armed Forces Radiobiology Research Institute, Bethesda, MD*): Regarding P. Randall's very elegant presentation, every time that we have ever tried to manipulate receptors and look at the change in behavior, we found that it is almost like an all or none thing. It seems like receptors reach critical points and then go. It is almost like a dichotomous thing rather than a continuous thing in our hands. It may be that what you want to try is to use DA receptor antagonists such as EEDQ. One of the things that we have been able to do with this is to uncouple the behavior from the receptor concentration; at least what you might call a critical level of dopamine receptor concentration. However, it may be that redundant systems take up the slack in the young animals and thereby get by with fewer receptors. In addition, DA receptor concentration could be less tied to behavior in young animals.

F. GAGE (*University of California, San Diego, CA*): There seems to be a bias here in terms of what we are calling an animal model. I work with rodents, but I would like to understand what the objective of this group is in working with rodents. Are we trying to model human aging by using rodents? If that is the case, then I think that we are missing steps in here. We ought to bring in the primatologists or do some primate work, unless, of course, our objective is just in looking at aging as a concept separately from us. Therefore, why is there not more emphasis on primate aging? What is the objective of the work with the rats? What is the objective in terms of aging?

R. SPROTT (*National Institute of Aging, NIH, Bethesda, MD*): NIA's point of view is that there is no best model and there is no better model; the model is determined by the research that you want to do and in the system that you are interested in. It may be that many people are interested in aging as a general phenomena within any particular species and that is fine. However, in the last five years, the political system has come to decide (to a far greater degree than any of us would care to admit) what is fundable science. Therefore, this has tended to translate into those things that have direct human applicability (even though study sections deny it and say that they are primarily interested in good science only). In fact, that consideration has gotten into our language and into our discussions of a great many things that we do. Thus, the bias is a very real one that we are all allowing to creep into the research that we do.

INGRAM: I would take a different attack to the question. For example, we now have an opportunity to develop an animal model of Parkinson's disease and we will see examples of that given in later sessions. The reason we call it a model is because we have a Parkinson disease entity. Now, even though this does not exist in rodents, we are still trying to study it to produce a model. Aging is a phenomenon that exists in virtually all organisms, so it is a phenomena that at least appears universal; thus, we do not need to model it because it exists.

Therefore, what we are attempting to understand is whether there are mechanisms that are shared in common by different species. We mostly look at rodents, but we could look at primates if we wanted to fine-tune the modeling somewhat. Thus, in regard to our objective, we are trying to understand the basic biology of aging as it exists and to the extent to which it exists as a universal phenomenon shared by many mammalian species.

UNIDENTIFIED DISCUSSANT: That is probably a minority viewpoint. Realistically, most of the models that are going on in experimental research are modeling specific disease states. The presentation that you are giving (and that the rest of the panel is presenting) is a purer position of interest in aging per se as opposed to the disease or pathology associated with aging. In that case, there really is not a model as you say because the models come when you try to make an analogue to the state in the human situation.

M. BRENNAN (*Revlon Health Care, Tuckahoe, NY*): I just want to amplify what was said about the models. If we move away from the motor system and start considering animal models of learning and memory disorder in aging (or with brain damage or whatever), we realize the problems of trying to force a model from one situation onto another. I think that the validation of the model in and of itself (rather than trying to sell it as a model for human aging) is where the merits of the research go.

TATE: Again, I think the effort to try to sell the model—to come up with a model that will fit the bill—causes us to lose sight of what we have in front of us. It is quite clear that there are a lot of complicated parts ignored in just trying to sell the model and we have to learn to look at these parts.

Dopaminergic Changes in the Basal Ganglia
A Generalized Phenomenon of Aging in Mammals[a]

DAVID G. MORGAN AND CALEB E. FINCH

Andrus Gerontology Center
and
Department of Biological Sciences
University of Southern California
Los Angeles, California 90089-0191

INTRODUCTION

The dopamine system in mammalian brain is one of the better understood central nervous system chemical pathways. This status results from the early demonstration of its anatomic loci by histochemical fluorescence techniques (see Lindvall and Bjorklund,[1] and references therein) and its putative involvement in two prevalent neuropsychiatric disorders, namely, schizophrenia[2,3] and Parkinson's disease.[4]

The major dopamine pathway in mammals originates from cell bodies in the midbrain (areas A9 and A10—the substantia nigra and the ventral tegmental area of Tsai, respectively) and terminates in the basal ganglia, chiefly the caudate nucleus, putamen, and nucleus accumbens, with smaller projections to the globus pallidus, olfactory tubercle, and frontal and entorhinal cortices.[1] In rodents, the caudate nucleus and putamen are melded together to form the neostriatum, which combined with the globus pallidus is called the striatum. Owing to the high concentrations of dopamine in the striatal regions, most studies of dopamine in aging have focused on this region; therefore, this review will highlight the nigrostriatal dopamine system. Other regions where dopamine changes with age have been reported are the hypothalamus[5] and retina.[6]

The dopaminergic synapse contains several useful biochemical markers (FIGURE 1). Primary among these is the level of dopamine itself. Dopamine levels are thought to represent the density of dopamine terminals within a region. They are relatively insensitive to physiological changes in the rate of dopamine release because of the tightly coupled negative feedback of intraterminal dopamine concentrations on tyrosine hydroxylase activity (the rate limiting enzyme for dopamine synthesis).[7] Thus, although alternate interpretations are feasible, a loss of dopamine levels within a structure is believed to reflect a loss of dopamine terminals. In addition to dopamine, tyrosine hydroxylase activity and synaptosomal [³H]dopamine uptake are markers for dopamine terminals. Tyrosine hydroxylase is also found in noradrenergic terminals and is not specific for dopamine (although very little noradrenaline is present in striatum). The metabolites of dopamine are more sensitive to changes in the activity of the dopamine system than the parent amine, and while useful for CSF measurements or studies of dopamine turnover, analysis of metabolic levels are less useful in determining the density of dopaminergic innervation.

[a] This research was supported by Grant No. AG-05142 to C. E. Finch. D. G. Morgan was supported by a fellowship from the John Douglas French Foundation for Alzheimer's Disease. C. E. Finch is the ARCO/William F. Keischnick Professor in the Neurobiology of Aging.

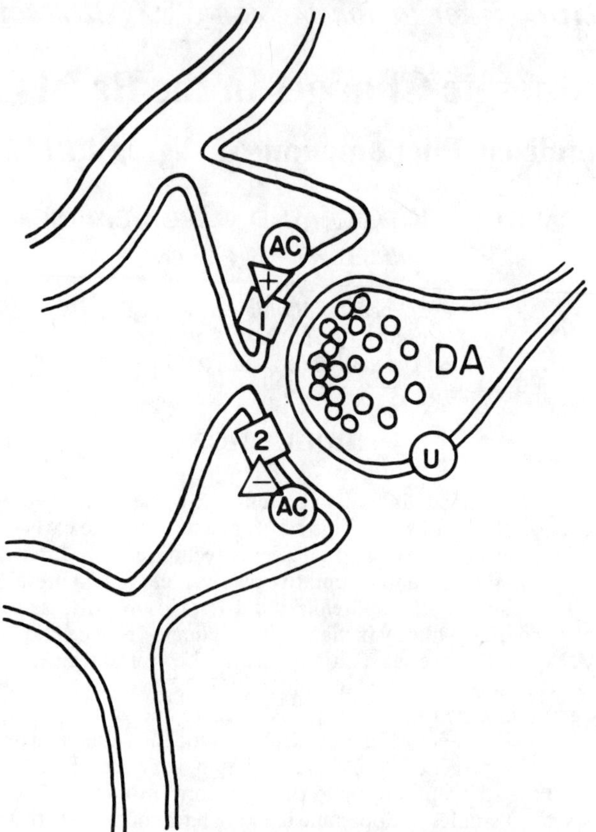

FIGURE 1. Model of the dopaminergic synapse in human striatum. Pre- and post-synaptic elements are indicated on the center and left of the figure, respectively. This model shows D-1 and D-2 binding sites on separate postsynaptic elements, but they may be colocalized on the same neuron in some instances. Tyrosine hydroxylase is located within the dopamine terminal. DA: dopaminergic terminal; 1: D-1 binding site; +: excitatory G/F protein; AC: adenylate cyclase; 2: D-2 binding site; −: inhibitory G protein; U: uptake site.

The postsynaptic receptors for dopamine consist of two types: D-1 and D-2 (FIGURE 1). The D-1 receptor is positively linked to adenylate cyclase activity, while the D-2 receptor appears, in at least some loci, to inhibit adenylate cyclase activity.[8] These opposing linkages allow for antagonism between these two receptors when localized on the same neurons.[9,10] Most [³H]agonist ligands for dopamine receptors bind to the high affinity state of both D-1 and D-2 sites.[11] Antagonist radioligands are generally more selective. The antagonist [³H]spiperone is an excellent ligand for labeling D-2 receptors (although some cautions apply; see Seeman *et al.*[12]) and most studies of D-2 receptors in aging have used this radioligand. Only recently have several D-1 selective radioligands become commercially available; thus, radioligand studies of D-1 receptors in aging brain are few. While examinations of dopamine-stimulated adenylate cyclase activity give some indication of D-1 receptor density, changes in this marker may also result from altered high affinity agonist states or receptor-cyclase coupling.

NONPATHOLOGICAL AGE-RELATED CHANGES IN THE DOPAMINE SYSTEM OF HUMAN BRAIN

The largest declines in dopamine levels are found in human brain, with a consensus reduction of "up to 50%" over the life span (TABLE 1). However, several studies[13-15] report no change with age in dopamine levels in human neostriatal structures. One study[16] finds a significant reduction in caudate nucleus, but not in putamen. The failure of some studies to report age-related declines in dopamine is not due to small sample sizes and (thus) low statistical power. In most respects, the inconsistencies cannot be explained.

The human literature on this topic differs in two respects from the rodent data. First, the individual variability in human dopamine levels is very large as compared to rodent studies, thereby reducing statistical power. This variability is not due to differences in postmortem time, but may be related to premorbid agonal conditions. Humans frequently die due to illness, whereas unhealthy rodents are usually culled from studies. A second difference is that human data are generally analyzed by regression analysis, while rodent data are analyzed by age groups using ANOVA or paired comparison range tests (t tests, Duncan's, Newman-Keul's).

The most extensive study of human striatal dopamine levels was done by Carlsson.[17] Carlsson and co-workers analyzed the sum of dopamine plus 3-methoxytyramine (3-MT) rather than dopamine alone. They have demonstrated that dopamine is catabolized into 3-MT in a time-dependent manner during the postmortem period. Thus, the sum of these two amines reflects the dopamine concentration at death. However, because Carlsson[17] claims similar results are obtained if dopamine levels alone are analyzed, this postmortem autolysis of dopamine is unlikely to explain the negative findings in the literature. A critical feature of Carlsson's data is that the rate of dopamine loss with aging accelerates after age 60. Therefore, an uneven distribution of ages may influence the analysis of age changes in the dopamine system.

We conclude that dopamine levels do decline with age in human neostriatum, but that the loss is variable amongst individuals. Moreover, this loss of dopamine may be secondary to degeneration of dopaminergic neurons in the human substantia nigra, where a 50% loss has been reported between 20 and 80 years.[18] Further support for reduced dopaminergic innervation of the human neostriatum with age is derived from a loss of tyrosine hydroxylase activity.[19,20] There appears to be a massive loss (80%) of tyrosine hydroxylase activity between 5 and 20 years, and a slower loss after that period.[20] However, one contradictory report has appeared.[14]

Postsynaptically, four independent studies confirm a loss of D-2 receptors in caudate nucleus (TABLE 1); one of these studies used healthy living subjects and a positron-emitting radioligand.[21] The loss of D-2 receptors, though, does not occur in putamen. The binding of [³H]agonist ligands to high affinity states of D-1 and D-2 receptors is also reduced in caudate nucleus, but not in putamen. We have recently reported a substantial increase in D-1 receptors in caudate nucleus and putamen.[22] The increase in D-1 sites was inversely related to the loss of dopamine in the putamen. However, a negative report has also appeared.[23]

TABLE 1. Changes in Dopamine Markers with Age: Human

(A) DOPAMINE CONCENTRATION

Study	Age Range[a]	n[b]	Region	Difference[c]
Bertler[33]	43–60; 73–87	11	caudate nucleus	↓30%
			putamen	↓40%
			subst. nigra	0
Bird & Iverson[13]	15–90	18	putamen	0
Carlsson & Winblad[34]	47–90	30	putamen	↓40%
Reiderer & Wuketich[35]	50–90	28	caudate nucleus	↓50%
Robinson et al.[14]	4–83	19	caudate nucleus	0
		10	subst. nigra	0
Adolfsson et al.[16]	24–90	23	caudate nucleus	↓50%
		24	putamen	0
			midbrain	↓?
Carlsson[17]	25–90	70	caudate nucleus	↓40% (late)
			putamen	↓?
			midbrain	↓?
MacKay et al.[15]	17–94	66	caudate nucleus	0
		56	nucleus accumbens	0
Hornykiewicz[36]	46–69; 70–93	18	caudate nucleus	↓40%

(B) TYROSINE HYDROXYLASE ACTIVITY

Study	Age Range	n	Region	Difference
McGeer et al.[19]	5–57	6	caudate nucleus	↓80%
McGeer & McGeer[20]	5–72	28	putamen	↓80% (early)
Robinson et al.[14]	4–83	18	caudate nucleus	0
		10	subst. nigra	0

TABLE 1. (continued)

(C) DOPAMINE RECEPTORS

Study	Age Range	n	Region	Difference; type[d]
Severson et al.[37]	1–100	13	caudate nucleus	↓60%; agonist
	19–80	11	caudate nucleus	↓50%; agonist
	19–60	12	caudate nucleus	0; agonist
	1–100	13	caudate nucleus	↓30%; D-2
	19–72	13	caudate nucleus	↓30%; D-2
	19–60	17	caudate nucleus	0; D-2
	1–94	12	subst. nigra	↓30%; D-2
	1–94	13	putamen	0; agonist
	19–80	11	putamen	0; agonist
	19–60	12	putamen	0; agonist
	1–94	13	putamen	0; D-2
	19–78	14	putamen	0; D-2
	19–60	12	putamen	0; D-2
Wong et al.[21]	19–72	43	caudate nucleus	↓35%; D-2
Bzowej & Seeman[23]	<40; 40–69; >70	81	caudate nucleus	↓?; D-2
		80	putamen	0; D-2
		34	striatum	0; D-1
Morgan et al.[22]	17–100	21	caudate nucleus	↓40%; D-2
		23	putamen	0; D-2
		23	caudate nucleus	↑80%; D-1
		23	putamen	↑150%; D-1

[a] Age ranges are in years of cases studied. If two or more groups are compared within the study, the age ranges of the groups are separated by semicolons.
[b] Total number of cases in the study.
[c] Difference between youngest and oldest groups examined, or the difference between the youngest and oldest cases in the age range—"↓": a decrease in the old group; "↑": an increase; "early": the greatest change occurred before mid-life; "late": the greatest change occurred after mid-life; "?": the extent of the difference could not be determined from the data presented.
[d] The type of radioligand used in the receptor study—"agonist": a [³H]agonist radioligand was used; "D-1": a D-1 selective radioligand was used; "D-2": a D-2 selective radioligand was used.

TABLE 2. Changes in Striatal Dopamine Levels

(A) RATS

Study	Strain[a]	Age Range[b]	Difference[c]
Joseph et al.[38]	Wistar (GRC)	6;25	↓55%
Ponzio et al.[39]	Wistar	3;36	0
Austin et al.[40]	Sprague-Dawley	3;6;12;18	↓35% (ant. forebrain)
Demarest et al.[5]	Long-Evans	5;24	↓20%
Joseph et al.[41]	Wistar (GRC)	6–8;24	0
Hirshhorn et al.[42]	F344	4;24	0
	F344	4;26	↓20%
Ponzio et al.[43]	Sprague-Dawley	4;18;29	↓40%
Strong et al.[44]	Sprague-Dawley (NIA)	6;16;26	↓20% (late, posterior)
Marshall et al.[45]	F344 (NIA)	4–5;27–28	↓20% (not significant)
Ponzio et al.[46]	Sprague-Dawley (Italy)	5;15;27	↓65%
Timiras et al.[47]	Long-Evans	2;4;6;12;24;30	↓20% (not significant)

(B) MICE

Study	Strain	Age Range	Difference
Finch[48]	C57BL/6J	10–12;28–30	↓25%
Papavasiliou et al.[49]	Swiss (Hale-Stoner)	2;5;17;21	0
Severson et al.[50]	C57BL/6J	8;21	0
		3;12;28	0
Osterburg et al.[51]	C57BL/6J	4;12;17;21;30	↓20% (late, variable)

TABLE 2. (continued)

(C) RABBITS

Study	Strain	Age Range	Difference
Makman *et al.*[52]	New Zealand	0.5; 5 years	0

(D) PRIMATES

Study	Strain	Age Range	Difference
Sladek & Sladek[53]	macaque	4; 20 years	↓60% (nigral fluorescence)
Goldman-Rakic & Brown[54]	rhesus	2–3;5;10;>18	↓35%

[a] Strain of the species used in that study—"GRC": strains obtained at the Gerontology Research Center, Baltimore, Maryland; "NIA": strains obtained from the National Institute on Aging colony administered by Charles River.

[b] As in TABLE 1. All ages are in months (except where otherwise indicated).

[c] As in TABLE 1—"ant. forebrain": the region included more than striatum; "posterior": the greatest changes were found in posterior striatum; "variable": not all experiments showed statistically significant changes; "nigral fluorescence": measurements of histochemical fluorescence in substantia nigra using quantitative spectral analysis.

AGE-RELATED DOPAMINERGIC CHANGES IN RATS, MICE, RABBITS, AND NONHUMAN PRIMATES

The loss of dopamine in rats and mice over the life span is smaller than that found in humans (TABLE 2). Again, several negative reports have appeared, as have reports of small, statistically not significant changes. Overall, dopamine levels decline by 20–25% in rats and mice, with the greatest loss found after mid-life. One report found no change in dopamine levels in rabbits (TABLE 2). Two studies in nonhuman primates indicate slightly greater losses than rodents.

The loss of dopamine in rodents is corroborated by studies of tyrosine hydroxylase activity (TABLE 3). This marker declines less in rodents than in humans when the entire ontogenetic spectrum is considered. However, none of the rodent studies have included reproductively immature subjects analogous to the age range where the major loss was reported in humans.

One marker that is consistently reported to change with aging in mice, rats, and rabbits is the D-2 receptor density (B_{max}) measured with [^{3}H]spiperone (TABLE 4B). These losses are typically 30–50% over the life span and they appear to be progressive with both early and late declines.[24–27] The D-2 receptor affinity (K_d) has rarely been reported to change during aging. Joyce *et al.*,[28] using *in vitro* autoradiographic techniques, found the receptor loss to be greatest (up to 60%) in the ventral and lateral portions of the striatum. While several exceptions to the D-2 loss with aging have been reported (TABLE 4), these studies used radioligands such as [^{3}H]haloperidol, [^{3}H]sulpiride, and [^{3}H]domperidone. While these drugs have selectivity for D-2 receptors similar to [^{3}H]spiperone, they have higher levels of nonspecific binding and the techniques for their use are less standardized. The weight of the presently available evidence strongly favors a substantial loss of D-2 receptors throughout the life span of all mammals studied.

The results of [^{3}H]agonist labeling studies are consistent with those obtained with [^{3}H]spiperone (TABLE 4C). The loss of high affinity agonist binding sites with age is somewhat greater than the loss of antagonist sites in studies making direct comparisons.[24,29] Severson and Randall[30] have recently used dopamine displacement curves of [^{3}H]spiperone binding to demonstrate that the high affinity component of the displacement curve is selectively lost with aging in mice.

The data concerning D-1 receptors is mixed. Two studies report no change, while two studies in press report losses. Obviously, more data are called for.

In rat brain, large reductions of dopamine-stimulated adenylate cyclase are reported consistently (with two exceptions; see TABLE 5). Generally, these reductions occur in the absence of changes in basal adenylate cyclase activity. Thus, even if D-1 receptors

TABLE 3. Changes in Striatal Tyrosine Hydroxylase with Aging

Study	Strain[a]	Age Range[b]	Difference[c]
McGeer *et al.*[55]	Wistar	2–29 (8 ages)	↓30%
Reis *et al.*[56]	F344	4;26	↓20%
	CB6F1 mice	4;28	0
Joseph *et al.*[41]	Wistar (GRC)	6–8;24	↓15%
Ponzio *et al.*[43]	Sprague-Dawley (Canada)	4;18;29	↓30% (early)

[a] All strains are rats unless indicated.
[b] All ages are in months. As in TABLE 1.
[c] As in TABLE 2.

TABLE 4. Changes in Striatal Dopamine Receptor Density with Aging

(A) D-1 Receptors

Study	Strain[a]	Age Range[b]	Difference[c]
O'Boyle & Waddington[57]	Sprague-Dawley (Wolfson)	4;22	0 ($\uparrow$ nonspecific)
Morgan et al.[22]	C57BL/6J mice	4;9–10;16–19;24–26	0
Giorgi et al.[58]	Sprague-Dawley (Italy)	3;26	$\downarrow$40%
Henry and Roth (unpubl.)	rats (GRC)	3;24	$\downarrow$30%

(B) D-2 Receptors

Study	Species/Strain	Age Range	Difference
Joseph et al.[38]	Wistar (GRC)	6;25	$\downarrow$35%
Govoni et al.[59]	Wistar	10;30	0 (5 × $\uparrow K_d$)
Severson & Finch[24]	C57BL/6J mice	3;8;20;28	$\downarrow$50%
Thal et al.[29]	New Zealand rabbits	0.5; 5 years	$\downarrow$30%
Govoni et al.[60]	Sprague-Dawley	3–4;24–30	0 ($\uparrow K_d$)
Memo et al.[61]	Sprague-Dawley	3–4;24–28	$\downarrow$35%
Randall et al.[25]	C57BL/6J mice	5;12;24–26	$\downarrow$30%
Misra et al.[62]	F344 (NIA)	7;25	$\downarrow$35%
Joseph et al.[63]	Wistar (GRC)	6–8;24	$\downarrow$30% (not significant)
Algeri et al.[26]	CD-COBS (Italy)	5;7;21;26	$\downarrow$20%
DeBlasi & Menini[64]	Sprague-Dawley (Italy)	3;21–23	$\downarrow$50%
Marquis et al.[65]	CD (Charles River)	6;26	$\uparrow$350 ($\uparrow K_d$)
	C57BL/6J mice	4;32 (6 ages)	$\uparrow$800%
Misra et al.[66]	F344 (NIA)	7;25	$\downarrow$14% (not significant)

(continued on next page)

TABLE 4. (continued)

Study	Species/Strain	Age Range	Difference
Cimino et al.[67]	rats	3;30	↓30%
Joseph et al.[68]	F344 (Harlan)	6–8;15–18;25	↓10%
Levin et al.[69]	Wistar (GRC)	4–6;24	↓30%
Marshall et al.[45]	F344 (NIA)	4–5;27–28	0
			(*in vivo* labeling)
Missale et al.[70]	rats	3;25	↑100%
Henry & Roth[71]	Wistar (GRC)	3–6;24–25	↓25%
O'Boyle & Waddington[57]	Sprague-Dawley (Wolfson)	4;22	↓25%
Roth et al.[27]	Wistar (GRC)	3;12;24	↓50%
Randall et al.[72]	C57BL/6J mice	6;13;27–30	↓25%
Severson & Randall[73]	C57BL/6J mice	3;12;24	↓35%
Joyce et al.[28]	F344 (NIA)	5–6;26–28	↓0–60%
			(autoradiography)

(C) AGONISTS

Study	Species/Strain	Age Range	Difference
Severson & Finch[24]	C57BL/6J mice	8;26	↓40%
Thal et al.[29]	New Zealand rabbits	0.5; 5 years	↓60%
Levin et al.[74]	Wistar (GRC)	4;24	↓40%
Hirschhorn et al.[42]	F344 (NIA)	6;24–26	↓35%
DeBlasi & Menini[64]	Sprague-Dawley (Italy)	3;21–23	0
Severson & Randall[73]	C57BL/6J mice	3;12;24	↓35%

[a] All strains are rats unless indicated. As in TABLE 2.

[b] All ages are in months unless indicated.

[c] "↑ nonspecific": Nonspecific binding of [^{3}H]piflutixol increased in the old rats. No change in specific binding; "↑ K_d": the dissociation constant increases; "*in vivo* labeling": radiotracer [^{3}H]spiperone was injected intravenously to label D-2 receptors; "autoradiography": results obtained using *in vitro* receptor autoradiography (see text). As in TABLE 2.

TABLE 5. Changes in Striatal Dopamine-Stimulated Adenylate Cyclase with Aging

Study	Strain[a]	Age Range[b]	Difference[c]
Walker & Walker[75]	Sprague-Dawley	3;24	↓70%
Puri & Volicer[76]	CD-F (Charles River)	4;12;24;30	↓75 (early)
Govini et al.[6]	Sprague-Dawley (Italy)	2–3;20–24	↓60%
Schmidt & Thornberry[77]	Wistar (Harlan)	3;12;24	↓30% (early)
Govoni et al.[59]	Wistar	10;30	↓60%
Makman et al.[52]	New Zealand (Rabbits)	0.5; 5 years	↓45%
Joseph et al.[63]	Wistar (GRC)	6–8;24	0
Papavasiliou et al.[49]	Swiss mice (Hale-Stoner)	2;5;17;21	↓50% (not significant)
Hirschhorn et al.[42]	F344	4;14;29	0
Cimino et al.[67]	rats	3;30	↓30%

[a] As in TABLE 3.
[b] As in TABLE 2.
[c] As in TABLE 2.

do not decline with aging, their coupling to adenylate cyclase is compromised. The loss of dopamine-stimulated adenylate cyclase activity is an early event in the aging striatum, with the greatest decline occurring before 12 months of age. The overall extent of this decline is 50–70% over the life span.

CONCLUSIONS

While certainly no revelation, the major conclusion that we draw from this survey of the literature is that individual studies of the dopamine system during aging produce divergent results and conclusions. At least in this field, it is critical to derive weighted averages of all studies before any results can be accepted as truth. Our impression from other literature surveys that we performed recently on the serotonin system in Alzheimer's disease[31] and on receptor changes in Alzheimer's disease[32] is very much the same. Two laboratories using the same techniques can obtain one positive and one negative result.

Fortunately, in the literature reviewed here, the positive findings (loss of dopamine, receptors, or cyclase activation with age) are always in the same direction and outnumber the studies reporting no change. Thus, we conclude that the dopamine system does degenerate with nonpathological aging in man and, to a lesser extent, in other mammals. The postsynaptic responsiveness to dopamine also declines as measured by dopamine-stimulated adenylate cyclase or D-2 receptor density. The end result is a substantial decrement in dopaminergic tone, which, as described in other chapters in this volume, will lead to impaired motor performance and reduced sensorimotor integration.

ACKNOWLEDGMENTS

We thank Diana Lerner for her expert assistance in preparing the manuscript.

REFERENCES

1. LINDVALL, O. & A. BJORKLUND 1983. Dopamine and norepinephrine containing neuron systems. Their anatomy in the rat brain. *In* Chemical Neuroanatomy. P. C. Emson, Ed.: 229–255. Raven Press. New York.

2. SNYDER, S. H. 1976. The dopamine hypothesis of schizophrenia: Focus on the dopamine receptor. Am. J. Psychiatry **133:** 197–202.

3. SEEMAN, P. 1980. Brain dopamine receptors. Pharmacol. Rev. **32:** 229–313.

4. BERNHEIMER, H., W. BIRKMAYER, O. HORNYKIEWICZ, K. JELLINGER & F. SEITELBERG. 1973. Brain dopamine and the syndromes of Parkinson and Huntington. Clinical, morphological and neurochemical correlations. J. Neurol. Sci. **20:** 415–455.

5. DEMAREST, K. T., G. D. RIEGLE & K. E. MOORE. 1980. Characteristics of dopaminergic neurons in the aged male rat. Neuroendocrinology **31:** 222–227.

6. GOVONI, S., P. LODDO, P. F. SPANO & M. TRABUCCHI. 1977. Dopamine receptor sensitivity in brain and retina of rats during aging. Brain Res. **138:** 565–570.

7. COOPER, J. R., F. E. BLOOM & R. H. ROTH. 1985. The Biochemical Basis of Neuropharmacology. Oxford University Press. London/New York.

8. STOOF, J. C. & J. W. KEBABIAN. 1984. Two dopamine receptors: Biochemistry, physiology, and pharmacology. Life Sci. **35:** 2281–2296.

9. STOOF, J. C. & J. W. KEBABIAN. 1981. Opposing roles for D-1 and D-2 dopamine receptors in efflux of cyclic AMP from rat neostriatum. Nature **294:** 366–368.

10. ONALI, P., M. C. OLIANAS & G. L. GESSA. 1984. Selective blockade of dopamine D-1 receptors by SCH 23390 discloses striatal dopamine D-2 receptors mediating the inhibition of adenylate cyclase in rats. Eur. J. Pharmacol. **99:** 127.

11. BACOPOULOS, N. G. 1983. (3H)Dopamine binds to D-1 and D-2 receptors in rat striatum. Eur. J. Pharmacol. **87:** 353–356.

12. SEEMAN, P., C. ULPIAN, K. A. WREGGET & J. W. WELLS. 1984. Dopamine receptor parameters detected by [³H]spiperone depend on tissue concentration: Analysis and examples. J. Neurochem. **43:** 221–227.

13. BIRD, E. D. & L. L. IVERSEN. 1974. Huntington's chorea: Post-mortem measurement of glutamic acid decarboxylase, choline acetyltransferase and dopamine in basal ganglia. Brain **97:** 457–472.

14. ROBINSON, D. S., R. L. SOURKES, A. NIES, L. S. HARRIS, S. SPECTOR, D. L. BARTLETT & I. S. KAYE. 1977. Monoamine metabolism in human brain. Arch. Gen. Psychiatry **34:** 89–92.

15. MACKAY, A. V. P., L. L. IVERSON, M. ROSSOR, E. SPOKES, E. BIRD, A. ARREGUI, I. CREESE & S. SNYDER. 1982. Increased brain dopamine and dopamine receptors in schizophrenia. Arch. Gen. Psychiatry **39:** 991–997.

16. ADOLFSSON, R., C. G. GOTTFRIES, B. E. ROOS, B. E. ROOS & B. WINBLAD. 1979. Changes in brain catecholamines in patients with dementia of Alzheimer type. Br. J. Psychiatry **135:** 216–223.

17. CARLSSON, A. 1981. Aging and brain neurotransmitters. *In* Funktionsstorurgen des Gehirns im Alter. D. Platt, Ed.: 67–81. Schattauer. Stuttgart.

18. McGEER, P. L., E. G. McGEER & J. S. SUZUKI. 1977. Aging and extrapyramidal function. Arch. Neurol. Chicago **34:** 33–35.

19. McGEER, E. G., P. L. McGEER & J. A. WADA. 1971. Distribution of tyrosine hydroxylase in human and animal brain. J. Neurochem. **18:** 1647–1658.

20. McGEER, P. L. & E. G. McGEER. 1976. Enzymes associated with the metabolism of catecholamines, acetylcholine and GABA in human controls and patients with Parkinson's disease and Huntington's chorea. J. Neurochem. **26:** 65–76.

21. WONG, D. F., H. N. WAGNER, R. F. DANNALS, J. M. LINKS, J. J. FROST, H. T. RAVERT, A. A. WILSON, A. E. ROSENBAUM, A. GJEDDE, K. H. DOUGLASS, J. D. PETRONIS, M. F. FOLSTEIN, J. K. TUONG, H. D. BURNS & M. J. KUHAR. 1984. Effects of age on dopamine and serotonin receptors measured by positron tomography in the living human brain. Science **226:** 1393–1396.

22. MORGAN, D. G., P. C. MAY & C. E. FINCH. 1986. Dopamine and serotonin systems in human and rodent brain: Effects of age and degenerative disease. J. Am. Geriatr. Soc. **35:** 334–345.

23. BZOWEJ, N. H. & P. SEEMAN. 1985. Age and dopamine D1 and D2 receptors in human brain. Neurosci. Abstr. **11:** 889 (#260.5).

24. SEVERSON, J. A. & C. E. FINCH. 1980. Reduced dopaminergic binding during aging in the rodent striatum. Brain Res. **192:** 147–162.

25. RANDALL, P. K., J. A. SEVERSON & C. E. FINCH. 1981. Aging and the regulation of striatal dopaminergic mechanisms in mice. J. Pharmacol. Exp. Ther. **219:** 690–700.

26. ALGERI, S., G. ACHILLI, M. CIMINO, C. PEREGO, F. PONZIO & G. VANTINI. 1982. Study on some compensatory responses of dopaminergic system in aging rats. Exp. Brain Res. Suppl. **5:** 146–152.

27. ROTH, G. S., D. K. INGRAM & J. A. JOSEPH. 1984. Delayed loss of striatal dopamine receptors during aging of dietarily restricted rats. Brain Res. **300:** 27–32.

28. JOYCE, J. N., S. K. LOESCHEN, D. W. SAPP & J. F. MARSHALL. 1986. Age-related regional loss of caudate-putamen dopamine receptors revealed by quantitative autoradiography. Brain Res. **378:** 158–163.

29. THAL, L. J., S. G. HOROWITZ, B. DVORKIN & M. H. MAKMAN. 1980. Evidence for loss of brain [³H]spiroperidol and [³H]ADTN binding sites in rabbit brain with aging. Brain Res. **152:** 626–632.

30. SEVERSON, J. A. & P. K. RANDALL. 1985. D-2 dopamine receptors in aging mouse striatum: Determination of high- and low-affinity agonist binding sites. J. Pharmacol. Exp. Ther. **233:** 361–368.

31. MORGAN, D. G. & C. E. FINCH. 1986. The role of serotonin deficiency in Alzheimer's Disease. Bull. Clin. Neurosci. In press.

32. MORGAN, D. G., P. C. MAY & C. E. FINCH. 1986. Neurotransmitter receptors in normal human aging and Alzheimer's disease. *In* Receptors and Ligands in Psychiatry and Neurology. A. K. Sen & T. Y. Lee, Eds. In press.

33. BERTLER, A. 1961. Occurrence and localization of catecholamines in the human brain. Acta Physiol. Scand. **51:** 97–107.

34. CARLSSON, A. & B. WINBLAD. 1976. The influence of age and time interval between death and autopsy on dopamine and 3-methoxytyramine levels in human basal ganglia. J. Neural Transm. **38:** 271–276.

35. REIDERER, P. & S. T. WUKETICH. 1976. Time course of nigrostriatal degeneration in Parkinson's disease. J. Neural Transm. **38:** 277–301.

36. HORNYKIEWICZ, O. 1983. Dopamine changes in the aging human brain: Functional considerations. *In* Aging, Vol. 23: Aging Brain and Ergot Alkaloids. A. Agnoli *et al.*, Eds.: 9–14. Raven Press. New York.

37. SEVERSON, J. A., J. MARCUSSON, B. WINBLAD & C. E. FINCH. 1982. Age-correlated loss of dopaminergic binding sites in human basal ganglia. J. Neurochem. **39:** 1623–1631.

38. JOSEPH, J. A., R. E. BERGER, B. T. ENGEL & G. S. ROTH. 1978. Age-related changes in the nigrostriatum: A behavioral and biochemical analysis. J. Gerontol. **33:** 643–649.

39. PONZIO, F., N. BRUNELLO & S. ALGERI. 1978. Catecholamine synthesis in brain of aging rat. J. Neurochem. **30:** 1617–1620.

40. AUSTIN, J. H., E. CONNOLE, K. DOUBRAVKA & J. COLLINS. 1978. Studies in aging of the brain. V. Reduced norepinephrine, dopamine, and cyclic AMP in rat brain with advancing age. Age **1:** 121–124.

41. JOSEPH, J. A., C. FILBURN, S. P. TZANKOFF, J. M. THOMPSON & B. T. ENGEL. 1980. Age-related neostriatal alterations in the rat: Failure of L-DOPA to alter behavior. Neurobiol. Aging **1:** 119–125.

42. HIRSCHORN, I. D., M. H. MAKMAN & N. S. SHARPLESS. 1982. Dopamine receptor sensitivity following nigrostriatal lesions in the aged rat. Brain Res. **234:** 257–368.

43. PONZIO, F., G. CALDERINI, G. LOMUSCIO, G. VANTINI, G. TOFFANO & S. ALGERI. 1982. Changes in monoamine and their metabolite levels in some brain regions of aged rats. Neurobiol. Aging **3:** 23–39.

44. STRONG, R., T. SAMORAJSKI & Z. GOTTESFELD. 1982. Regional mapping of neostriatal neurotransmitter systems as a function of aging. J. Neurochem. **39:** 831–836.

45. MARSHALL, J. F., M. C. DREW & K. A. NEVE. 1983. Recovery of function after mesotelencephalic dopaminergic injury in senescence. Brain Res. **259:** 249–260.

46. PONZIO, F., G. ACHILLI, G. CALDERINI, P. FERRETTI, C. PEREGO, G. TOFFANO & S. ALGERI. 1984. Depletion and recovery of neuronal monoamine storage in rats of different ages treated with reserpine. Neurobiol. Aging **5:** 101–104.

47. TIMIRAS, P. S., D. B. HUDSON & P. E. SEGALL. 1984. Lifetime brain serotonin: Regional effects of age and precursor availability. Neurobiol. Aging **5:** 235–242.

48. FINCH, C. E. 1973. Catacholamine metabolism in the brains of aging male mice. Brain Res. **52:** 261–276.

49. PAPAVASILIOU, P. S., S. T. MILLER, L. S. THAL, L. J. NERDER, G. HOULIHAN, S. N. RAO & J. M. STEVENS. 1981. Age-related motor and catecholamine alterations in mice on levodopa supplemented diet. Life Sci. **28:** 2945–2952.

50. SEVERSON, J. A., H. H. OSTERBURG & C. E. FINCH. 1981. Aging and haloperidol-induced dopamine turnover in the nigro-striatal pathway of C57BL/6J mice. Neurobiol. Aging **2:** 193–197.

51. OSTERBURG, H. H., H. G. DONAHUE, J. A. SEVERSON & C. E. FINCH. 1981. Catecholamine levels and turnover during aging in brain regions of male C57BL/6J mice. Brain Res. **224:** 337–352.

52. MAKMAN, M. H., E. L. GARDNER, L. J. THAL, I. D. HIRSCHHORN, T. F. SEEGER & G. BHARGAVA. 1980. Central monoamine receptor systems. Influence of aging, lesion, and drug treatment. *In* Neural Regulatory Mechanisms during Aging, p. 91–127. Alan R. Liss. New York.

53. SLADEK, J. R. & C. D. SLADEK, 1979. Relative quantitation of monoamine histofluorescence in young and old non-human primates. Parkinson's Disease II, Aging and Neuroendocrine Relationships. C. E. Finch, D. E. Potter & A. D. Kenny, Eds.: 241–250. Plenum. New York.

54. GOLDMAN-RAKIC, P. S. & R. M. BROWN. 1981. Regional changes of monoamines in cerebral cortex and subcortical structures of aging rhesus monkeys. Neuroscience **6:** 177–187.

55. MCGEER, E. G., H. C. FIBIGER, P. L. MCGEER & V. WICKSON. 1971. Aging and brain enzymes. Exp. Gerontol. **6:** 391–396.

56. REIS, D. J., R. A. ROSS & T. H. JOH. 1977. Changes in the activity and amounts of enzymes synthesizing catecholamines and acetylcholine in brain, adrenal medulla, and sympathetic ganglia of aged rat and mouse. Brain Res. **136:** 465–474.

57. O'BOYLE, K. M. & J. L. WADDINGTON. 1984. Loss of rat striatal dopamine receptors with aging is selective for D-2 but not D-1 sites: Association with increased nonspecific binding of the D-1 ligand [^{3}H]piflutixol. Eur. J. Pharmacol. **105:** 171–174.

58. GIORGI, O., G. CALDERINI, G. TOFFANO & G. BIGGIO. 1986. D-1 dopamine receptors labelled with [^{3}H]SCH-23390: Decrease in the striatum of aged rats. Neurobiol. Aging. In press.

59. GOVONI, S., P. F. SPANO & M. TRABUCCHI. 1978. [^{3}H]Haloperidol and [^{3}H]spiroperidol binding in rat striatum during aging. J. Pharm. Pharmacol. **30:** 448–449.

60. GOVONI, S., M. MEMO, L. SAIANI, P. F. SPANO & TRABUCCI. 1980. Impairment of brain neurotransmitter receptors in aged rats. Mech. Aging Dev. **12:** 39–46.

61. MEMO, M., L. LURCHI, P. F. SPANO & M. TRABUCCHI. 1980. Aging process affects a single class of dopamine receptors. Brain Res. **202:** 488–492.

62. MISRA, C. H., H. SHELAT & R. C. SMITH. 1981. Influence of age on the effects of chronic fluphenazine on receptor binding in rat brain. Eur. J. Pharmacol. **76:** 317–324.

63. JOSEPH, J. A., C. R. FILBURN & G. S. ROTH. 1981. Development of dopamine receptor denervation supersensitivity in the neostriatum of the senescent rat. Life Sci. **29:** 575–584.

64. DEBLASI, A. & T. MENNINI. 1982. Selective reduction of one class of dopamine receptor binding sites in the corpus striatum of aged rats. Brain Res. **242:** 361–364.

65. MARQUIS, J. K., A. S. LIPPA & R. W. PELHAM. 1982. Dopamine receptor alterations with aging in mouse and rat corpus striatum. Biochem. Pharmacol. **30:** 1876–1878.

66. MISRA, C. H., H. SHELAT & R. C. SMITH. 1982. Age affects dopamine receptor changes during chronic administration of fluphenazine. Eur. J. Pharmacol. **85:** 343–346.

67. CIMINO, M., G. CURATOLA, C. PEZZOLI, G. STRAMENTINOLI, G. VANTINI & S. ALGERI. 1983.

Age-related modification of dopaminergic and B-adrenergic receptor system: Restoration of normal activity by modifying membrane fluidity with S-adenosyl methionine. Aging **23:** 79–86.

68. JOSEPH, J. A., R. T. BARTUS, D. CLODY, D. MORGAN, C. FINCH, B. BEER & S. SESACK. 1983. Psychomotor performance in the senescent rodent: Reduction of deficits via striatal dopamine receptor up-regulation. Neurobiol. Aging **4:** 313–319.

69. LEVIN, P., M. HAJI, J. A. JOSEPH & G. S. ROTH. 1983. Effect of aging on prolactin regulation of rat striatal dopamine receptor concentrations. Life Sci. **32:** 1743–1749.

70. MISSALE, C., S. GOVONI, L. CASTELLETTI, P. F. SPANO & M. TRABUCCHI. 1983. Brain neurotransmitter changes in brains of aged rats. Aging **23:** 15–22.

71. HENRY J. M. & G. S. ROTH. 1984. Effect of aging on recovery of striatal dopamine receptors following *n*-ethoxycarbonyl-2-ethoxy-1, 2-dihydroquinoline (EEDQ) blockade. Life Sci. **35:** 899–904.

72. RANDALL, P. K., J. A. SEVERSON, S. M. HURD & W. O. MCCLURE. 1985. Effect of duration of haloperidol treatment on DA receptor supersensitization in aging C57BL/6J mice. Brain Res. **333:** 85–95.

73. SEVERSON J. A. & P. K. RANDALL. 1985. D-2 dopamine receptors in aging mouse striatum: Determination of high- and low-affinity agonist binding sites. J. Pharmacol. Exp. Ther. **233:** 361–368.

74. LEVIN, P., J. K. JANDA, J. A. JOSEPH, D. K. INGRAM & G. S. ROTH. 1981. Dietary restriction retards the age-associated loss of rat striatal dopaminergic receptors. Science **214:** 561–562.

75. WALKER, J. B. & J. P. WALKER. 1973. Properties of adenylate cyclase from senescent rat brain. Brain Res. **54:** 391–396.

76. PURI, S. K. & L. VOLICER. 1977. Effects of aging on cyclic AMP levels and adenylate cyclase and phosphodiesterase activities in the rat corpus striatum. Mech. Aging Dev. **6:** 53–58.

77. SCHMIDT, M. J. & J. F. THORNBERRY. 1978. Cyclic AMP and cyclic GMP accumulation *in vitro* in brain regions from young, old and aged rats. Brain Res. **139:** 159–177.

DISCUSSION OF THE PAPER

D. INGRAM (*NIA, Baltimore, MD*): What do you mean by dopamine tone, particularly in regard to the fact that the evidence for loss of dopamine per se was not overwhelming as the loss of dopamine receptors was?

D. MORGAN (*University of Southern California, Los Angeles, CA*): Tone is kind of a general term; however, I think of it in the same sense as muscle tone, that is, tension in that system. I consider it an integrated aspect of both the input to that system and the number of receptors on the output side. We know that the D-2 receptors are going down. Perhaps the D-1 receptors are going up, but there is contrary evidence that has not been published yet. Thus, the overall change postsynaptically (at least for the D-2 receptors) appears to be downward in the dopamine system. In addition, the dopamine-sensitive adenylate cyclase activity, which should be a measure of D-1 function, declines as an early event in aging (that is, up to about 12 months) and is stable thereafter.

A. ALTAR (*CIBA–GEIGY Corporation, Summit, NJ*): You mentioned that you did not see an age-related decrease in D-1 receptors in the striatum and in mouse brain. Have you looked in the substantia nigra? The evidence there is very clear that virtually all of the D-1 sites in the substantia nigra are on the terminals of nigrostriatal neurons. It would be interesting if there were losses there—not only because of the fact that they would show the loss of D-1 receptors, but also because it may start implicating some of those nigrostriatal neurons that represent the output pathway as contributing to age-related impairments.

MORGAN: I would like to do it, but the nigra in a mouse is so small that it would be rather difficult for us to do that using our *in vitro* techniques. Certainly, the autoradiographic approach might be able to pick up those receptors, at least much easier than we could. Jim Severson also did some work with D-2 in nigra in human brain, but we just have not looked in nigra at this time for D-1.

Regionally Selective Manifestations of Neostriatal Aging

RANDY STRONG

Geriatric Research, Education, and Clinical Center
Veterans Administration Medical Center
and
Departments of Pharmacology and Medicine
St. Louis University School of Medicine
St. Louis, Missouri 63125

INTRODUCTION

Deterioration of the speed and precision of motor performance is a major attribute of aging.[1] Neurochemical and morphological changes in several brain areas, including the motor cortex,[2-4] cerebellum,[5-7] and basal ganglia,[8-12] may underlie motor deficits associated with advanced age. However, research has concentrated largely on the basal ganglia because a variety of neurological disorders involve pathological changes in these nuclei.[13] Basal ganglia pathology is present in at least two major age-associated disorders — Parkinson's disease and Huntington's chorea. Less severe symptoms of these diseases, including senile tremors and chorea, frequently develop in otherwise healthy older persons.[1,13,14] The elderly also have a greater risk of developing drug side effects involving the basal ganglia. Furthermore, the incidence of drug-induced parkinsonism and tardive dyskinesia increases with age.[15-17] Interestingly, the age distribution for drug-induced extrapyramidal disorders overlaps considerably with that of Parkinson's symptomatology.[8,16,18] This suggests an interaction between the pathophysiology underlying these conditions and the physiological changes occurring during the normal aging process.

Present evidence indicates that many of the behavioral abnormalities that occur during the normal aging process result from a reduced capacity for neurotransmission in the brain. The deficits in neurotransmission are inferred from decreases in various presynaptic and postsynaptic neurochemical parameters in a variety of brain regions.[2,5,7-9,11,12,19,20] Pharmacological studies of the striatum of rodent brain demonstrate that neurochemical deficits may underlie some motor malfunctions associated with aging.[8,11,18,21-24] In this regard, the cholinergic and dopaminergic systems seem particularly susceptible.

Until recently, few studies considered the functional and neurochemical organization of the striatum with respect to age-related changes. Numerous reports provide evidence that discrete regions of the neostriatum are both neurochemically and functionally distinct from each other.[25-27] Neurochemical studies reveal that cholinergic, dopaminergic, glutamatergic, GABAergic, serotonergic, and various peptidergic systems have a heterogeneous distribution in the striatum.[28-34] This fact supports the idea that functionally independent regions exist within the neostriatum. In the following sections, we will discuss the evidence for functional heterogeneity of the striatum. We will review the data showing that disruption of neurotransmitter systems within discrete regions of the striatum produces specific behavioral effects. Then, we will describe results of experiments carried out in our laboratory that reveal the neurochemical topography of the striatum and how it changes with age. The emphasis in these experiments is on the cholinergic and dopaminergic systems. We choose these systems for study because they are particularly vulnerable to the effects of aging. Additionally, their relationship to basal ganglia function is relatively well known.

Functional Heterogeneity of the Neostriatum

Studies employing pharmacological and behavioral techniques combined with stereotaxic methods provide compelling evidence that various parts of the neostriatum subserve different functions. These functions may be specifically disrupted by interruption of neurotransmission within discrete regions. Functional distinctions exist between the medial and lateral striatum. For example, injection of atropine, a cholinergic antagonist, into the anterior medial striatum produces retrograde amnesia for acquisition of spatial alternation performance.[35] Injections into other regions do not affect this behavior.[35] On the other hand, destruction of cell bodies in the ventral-lateral striatum with kainic acid causes sensorimotor impairment and impaired limb use.[36] Lesions of other striatal areas are ineffective on these behaviors.[36] Disruption of dopaminergic neurotransmission also has region-dependent behavioral effects. Destruction of dopaminergic nerve terminals in the lateral striatum with 6-hydroxydopamine (6-OHDA) is critical for the occurrence of stress-induced akinesia.[37] Lesions of the central or medial regions of the striatum are ineffective in this behavioral paradigm.[37] These studies provide evidence that the medial striatum plays a role in the acquisition of learned performance, while the lateral striatum is necessary for motor function.

Functional distinctions also exist between dorsal and ventral neostriatum. Lesions in the ventral striatum made with 6-OHDA block amphetamine-induced stereotyped behavior.[38] In contrast, lesions with 6-OHDA in the dorsal striatum are without effect.[38] Lesions of the dorsal striatum with kainic acid enhance the stereotypy-inducing effect of amphetamine without affecting apomorphine-induced stereotyped behavior.[39] Alternatively, kainic acid lesions of the ventral striatum do not influence this behavior.[39] Functional dissociation of striatal regions is also manifested in other behavioral paradigms, including the modulation of blood pressure,[27] consummatory behavior,[40] and active avoidance behavior.[41]

Neurochemical Deficits in Striatal Subregions
in Huntington's and Parkinson's Diseases

Discrete regional deficits in striatal neurotransmitter systems are manifested in Huntington's and Parkinson's diseases. The changes in discrete striatal areas may underlie specific cognitive and motor impairments that are symptomatic of these disorders. The enzyme marker of striatal cholinergic neurons, choline acetyltransferase (ChAT), is markedly depleted in Huntington's disease. McGeer and co-workers reported that loss of ChAT activity was "patchy" in the striatum of individuals who had Huntington's chorea.[42,43] They also found that the caudate was more vulnerable than the putamen to loss of ChAT activity.[43] Aquilonius and co-workers confirmed the uneven loss of ChAT in Huntington's disease.[44] Furthermore, they found that the rostromedial part of the caudate nucleus was the most severely affected area. This is noteworthy because interruption of cholinergic transmission in the rostromedial striatum interferes with memory processes.[35] Possibly, the destruction of cholinergic neurons in the rostromedial striatum contributes to the dementia that develops during this disease.

A few studies also provide evidence that neurochemical deficits in Parkinson's disease are not uniform within the striatum. Dopamine and its metabolites are severely depleted in the substantia nigra and striatum of Parkinson patients.[45] Associated with this loss of dopamine is a loss of cells from the pars compacta of the substantia nigra.[45] Gaspar and co-workers reported a study of the topographical distribution of tyrosine hydroxylase (TH) in the caudate and putamen of Parkinson's patients.[46] That study showed that TH was more severely decreased in the putamen than in the caudate nucleus. Additionally, the magnitude of the loss of TH was greatest in the rostral regions as compared to the caudal regions of the putamen. Because the nigrostriatal projections are topographically organized,[25,47] the patchy decrease in TH may reflect the uneven regional cell loss found in the substantia nigra of Parkinson's patients.[45]

The dopaminergic system is also not the only system to manifest regional differences in the effects of Parkinson's disease on the basal ganglia. Decreases in met- and leu-enkephalin occur in the putamen, but not in the caudate nucleus.[48] Taken together, the studies cited above indicate that selected regions of the caudate nucleus are most vulnerable in Huntington's disease, while the putamen, particularly the rostral region, is more susceptible to alterations in Parkinson's disease.

AGE-RELATED CHANGES IN STRIATAL SUBREGIONS

There are functionally discrete regions within the striatum and pathological changes in the striatum occur in particular subregions. We hypothesized that if some regions are particularly prone to disease, then discrete areas within the striatum might also be uniquely susceptible to the effects of aging. Our laboratory initiated studies to discover possible age-related alterations in the distribution of presynaptic and postsynaptic "markers" of striatal transmitter systems, with particular emphasis on the cholinergic and dopaminergic systems.

Cholinergic System

Choline acetyltransferase is the enzyme that synthesizes acetylcholine. It is a very useful marker of the distribution of the cholinergic system in the brain because it is restricted to cholinergic neurons.[49] Many investigators have reported that striatal choline acetyltransferase (ChAT) activity declines with age in several strains of rodents.[2,11,50-52] However, all of these laboratories assayed ChAT in grossly dissected striatal tissue. To determine if these age-associated changes in ChAT occurred in discrete striatal regions, we measured ChAT in tissue punches taken from medial and lateral striatum in 11 consecutive frozen sections of the brain of Sprague Dawley rats of three different ages (see FIGURE 1).[53]

FIGURE 2 demonstrates the fact that the cholinergic system is heterogeneously distributed in the striatum. In general, ChAT activity was higher in the rostral levels relative to the caudal levels of the striatum in all age groups. In addition, enzyme activity was lower in the medial regions (FIGURE 2A) as compared to the lateral regions (FIGURE 2B).

Age-related decreases in ChAT were evident in several discrete striatal regions. ChAT activity was lower in a few medial striatal regions of rats that were 16 months old as compared to younger rats (FIGURE 2A). No reduction in ChAT occurred in the lateral

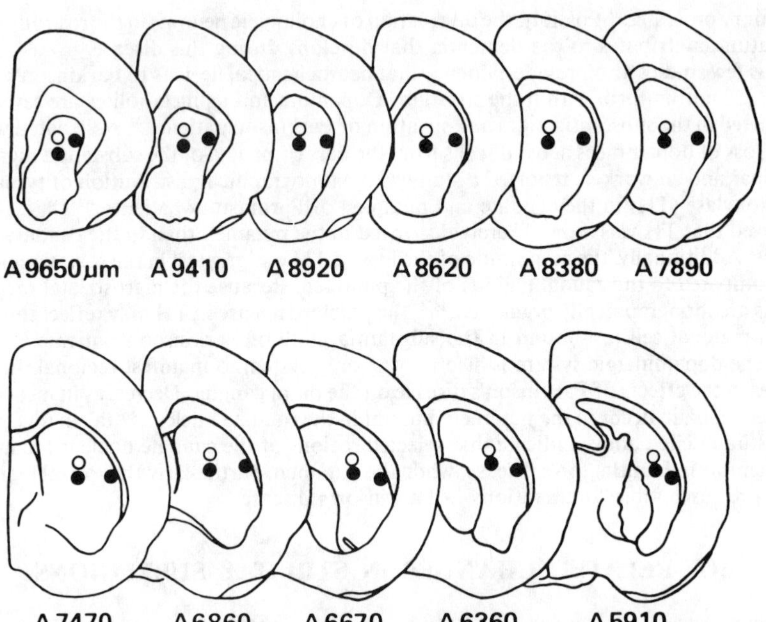

FIGURE 1. Coordinates (according to Konig and Klippel[68]) of serial frontal sections through the neostriatum of Sprague Dawley rats. The light circles represent punches assayed for dopamine and norepinephrine. The dark circles represent punches that were removed for measuring GAD and ChAT.

aspect of the striatum in this age group (FIGURE 2B). Decreases in ChAT activity were more extensive in the 26-month-old group, which showed a marked reduction in selected medial regions, especially at the caudal levels (7470–5910). In contrast, reductions in ChAT activity were manifested in only half as many lateral striatal regions (FIGURE 2B). Thus, the age-related changes in the striatum were not ubiquitous, but were confined to discrete regions. FIGURE 3 shows the distribution of glutamic acid decarboxylase (GAD) activity (the enzyme that synthesizes GABA). This figure serves to illustrate that the pattern of distribution of each neurotransmitter system in the neostriatum is unique. The distribution of GAD was markedly different from that of ChAT. Furthermore, there were no age-related decreases in GAD. Because both ChAT and GAD were measured in portions of the same tissue punches, it is unlikely that decreases in ChAT were the result of nonspecific factors such as changes in tissue composition.

One explanation for the age-linked decline in ChAT is that the neurochemical change is secondary to cell loss. Indeed, reduced numbers of neurons and synapses occur in the neostriatum of old rats and mice (see references 10 and 54–56; also see McNeill in this volume). We tested this hypothesis using high-affinity sodium-dependent choline uptake (HACU) as an indirect measure of the number of cholinergic neurons. Like ChAT, HACU is a specific marker for cholinergic neurons, particularly the axon terminal.[57] In addition, HACU is the rate-limiting step in the formation of acetylcholine and, therefore, it may be a better indicator of the functional capacity of the neuron.[58] Because the National Institute on Aging discontinued the Sprague Dawley rat strain

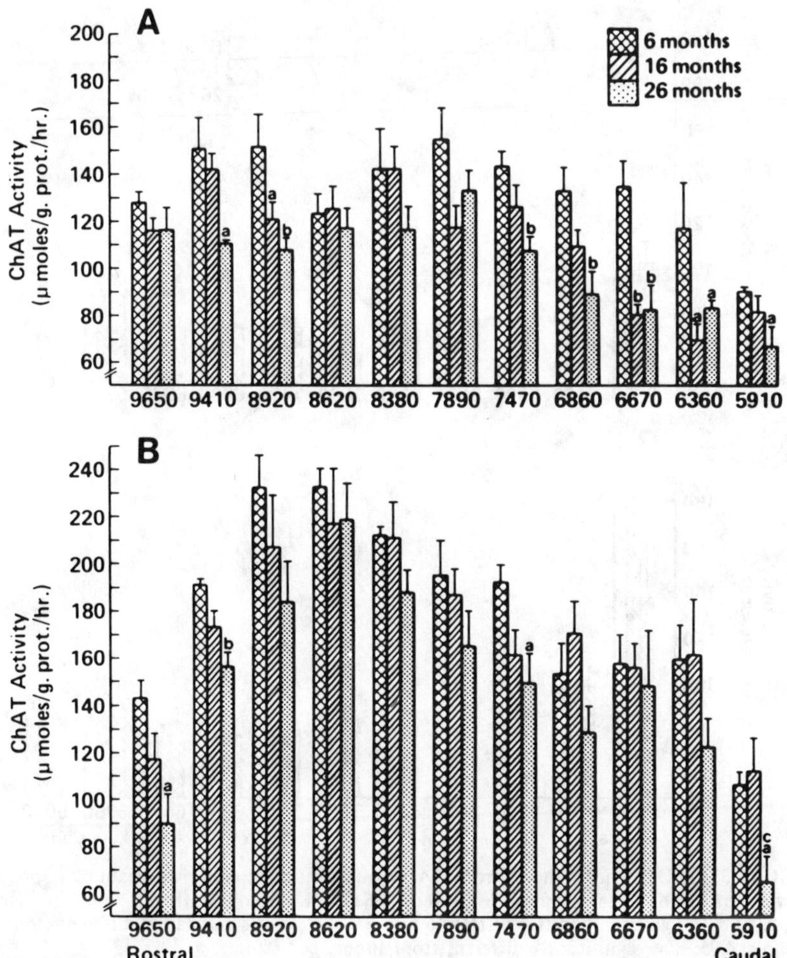

FIGURE 2. ChAT activity in the centromedial (A) and centrolateral (B) neostriatum of Sprague Dawley rats. Each value is the mean ± SEM of 3–6 rats: a = significantly different from 6 mo, $p < 0.05$; b = significantly different from 6 mo, $p < 0.01$; c = significantly different from 16 mo, $p < 0.05$; d = significantly different from 16 mo, $p < 0.01$.

from their contract colonies, we performed these experiments with Fischer 344 rats. We measured HACU in synaptosomes prepared from four regions of the neostriatum of three age groups of Fischer 344 rats (see FIGURE 4).[59] We also assayed ChAT activity because age differences in this parameter may be strain- and species-dependent.[11,60,61] Moreover, if decreases in HACU result from cell loss, then ChAT should be reduced by the same amount.

The pattern of distribution of HACU and ChAT in the striatum of the Fischer 344 rat (FIGURES 5 and 6) was comparable to that of ChAT in the Sprague Dawley

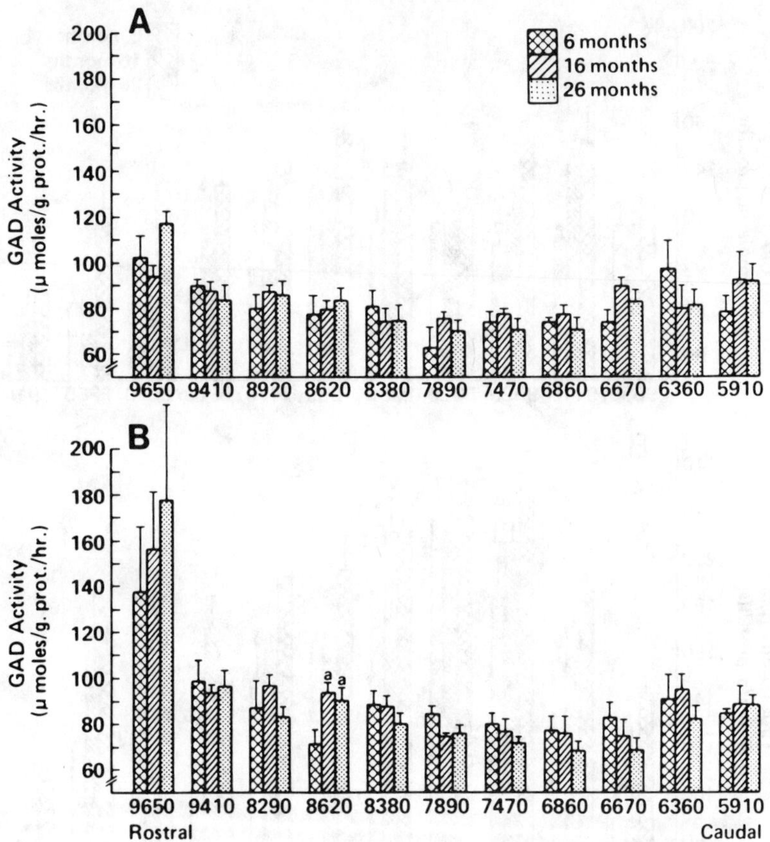

FIGURE 3. GAD activity in the centromedial (A) and centrolateral (B) neostriatum of Sprague Dawley rats. Each value is the mean ± SEM of 3–6 rats: a = significantly different from 6 mo, $p < 0.05$; b = significantly different from 6 mo, $p < 0.01$; c = significantly different from 16 mo, $p < 0.05$; d = significantly different from 16 mo, $p < 0.01$.

rat (FIGURE 2). Both cholinergic markers were higher laterally than medially and there was a rostrocaudal gradient for both markers in the medial regions. Age-related decreases in HACU were also regionally dependent. Significant age-correlated decreases in HACU were restricted to the rostromedial and caudolateral striatum (TABLE 1 and FIGURE 5). However, in contrast to findings in Sprague Dawley rats (FIGURE 2), ChAT did not differ between age groups (FIGURE 6). This is taken as evidence that the decrease in HACU was not due to the loss of cholinergic neurons. The lack of change in ChAT in the Fischer 344 rat is in accord with a previous study using this rat strain.[60] The difference between the results for Fischer 344 and Sprague Dawley rats agrees with studies showing that the effect of age on ChAT is species- and strain-dependent.[11,60,61]

The changes in HACU in Fischer 344 rats probably reflect regionally selective decreases in the activity of cholinergic neurons *in vivo*. It is well established that ex-

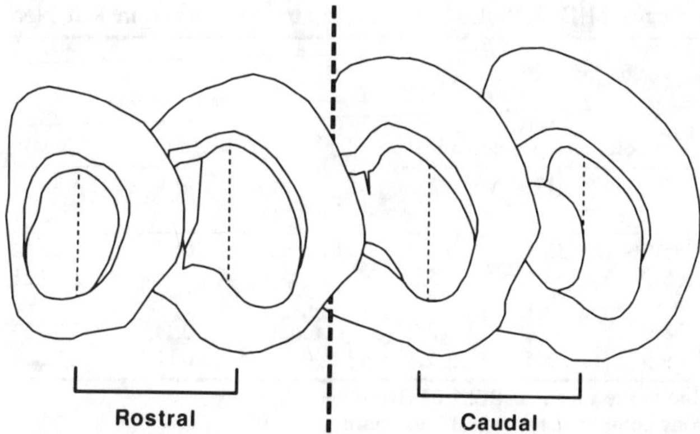

FIGURE 4. The anterior and posterior extent of each of two fresh tissue sections (rostral and caudal) from which striatal tissue was dissected from Fischer 344 rats to make synaptosomes. The striatum was bisected (dotted line) into medial and lateral parts and then carefully dissected from the surrounding tissue.

perimental conditions that affect the activity of cholinergic neurons *in vivo* alter HACU *in vitro*. Thus, it was suggested that *in vitro* HACU is useful as a measure of *in vivo* cholinergic activity.[62] The age-associated decreases in HACU may reflect decreases in the activity of cholinergic neurons in response to regionally selective changes in afferent neurotransmitter systems.

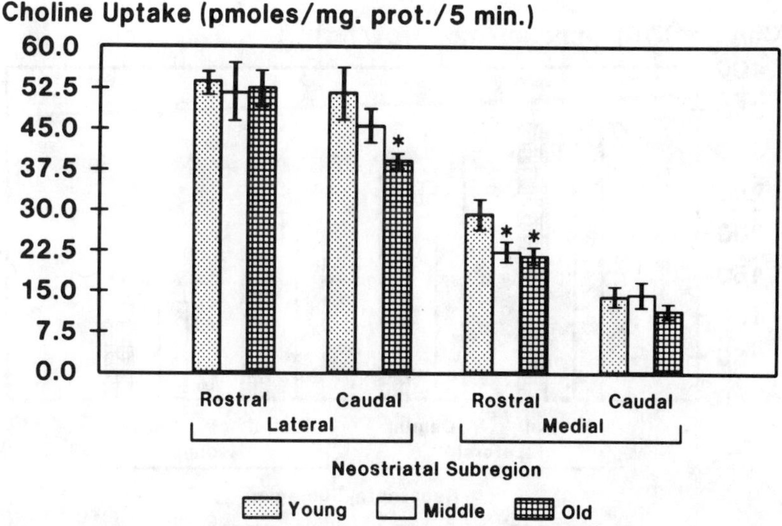

FIGURE 5. Distribution of sodium-dependent, high-affinity choline uptake in striatum of Fischer 344 rats. Values are the mean ± SEM of 7–8 individual determinations performed in triplicate. All medial-lateral differences were significant ($p < 0.05$). All rostrocaudal differences in the medial striatum were significant ($p < 0.05$). The asterisk stands for significantly different from the six-month-old group, $p < 0.05$.

TABLE 1. Regional Distribution of ³H-Dopamine Uptake in Rat Neostriatum

	V_{max} (pmoles/mg protein/min)				K_t (μM)		
					Age (months)		
Region	7	17	27	Region	7	17	27
Rostral	45.2 ± 5.9	53.4 ± 6.3	41.4 ± 5.5	Rostral	0.105 ± 0.008	0.142 ± 0.021	0.109 ± 0.013
Caudal	38.0[b] ± 9.9	34.0[b] ± 5.5	28.2[b] ± 5.4	Caudal	0.115 ± 0.004	0.120 ± 0.009	0.110 ± 0.13

[a] Each value is the mean ± SEM of five determinations.
[b] $p < 0.05$ as compared to rostral neostriatum.

We also measured the density of muscarinic cholinergic receptors in striatal regions in three age groups of Sprague Dawley rats (FIGURE 7) and in striatal regions of Fischer 344 rats (FIGURE 4).[59,63] The distribution of receptors was similar for the two rat strains and corresponded with the other markers of the cholinergic system (FIGURES 8 and 9). Age-related decreases in binding were detected in both strains of rats (TABLE 1 and FIGURES 8 and 9). However, the two strains differed in the regional distribution of the age changes. Binding in the oldest Fischer rats was about 20% less than that in the youngest group in each region of the striatum (FIGURE 9). In contrast, age differ-

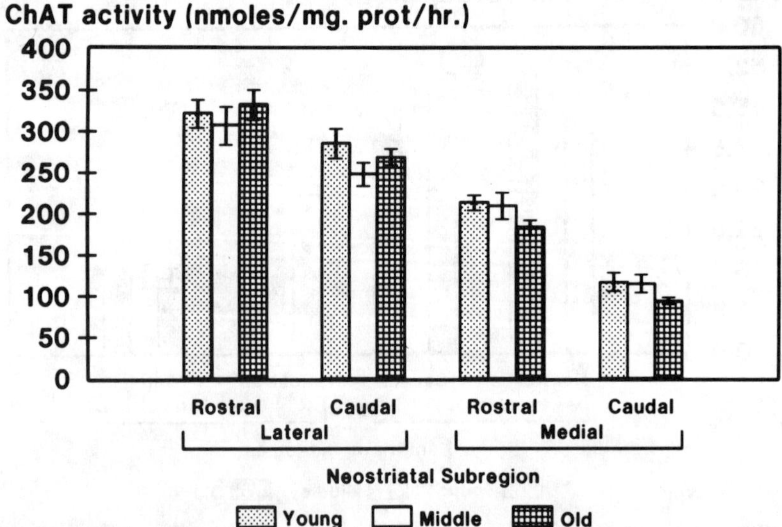

FIGURE 6. Distribution of choline acetyltransferase activity in striatum of Fischer 344 rats. Values are the mean ± SEM of 7–8 individual determinations performed in duplicate. All medial-lateral differences were significant ($p < 0.05$). All rostrocaudal differences in the medial striatum were significant ($p < 0.05$).

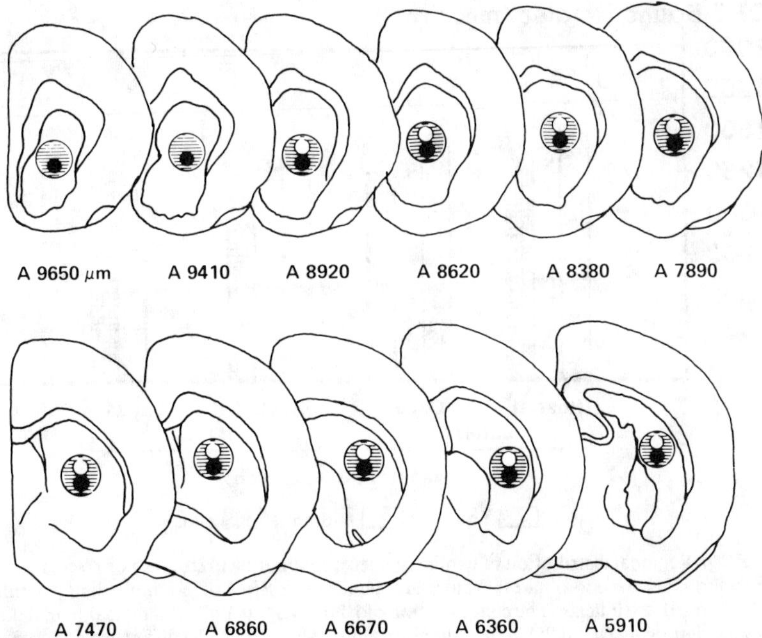

FIGURE 7. Coordinates (according to Konig and Klippel[68]) of serial frontal sections through the neostriatum of Sprague Dawley rats. The light circles represent punches removed for tyrosine hydroxylase assays. The dark circles represent punches that were removed for measuring [³H]QNB binding. The hatched circles represent sites where tissue was removed for [³H]spiroperidol binding assays.

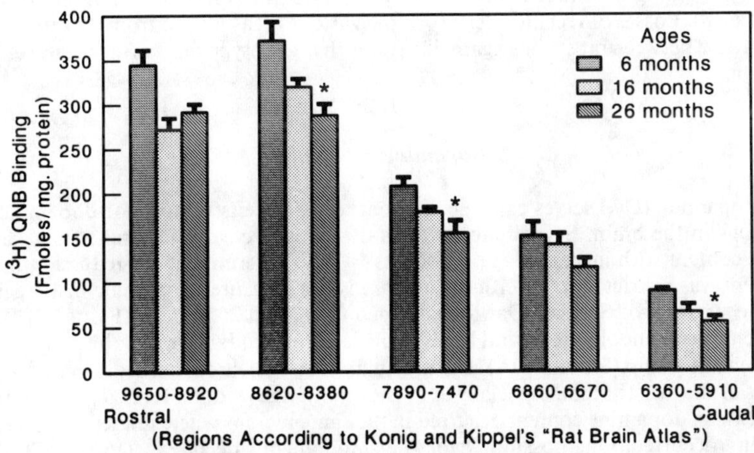

FIGURE 8. Regional distribution of cholinergic muscarinic receptor binding in striatum of Sprague Dawley rats (refer to FIGURE 7 for coordinates). Each value represents the mean ± SEM of 6 individual determinations in duplicate. The concentration of [³H]QNB was 0.15 nM. The asterisk stands for significantly different from the youngest age group, $p < 0.05$.

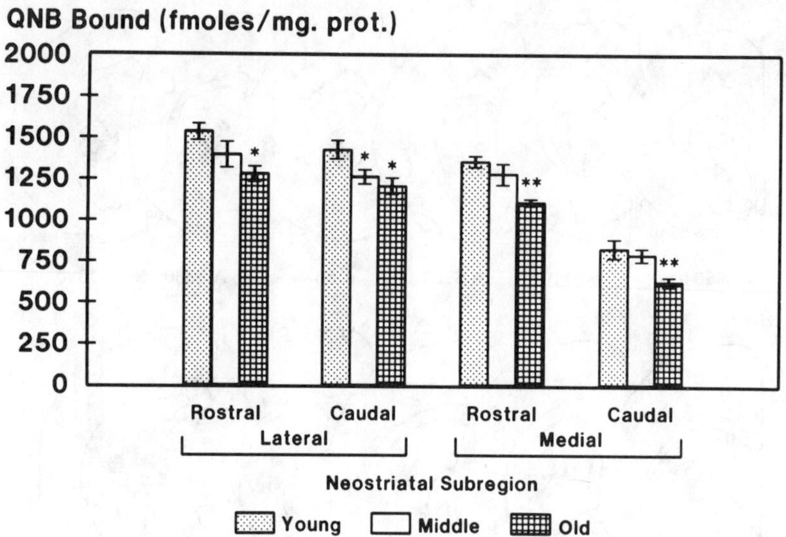

FIGURE 9. Regional distribution of cholinergic receptor binding in striatum of Fischer 344 rats (refer to FIGURE 4 for coordinates). Values are the mean ± SEM of 7–8 individual determinations performed in triplicate. The concentration of [³H]QNB was 1 nM. All medial-lateral differences were significant ($p < 0.05$) in the caudal striatum. All rostrocaudal differences in the medial striatum were significant ($p < 0.05$). (* stands for significantly different from the 6-month-old group, $p < 0.05$; ** stands for significantly different from the 6- and 18-month-old groups, $p < 0.05$.)

ences in binding in Sprague Dawley rats were regionally variable within the striatum (FIGURE 8). Losses of receptor density in the various areas ranged from 0 to 50%. This difference between rat strains again illustrates that genotype may influence the effects of aging.

Dopaminergic System

Dopamine (DA) serves as a specific marker of the distribution of dopaminergic neurons in the brain. Several laboratories observed decreases in total striatal dopamine content with increased age in rodents.[8,9,19] To determine if the reduction in DA content was restricted to specific striatal areas, we measured dopamine in 11 regions of the striatum of Sprague Dawley rats aged 6, 16, and 26 months (FIGURE 1).[53] DA content was higher in the rostral levels relative to the caudal levels of the neostriatum in each age group (FIGURE 10A). During aging, DA decreased markedly in the caudal levels of the neostriatum, especially at 26 months of age (FIGURE 10A). The age-related decrease in dopamine content occurred in the same regions where reductions in ChAT activity occurred. One possibility for the simultaneous decline in DA and ChAT is that there is a nonspecific loss of neuronal elements in this brain region. We measured noradrenaline (NA) in the same tissue punches used to measure dopamine and we found that the distribution of NA was more homogeneous within the striatum than dopamine (FIGURE 10B). NA was slightly, but significantly higher in the three most rostral

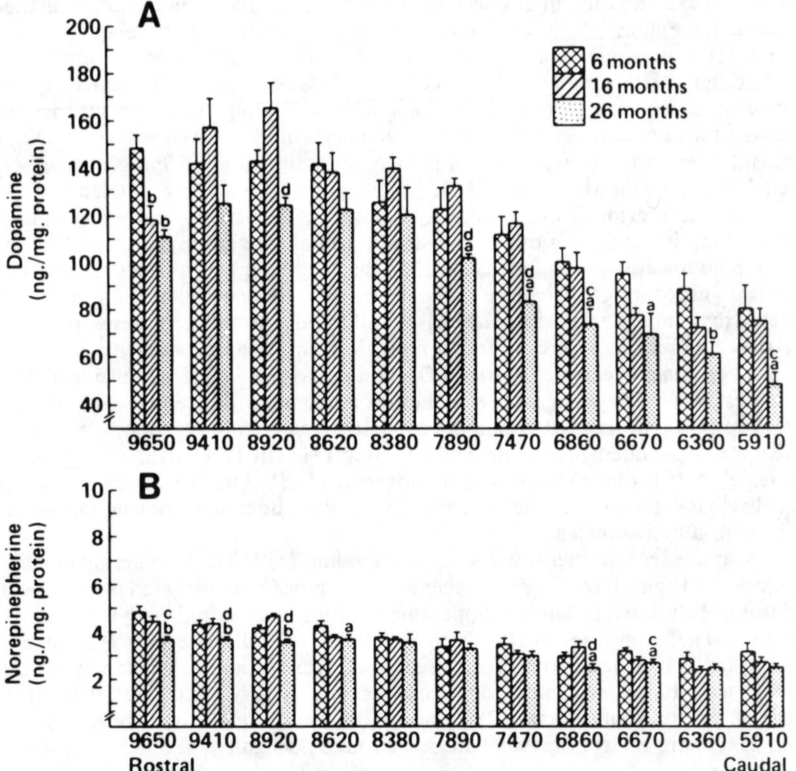

FIGURE 10. Dopamine and norepinephrine levels in the striatum of Sprague Dawley rats (refer to FIGURE 1 for coordinates). Each value is the mean ± SEM of 4–6 rats: a = significantly different from 6 mo, $p < 0.05$; b = significantly different from 6 mo, $p < 0.01$; c = significantly different from 16 mo, $p < 0.05$; d = significantly different from 16 mo, $p < 0.01$.

regions as compared to the three most caudal regions. This again illustrates the uniqueness of the neurochemical topography of each neurotransmitter system in the striatum. However, contrary to the findings for DA, NA was affected by aging primarily in the four most rostral areas (FIGURE 10B). This provided evidence that decreases in DA did not arise from nonspecific factors.

A possible cause of age-associated decreases in dopamine content is degeneration of dopamine-containing axon terminals. To determine if this explained our results, ·we used DA accumulation by synaptosomes as a measure of the functional integrity of dopaminergic axon terminals. High-affinity sodium-dependent DA uptake was measured in synaptosomes prepared from rostral and caudal striatum of rats aged 7, 17, and 27 months.[64] Data in TABLE 1 show that the apparent number of DA uptake sites (V_{max}) was greater in the rostral striatum as compared to the caudal striatum. These data are in agreement with the findings on distribution of DA. However, neither the apparent number of uptake sites (V_{max}) nor the transport affinity (K_t) differed between age groups. These findings agree with those of Thompson *et al.*,[65] who reported that the rate and amount of DA accumulation by rat striatal slices remained unaltered by aging. It is unlikely, therefore, that age-related reductions in dopamine content resulted from fewer axon terminals or reduced capacity for reuptake of released neurotransmitter.

Another possible reason for the age-related loss of dopamine is reduced tyrosine hydroxylase. Tyrosine hydroxylase (TH) is the rate-limiting enzyme in the metabolic pathway for dopamine. A decrease in its activity would result in reduced dopamine content. Therefore, we measured TH in eight striatal regions of Sprague Dawley rats aged 7, 17, and 27 months (FIGURE 7).[63] The regions chosen corresponded to regions where we had previously measured DA (FIGURE 1). TH activity was higher in rostral regions than in caudal regions of the striatum in all age groups (FIGURE 11). There was a trend toward age-related decreases in the caudal regions of the striatum. However, a significant age difference was detected in only one region (FIGURE 11). It is noteworthy that the areas where decreases and trends toward decreases were detected are the same regions where we found reductions in dopamine content.

An age-related decrease in striatal DA and no change in TH was also reported by Demarest *et al.*[66] They concluded that the lack of change in TH represented a compensatory response to reduced dopamine content. Experimentally induced decreases in catecholamine content are followed by increased TH activity relative to catecholamine content.[37,66] This phenomenon was first observed in Parkinson's disease.[45] Increases in TH activity may compensate for decreases in striatal dopamine content during aging, at least to a limited extent.

Dopamine receptor density is affected by aging.[12,22-24] Most studies on dopamine receptors and aging have measured receptors in homogenates prepared from the whole striatum. We wanted to know if dopamine receptor loss during aging is restricted to specific striatal subregions. We thus measured butaclamol-displaceable [³H]spiroperidol binding in tissue punches from five consecutive frozen sections of striatum (see FIGURE 7).[63] As with dopamine content, dopamine receptor density was greatest in the rostral areas of the striatum (FIGURE 12). However, although trends toward decreases (less than 25%) were evident in several areas, we found no significant differences between

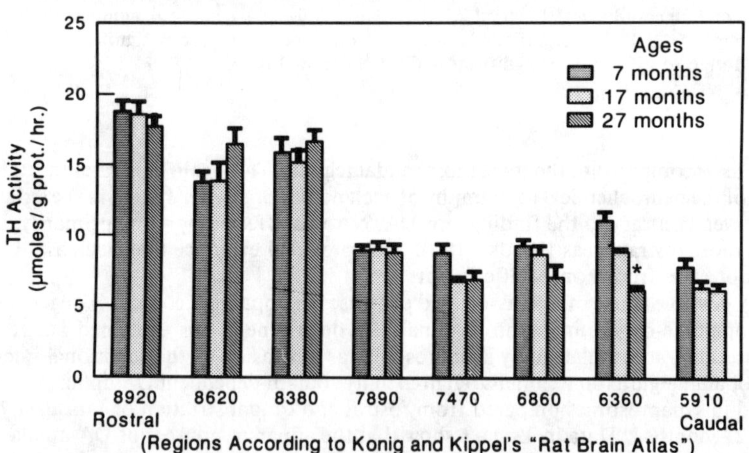

FIGURE 11. Regional distribution of tyrosine hydroxylase activity in striatum of Sprague Dawley rats (refer to FIGURE 7 for coordinates). Each value represents the mean ± SEM of six animals per group. The asterisk stands for significantly different from the six-month-old group, $p < 0.05$.

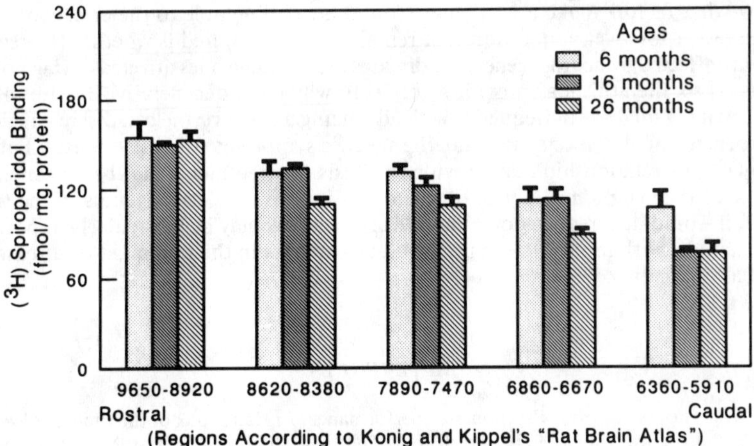

FIGURE 12. Regional distribution of dopamine receptor binding in striatum of Sprague Dawley rats (refer to FIGURE 7 for coordinates). Each value represents the mean ± SEM of six animals per group. The concentration of [³H]spiroperidol was 0.2 nM.

age groups in any area (FIGURE 12). These results are in contrast to many studies carried out on whole striatum. However, one recent aging study used quantitative dopamine receptor autoradiography to search for regional differences in striatum of Fischer 344 rats.[67] They found that the age-associated loss (30–60%) of dopamine receptors was restricted to the lateral caudal region of the striatum. This region showed the densest binding in young rats. We failed to sample that area using the tissue punch scheme in our study. Therefore, it is highly probable that we failed to find evidence for decreases in dopamine receptors because we did not examine the affected areas.

SUMMARY

Presynaptic and postsynaptic markers of the cholinergic and dopaminergic systems have characteristic topographical distributions within the striatum. Aside from the dopaminergic afferents, several other afferent systems exhibit a heterogeneous distribution in the striatum. The net result is that each part of the striatum receives a specific and unique combination of afferents. Moreover, the intrinsic striatal systems also have unique distributions, so each part of the striatum consists of a unique combination of afferent and intrinsic neurotransmitter systems. In view of these points, one may expect that the striatum is functionally very complex, integrating information from a wide variety of brain areas. One may also assume from these facts that the striatum is a functionally heterogeneous structure. Consistent with that conclusion, behavioral and pharmacological studies show that interruption of neurotransmission in localized regions of the striatum produces very specific behavioral and physiological effects.

Age-related neurochemical changes are also confined to specific striatal regions. Which regions are affected will depend on a variety of factors, including the neurochemical parameter studied and the species or strain of animal. However, we still do not know what factors make a particular striatal area vulnerable to the effects of aging or disease. Moreover, a question that remains to be answered is whether the regions that are affected by neurodegenerative diseases are the same ones affected during normal aging. If so, then this may provide a clue as to why neurodegenerative diseases of the basal ganglia increase in frequency with advancing age. Nevertheless, discrete regional neurochemical alterations may underlie specific symptoms of these diseases. Further study of this relationship may provide the basis for treatments that better target the source of the symptoms. Not only would this increase the effectiveness of the treatment, it would help reduce potential side effects. This may be particularly important, for example, with respect to the use of tissue explants in the treatment of diseases of the basal ganglia.

REFERENCES

1. WELFORD, A. T. 1959. Psychomotor performance. *In* Handbook of the Biology of Aging and the Individual. J. E. Birren, Ed.: 562–613. Univ. of Chicago Press. Chicago.
2. ALLEN, S. J., J. S. BENTON, M. J. GOODHARDT, E. A. HAAN, N. R. SIMS, C. C. T. SMITH, J. A. SPILLANE, D. M. BOWEN & A. M. DAVISON. 1983. Biochemical evidence of selective nerve cell changes in the normal aging human and rat brain. J. Neurochem. **41:** 256–265.
3. SCHEIBEL, A. B. 1981. The gerohistology of the aging human forebrain: Some structuro-functional considerations. *In* Brain Neurotransmitters and Receptors in Aging and Age-Related Disorders. S. J. Enna, T. Samorajski & B. Beer, Eds.: 31–42. Raven Press. New York.
4. SCHEIBEL, M. E., U. TOMIYOSA & A. B. SCHEIBEL. 1977. The aging human betz cell. Exp. Neurol. **56:** 598–609.
5. ENNA, S. J. & R. STRONG. 1981. Age-related alterations in central nervous system neurotransmitter receptor binding. *In* Brain Neutrotransmitters and Receptors in Aging and Age-Related Disorders. S. J. Enna, T. Samorajski & B. Beer, Eds.: 31 –42. Raven Press. New York.
6. ROGERS, J., M. A. SILVER, W. J. SHOEMAKER & F. E. BLOOM. 1980. Senescent changes in a neurobiological model system: Cerebellar Purkinje cell electrophysiology and correlative anatomy. Neurobiol. Aging **1:** 3–11.
7. KENDALL, D. A., R. STRONG & S. J. ENNA. 1982. *In* Modifications of Rat Brain GABA Receptor Binding as a Function of Age. A. Giacobini, G. Filogama & A. Vernadakis, Eds.: 211–221. Raven Press. New York.
8. FINCH, C. E., P. K. RANDALL & J. F. MARSHALL. 1981. Aging and basal gangliar functions. Ann. Rev. Gerontol. Geriatr. **2:** 47–49.
9. OSTERBURG, H. H., H. G. DONAHUE, J. A. SEVERSON & C. E. FINCH. 1981. Catecholamine levels and turnover during aging in brain regions of male C57Bl/6J mice. Brain Res. **161:** 303–310.
10. BUGIANI, O., S. SALVARINI, F. PERDELLI, G. L. MANCARDI & A. LEONARDI. 1978. Nerve cell loss with aging in the putamen. Eur. Neurol. **17:** 286–291.
11. STRONG, R., P. HICKS, L. HSU, R. T. BARTUS & S. J. ENNA. 1980. Age-related alterations in the rodent brain cholinergic system and behavior. Neurobiol. Aging **1:** 59–63.
12. SEVERSON, J. A., J. MARCUSSON, B. WINBLAD & C. E. FINCH. 1982. Age-correlated loss of dopaminergic binding sites in human basal ganglia. J. Neurochem. **39:** 1623–1631.
13. KRAMER, J. & H. L. KLAWANS. 1979. Involuntary movement disorders—each has a meaning of its own. Geriatrics **34:** 63–71.
14. CRITCHLEY, M. 1956. Neurologic changes in the aged. J. Chr. Dis. **3:** 459–477.
15. CRANE, G. E. 1968. Tardive dyskinesia in patients treated with chronic neuroleptics. Am. J. Psychiatry **124:** 40–48.
16. AYD, F. J. 1961. A survey of drug induced extrapyramidal reactions. J. Am. Med. Assoc. **175:** 1054–1060.

17. KLETT, C. J. & E. CAFFEY. 1972. Evaluating the long-term need for antiparkinson's drugs by chronic schizophrenics. Arch. Gen. Psychiatry **26**: 374–379.

18. RANDALL, P. K. 1980. Functional aging of the nigro-striatal system. Peptides **1**: 177–184 (suppl. 1).

19. PRADHAN, S. N. 1980. Minireview: Central neurotransmitters and aging. Life Sci. **26**: 1643–1656.

20. STRONG, R. 1985. Neurochemistry of aging: 1982–1984. *In* Review of Biological Research in Aging. M. Rothstein, Ed.: 181–196. Alan R. Liss. New York.

21. HICKS, P., R. STRONG, J. C. SCHOOLAR & T. SAMORAJSKI. 1980. Aging alters amphetamine-induced stereotyped gnawing and neostriatal elimination of amphetamine in mice. Life Sci. **27**: 715–722.

22. JOSEPH, J. A., R. E. BERGER, B. T. ENGLE & G. S. ROTH. 1978. Age-related changes in the nigrostriatum: a behavioral and biochemical analysis. J. Gerontol. **33**: 643–649.

23. MARSHALL, J. F. & N. BERRIOS. 1979. Movement disorders of aged rats: reversal by dopamine receptor stimulation. Science **206**: 477–479.

24. CUBELLS, J. F. & J. A. JOSEPH. 1981. Neostriatal dopamine receptor loss and behavioral deficits in the senescent rat. Life Sci. **28**: 1215–1218.

25. REDGRAVE, P. & I. MITCHELL. 1982. Functional validation of projection topography in the nigrostriatal dopamine system. Neuroscience **7**: 885–894.

26. GUYENET, P., C. EUVARD, F. JAVOY, A. HERBET & J. GLOWINSKI. 1977. Regional differences in the sensitivity of cholinergic neurons to dopaminergic drugs and quipazine in the rat striatum. Brain Res. **136**: 487–500.

27. PAZO, J. H. & J. H. MEDINA. 1983. Cholinergic mechanisms within the caudate nucleus mediate changes in blood pressure. Neuropharmacology **22**: 717–720.

28. FONNUM, F., Z. GOTTESFELD & I. GRAFOVA. 1978. Distribution of glutamate decarboxylase, cholineacetyltransferase and aromatic amino acid decarboxylase in the basal ganglia of normal and operated rats. Evidence for striatopallidal, striatoentopeduncular and striatonigral GABAergic fibers. Brain Res. **143**: 125–138.

29. SCALLY, M. C., I. H. ULUS, R. J. WURTMAN & D. J. PETTIBONE. 1978. Regional distribution of neurotransmitter-synthesizing enzymes and substance P within the rat corpus striatum. Brain Res. **143**: 556–560.

30. REA, M. A. & J. R. SIMON. 1981. Regional distribution of cholinergic parameters within the rat striatum. Brain Res. **219**: 317–326.

31. GRAYBIEL, A. M., C. W. RAGSDALE, E. S. YONEOKA & R. P. ELDE. 1981. An immuno-histochemical study of enkephalins and other neuropeptides in the striatum of the cat with evidence that the opiate peptides are arranged to form mosaic patterns in register with the striosomal compartments visible by acetylcholinesterase staining. Neuroscience **6**: 377–397.

32. CARTER, C. J. 1982. Topographical distribution of possible glutamatergic pathways from the frontal cortex to the striatum and substantia nigra in rats. Neuropharmacology **21**: 379–383.

33. TAKANO, Y., K. UCHIMURA, Y. KOHJIMOTO & H. O. KAMIYA. 1981. Properties and distribution of muscarinic cholinergic receptors in rat striatal micropunched tissue homogenates. Eur. J. Pharmacol. **70**: 559–564.

34. TAKANO, Y., K. UCHIMURA, Y. KOHJIMOTO & H. O. KAMIYA. 1980. Mapping of the distribution of high affinity choline uptake and choline acetyltransferase in the striatum. Brain Res. **194**: 583–587.

35. PRADO-ALCALA, R. A., F. BERMUDEZ-RATTONI, D. N. VELAZQUEZ-MARTINEZ & M. G. BACHA. 1978. Cholinergic blockade of the caudate nucleus and spatial alternation performance in rats: overtraining induced protection against behavioral deficits. Life Sci. **23**: 889–896.

36. DUNNETT, S. B. & S. D. IVERSEN. 1982. Sensorimotor impairments following localized kainic acid and 6-hydroxydopamine lesions of the striatum. Brain Res. **248**: 121–127.

37. SNYDER, A. M., E. M. STRICKER & M. J. ZIGMOND. 1985. Stress-induced neurological impairments in an animal model of parkinsonism. Ann. Neurol. **18**: 544–551.

38. DUNNETT, S. & S. D. IVERSEN. 1982. Regulatory impairments following selective 6-OHDA lesions of the neostriatum. Behav. Brain Res. **4**: 195–202.

39. MASON, S. T., P. F. SANBERG & H. C. FIBIGER. 1978. Kainic acid lesions of the striatum dissociate amphetamine and apomorphine stereotypy: Similarities to Huntington's chorea. Science **201:** 352–355.

40. NEILL, D. B. & C. L. LINN. 1975. Deficits in consummatory responses to regulatory challenges following basal ganglia lesions in rats. Physiol. Behav. **14:** 617–624.

41. NEILL, D. B. & S. P. GROSSMAN. 1970. Behavioral effects of lesions or cholinergic blockade of the dorsal and ventral caudate of cats. J. Comp. Physiol. Psychol. **71:** 311–317.

42. McGEER, P. L., E. G. McGEER & H. C. FIBIGER. 1973. Choline acetylase and glutamic acid decarboxylase in Huntington's chorea. A preliminary study. Neurology **23:** 912–917.

43. McGEER, P. L. & E. G. McGEER. 1976. Enzymes associated with the metabolism of catecholamines, acetylcholine and GABA in human controls and patients with Parkinson's disease and Huntington's chorea. J. Neurochem. **26:** 65–76.

44. AQUILONIUS, S. M., S. A. ECKERNIS & A. SUNDWALL. 1975. Regional distribution of choline acetyltransferase in the human brain: Changes in Huntington's chorea. J. Neurol. Neurosurg. Psychiatry **38:** 669–677.

45. BERNHEIMER, H., W. BIRKMAYER, O. HORNYKIEWICZ, K. JELLINGER & F. SEITLBIRGER. 1973. Brain dopamine and the syndrome of Parkinson and Huntington. Clinical, morphological and neurochemical correlates. J. Neurosurg. Sci. **20:** 61–67.

46. GASPAR, P., F. JAVOY-AGID, A. PLOSKA & Y. AGID. 1980. Regional distribution of neurotransmitter synthesizing enzymes in the basal ganglia of human brain. J. Neurochem. **34:** 278–283.

47. VEENING, J. G., F. M. CORNELISSEN & P. A. J. M. LIEVEN. 1980. The topical organization of the afferents to the caudatoputamen of the rat. A horseradish peroxidase study. Neuroscience **5:** 1253–1268.

48. TAQUET, H., F. JAVOY-AGID, M. HAMON, J. C. LEGRAND, Y. AGID & F. CESSELIN. 1983. Parkinson's disease affects differently met- and leu-enkephalin in the human brain. Brain Res. **280:** 379–382.

49. FONNUM, F. 1973. Recent developments in biochemical investigations of cholinergic transmission. Brain Res. **62:** 497–507.

50. MEEK, J. L., L. BERTILSSON, D. L. CHENEY, G. ZSILLA & E. COSTA. 1977. Aging induced changes in acetylcholine and serotonin content of discrete brain nuclei. J. Gerontol. **32:** 129–131.

51. LAI, J. C. K., T. K. C. LEING & L. LIM. 1981. Brain regional distribution of glutamic acid decarboxylase, choline acetyltransferase and acetylcholinesterase in the rat. Effects of chronic manganese chloride administration after two years. J. Neurochem. **36:** 1443–1448.

52. McGEER, E. G., H. C. FIBIGER, P. L. McGEER & V. WICKSON. 1971. Aging and brain enzymes. Exp. Gerontol. **6:** 391–396.

53. STRONG, R., T. SAMORAJSKI & Z. GOTTESFELD. 1982. Regional mapping of neostriatal neurotransmitter systems as a function of aging. J. Neurochem. **39:** 831–836.

54. BRIZZEE, K. R., T. SAMORAJSKI, R. C. SMITH & D. L. BRIZZEE. 1981. The effect of age and chronic neuroleptic drug treatment on cell populations in the neostriatum of Fischer 344 rats. *In* Brain Neurotransmitters and Receptors in Aging and Age-Related Disorders. S. J. Enna, T. Samorajski & B. Beer, Eds.: 59–80. Raven Press. New York.

55. MENSAH, P. 1979. The effects of aging on neuron "cell islands" in mouse striatum. Proc. Soc. Neurosci. **5:** 76.

56. BRIZZEE, K. R., T. SAMORAJSKI, D. L. BRIZZEE, J. M. ORDY, W. DUNLAP & R. C. SMITH. 1983. Age pigments and cell loss in the mammalian nervous system: Functional implications. *In* Brain Aging: Neuropathology and Neuropharmacology. J. Cervos-Navarro & H-I. Sarkander, Eds.: 211–229. Raven Press. New York.

57. YAMAMURA, H. I. & S. H. SNYDER. 1972. Choline: High affinity uptake by synaptosomes. Science **178:** 626–628.

58. SIMON, J. R., S. ATWEH & M. J. KUHAR. 1976. Sodium-dependent high affinity choline uptake: A regulatory step in the synthesis of acetylcholine. J. Neurochem. **26:** 909–922.

59. STRONG, R., C. REHWALDT & W. G. WOOD. 1986. Intra-regional variations in the effect of aging on high-affinity choline uptake, choline acetyltransferase and muscarinic cholinergic receptors in rat neostriatum. Exp. Gerontol. **21:** 177–186.

60. REIS, D. J., R. A. ROSS & T. H. JOH. 1977. Changes in the activities and amounts of en-

zymes synthesizing catecholamines and acetylcholine in the brain, adrenal medulla and sympathetic ganglia of aged rat and mouse. Brain Res. **64:** 345–353.

61. WALLER, S. B., D. K. INGRAM, M. A. REYNOLDS & E. D. LONDON. 1983. Age and strain comparisons of neurotransmitter synthetic enzyme activities in the mouse. J. Neurochem. **41:** 1421–1428.

62. ATWEH, S., J. R. SIMON & M. J. KUHAR. 1976. Utilization of sodium-dependent high affinity choline uptake *in vitro* as a measure of the activity of cholinergic neurons *in vivo*. Life Sci. **17:** 1535–1544.

63. STRONG, R., J. C. WAYMIRE, T. SAMORAJSKI & Z. GOTTESFELD. 1984. Regional analysis of neostriatal cholinergic and dopaminergic receptor binding and tyrosine hydroxylase activity as a function of aging. Neurochem. Res. **9:** 1641–1652.

64. STRONG, R., T. SAMORAJSKI & Z. GOTTESFELD. 1984. High-affinity uptake of neurotransmitters in rat neostriatum: Effects of aging. J. Neurochem. **43:** 1766–1768.

65. THOMPSON, J. M., J. R. WHITTAKER & J. A. JOSEPH. 1981. [³H]Dopamine accumulation and release from striatal slices in young, mature and senescent rats. Brain Res. **224:** 436–440.

66. DEMAREST, K. T., G. D. REIGLE & K. E. MOORE. 1980. Characteristics of dopamine neurons in the aged male rat. Neuroendocrinology **31:** 222–227.

67. JOYCE, J. N., S. K. LOESCHEN, D. W. SAPP & J. F. MARSHALL. 1986. Age-related regional loss of caudate-putamen dopamine receptors revealed by quantitative autoradiography. Brain Res. **378:** 158–163.

68. KONIG, J. F. R. & R. A. KLIPPEL. 1963. The Rat Brain: A Stereotaxic Atlas of the Forebrain and Lower Parts of the Brain Stem. Krieger. Huntington, New York.

DISCUSSION OF THE PAPER

G. S. ROTH (*NIA, Baltimore, MD*): There are a couple of questions that those of us who deal with the striatal dopamine receptors have been concerned with—one is whether the mechanism is by means of cell loss and another one is where exactly are the D-2 receptors localized; that is, are they on the cholinergic interneurons or are they on the neurons projected to the cortex? Assuming that a substantial portion of these receptors are on the cholinergic interneurons, would you conclude that at least part of the change in dopamine receptors is not due to cell loss based on your data?

R. STRONG (*Veterans Administration Medical Center, St. Louis, MO*): Yes, the changes in dopamine receptors may be due to other factors. It is well known that there are changes in membranes with aging. The membrane becomes more rigid (at least in certain preparations). In addition, the change in the physical state of the membrane may affect the expression (or the insertion perhaps) of receptors into the membrane.

Agonist Binding to Striatal Dopamine Receptors in Aging

The Ternary Complex of Receptor and Guanine Nucleotide Binding Regulatory Protein

JAMES A. SEVERSON[a] AND RICHARD E. WILCOX[b]

[a]Amersham Corporation
Arlington Heights, Illinois 60005

[b]Department of Pharmacology
College of Pharmacy
University of Texas
Austin, Texas 78712

INTRODUCTION

Early theoretical studies[1,2] offered models of receptor action to explain receptor binding patterns that differed from those expected from mass-action principles. These models proposed that (a) some receptors and their limited effectors were separate entities with mobility in the plane of the membrane, and (b) receptor-effector complexes associated and transduced extracellular signals into intracellular events only when the receptor was activated by agonist. Such models were confirmed for the hepatic glucagon receptor[3] and the β-adrenergic receptor systems.[4] Present evidence suggests that all hormones and neurotransmitters that modulate adenylate cyclase activity through cell-surface receptors act through a ternary complex of agonist, receptor, and transducing element.[3,5]

It is known that the transducing effector-associated proteins are guanine nucleotide binding regulatory proteins (G-proteins). G-proteins that regulate adenylate cyclase are referred to as Gs and Gi, respectively, for their stimulatory and inhibitory effects. However, other G-proteins are involved in other signal pathways, such as phototransduction, olfactory transduction, and receptor-mediated phosphatidylinositol hydrolysis.

In addition to regulation of adenylate cyclase activity, Gs and Gi also regulate agonist binding to receptors. Coupling of a receptor with an appropriate G-protein results in high-affinity (nM range) agonist binding. Conversely, in the absence of coupling to a G-protein, the receptor maintains a low affinity for agonists (μM range) (reviewed in references 4–6). Physiologic and biochemical studies support the high-affinity agonist binding complex of agonist, receptor, and G-protein as a physiologically relevant intermediate in receptor signal transduction.[5,7–11]

The description of dopamine (DA) receptors as D-1 and D-2 based on coupling or noncoupling, respectively, to adenylate cyclase[12] has been enhanced by a further subdivision based on the interaction of the receptor with G-proteins[13] and the apparent negative coupling of at least some D-2 receptors to adenylate cyclase.[14–16] The ternary complex model is consistent with these interactions; D-1 and D-2 DA receptors exist in either a high- or low-affinity agonist binding configuration that is dependent upon the presence or absence, respectively, of coupling of the receptor with its respective G-protein.[17,18]

Such general mechanisms imply that (a) the receptor does not define end-organ responsiveness exclusively, and (b) a second, membrane-bound factor must also be considered in biological response production. Thus, new questions must be formulated to address the molecular mechanisms that mediate age-related changes in biological response. These new questions include:

(1) What is the nature of the coupling mechanism between cell-surface receptors and the intracellular amplification system?

Transfer of the agonist signal across the membrane is initiated by high-affinity agonist binding, which is a product of the ternary complex. Age-associated changes in the interaction of receptor and G-protein could occur that are independent of a change in receptor number. Thus, investigation of the formation or dissociation of the ternary complex could indicate changes in signal transduction pathways that are not apparent from binding studies alone, particularly from antagonist binding profiles.

(2) How do changes in the signal transduction pathway affect the flow of information through the cascade amplifier system?

If changes in high-affinity agonist binding are observed in aging, functional studies are important to determine the impact of these changes on physiologic responses mediated by receptor stimulation.

(3) How do age-associated changes in receptor systems with complementary actions on signal transduction or amplification affect the regulation of physiologic function?

Different receptor types may regulate adenylate cyclase,[6,14,15] so changes in the enzymatic regulation by one factor may affect the balanced response of competing systems. For instance, age-related alterations in the proportion of D-1 to D-2 DA receptors are proposed to result in repetitive jaw movements in rats[19] that may be analogous to oral behaviors observed in humans with either age or long-term treatment with antipsychotics.

(4) What is the brain regional and neurotransmitter system specificity of age-related changes in the receptor-effector coupling mechanism?

Characterization of the interaction of receptors and G-proteins with age is the first step to determine if age-related changes in these mechanisms are a general observation or if they are restricted to specific neurotransmitter systems.

STRIATAL D-2 DA RECEPTORS

The D-2 DA receptor antagonist [3H]spiperone ([3H]SP) is recognized with equal affinity by both agonist binding components of the receptor; thus, this defines the entire population of D-2 receptors.[18,20] In contrast, dopaminergic [3H]agonists bind primarily to the high-affinity agonist binding component of the D-2 receptor and, under certain assay conditions, to the high-affinity agonist binding component of the D-1 receptor.[21] In addition, [3H]agonist binding to DA receptors is difficult to control.[22,23] Thus, displacement of labeled antagonist binding by an unlabeled agonist offers an alternative method to examine high-affinity agonist binding sites, along with the opportunity for simultaneous analysis of low-affinity sites that cannot be examined by direct binding methods.[24]

Displacement of [³H]SP binding by DA was modeled using LIGAND.[25] This interactive computer program derives least squares estimates of the affinities of binding sites for ligands and the concentrations of these sites using mass-action formulae[26] in a nonlinear model.[25,27] LIGAND operates on the assumption that receptor populations are independent (i.e., noninteractive) and obey Michaelis-Menten kinetics. Agonist binding configurations of the ternary complex probably do not conform to this assumption. However, our studies[28] and others[29] have compared [³H]agonist binding to high-affinity agonist binding derived by nonlinear regression analysis and they suggest that the data are comparable. In addition, within the experimental error observed in our studies, computer simulation studies[30] suggest that estimates obtained from two-site analysis are close approximations of the actual parameters.

DA displacement of [³H]SP binding to striatal homogenates from C57BL/6J mice (ages 3, 12, and 24 months) was best described by a two-site model. There were no age-related differences in the affinities of either site for DA: DA bound to the high-affinity site with a dissociation constant (K_H) of approximately 12 nM, while the low-affinity site had a K_L for DA of about 1200 nM (TABLE 1, FIGURE 1). These affinities are similar to those observed in young adult rat,[18,31–33] dog,[34] and calf[35,36] striatum using similar assay conditions and data analysis.

The percent of the total D-2 receptor population in the high-affinity agonist binding complex ($\%R_H$) was less in membranes from 12-month-old mice compared to 3-month-old mice and did not change between 12 and 24 months of age (TABLE 2). The density of R_L was also unchanged between 12 and 24 months of age. The density of R_L peaked at 12 months of age: R_L was 20% higher than at 3 months of age and declined between 12 and 24 months of age. The increase in the density of R_L between

TABLE 1. D-2 DA Receptor Affinities from One- and Two-Site Receptor Binding Analyses[a]

Age (months)	One-Site K_d (nM)	Two-Site K_H (nM)	K_L (nM)
3	200 ± 10	14 ± 4	1430 ± 360
12	190 ± 10	10 ± 2	980 ± 100
24	230 ± 20	14 ± 1	1220 ± 110

[a] Homogenates prepared from striata of two C57BL/6J mice were assayed in duplicate for [³H]SP binding (500 pM) in the presence of 20 concentrations of DA (10^{-9} to 10^{-4} M). Displacement curves were modeled to one- and two-site models; a two-site model significantly reduced the sums of squares of the deviations from regression in all curves.

The following parameters were estimated by nonlinear regression analysis:[25] equilibrium dissociation constants of the binding sites for DA (K_H and K_L), their respective capacities (R_H and R_L), and nonspecific binding of the radioligand. Curves were modeled first to a one-site model and then to a two-site model. The two-site model was accepted only if addition of the second site reduced the residual sums of squares of deviations from regression (as judged by a significant F-statistic).

Data are the geometric mean ± SEM of 13 individual determinations for 3- and 12-month-old mice and of 10 individual determinations for 24-month-old mice. Statistical significance was tested using Newman-Keuls' test for multiple comparisons. No significant differences were found.

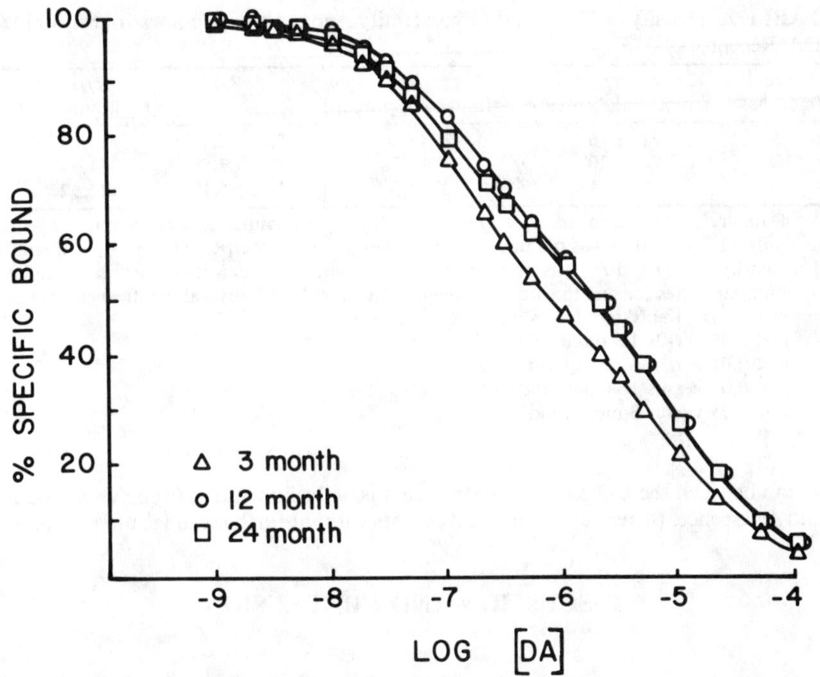

FIGURE 1. Displacement of striatal [³H]SP binding by DA. Data are the mean of the determinations summarized in TABLES 1 and 2. These curves were best described by a two-site model. Data are plotted as the percent of specific binding versus the logarithm of the concentration of DA. (Republished from *J. Pharmacol. Exp. Ther.* **233**: 361–368 (1985), by permission of the American Society for Pharmacology and Experimental Therapeutics.)

3 and 12 months of age may indicate that the relative decline in $\%R_H$ that occurred during this period was more rapid than the decline in total D-2 receptor density.

The maximum density (B_{max}) of [³H]SP binding to mouse striatal homogenates declined progressively with age; B_{max} was less in homogenates from 12-month-old mice compared to 3-month-old mice, and in homogenates from 24-month-old mice compared to 12-month-old mice (TABLE 3). Total D-2 receptor density, obtained by either Scatchard analysis (B_{max}) or the displacement analysis ($R_H + R_L$), was similar (TABLES 2 and 3). Similar to our previous data for the aging mouse,[38–40] there was no change in the equilibrium dissociation constant (K_d) with age (TABLE 3).

The decline of high-affinity agonist binding (R_H) before mid-life (and changing little thereafter) is consistent with the DA [³H]agonist binding observed by us[28] and others.[37] Striatal DA agonist binding declines more rapidly with age than antagonist binding in mouse, rabbit,[41] and human striatum[42] and is consistent with apparent independent loss of the receptor and the Gi (the G-protein that is required for high-affinity agonist binding to the D-2 receptor).[43,44]

Two mechanisms may act during aging to decrease apparent D-2 receptor binding: (a) before mid-life, there is a loss of D-2 receptors and a decline in the functional inter-

TABLE 2. Density of High- and Low-Affinity Agonist Binding Sites for Striatal D-2 DA Receptors[a]

Age (months)	R_H (fmole/mg protein)	R_L (fmole/mg protein)	$\%R_H$	$R_H + R_L$ (fmole/mg protein)
3	319 ± 16	270 ± 24^b	55.0 ± 2.7	589 ± 27
12	240 ± 20^c	324 ± 26	42.4 ± 2.8^c	564 ± 37
24	195 ± 31^c	232 ± 22^d	44.2 ± 5.1^e	$427 \pm 27^{b,d}$

[a] Data are arithmetic mean ± SEM of the number of individual assays given in the legend to FIGURE 1. The $\%R_H$ was obtained by the following equation: $[R_H/(R_H + R_L)] \times 100\%$. The density of R_H and R_L was obtained as the quotient of the density of each site estimated by nonlinear regression and the protein content of the sample.[72] Statistical significance was tested using Newman-Keuls' test for multiple comparisons.

[b] $p < 0.05$ versus 12-month-old mice.

[c] $p < 0.01$ versus 3-month-old mice.

[d] $p < 0.01$ versus 12-month-old mice.

[e] $p < 0.05$ versus 3-month-old mice.

action between the D-2 receptor and Gi, that is, a decline in R_H; (b) between mid-life and senescence, there is a loss of D-2 receptors without further change in $\%R_H$ or R_H.

DISCUSSION AND CONCLUSIONS

Mechanisms for Impaired Formation of the Ternary Complex

Binding studies such as those described here cannot determine the nature of the impaired coupling of D-2 receptor and G-protein in aged mouse striatum. This impairment could be the result of (a) an age-related loss of G-protein or (b) modifications of the receptor or G-protein that prevent formation of the high-affinity agonist binding complex.

However, computer modeling studies raise other questions relating to formation

TABLE 3. Scatchard Analysis of [³H]SP Binding Isotherms in Aged Mouse Striatal Membranes[a]

Age (months)	B_{max} (fmole/mg protein)	K_d (pM)
3	608 ± 20	82 ± 3
12	532 ± 17^b	79 ± 3
24	$459 \pm 38^{b,c}$	84 ± 4

[a] Binding isotherms were obtained by incubation of six concentrations of [³H]SP (30–1000 pM) in duplicate for total and nonspecific binding (2 μM d-butaclamol). Data were linearized by the Scatchard transformation[73] and the total binding density (B_{max}) and the equilibrium dissociation constant (K_d) were determined by least squares linear regression. Data are the arithmetic mean ± SEM for B_{max} and the geometric mean ± SEM for K_d of the number of individual experiments given in the legend to FIGURE 1. Statistical significance was tested using Newman-Keuls' test for multiple comparisons.

[b] $p < 0.01$ versus 3-month-old mice.

[c] $p < 0.05$ versus 12-month-old mice.

of high-affinity agonist binding complexes: (a) is the concentration of G-protein a limiting factor in signal transduction?; and (b) are the effects of age on receptor density greater than the effects on G-protein?

If the concentration of G-protein initially is less than that of the receptor, a decrease in receptor concentration without an accompanying change in the concentration of the G-protein results in a decrease in the $\%R_H$.[30,45] Thus, the decrease in $\%R_H$ that we observe with age (TABLE 2) may reflect primarily a decrease in total receptor density and, hence, a reduced coupling to Gi rather than an actual decrease in the concentration of Gi. Alternatively, in reconstitution studies,[46] G-protein in excess of the concentration of receptor is required for full expression of high-affinity agonist binding and the percent of high-affinity agonist binding is directly proportional to the concentration of G-protein. In that case, the decrease in $\%R_H$ that we observed with age (TABLE 2) may reflect limiting association kinetics for formation of the ternary complex[47,48] plus the documented decrease in D-2 receptor density (TABLES 2 and 3) rather than an actual decrease in G-protein. Finally, our data and those of Haga *et al.*[46] are compatible with either an age-associated reduction in total D-2 receptor density alone or in combination with a decrease in the concentration of Gi.

The implication that G-protein may be limiting for formation of the ternary complex is surprising given the above-cited papers and findings of a molar excess of G-proteins in brain.[49,50] However, Gi that is accessible to D-2 receptors may be limited by cellular content or by cellular compartmentalization. Cellular content is a plausible explanation; in some cultured cell lines, Gi may be limiting for formation of high-affinity agonist binding complexes with receptors.[51] An alternative possibility raised in reconstitution studies is that the receptor activates multiple Gi molecules as part of the signal amplification system[52] so that a molar excess of G-protein is required for a fully functional response system.

These data suggest that the measurement of total striatal Gi content may quantitate gross changes in Gi with age, but probably would not detect changes in Gi accessible to D-2 receptors. An alternative approach would be to measure high-affinity agonist binding in homogenates from aged mice after addition of purified Gi. This indirect approach might determine if additional Gi can increase high-affinity agonist binding to the level seen in the young. A similar approach reconstituted receptor-effector coupling to cultured cells in which Gi had been inactivated.[53]

Receptor-Effector Coupling

Coupling of striatal D-1 receptors to adenylate cyclase appears to be enhanced in postmortem samples of caudate nucleus and nucleus accumbens from schizophrenics.[54] However, platelets derived from schizophrenic patients have decreased adenylate cyclase response to prostaglandin E_1 (PGE_1),[55,56] which is a defect that appears to involve signal transduction from the receptor rather than a change in receptor number. If consonant, these data suggest a disease-associated imbalance of complementary modulator systems. Similar deficits in PGE_1-stimulated adenylate cyclase activity occur in platelets from individuals with unipolar depression.[57] In addition, α_2-adrenergic receptor inhibition of PGE_1-stimulation of adenylate cyclase activity is impaired in unipolar depression even though there is no change in α_2-adrenergic receptor density. Thus, the adenylate cyclase response to receptor stimulation is affected independent of change in receptor density.

In aged rat heart[58] and leukocytes from aged humans,[59] the density of β-adrenergic receptors does not change with age; however, stimulation of adenylate cyclase by β-

receptor agonists is impaired. Complementation of Gs-deficient cyc⁻ S49 lymphoma cells with Gs derived from young and aged heart suggests 25% less Gs in this organ in aged rats.[58] Thus, the reduced cardiac cascade with age appears to be due to impaired β-adrenergic receptor-effector coupling. In contrast, complementation assays suggest normal concentrations of Gs in lymphocytes from aged humans, but with impaired catalytic unit activity of the adenylate cyclase enzyme.[60]

The β-adrenergic receptor displacement by the agonist isoproterenol indicates fewer high-affinity agonist binding sites on human lymphocytes during aging without change in total β-receptor density.[59] Muscarinic cholinergic receptors form fewer high-affinity agonist binding complexes (dependent upon coupling to Gi[46,52]) in aged heart even though there is no change in the density of muscarinic cholinergic receptors with age.[62] This is similar to the effects of age on β-adrenergic receptors and the coupling to Gs. As a result, inhibition of β-adrenergic receptor-stimulated adenylate cyclase activity by muscarinic agonists is impaired.[63]

Inhibition of acetylcholine release from striatal slices by apomorphine is mediated by D-2 receptors that are located on striatal nerve terminals.[64,65] The age-related pattern of that inhibition[66] differs from that of D-2 high-affinity agonist binding: decreased inhibition of acetylcholine release was found only between mid-life and old age; no changes were found prior to mid-life. Thus, impaired regulation of neurotransmitter release mediated by the high-affinity agonist binding state of the D-2 dopamine receptor may occur during aging because of reduced efficiency of receptor-effector coupling on striatal DA target neurons. However, further studies are required to determine the extent of age-related changes in receptor responses mediated by the ternary complex of the D-2 receptor and Gi.

To summarize, changes in signal transduction pathways mediated by Gs and Gi occur in several psychiatric conditions and in aging. As predicted by modeling studies, impaired receptor-effector coupling decreases the physiologic responses mediated by receptor stimulation. The lack of an apparent trend in the available data suggests that age-related changes in the interaction of G-proteins and receptors may be both tissue-dependent and receptor-dependent. Alternatively, a similar sequence of age-associated changes may occur within a number of mediator systems, but these are masked by the limited age span typically examined (3 to 24 months). Thus, receptor-effector coupling changes (reflected in decreased functional response and decreased $\%R_H$) may always occur prior to detectable decreases in total receptor number.

Localization of Age Changes in Striatal DA Receptors

The decline in high-affinity agonist binding to D-2 receptors (R_H) and other age-related declines in striatal DA [³H]agonist binding[28,37,38,41,42] may be localized to D-2 receptors on neurons with cell bodies intrinsic to the striatum. D-2 receptors are localized to striatal intrinsic neurons and projection neurons, and to the glutamatergic projection from the cerebral cortex.[17,67] The high-affinity component of the DA displacement of striatal [³H]SP binding was eliminated after striatal kainic acid lesions,[68] while agonist binding after frontal cortical deafferentation[69-71] was unaltered. These data suggest that high-affinity agonist binding to the D-2 receptor on frontal cortical neurons terminating in the striatum does not occur, even though about 35% of the striatal [³H]SP B_{max} is localized to this projection in the mouse.[70]

Data Analysis

The suggestion arises from this discussion: Why not analyze the data using the correct biological and mathematical model? This question is reasonable, particularly because the ternary complex equations would estimate the G-protein that is available to the receptor. Unfortunately, modeling studies suggest that modeling of receptor binding displacement curves to the ternary complex equations does not give reliable results when only one displacement curve is analyzed.[30]

Another approach may be the simultaneous analysis of a family of curves generated from a single tissue homogenate,[45] with the concentration of GTP and age as variables in the analysis. The combination of multiple curves, and the dissociation of the ternary complex by increasing concentrations of GTP, would favor more precise estimation of the dissociation constants for the reactions of the ternary complex. These experiments are feasible given current technology, but would be five times larger than the present experiments that were analyzed by the two-site model.

Conclusions

We can return to the questions posed in the introduction:

(1) What is the nature of the coupling mechanism?

High-affinity agonist binding to striatal D-2 DA receptors declines with age. However, not all receptor systems that act through G-proteins have impaired formation of high-affinity agonist binding complexes with age.

(2) How do changes in the signal transduction pathway affect the flow of information through the cascade?

Initial reports suggest that changes in high-affinity agonist binding may result in impaired response, but more data are required. The regulation of striatal cyclic AMP production by D-1 and D-2 receptors[14-16] would extend the initial studies by inclusion of the interaction of the two receptor sites.

(3) How do changes in competing receptor systems affect the regulation of physiological function?

Few data are available, but the initial suggestion is that receptor regulatory patterns are altered by changes in the ratios of equi-effective agonist concentrations in competing receptor-effector systems. This represents a promising area for continued experimentation.

(4) What is the specificity of age-related changes in the coupling mechanism?

Examples of impaired coupling are available from a number of receptor systems that use both Gs and Gi. Thus, receptor coupling to G-proteins is another major factor to consider in cellular responsiveness with age.

REFERENCES

1. BOEYNAEMS, J. M. & J. E. DUMONT. 1975. Quantitative analysis of the binding of ligands to their receptors. J. Cyclic Nucleotide Res. **1:** 123–142.

2. JACOBS, S. & P. CUATRECASAS. 1976. The mobile receptor hypothesis and "cooperativity" of hormone binding: Application to insulin. Biochim. Biophys. Acta **433:** 482–495.

3. RODBELL, M. 1980. The role of hormone receptors and GTP regulatory proteins in membrane transduction. Nature (London) **284:** 17–22.

4. LEFKOWITZ, R. J., J. M. STADEL & M. G. CARON. 1983. Adenylate cyclase-coupled beta-adrenergic receptors: Structure and mechanisms of activation and deactivation. Annu. Rev. Biochem. **52:** 159–186.

5. LIMBIRD, L. E. 1984. GTP and Na$^+$ modulate receptor adenyl cyclase coupling and receptor-mediated function. Am. J. Physiol. **247** (Endocrinol. Metab. **10**): E59–E68.

6. BIRNBAUMER, L., J. CODINA, R. MATTERA, R. A. CERIONE, J. D. HILDEBRANDT, T. SUNYER, F. J. ROJAS, M. G. CARON, R. J. LEFKOWITZ & R. IYENGAR. 1985. Regulation of hormone receptors and adenylyl cyclases by guanine nucleotide binding N proteins. Recent Progr. Horm. Res. **41:** 41–99.

7. KENT, R. S., A. DELEAN & R. J. LEFKOWITZ. 1980. A quantitative analysis of beta-adrenergic receptor interactions: Resolution of high and low affinity states of the receptor by computer modeling of ligand binding data. Mol. Pharmacol. **17:** 14–23.

8. DELEAN, A., B. F. KILPATRICK & M. G. CARON. 1982. Dopamine receptor of the anterior pituitary gland: Evidence for two affinity states discriminated by both agonists and antagonists. Mol. Pharmacol. **22:** 290–297.

9. MCDONALD, W. M., D. R. SIBLEY, B. F. KILPATRICK & M. G. CARON. 1984. Dopaminergic inhibition of adenylate cyclase correlates with high affinity agonist binding to anterior pituitary D$_2$ dopamine receptors. Mol. Cell. Endocrinol. **36:** 201–209.

10. GEORGE, S. R., M. WATANABE, T. DIPAOLO, P. FALARDEAU, F. LABRIE & P. SEEMAN. 1985. The functional state of the dopamine receptor in the pituitary is in the high affinity form. Endocrinology **117:** 690–697.

11. BORGUNDVAAG, B. & S. R. GEORGE. 1985. Dopamine inhibition of anterior pituitary adenylate cyclase is mediated through the high-affinity state of the D$_2$ receptor. Life Sci. **37:** 379–386.

12. KEBABIAN, J. W. & D. B. CALNE. 1979. Multiple receptors for dopamine. Nature (London) **277:** 93–96.

13. CREESE, I., D. R. SIBLEY & S. E. LEFF. 1984. Agonist interactions with dopamine receptors: Focus on radioligand binding studies. Fed. Proc. Fed. Am. Soc. Exp. Biol. **43:** 2779–2784.

14. STOOF, J. C. & J. W. KEBABIAN. 1981. Opposing roles for D-1 and D-2 dopamine receptors in efflux of cyclic AMP from rat neostriatum. Nature (London) **294:** 366–368.

15. STOOF, J. C. & J. W. KEBABIAN. 1982. Independent *in vitro* regulation by the D-2 dopamine receptor of dopamine-stimulated efflux of cyclic AMP and K$^+$-stimulated release of acetylcholine from rat neostriatum. Brain Res. **250:** 263–270.

16. BATTAGLIA, G., A. B. NORMAN, E. J. HESS & I. CREESE. 1985. D$_2$ dopamine receptor-mediated inhibition of forskolin-stimulated adenylate cyclase activity in rat striatum. Neurosci. Lett. **59:** 177–182.

17. CREESE, I., D. R. SIBLEY, M. W. HAMBLIN & S. E. LEFF. 1983. The classification of dopamine receptors: Relationship to radioligand binding. Annu. Rev. Neurosci. **6:** 43–71.

18. HAMBLIN, M. W., S. E. LEFF & I. CREESE. 1984. Interactions of agonists with D-2 dopamine receptors: Evidence for a single receptor population existing in multiple agonist affinity-states in rat striatal membranes. Biochem. Pharmacol. **33:** 877–887.

19. ROSENGARTEN, H., J. W. SCHWEITZER & A. J. FRIEDHOFF. 1986. Selective dopamine D$_2$ receptor reduction enhances a D$_1$ mediated oral dyskinesia in rats. Life Sci. **39:** 29–35.

20. HUFF, R. M. & P. B. MOLINOFF. 1982. Quantitative determination of dopamine receptor subtypes not linked to activation of adenylate cyclase in rat striatum. Proc. Natl. Acad. Sci. (USA) **79:** 7561–7565.

21. HAMBLIN, M. W. & I. CREESE. 1982. ^{3}H-Dopamine binding to rat striatal D-2 and D-3 sites: Enhancement by magnesium and inhibition by guanine nucleotides and sodium. Life Sci. **30:** 1587–1595.

22. HADJICONSTANTINOU, M. & N. H. NEFF. 1983. Ascorbic acid could be hazardous to your experiments: a commentary on dopamine receptor binding studies with speculation on a role for ascorbic acid in neuronal function. Neuropharmacology **22:** 939–943.

23. HEIKKILA, R. E., F. S. CABBAT & L. MANZINO. 1983. Stereospecific binding of ^{3}H-dopamine

in neostriatal membrane preparations: inhibitory effects of sodium ascorbate. Life Sci. **32:** 2183–2191.

24. BENNETT, J. P., JR. & H. I. YAMAMURA. 1985. Neurotransmitter, hormone or drug receptor binding methods. *In* Neurotransmitter Receptor Binding (2nd edition). H. I. Yamamura, S. J. Enna & M. J. Kuhar, Eds.: 61–89. Raven Press. New York.

25. MUNSON, P. J. & D. RODBARD. 1980. LIGAND: A versatile computerized approach for characterization of ligand binding systems. Anal. Biochem. **107:** 220–239.

26. FELDMAN, H. A. 1982. Mathematical theory of complex ligand-binding systems at equilibrium: Some methods for parameter fitting. Anal. Biochem **48:** 317–338.

27. DeLEAN, A., A. A. HANCOCK & R. J. LEFKOWITZ. 1982. Validation and statistical analysis of a computerized modeling method for quantitative analysis of radioligand binding data for mixtures of pharmacological receptor subtypes. Mol. Pharmacol. **21:** 15–16.

28. SEVERSON, J. A. & P. K. RANDALL. 1985. D-2 dopamine receptors in aging mouse striatum: Determination of high- and low-affinity agonist binding sites. J. Pharmacol. Exp. Ther. **233:** 361–368.

29. SIBLEY, D. R., L. C. MAHAN & I. CREESE. 1983. Dopamine receptor binding on intact cells: Absence of high-affinity agonist-receptor binding state. Mol. Pharmacol. **23:** 295–302.

30. ABRAMSON, S. N., P. McGONIGLE & P. B. MOLINOFF. 1987. Evaluation of models for analysis of radioligand binding data. Mol. Pharmacol. **31:** 103–111.

31. SOKOLOFF, P., M. P. MARTRES & J. C. SCHWARTZ. 1980. Three classes of dopamine receptor (D-2, D-3, D-4) identified by binding studies with ^{3}H-apomorphine and ^{3}H-domperidone. Naunyn-Schmiedebergs Arch. Pharmacol. **315:** 89–102.

32. SIBLEY, D. R., S. E. LEFF & I. CREESE. 1982. Interactions of novel dopaminergic ligands with D-1 and D-2 dopamine receptors. Life Sci. **31:** 637–645.

33. MARTRES, M. P., P. SOKOLOFF, M. DELANDRE, J. C. SCHWARTZ, P. PROTIAS & J. COSTENIN. 1984. Selection of dopamine antagonists discriminating various behavioral responses and radioligand binding sites. Naunyn-Schmiedebergs Arch. Pharmacol. **325:** 102–115.

34. LEFF, S. E. & I. CREESE. 1982. Solubilization of D-2 dopamine receptors from canine caudate: Agonist occupation stabilizes guanine nucleotide sensitive receptor complexes. Biochem. Biophys. Res. Commun. **108:** 1150–1157.

35. WREGGETT, K. A. & P. SEEMAN. 1984. Agonist high- and low-affinity states of the D_2-dopamine receptor in calf brain: partial conversion by guanine nucleotides. Mol. Pharmacol. **25:** 10–17.

36. DE KEYSER, J., J-P. DEBACKER, A. CONVENTS, G. EBINGER & G. VAUQUELIN. 1985. D_2 dopamine receptors in calf globus pallidus: Agonist high- and low-affinity sites not regulated by guanine nucleotide. J. Neurochem. **45:** 977–979.

37. LEVIN, P., J. JANDA, J. A. JOSEPH, D. K. INGRAM & G. S. ROTH. 1981. Dietary restriction retards the age-associated loss of rat striatal dopaminergic receptors. Science (Wash., D.C.) **214:** 516–562.

38. SEVERSON, J. A. & C. E. FINCH. 1980. Reduced dopaminergic binding during aging in the rodent striatum. Brain Res. **192:** 147–162.

39. RANDALL, P. K., J. A. SEVERSON & C. E. FINCH. 1981. Aging and the regulation of striatal dopaminergic mechanisms in mice. J. Pharmacol. Exp. Ther. **219:** 695–700.

40. RANDALL, P. K., J. A. SEVERSON, S. M. HURD & W. O. McCLURE. 1985. Effect of duration of haloperidol treatment on dopamine receptor supersensitization in aging C57BL/6J mice. Brain Res. **333:** 85–95.

41. THAL, L. J., S. G. HOROWITZ, B. DVORKIN & M. H. MAKMAN. 1980. Evidence for loss of brain [^{3}H]spiroperidol and [^{3}H]ADTN binding sites in rabbit brain with aging. Brain Res. **192:** 185–194.

42. SEVESON, J. A., J. MARCUSSON, B. WINBLAD & C. E. FINCH. 1982. Age-correlated loss of dopaminergic binding sites in human basal ganglia. J. Neurochem. **39:** 1623–1631.

43. KUNO, T., O. SHIRAKAWA & C. TANAKA. 1983. Selective decrease in the affinity of D_2 dopamine receptor for agonist induced by islet-activating protein, pertussis toxin, associated with ADP-ribosylation of the specific protein of bovine striatum. Biochem. Biophys. Res. Commun. **115:** 325–330.

44. FUJITA, N., M. NAKAHIRO, I. FUKUCHI, K. SAITO & H. YOSHIDA. 1985. Effects of pertussis toxin on D_2 dopamine receptor in rat striatum: Evidence for coupling of Ni regulatory protein with D_2-receptor. Brain Res. **333:** 231–236.

45. WREGGETT, K. A. & A. DeLEAN. 1984. The ternary complex model: Its properties and application to ligand interactions with the D_2 dopamine receptor of the anterior pituitary gland. Mol. Phamacol. **26:** 214–227.

46. HAGA, K., T. HAGA & A. ICHIYAMA. 1986. Reconstitution of the muscarinic acetylcholine receptor: Guanine nucleotide-sensitive high affinity binding of agonists to purified muscarinic receptors reconstituted with GTP-binding proteins (G_1 and G_0). J. Biol. Chem. **261:** 10133–10140.

47. DeLEAN, A., J. M. STADEL & R. J. LEFKOWITZ. 1980. A ternary complex model explains agonist-specific binding properties of the adenylate cyclase-coupled β-adrenergic receptor. J. Biol. Chem. **255:** 7108–7117.

48. SIBLEY, D. R. & I. CREESE. 1983. Regulation of ligand binding to pituitary D-2 dopamine receptors. Effects of divalent cations and functional group modification. J. Biol. Chem. **258:** 4957–4965.

49. STERNWEIS, P. C. & J. D. ROBISHAW. 1984. Isolation of two proteins with high affinity for guanine nucleotides from membranes of bovine brain. J. Biol. Chem. **259:** 13806–13813.

50. GIERSCHIK, P., G. MILLIGAN, M. PINES, P. GOLDSMITH, J. CODINA, W. KLEE & A. SPIEGEL. 1986. Use of specific antibodies to quantitate the guanine nucleotide-binding protein G_0 in brain. Proc. Natl. Acad. Sci. (USA) **83:** 2258–2262.

51. MILLIGAN, G., P. GIERSCHIK, A. M. SPIEGEL & W. A. KLEE. 1986. The GTP-binding regulatory proteins of neuroblastoma × glioma, NG108-15, and glioma, C6, cells. FEBS Lett. **195:** 225–230.

52. KUROSE, H., T. KATADA, T. HAGA, K. HAGA, A. ICHIYAMA & M. UI. 1986. Functional interaction of purified muscarinic receptors with purified inhibitory guanine nucleotide regulatory proteins reconstituted in phospholipid vesicles. J. Biol. Chem. **261:** 6423–6428.

53. HIGASHIDA, H., R. A. STREATY, W. KLEE & M. NIRENBERG. 1986. Bradykinin-activated transmembrane signals are coupled via N_0 or N_1 to production of inositol 1,4,5-trisphosphate, a second messenger in NG108-15 neuroblastoma-glioma hybrid cells. Proc. Natl. Acad. Sci. (USA) **83:** 942–946.

54. MEMO, M., J. E. KLEINMAN & I. HANBAUER. 1983. Coupling of dopamine D_1 recognition sites with adenylate cyclase in nuclei accumbens and caudatus of schizophrenics. Science (Wash., D.C.) **221:** 1304–1307.

55. GARVER, D. L., C. JOHNSON & D. R. KANTER. 1982. Schizophrenia and reduced cyclic AMP production: Evidence for the role of receptor-linked events. Life Sci. **31:** 1987–1992.

56. KAFKA, M. S. & D. P. VAN KAMMEN. 1983. α-Adrenergic receptor function in schizophrenia. Arch. Gen. Psychiatry **40:** 264–270.

57. KAFKA, M. S., J. I. NURNBERGER, L. SIEVER, S. TARGUM, T. W. UHDE & E. S. GERSHON. 1986. Alpha₂-adrenergic receptor function in patients with unipolar and bipolar affective disorders. J. Affective Disorders **10:** 163–169.

58. O'CONNER, S. W., P. J. SCARPACE & I. B. ABRASS. 1983. Age-associated decrease in the catalytic unit activity of rat myocardial adenylate cyclase. Mech. Ageing Dev. **21:** 357–363.

59. FELDMAN, R. D., L. E. LIMBIRD, J. NADEAU, D. ROBERTSON & A. J. J. WOOD. 1984. Alterations in leukocyte β-adrenergic affinity with aging. A potential explanation for altered β-adrenergic sensitivity in the elderly. N. Engl. J. Med. **310:** 815–819.

60. ABRASS, I. B. & P. J. SCARPACE. 1982. Catalytic unit of adenylate cyclase: Reduced activity in aged-human lymphocytes. J. Clin. Endocrinol. Metab. **55:** 1026–1028.

61. LIANG, B. T., M. R. HELLMICH, E. J. NEER & J. B. GALPER. 1986. Development of muscarinic cholinergic inhibition of adenylate cyclase in embryonic chick heart: Its relationship to changes in the inhibitory guanine nucleotide regulatory protein. J. Biol. Chem. **261:** 9011–9021.

62. BAKER, S. P., S. MARCHAND, E. O'NEIL, C. A. NELSON & P. POSNER. 1985. Age-related changes in cardiac muscarinic receptors: Decreased ability of the receptor to form a high affinity agonist binding state. J. Gerontol. **40:** 141–146.

63. NARAYANAN, N. & L. TUCKER. 1986. Autonomic interactions in the aging heart: Age-associated decrease in muscarinic cholinergic receptor mediated inhibition of β-adrenergic activation of adenylate cyclase. Mech. Ageing Dev. **34:** 249–259.

64. KAMAL, L. A., S. ARBILLA & S. Z. LANGER. 1981. Presynaptic modulation of the release

of dopamine from the rabbit caudate nucleus: Differences between electrical stimulation, amphetamine and tyramine. J. Pharmacol. Exp. Ther. **216:** 592–598.

65. HOFFMANN, I. S. & L. X. CUBBEDU. 1984. Differential effects of bromocriptine on dopamine and acetylcholine release modulatory receptors. J. Neurochem. **42:** 278–282.

66. THOMPSON, J. M., C. L. MAKINO, J. R. WHITAKER & J. A. JOSEPH. 1984. Age-related decrease in apomorphine modulation of acetylcholine release from rat striatal slices. Brain Res. **299:** 169–173.

67. SEEMAN, P. 1980. Brain dopamine receptors. Pharmacol. Rev. **32:** 229–313.

68. CREESE, I., T. USDIN & S. H. SNYDER. 1979. Guanine nucleotides distinguish between two dopamine receptors. Nature (London) **278:** 577–578.

69. FUXE, K., H. HALL & C. KÖHLER. 1979. Evidence for an exclusive localization of [3H]-ADTN binding sites to postsynaptic nerve cells in the striatum of the rat. Eur. J. Pharmacol. **58:** 515–517.

70. SEVERSON, J. A. & P. K. RANDALL. 1983. Localization of [3H]N-propylnorapomorphine binding in mouse striatum. Brain Res. **279:** 295–298.

71. HALL, M. D., P. JENNER, E. KELLY & C. D. MARSDEN. 1983. Differential anatomical location of [3H]-*N,n*-propylnorapomorphine and [3H]spiperone binding sites in the striatum and substantia nigra of the rat. Br. J. Pharmacol. **79:** 599–610.

72. BRADFORD, M. M. 1976. A rapid and sensitive method for the quantification of microgram quantities of protein utilizing the principle of protein-dye binding. Anal. Biochem. **72:** 248–254.

73. SCATCHARD, G. 1949. The attractions of proteins for small molecules and ions. Ann. N.Y. Acad. Sci. **51:** 660–672.

DISCUSSION OF THE PAPER

A. ALTAR (*CIBA–GEIGY Corporation, Summit, NJ*): In the last slide, you showed that treatment ahead of time with an agonist increased the proportion of low-affinity sites and decreased the proportion of high-affinity sites. What reaction do you think occurs as a result of the normal age-related loss of the endogenous ligand for the dopamine receptor? How about for dopamine itself? Do you also think that these 20–30% losses of dopamine could in some way shift the proportion of these sites to a lower affinity site?

J. SEVERSON (*Amersham Corporation, Arlington Heights, IL*): The argument would probably be in the opposite direction. There is evidence from some *in vivo* work done in humans where lymphocytes are obtained from individuals and high-affinity beta-agonist binding is measured (as well as cyclase itself). The data show that if the individual is allowed to rest overnight in a clinical ward in a hospital and blood is drawn before the individual has a chance to get up in the morning, then somewhere around 40% high-affinity beta binding can be obtained. However, if you allow the individual to stand up and walk around for 30 minutes or so, the plasma norepinephrine doubles and the percent of beta receptors goes down by half.

In elderly individuals, though, that shift does not occur; you cannot force them down any farther. Thus, if there is indeed loss of dopamine in the caudate with age, that loss is occurring in the opposite direction. You might, though, expect a compensatory reaction for an increased number of high-affinity agonist binding sites.

ALTAR: I would be surprised if that occurred because you normally need such a large dopamine loss to induce an increase in the high-affinity component of D-2 binding.

SEVERSON: No one has demonstrated that a loss of dopamine in a lesion paradigm or even in a chronic drug treatment paradigm increases high-affinity agonist binding. However, I cannot explain the loss of high-affinity agonist binding to the dopamine receptor on the basis of changes in dopamine concentrations. It is, though, in the opposite direction from what we would expect.

L. ANTONIAN (*Matrix Research Laboratories, New York, NY*): I want to make a comment about the point you brought up about the loss of coupling of the D-2 receptor to the Gi protein in the older animals. You mentioned two possibilities—one is loss of G-protein, while the other one is membrane fluidity.

SEVERSON: Yes, that is true in a broader category of thermodynamic changes.

ANTONIAN: Exactly. There is thermodynamic evidence showing that the conversion of the hyposensitive state is not completed as the temperature is increasing, that is, as you are polarizing the membrane. We have some evidence that suggests a second possibility—that by induction of membrane fluidity, you can induce affinity changes in the dopamine receptor. This then perhaps could account for the loss of coupling of the D-2 receptor to the Gi protein.

D. MORGAN (*University of Southern California, Los Angeles, CA*): There are two ways to really get at high-affinity agonist states. One way is to do what you have done with the displacement curves, whereas the other is to do what you have done previously—that is, to only use the actual agonist binding itself that will bind to high-affinity agonist conditions. However, have you ever looked at high-affinity agonist bindings and then discriminated (much like we did with fluphenazine) to get a handle on that D-1 high-affinity state?

SEVERSON: We see a very good correspondence between binding of agonists (in our case, *N*-propylnorapomorphine) in aging animals and between the high-affinity agonist binding sites that are stripped out of these displacement curves by the computer program. However, we have not done precise direct comparisons.

MORGAN: Do you think your NPA binding is to both D-1 and D-2 sites under either of the conditions used?

SEVERSON: I suspect that it is.

MORGAN: You also mentioned that assay conditions have some influence on high-affinity agonist binding. In your aging studies, have you really tried to maximize as much as possible these sites? Can you get the same proportion of high-affinity agonist sites in the old animals?

SEVERSON: That is another line of experimentation and there are a couple of ways to approach that. I alluded to it when I talked about preincubation conditions; that is, if you preincubate tissue before the binding studies in high magnesium buffers, then you force more receptors (thus forcing the equilibrium) towards the high-affinity binding site. Therefore, one experimental approach would be to load up a buffer with magnesium, preincubate the tissue, and then seen how many receptors in the old you could push into the high-affinity state for agonists. That is one possibility.

The other possibility (which I did not think was possible until I had seen some recent experiments) is that you can probably take purified G-protein and incubate it with the homogenate. Once there, it seems to incorporate. More importantly, though, it seems to restore high-affinity agonist binding and function in tissues where G-proteins have been inactivated by treatment with either cholera or pertussis toxin. Therefore, we may be able to take homogenates from old animals, incubate with Gi, and supplement them to see if we can force the equilibrium that way. I would see those experiments as being complementary to each other.

One other alternative, of course, is to actually use a ternary complex equation to fit the model. The experiments would probably be five times larger than the experiments I mentioned here and they would be more difficult enterprises, but that is still another possibility.

Dopamine, Acetylcholine, and Glutamate Interactions in Aging

Behavioral and Neurochemical Correlates

GARY B. FREEMAN[a] AND GARY E. GIBSON[b]

Cornell University Medical College
Burke Rehabilitation Center
White Plains, New York 10605

INTRODUCTION

Differential alteration of neurotransmitter function may underlie age-related deficits in psychomotor performance[1] and cognition.[2] The multiple neurotransmitter changes that likely are involved in the production of age-related deficits in motor performance were assessed in aged animals and in animal models of hypoxia (i.e., diminished oxygen availability) and thiamin deficiency. In the latter two, neurotransmitter systems can be readily manipulated and their interactions in the production of motor deficits can be investigated. Normal aging and mild acute hypoxia produce similar alterations of behavior in man[3] and animals; in mice, both reduce open field behavior and tightrope test performance. Pharmacological and neurochemical studies suggest that alterations in the synthesis and release of dopamine (DA), acetylcholine (ACh), and glutamate may underlie the psychomotor performance deficits that accompany aging, hypoxia, and thiamin deficiency. In addition, aged animals are more sensitive to hypoxia and thiamin deficiency. Each aspect of these interactions will be discussed in detail in the following sections.

BEHAVIORAL AND NEUROCHEMICAL CHANGES DURING HYPOXIA

Mild acute hypoxia is a useful model of multiple neurotransmitter changes that lead to deficits in motor performance resembling those of normal aging. Hypoxia diminishes behavioral performance on a variety of tasks.[4] Tightrope test performance is a sensitive indicator of hypoxic-induced deficits of motor behavior. Chemical hypoxia induced with sodium nitrite impairs tightrope test performance by 20% (37.5 mg/kg), 40% (75 mg/kg), or 78% (150 mg/kg).[5] Hypoxic-induced decreases in tightrope performance and increased brain lactate are highly correlated.[6] Because the nature of the age-related deficits in psychomotor performance may vary between tasks, more than one task needs to be used. Open field behavior in an automated activity monitor decreases in a dose-dependent manner during chemical hypoxia (TABLE 1).[7]

---

[a] Current address: Battelle, Columbus Division, 505 King Avenue, Columbus, Ohio 43201-2693.
[b] To whom correspondence should be addressed.

TABLE 1. Open Field Activity[a] during Chemical Hypoxia

NaNO$_2$ (mg/kg)	Total Distance (inches)	Vertical Movements
saline	679 ± 47	87 ± 8
75	444 ± 67[b]	57 ± 6[b]
100	237 ± 35[c]	31 ± 7[c]
125	127 ± 23[c]	9 ± 3[d]
150	71 ± 7[d]	3 ± 1[d]

[a] Activity was measured for 10 min after 30 min of sodium nitrite–induced chemical hypoxia.[7]
[b] The value differs significantly ($p < 0.05$) from saline.
[c] The value differs significantly ($p < 0.05$) from 75 mg/kg.
[d] The value differs significantly ($p < 0.05$) from 100 mg/kg.

The interaction of behavioral deficits and neurotransmitter metabolism can be examined by pharmacological manipulation and by correlation to rates of neurotransmitter synthesis. The beneficial effects of central and peripheral cholinergic agonists and antagonists on tightrope behavior suggest a central muscarinic and nicotinic component of the hypoxic-induced deficit that is physiologically important. At the appropriate dosage, physostigmine (+182%), nicotine (+175%), and the muscarinic agonist, arecoline (+116%), improve the tightrope test performance of hypoxic mice.[5] Alterations in neurotransmitter metabolism during hypoxia are well documented and may underlie the impaired brain function.[8] Hypoxia impairs the *in vivo* synthesis of ACh,[9-11] DA and serotonin (5-HT),[7,12-15] and the amino acids.[11] Although the cholinergic system seems the most sensitive to hypoxia, when expressed as percent of control, this may not necessarily reflect physiological significance.

If decreased neurotransmitter formation underlies hypoxic-induced decreases in tightrope performance and open field behavior,[4,7] then stimulation of neurotransmitter synthesis should ameliorate behavioral deficits. During hypoxia, 3,4-diaminopyridine (3,4-DAP) partially reverses the deficit in ACh synthesis in the striatum and hippocampus and improves tightrope performance.[16] However, the behavioral improvement with DAP exceeds the increased ACh turnover *in vivo*, which suggests that other neurotransmitters are also important in the production of hypoxic-induced deficits. The behavioral effects of morphine, sodium nitrite, and their combination closely reflect neurochemical changes in DA in the striatum.[17] Morphine stimulates DA formation and behavioral activity, while hypoxia impairs both. Morphine also increases DA synthesis and activity in hypoxic animals. Thus, open field activity and neurochemical changes in DA are highly correlated (FIGURE 1). Such consistent interactions do not occur between 5-HT synthesis and behavior.[17]

BEHAVIORAL AND NEUROCHEMICAL CHANGES DURING THIAMIN DEFICIENCY

Thiamin deficiency is a model of age-related disorders that diminish psychomotor performance. It is thus useful for investigating the interaction between neurochemistry and behavior. Thiamin-induced behavioral alterations in maze learning ability, avoidance tasks, and motor performance have been extensively investigated in young rats.[18] Other than a few studies that demonstrate gross neurological changes with thiamin deficiency in mice,[19,20] behavioral changes in a mouse model of thiamin deficiency have not been well studied. Thiamin deficiency induced by an injection of pyrithiamin

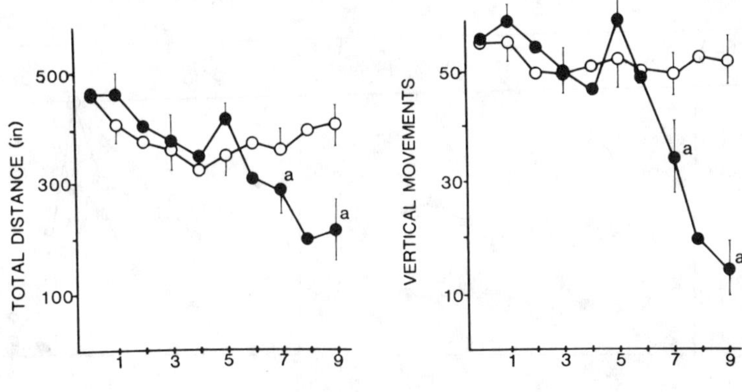

FIGURE 1. Mouse striatal dopamine metabolism and open field behavior. Values for estimated conversion rates are in pmol/mg per minute $\times$ 100 and total distance is in inches per 10-minute session. The letters denote that the value differs significantly ($p < 0.05$) from (a) control, (b) morphine, and (c) $NaNO_2$.

hydrobromide and subsequent maintenance on a thiamin-deficient diet alters open field behavior of CD-1 mice (FIGURE 2).[21] Total distance declines 37% and 54% by days 7 and 9, respectively, while the controls show no significant change. The number of vertical movements (rearing) declined (39%) by day 7 in the thiamin-deficient group and was further decreased (75%) by the final day of testing; controls, on the other hand, were not changed.

Altered neurotransmitter function may underlie the behavioral effects of thiamin

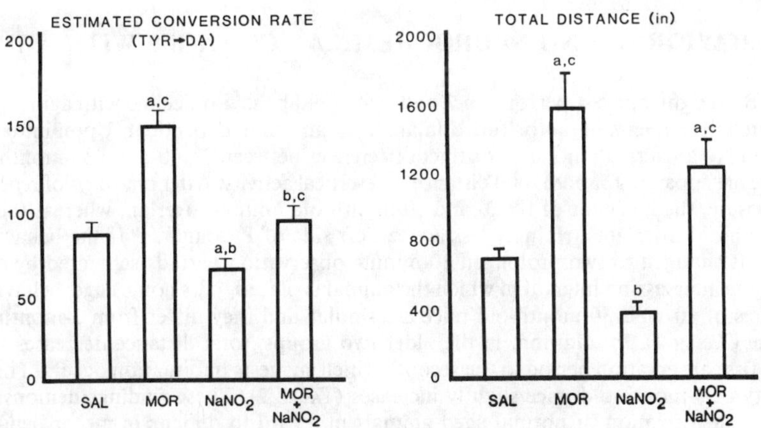

FIGURE 2. Open field activity in young CD-1 control (open circles) or thiamin-deficient (closed circles) mice. Activity was monitored for 5 min each day for 9 days. The "a" denotes that the value differs from day 1 of the corresponding treatment.

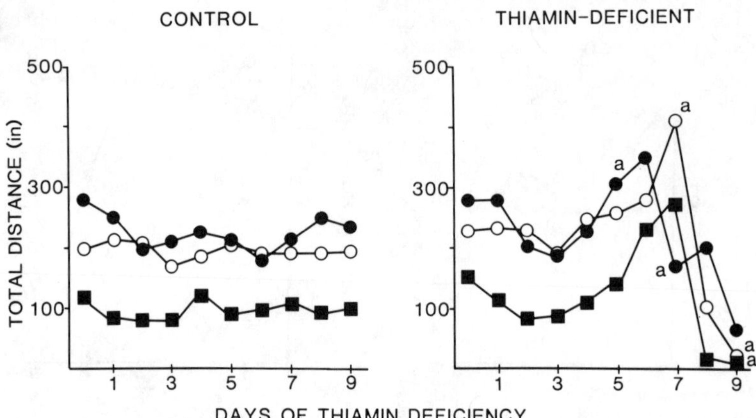

FIGURE 3. Age-related changes in open field activity of control and thiamin-deficient Balb/c mice (3 months, closed circles; 10 months, open circles; 30 months, closed squares). Activity was monitored for 5 min each day. The "a" denotes that the value differs from the preceding odd-day score.

deficiency. Pharmacological studies during thiamin deficiency demonstrate a physiologically significant cholinergic muscarinic deficit.[22-24] Cholinergic drug therapy,[23,24] in addition to treatment with thiamin,[25,26] partially reverses neurological symptoms as well as deficits in ACh synthesis. *In vitro* and *in vivo* studies demonstrate that thiamin deficiency alters ACh metabolism.[23,25] Catecholamine synthesis is also inhibited in thiamin-deficient rats.[27] Thiamin deficiency reduces whole brain levels of glutamate[28,29] and reduces concentrations in some, but not all brain regions.[30] Formation of [14C]glutamate from radioactive glucose decreases in thiamin deficiency,[29,31] while high-affinity uptake of glutamate may be enhanced.[30]

BEHAVIORAL AND NEUROCHEMICAL CHANGES WITH AGING

Both tightrope test performance and open field behavior decline with aging. Age-related decrements in motor function are task- and time-dependent. Upon initial exposure to an activity monitor, distinct differences between 3-, 10-, and 30-month-old mice are apparent for both total distance and vertical activity. After nine days of repeated exposure, the behavior of the 3- and 10-month-old animals overlap, whereas the 30-month-old mice are strikingly less active (left side of FIGURE 3).[21] If the behavioral task is changed to two prolonged 30-minute observation periods separated by a 15-minute intersession interval in which the animal is placed in its home cage, behavioral scores of 10- and 30-month-old mice are similar and they differ from 3-month-old mice (TABLE 2). In addition, in the older two groups, total distance decreases from the first observation period to the second, which suggests habituation occurs. The activity of 3-month-old mice slightly increases (TABLE 2). These findings demonstrate that categorization of normal aged animals in regard to deficits in motor behavior may vary according to the nature of the task as well as its length. Thus, the determination of the importance of individual neurochemical variables involved in motor function and age-related decline is complex.

TABLE 2. Effect of Age on Locomotor Activity[a] of Balb/c Mice during Two Prolonged Exposures to the Test Apparatus

Age (mo)	Total Distance Traveled	
	First 30 Min	Second 30 Min
3	635 ± 75	715 ± 45
10	486 ± 116	300 ± 15
30	453 ± 51	296 ± 62

[a] Activity was monitored for two 30-minute sessions separated by a 15-minute intersession interval.

Just as with hypoxia and thiamin deficiency, selective alteration of neurotransmitter function accompanies aging and may underlie age-related decreases in motor and cognitive function. Biochemical and pharmacological evidence supports the hypothesis that deficits in the cholinergic system may underlie geriatric cognitive dysfunction.[2] Nonhuman primates with decreased cognition show improved memory when they are treated with the acetylcholinesterase inhibitor, physostigmine, or the cholinergic agonist, arecoline. The synthesis of whole brain ACh is reduced in senescent mice.[6] Incorporation of [U-^{14}C]glucose into ACh declines 40% at 10 months and approximately 60% at 30 months (as compared to 3-month-old mice) without a corresponding reduction in ACh concentration. The depressed ACh synthesis correlates with behavioral deficits as measured with a string test. Turnover rates of DA decline in aged rats[32] and mice,[33,34] with either decreased[32,35–37] or unchanged levels.[38,39] Studies on the alteration of glutamate metabolism with aging are less conclusive. Decreased glutamate levels have been reported in aged rats,[40–43] but not in aged mice.[11,44] Synthesis of glutamate *in vivo* from radiolabeled glucose either decreases[45] or remains unchanged[11,41] with age.

INTERACTION OF AGING WITH HYPOXIA AND THIAMIN DEFICIENCY

Few studies have examined the relative susceptibility of the aged brain to metabolic insults. The synthesis of ACh in aged animals appears to be particularly vulnerable to hypoxic insults; the rate in 30-month-old mice is 10% of that in a 3-month-old nonhypoxic mouse.[46] Aging alters the biochemical sensitivity of the brain to thiamin deficiency.[21] Because, in man, the memory deficits due to thiamin deficiency occur mainly in the elderly, thiamin deficiency was examined in mice of various ages. The activity of 2-oxoglutarate dehydrogenase (KGDH) in 30-month-old control Balb/c mice was significantly lower (−16%) than that of 10-month-mice. In addition, KGDH in the aged brain was more sensitive than in the young brain to thiamin deficiency; KGDH activity declined 41% (3 month), 57% (10 month), and 74% (30 month).[21] These results suggest that the aged animal is more sensitive to metabolic insults.

Aging also alters the behavioral response of animals to thiamin deficiency. The large genetic diversity in mice[47] makes the mouse model of thiamin deficiency useful for investigating genetic interactions in the susceptibility to nutritional disorders. These may be important in the characterization of age-related deficits in motor performance. In addition, the considerable cost benefit of using aged mice rather than aged rats further enhances the attractiveness of a mouse model of thiamin deficiency for studies related to aging. The early changes and patterns of the behavioral response of mice to thiamin deficiency varied with age (right side of FIGURE 3).[21] Total distance decreased slightly, but then increased. The time and extent of this rise in total distance differed with age. The activity of 3-month-old mice peaked on day 6 (126% of initial score), whereas 10- and 30-month-old animals showed their highest activity on day 7 (179% and 174% of initial score, respectively). A decline in total distance followed. The behavioral outcome by the last day of treatment was similar at all ages. The sensitivity of the activity measures to thiamin depletion and the use of a repeated measures design were important in assessment because weight loss curves did not suggest age-related differences.

MOLECULAR BASIS OF THE NEUROCHEMICAL AND BEHAVIORAL CHANGES WITH AGING, HYPOXIA, AND THIAMIN DEFICIENCY

In vivo, similar behavioral and neurochemical deficits are seen in hypoxia, thiamin deficiency, and aging (decreased motor activity and decreased turnover). This suggests that similar molecular mechanisms may be involved. A larger decrease in synthetic rates than in levels suggests that release mechanisms may be altered. The striatum is an attractive area for investigating the sensitivity of glutamate and ACh as well as DA metabolism because high concentrations of each are present.[48] Furthermore, the interactions among transmitters in the striatum have been studied extensively. Thus, a sensitive *in vitro* model in mouse brain striatal slices was developed that allows determination of glutamate, ACh, and DA release in a single system.

Anoxia increases the extracellular concentration of DA and glutamate, but decreases that of ACh.[49] Hypoxia reduces the calcium-dependent release of ACh (-23%), and this impairment may underlie the subsequent decrease of *in vivo* synthesis and the subsequent decline in behavioral performance. Diminished oxygen availability during high K^+ conditions (31 mM) increases extracellular glutamate (200%) in the striatum. Anoxia also stimulates DA release and increases DA reuptake, but to a lesser extent than release.[50] This combination produces a 487% increase in extracellular DA. Extracellular DA is also increased during hypoxia *in vivo*.[51] The increase in extracellular DA may impair subsequent synthesis because striatal DA nerve terminals possess distinct synthesis- and release-modulating autoreceptors.[52-54] The increase in extracellular dopamine release is difficult to reconcile with the impairment of motor performance during hypoxia[7] because increased dopamine is normally associated with increased behavioral activity.[55] Thus, the functional significance of the presynaptic deficit in release to altered behavior and synthesis requires further investigation.

Previous studies suggest that the hypoxic-induced alterations of neurotransmitter metabolism are related to altered calcium homeostasis. The hypoxic-induced impairment of ACh release and calcium uptake are highly correlated.[56] In addition, omission of calcium from an anoxic incubation enhances the stimulation of DA and glutamate release and further depresses ACh release.[49] The stimulation of DA and glutamate release by anoxia would appear to contradict an integral role of diminished calcium uptake in hypoxic-induced changes. However, nimodipine, a calcium channel antagonist, enhances DA release and decreases ACh release.[57] The inhibition of ACh release by nimodipine may be explained by the inhibition of presynaptic calcium influx by nimodipine. Enhancement of DA release, on the other hand, may reflect an unknown mode of action. The differential effects of anoxia on DA, glutamate, and ACh release in the same tissue suggest that calcium's role in the release of these neurotransmitters varies.

The underlying mechanisms that lead to altered neurotransmitter metabolism and behavior during thiamin deficiency may be similar. The activities of the thiamin pyrophosphate (TPP) dependent enzymes—transketolase (TK) and 2-oxoglutarate dehydrogenase (KGDH)—decrease during thiamin deficiency.[25,58,59] A lesion in KGDH is correlated to impaired oxidative metabolism and is thus a form of histoxic hypoxia. The deficiencies in KGDH are also related to thiamin-induced behavioral deficits and the impairment of ACh release that accompanies thiamin deficiency.[25] The relationship between these enzymatic deficiencies and open field activity were examined during thiamin deficiency in mice. KGDH and TK activities of CD-1 mice decreased with thiamin deficiency (45% and 54%, respectively).[21] Significant correlations between various aspects of open field behavior and KGDH activity in CD-1 mice[21] support the suggestion that the reversible behavioral symptoms of thiamin deficiency are related to diminished activity of KGDH.[25]

Altered release mechanisms may also underlie neurochemical and behavioral changes during aging. The release of DA, glutamate, and ACh in young (3 month) and old (30 month) Balb/c mice was examined in a single release system. Aging increases the basal release of glutamate (77%) and DA (29%) in the striatum, but does not alter the concentration of these neurotransmitters in the media after K[+] stimulation; however, the K[+]-stimulated release of ACh is reduced.[60] Selective alteration of release in the striatum strengthens the hypothesis that presynaptic changes in neurotransmitter metabolism may underlie the motor deficits with aging.

IMPLICATIONS OF ALTERED RELEASE IN AGING AND NEUROLOGICAL DISEASE

Increased extracellular DA and glutamate may play a role in mediating degenerative changes that occur postsynaptically[61] through an excitotoxin mechanism. This has been proposed for glutamate during hypoxia/ischemia.[62] Thus, if the tissue damage is related to the large increases in DA and glutamate, the ischemic damage may be ameliorated by treatment of presynaptic deficits. 3,4-DAP, which reverses *in vivo* hypoxic-induced deficits in behavior and turnover, significantly reduces the K[+]-stimulated release of DA and glutamate (−20%) during an anoxic incubation.[49] Therefore, decreasing the release of DA and glutamate may be an effective means to ameliorate anoxic or ischemic injury.

Age-related differences in the sensitivity to thiamin deficiency and alterations of glutamate release in normal aged mice may have important implications in the pathophysiology of age-related neurodegenerative disorders. KGDH and TK activities are reduced in brain and peripheral tissue in Alzheimer's disease.[63] Diminished activity of the thiamin-dependent enzyme KGDH would impair oxidative metabolism and thus cholinergic activity because cholinergic cells are exquisitely vulnerable to conditions that impair oxidative metabolism.[64] Pearce *et al.*[65] proposed that glutamate neurotransmission is altered in Alzheimer's disease. Excessive glutamatergic stimulation may underlie the loss of other cells in Alzheimer's disease (i.e., an excitotoxic lesion), and KGDH deficiency would impair the metabolic removal of glutamate and would, through histotoxic hypoxia, stimulate its release.[49,66] Altered glutamate metabolism has also been implicated in Huntington's disease, which is a neurodegenerative disorder with severe motor as well as memory impairments.[67-69]

SUMMARY

Aging, hypoxia, and thiamin deficiency diminish motor performance. Similar alterations of ACh, DA, and glutamate metabolism accompany hypoxia, thiamin deficiency, and aging. Both aging and hypoxia reduce ACh release and stimulate DA and glutamate release. Presynaptic enhancement of DA and glutamate release may be important in the production of cell damage that may contribute, in part, to age-related deficits in motor as well as cognitive function. The decline in ACh release may be important in the production of the cognitive deficits. An understanding of the interactions of neurotransmitters in hypoxia and thiamin deficiency aids our understanding of normal aging and increases the possibility of developing better treatments for the multiple neurotransmitter deficiencies that accompany many metabolic, age-related, and chronic degenerative disorders.

REFERENCES

1. JOSEPH, J. A., R. T. BARTUS, D. CLODY, D. MORGAN, C. FINCH, B. BEER & S. SESACK. 1983. Psychomotor performance in the senescent rodent: reduction of deficits via striatal dopamine receptor up-regulation. Neurobiol. Aging **4:** 313–319.
2. BARTUS, R. T., R. L. DEAN, B. BEER & A. S. LIPPA. 1982. The cholinergic hypothesis of geriatric memory dysfunction. Science **217:** 408–417.
3. McFARLAND, R. A. 1952. *In* The Biology of Mental Health and Disease. Harper & Row (Hoeber). New York.
4. GIBSON, G. E. 1985. Hypoxia. *In* Cerebral Energy Metabolism and Metabolic Encephalopathy. D. W. McCandless, Ed.: 43–78. Plenum. New York.
5. GIBSON, G. E., C. J. PELMAS & C. PETERSON. 1983. Cholinergic drugs and 4-aminopyridine alter hypoxic-induced behavioral deficits. Pharmacol. Biochem. Behav. **18:** 909–916.
6. GIBSON, G. E., C. PETERSON & D. J. JENDEN. 1981. Whole brain acetylcholine synthesis declines with senescence. Science **213:** 674–676.
7. FREEMAN, G. B., P. NIELSEN & G. E. GIBSON. 1986. Monoamine neurotransmitter metabolism and locomotor activity during chemical hypoxia. J. Neurochem. **46:** 733–738.
8. GIBSON, G. E., W. PULSINELLI, J. P. BLASS & T. E. DUFFY. 1981. Brain dysfunction in mild to moderate hypoxia. Am. J. Med. **70:** 1247–1254.
9. GIBSON, G. E. & J. P. BLASS. 1976. Impaired synthesis of acetylcholine in brain accompanying mild hypoxia and hypoglycemia. J. Neurochem. **27:** 37–42.
10. GIBSON, G. E. & T. E. DUFFY. 1981. Impaired synthesis of acetylcholine by mild hypoxic hypoxia or nitrous oxide. J. Neurochem. **36:** 28–33.
11. GIBSON, G. E., C. PETERSON & J. SANSONE. 1981. Decreases in amino acid and acetylcholine metabolism during hypoxia. J. Neurochem. **37:** 192–201.
12. BROWN, R. M., S. R. SNIDER & A. CARLSSON. 1974. Changes in biogenic amine synthesis and turnover induced by hypoxia and/or footshock stress. II. The central nervous system. J. Neural Transm. **35:** 293–305.
13. BROWN, R. M., W. KEHR & A. CARLSSON. 1975. Functional and biochemical aspects of catecholamine metabolism in brain under hypoxia. Brain Res. **85:** 491–509.
14. DAVIS, J. N. & A. CARLSSON. 1973. Effect of hypoxia on tyrosine and tryptophan hydroxylation in unanesthesized rat brain. J. Neurochem. **20:** 913–915.
15. DAVIS, J. N. & A. CARLSSON. 1973. The effect of hypoxia on monoamine synthesis, levels and metabolism in rat brain. J. Neurochem. **21:** 783–790.
16. PETERSON, C. & G. E. GIBSON. 1982. 3,4-Diaminopyridine alters acetylcholine metabolism and behavior during hypoxia. J. Pharmacol. Exp. Ther. **222:** 576–582.
17. FREEMAN, G. B., P. NIELSEN & G. E. GIBSON. 1986. Behavioral and neurochemical correlates of morphine and hypoxia interactions. Pharmacol. Biochem. Behav. **24:** 1687–1693.
18. GIBSON, G., L. BARCLAY & J. BLASS. 1982. The role of the cholinergic system in thiamin deficiency. *In* Thiamin. Volume 378. H. Z. Sable & C. J. Gubler, Eds.: 382–403. N.Y. Acad. Sci. New York.
19. OGUCHI, E. & K. SAKAMOTO. 1982. Effect of a single, large dose injection of pyrithiamin on the thiamin deficiency of the mouse. Jpn. J. Pharmacol. **32:** 775–783.

20. WATANABE, I. 1978. Pyrithiamin-induced acute thiamin-deficient encephalopathy in the mouse. Exp. Mol. Pathol. **28:** 381–394.

21. FREEMAN, G. B., P. E. NIELSEN & G. E. GIBSON. 1987. Behavioral and enzymatic changes during thiamin deficiency: strain and age interactions. Submitted.

22. BARCLAY, L. L., G. E. GIBSON & J. P. BLASS. 1981. The string test: an early behavioral change in thiamine deficiency. Pharmacol. Biochem. Behav. **14:** 153–157.

23. BARCLAY, L. L., G. E. GIBSON & J. P. BLASS. 1981. Impairment of behavior and acetylcholine metabolism in thiamine deficiency. J. Pharmacol. Exp. Ther. **217:** 537–543.

24. BARCLAY, L. L., G. E. GIBSON & J. P. BLASS. 1982. Cholinergic therapy of abnormal open-field behavior in thiamin-deficient rats. J. Nutr. **112:** 1906–1913.

25. GIBSON, G. E., H. KSIEZAK-REDING, K. F. R. SHEU, V. MYKYTYN & J. P. BLASS. 1984. Correlation of enzymatic, metabolic, and behavioral deficits in thiamin deficiency and its reversal. Neurochem. Res. **9:** 803–814.

26. GIBSON, G. E., C. PELMAS & J. P. BLASS. 1983. A central cholinergic deficit in rats with dietary thiamin deficiency. Neurochem. Pathol. **1:** 125–135.

27. IWATA, H., T. NISHIKAWA & A. BABA. 1970. Catecholamine accumulation in tissues of thiamin-deficient rats after inhibition of monoamine oxidase. Eur. J. Pharmacol. **12:** 253–256.

28. GAITONDE, M. K. & N. A. FAYEIN. 1975. Decreased metabolism *in vivo* of glucose into amino acids of the brain of thiamin-deficient rats after treatment with pyrithiamine. J. Neurochem. **24:** 1215–1223.

29. GUBLER, C. J., B. L. ADAMS, B. HAMMOND, E. C. YUAN, S. M. GUO & M. BENNION. 1974. Effect of thiamine deprivation and thiamine antagonists on the level of γ-aminobutyric acid and on 2-oxoglutarate metabolism in rat brain. J. Neurochem. **22:** 831–836.

30. PLAITAKIS, A., E. C. HWANG, M. H. VAN WOERT, P. I. A. SZILAGYI & S. BERL. 1982. Effect of thiamin deficiency on brain neurotransmitter systems. *In* Thiamin. Volume 378. H. Z. Sable & C. J. Gubler, Eds.: 382–403. N.Y. Acad. Sci. New York.

31. GAITONDE, M. K., R. W. K. NIXEY & I. M. SHARMAN. 1974. The effect of deficiency of thiamine on the metabolism of [U-^{14}C]glucose and [U-^{14}C]ribose and the levels of amino acids in rat brain. J. Neurochem. **22:** 53–61.

32. CARFAGNA, N., F. TRUNZO & A. MORETTI. 1985. Brain catecholamine content and turnover in aging rats. Exp. Gerontol. **20:** 265–269.

33. FINCH, C. E. 1973. Catecholamine metabolism in the brains of aging male mice. Brain Res. **52:** 261–276.

34. FINCH, C. E., V. JONEC, G. HODY, J. P. WALKER, W. MORTON-SMITH, A. ALPER & G. J. DOUGHER. 1975. Aging and the passage of L-tyrosine, L-DOPA, and insulin into mouse brain slices *in vitro*. J. Gerontol. **30:** 33–40.

35. ADOLFSSON, R., C. G. GOTTFRIES, B-E. ROOS & B. WINBLAD. 1979. Post-mortem distribution of dopamine and homovanillic acid in human brain, variation related to age, and a review of the literature. J. Neural Trans. **45:** 81–105.

36. BHASKARAN, D. & E. RADHA. 1984. Circadian variation in the monoamine levels and monoamine oxidase activity in different regions of the rat brain as a function of age. Exp. Gerontol. **19:** 153–170.

37. STRONG, R., T. SAMORAJSKI & A. GOTTESFELD. 1982. Regional mapping of neostriatal neurotransmitter systems as a function of aging. J. Neurochem. **39:** 831–836.

38. JOSEPH, J. A., C. FILBURN, S. TZANKOFF, J. M. THOMPSON & B. T. ENGEL. 1980. Age-related neostriatal alterations in the rat: failure of L-DOPA to alter behavior. Neurobiol. Aging **1:** 119–125.

39. PONZIO, F., N. BRUNELLO & S. ALGERI. 1978. Catecholamine synthesis in brains of aging rats. J. Neurochem. **30:** 1617–1620.

40. DAVIS, J. & W. A. HIMWICH. 1975. Neurochemistry of the developing and aging mammalian brain. *In* Advances in Behavioural Biology [Neurobiology of Aging]. Volume 16. J. M. Ordy & K. R. Brizzee, Eds.: 329–357. Plenum. New York.

41. DEKONING-VEREST, I. F. 1980. Glutamate metabolism in aging rat brain. Mech. Aging Dev. **13:** 83–92.

42. HIMWICH, W. A. 1973. Neurochemical patterns in the developing and aging grain. *In* De-

velopment and Aging in The Nervous System. M. Rockstein, Ed.: 151–170. Academic Press. New York.

43. TIMARAS, P. S., D. B. HUDSON & S. OKLUND. 1973. Changes in central nervous system free amino acids with development and aging. *In* Neurobiological Aspects of Maturation and Aging [Progress in Brain Research]. Volume 40. D. H. Ford, Ed.: 267–275. Elsevier. Amsterdam/New York.

44. KIRZINGER, S. S. & M. L. FONDA. 1978. Glutamine and ammonia metabolism in the brains of senescent mice. Exp. Gerontol. **13:** 255–261.

45. TYCE, G. M. & K-L. WONG. 1980. Conversion of glucose to neurotransmitter amino acids in the brains of young and aging rats. Exp. Gerontol. **15:** 527–532.

46. GIBSON, G. E., C. PETERSON & J. SANSONE. 1981. Neurotransmitter and carbohydrate metabolism during aging and mild hypoxia. Neurobiol. Aging **2:** 165–172.

47. ALTMAN, P. L. & D. D. KATZ, Eds. 1979. Biological Handbooks III. Inbred and Genetically Defined Strains of Laboratory Animals. Part I. Mouse and Rat. Fed. Amer. Soc. Exp. Biol. Maryland.

48. JOHNSTON, M. V. 1983. Neurotransmitter alterations in a model of perinatal hypoxic-ischemic brain injury. Ann. Neurol. **13:** 511–518.

49. FREEMAN, G. B., V. MYKYTYN & G. E. GIBSON. 1987. Selective alteration of dopamine, acetylcholine and glutamate release during anoxia and/or 3,4-diaminopyridine treatment. Neurochem. Res. In press.

50. FREEMAN, G. B. & G. E. GIBSON. 1986. Effect of decreased oxygen on *in vitro* release of endogenous 3,4-dihydroxyphenylethylamine from mouse striatum. J. Neurochem. **47:** 1924–1931.

51. BRODERICK, P. A. & G. E. GIBSON. 1986. Extracellular dopamine and serotonin *in vivo* during repeated episodes of hypoxic-hypoxia. Soc. Neurosci. Abstr. No. 156.7.

52. FARNEBO, L. O. & B. HAMBERGER. 1971. Drug-induced changes in the release of ^{3}H-monoamines from field-stimulated rat brain slices. Acta Physiol. Scand. Suppl. **371:** 35–44.

53. PARKER, E. M. & L. X. CUBEDDU. 1985. Evidence for autoreceptor modulation of endogenous dopamine release from rabbit caudate nucleus *in vitro*. J. Pharmacol. Exp. Ther. **232:** 492–500.

54. WOLF, M. E., M. P. GALLOWAY & R. H. ROTH. 1986. Regulation of dopamine synthesis in the medial prefrontal cortex: studies in brain slices. J. Pharmacol. Exp. Ther. **236:** 699–707.

55. CARROLL, B. J. & P. T. SHARP. 1972. Monoamine mediation of the morphine-induced activation of mice. Br. J. Pharmacol. **46:** 124–139.

56. PETERSON, C. & G. E. GIBSON. 1984. Synaptosomal calcium metabolism during hypoxia and 3,4-diaminopyridine treatment. J. Neurochem. **42:** 248–253.

57. NORDSTROM, O., S. BRAESCH ANDERSEN & T. BARTFAI. 1986. Dopamine release is enhanced while acetylcholine release is inhibited by nimodipine (Bay e 9736). Acta Physiol. Scand. **126:** 115–120.

58. BENNETT, C. D., J. H. JONES & J. NELSON. 1966. The effect of thiamin deficiency on the metabolism of the brain. Oxidation of various substrates *in vitro* by the brain of normal and pyrithiamin fed rats. J. Neurochem. **13:** 449–459.

59. HOLOWACH, J., F. KAUFFMAN, M. G. IKOSSI, C. THOMAS & D. B. MCDOUGAL. 1968. The effects of a thiamin antagonist, pyrithiamin, on levels of selected metabolic intermediates and on activities of thiamin dependent enzymes in brain and liver. J. Neurochem. **15:** 621–631.

60. FREEMAN, G. B. & G. E. GIBSON. 1987. Selective alteration of mouse brain neurotransmitter release with age. Neurobiol. Aging **8:** 147–152.

61. SIMON, R. P., J. H. SWAN, T. GRIFFITHS & B. S. MELDRUM. 1984. Blockade of *n*-methyl-*d*-aspartate receptors may protect against ischemic-damage in the brain. Science **226:** 850–852.

62. ROTHMAN, S. M. & J. W. OLNEY. 1986. Glutamate and the pathophysiology of hypoxic-ischemic brain damage. Ann. Neurol. **19:** 105–111.

63. GIBSON, G. E., K. F. R. SHEU, J. P. BLASS, A. BAKER, K. C. CARLSON, J. DALE, B. HARDING & P. PERRINO. 1985. Thiamin-dependent enzymes in brains and peripheral tissues from Alzheimer's patients. Soc. Neurosci. Abstr. **11:** 54.6.

64. GIBSON, G. E. & J. P. BLASS. 1983. Metabolism and neurotransmission. *In* Handbook of Neurochemistry. Volume 3. A. Lajtha, Ed.: 633–651. Plenum. New York.
65. PEARCE, B. R., A. M. PALMER, D. M. BOWEN, G. K. WILCOCK, M. M. ESIRI & A. N. DAVISON. 1984. Neurotransmitter dysfunction and atrophy of the caudate nucleus in Alzheimer's Disease. Neurochem. Pathol. **2:** 221–232.
66. HIRSCH, J. A. & G. E. GIBSON. 1984. Selective alteration of neurotransmitter release by low oxygen *in vitro*. Neurochem. Res. **9:** 1037–1047.
67. COYLE, J. T. & R. SCHWARCZ. 1976. Lesions of striatal neurones with kainic acid provides a model of Huntington's chorea. Nature **263:** 244–246.
68. McGEER, E. G. & P. L. McGEER. 1976. Duplication of biochemical changes of Huntington's chorea by intrastriatal injections of glutamic and kainic acids. Nature **262:** 517–519.
69. OLNEY, J. W. & T. S. DE GUBAREFF. 1978. Glutamate neurotoxicity and Huntington's chorea. Nature **271:** 557–559.

DISCUSSION OF THE PAPER

D. MORGAN (*University of Southern California, Los Angeles, CA*): One of the major enzymes that thiamin is regulating (or is a cofactor for) that you have not mentioned is pyruvate hydrogenase, which is the major enzyme in regulating energy metabolism in the central nervous system. Do you have any evidence, one way or the other, as to how that might be mediating some of these effects that you have actually looked at?

G. FREEMAN (*Burke Rehabilitation Center, White Plains, NY*): Our laboratory has looked into PDH, but not in this same context.

MORGAN: Have you looked at the energy change in this system to find out if there were any changes in ATP ratios or anything like that?

FREEMAN: No, I have not looked at those yet.

B. HOFFER (*University of Colorado Health Science Center, Denver, CO*): One of the transmitter systems that is exquisitely sensitive to transient hypoxia is that of GABAergic interneurons. Have you done anything with GABA release or GABA turnover to determine how this might influence your other measurements?

FREEMAN: No, we have just basically looked at these three.

G. S. ROTH (*NIA, Baltimore, MD*): You are probably aware that many individuals now favor an oxygen-radical damage theory of aging, yet you still have hypoxia currently mimicking the aging situation. Do you think this argues against the free radical theory of aging?

FREEMAN: Based on the correlates that I have shown here, it would not seem to go along with that theory.

ROTH: Have you in any way tried to measure whether there is any oxidative damage? Sometimes, you can induce oxidative damage with low oxygen tension as well as with high. Have you tried to do any of that?

FREEMAN: No.

J. A. JOSEPH (*Armed Forces Radiobiology Research Institute, Bethesda, MD*): Indications from the released data on dopamine, etc., are starting to look about as bad as the data that David Morgan presented earlier today on striatal DA levels and aging. Could you discuss a little more of your methodology concerning release from slices and how release is measured, especially in regard to how this might account for some of these differences? I do not see any decrease in DA release with age. In fact, K⁺-evoked release is about the same in the young and the old. Didn't B. Hoffer see this?

HOFFER: We saw two subpopulations and we saw it at 29 months; usually, though, it is at 24 months when you see clear subpopulations.

J. SEVERSON (*Amersham Corporation, Arlington Heights, IL*): Were these Fischer rats that were used?

HOFFER: Yes.

FREEMAN: We measured the release in an incubation system rather than in a superfusion-type system. We looked at the endogenous dopamine release after both the dopamine and our supernatant were put on an HPLC, and we measured the total endogenous dopamine release induced by potassium stimulation. We did not subtract the normal K^+ from the high K^+, so we measured the total release after potassium stimulation. In the aging experiment, there was not any difference in the total release. However, there was a small difference in the basal release that was still statistically significant. We are now pursuing that difference and looking at synaptosomes to see if that is a real presynaptic event.

JOSEPH: Do you make striatal prisms or slices?

FREEMAN: Prisms.

HOFFER: Are we talking about fractional release in terms of measuring the total amount of dopamine or is this some absolute level of dopamine that is coming out?

FREEMAN: When I said low K^+ and high K^+, it was the amount of dopamine under normal conditions versus the amount of dopamine after potassium stimulation. I did not show it, but when the high is subtracted from the low, that difference is seen.

HOFFER: However, are you looking at release as the amount of dopamine that is in the tissue or is it the absolute amount of dopamine?

FREEMAN: No, it is the absolute.

In Vivo Measurement of Dopamine Receptors in Human Brain by Positron Emission Tomography
Age and Sex Differences[a]

DEAN F. WONG,[b] EMMANUEL P. BROUSSOLLE,[b,c] GARY WAND,[d]
VICTOR VILLEMAGNE,[b] ROBERT F. DANNALS,[b]
JONATHAN M. LINKS,[b] HOWARD A. ZACUR,[e] JAMES HARRIS,[f]
SAKKUBAI NAIDU,[g] CLAUS BRAESTRUP,[h]
HENRY N. WAGNER, JR.,[b] AND ALBERT GJEDDE[i]

[b]Division of Nuclear Medicine
Department of Radiology
The Johns Hopkins University School of Medicine
and
Division of Radiation Health Sciences
Department of Environmental Health Sciences
The Johns Hopkins University School of Hygiene and Public Health
Baltimore, Maryland 21205

[c]Neuropharmacology Laboratory
Addiction Research Center
National Institute of Drug Abuse
Baltimore, Maryland 21224

[d]Division of Endocrinology
Department of Medicine
The Johns Hopkins University School of Medicine
Baltimore, Maryland 21205

[e]Division of Reproductive Endocrinology
Department of Gynecology and Obstetrics
The Johns Hopkins University School of Medicine
Baltimore, Maryland 21205

[f]Department of Psychiatry and Pediatrics
The Johns Hopkins University School of Medicine
and
Kennedy Institute
Baltimore, Maryland 21205

[a] This work was supported by United States Public Health Service Grant No. NS15080.

gDepartment of Neurology and Pediatrics
The Johns Hopkins University School of Medicine
and
Kennedy Institute
Baltimore, Maryland 21205

hNovo Industries
Copenhagen, Denmark 2200

iMedical Physiology Department A
Panum Institute
Copenhagen University
Copenhagen, Denmark 2200

INTRODUCTION

Human and animal studies have indicated age-related declines in many behavioral functions, including motor activity, motivation, learning and short-term memory, sexual activity, food intake, and sleep.[1] Aging has also been associated with an increased frequency in the occurrence of Parkinson's disease and senile dementia. It seems reasonable that these sequelae of aging have a neurochemical basis. *In vitro* studies of animal and human postmortem brains have revealed age differences in several neurotransmitters, in their associated enzymes, and in their receptors.[2-5] Of particular interest is the reported age-related decline of D_2 dopamine receptor density (but not affinity) in the striatum.[6-15]

The recent advent of specific chemical ligands labeled with positron emitting radioisotopes has allowed external imaging of some neurochemical markers *in vivo* by positron emission tomography (PET). PET permits noninvasive *in vivo* imaging of ligands specific for neurochemical elements such as receptors (in normal physiological states) and does this as a function of disease and therapy. We demonstrated the feasibility of *in vivo* visualization of neuroreceptors[16] with the successful imaging of D_2 dopamine and S_2 serotonin receptors in a normal adult using a potent ligand, (3-N-[11C]-methyl)spiperone ([11C]NMSP). We then began to assess possible age and sex differences in D_2 dopamine receptors using this procedure.

RELATIVE D_2 DOPAMINE RECEPTOR COMPARISON: THE CAUDATE/CEREBELLUM RATIO INDEX

A preliminary study[17] included 22 male and 22 female volunteers who were healthy as determined by medical, neurological, and neuropsychological examinations. Their ages ranged from 19 to 73 years in the case of the males and from 19 to 67 years for the females (mean age ± standard deviation was 39 ± 17 years for males and 36 ± 14 years for females). All subjects gave informed consent in compliance with the Johns Hopkins Human Investigation Committee. A noncontrast X-ray CT scan was performed to verify the absence of pathological processes and to determine the appropriate transaxial slices for maximum delineation of the caudate, putamen, cerebellum, and frontal cortex. The PET scan technique consisted of the intravenous injection of 15–20 mCi of [11C]NMSP and the subsequent acquisition of multiple PET images for 90 minutes (FIGURE 1). Binding to the D_2 dopamine receptor was estimated by the ratio of radioactivity in the caudate to that in the cerebellum. Binding to the S_2 serotonin receptor was estimated by the ratio of radioactivity in the frontal cortex to that in the cerebellum.

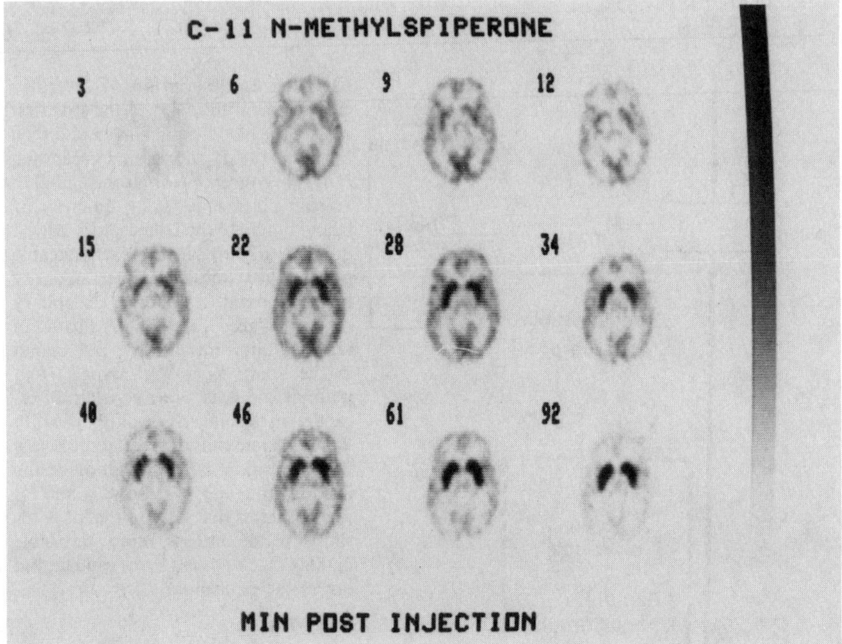

FIGURE 1. PET images of the human brain at various times (3 to 92 min) after intravenous injection of [¹¹C]NMSP at 40 mm above the cantho-meatal line. This middle slice of the PET scan passes through the frontal horn and permits maximum visualization of the caudate and putamen. These images show a high accumulation of the tracer in the basal ganglia over time.

In all of the subjects, the caudate/cerebellum ratio increased linearly with time after the radiotracer injection. This is a finding that has been consistent in further studies involving 400 normal volunteers and patients. Under certain circumstances, the slope of caudate/cerebellum ratio was considered (*vide infra*) to reflect the rate constant of [¹¹C]NMSP binding to the D_2 receptor (k_3). This ratio index had been previously used by other investigators, specifically in *in vivo* rodent studies,[18-21] to demonstrate the pharmacokinetics of [³H]spiperone binding and the effects of blocking drugs. Using this approach, we described an age-related decline in the caudate/cerebellum ratio and in the frontal/cerebellum ratio.[17] In addition, the slope of the caudate/cerebellum ratio versus time changed with age in a similar manner, but a statistically significant difference was found between men and women in the distribution of the caudate/cerebellum ratio as a function of age.

D_2 DOPAMINE RECEPTOR DENSITY: THE THREE COMPARTMENT MODEL

In this initial study of aging, using a three compartment model, we argued that the ratio index reflected receptor binding and was less related to the effect of blood flow (FIGURE 2). This interpretation depended upon a relatively low value of the rate constant of binding to the receptor (k_3) as compared to the reverse binding from brain

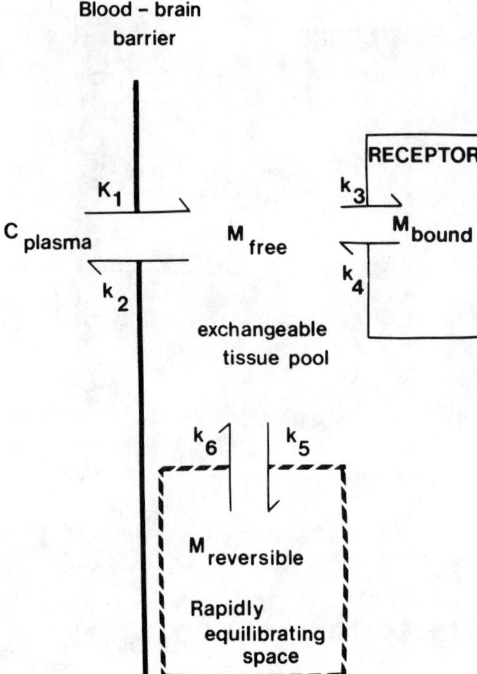

FIGURE 2. Description of the three compartment model. [^{11}C]NMSP first crosses the blood-brain barrier and then binds to the D_2 dopamine receptors. C_{plasma}: concentration of the ligand in arterial plasma. M_{bound}: quantity of ligand bound to the D_2 receptors. M_{free}: quantity of drug in the exchangeable pool of the tissue. $M_{reversible}$: quantity of drug bound to the other secondary or non-D_2 receptors assumed to be in rapid equilibrium with the free ligand in the brain. K_1 is a clearance (from plasma) and k_2 is a rate constant of escape from the brain tissue of [^{11}C]NMSP; k_3 and k_4: rate constants for, respectively, the association and dissociation of the ligand with the D_2 receptors; k_5 and k_6: rate constants that refer to the lower affinity or secondary rapid reversible binding that is present in the caudate, but not in the cerebellum.

back to plasma (k_2). Such a condition would be the case in low receptor densities. The lower the receptor density, the more the ratio is representative of k_3, which is the product of B'_{max} (the available number of receptors) and k_{on} (the *in vivo* rate of association to the receptor). Because affinity changes have not been previously demonstrated during the aging process from *in vitro* studies, our preliminary interpretation was that the caudate/cerebellar ratio was related to receptor binding and that the decrease in the ratio with age was more representative of receptor number than of affinity changes.

The complication that exists with the use of [^{11}C]NMSP is that its short half-life (20 minutes) and its high affinity to the D_2 dopamine receptors do not allow equilibrium to occur during the PET scan imaging period; that is, the ratio between the bound and unbound brain concentrations and that in the blood is not a constant, as it is in full equilibrium. However, a steady-state analysis can be carried out if the ligand reaches a steady state between nonspecifically bound ligand in brain and plasma by measuring the kinetics in the cerebellum, where there are no D_2 receptors present. Thus, by using a three compartment analysis,[22-24] the rate constant of binding to the dopamine receptor from free and nonspecifically bound tissue to receptor bound (k_3) tissue can be directly measured. This approach requires the plasma input function and the brain time-activity curves, which are recorded over the 90-minute imaging period.

We have calculated the binding rate constant k_3 in 18 male and 18 female normal volunteers (FIGURE 3). Their ages ranged from 19 to 67 and from 19 to 71, respectively (mean age ± SD was 37.1 ± 16.6 years for males and 34.0 ± 13.9 years for females).

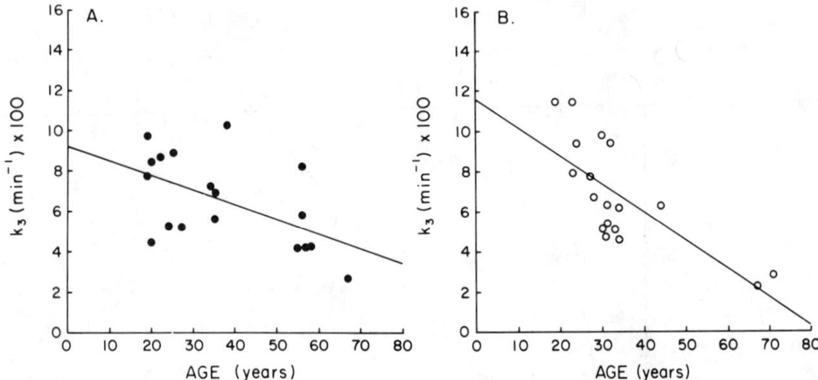

FIGURE 3. Decrement with age of the binding rate constant k_3 (per minute $\times$ 100) to D_2 dopamine receptors in the human caudate in 18 males (A) and in 18 females (B). The regression coefficients were 0.54 and 0.73 and the slopes of the regression line were -0.072 and -0.141 for males and females, respectively. A multiple linear regression analysis of the pooled male/female data (dependent variable: k_3; independent variables: age, sex, and product of age and sex) demonstrated a significant age effect ($p < 0.05$) for either sex with k_3, while the difference in slopes and intercepts between the sexes did not quite reach the statistical level ($p = 0.11$).

The results show a significant decrease in k_3 as a function of age in both sexes. This decrease is more pronounced in females than in males (but the difference was not significant at $p = 0.11$). This differs somewhat from our initial findings using the caudate/cerebellum ratio index,[17] where the male ratio fell faster and exponentially. This apparent difference from previous studies can be partly explained by the fact that the ratio index may be influenced by cerebral blood flow, especially in young subjects with higher receptor density. A larger number of subjects (particularly in the middle ages), the development of multiple PET scans for receptor density (*vide infra*), and control for menstral cycle (*vide infra*) are necessary to further investigate these possible sex differences.

The recent development of blocking studies with haloperidol — a potent D_2 dopamine receptor antagonist that reduces the number of receptors available for binding by [11C]NMSP — makes it possible to carry out something analogous to an *in vivo* Scatchard plot. A direct computation of the receptor density B'_{max} can be obtained from the slope of the reciprocal of the receptor binding rate constant ($1/k_3$) plotted against serum haloperidol levels (FIGURE 4). Brain haloperidol levels are in turn computed from a partition coefficient estimated for serum haloperidol by a procedure that has undergone other experimental validation (FIGURE 4).[22-24]

By using this method, we have now been able to determine receptor densities in three subjects over the age of 58 and in nine subjects between the ages of 18 and 30. Each subject received two PET scans, with the second one preceded by oral administration of 7.5 mg of haloperidol four hours prior to [11C]NMSP injection. Multiple PET images and arterialized blood samples were taken for 90 minutes after injection of tracer. Haloperidol plasma samples were obtained throughout the PET procedure.[22-24] The receptor densities determined by the full kinetic model showed a marked (50%) decrease in receptor density with age. The B_{max} ($\pm$ SD) was 18.4 $\pm$ 8 (pmol/g) in young subjects as compared to 9 $\pm$ 1 in old subjects. These results, although preliminary, are in contrast with our recent findings of elevated D_2 dopamine receptor density

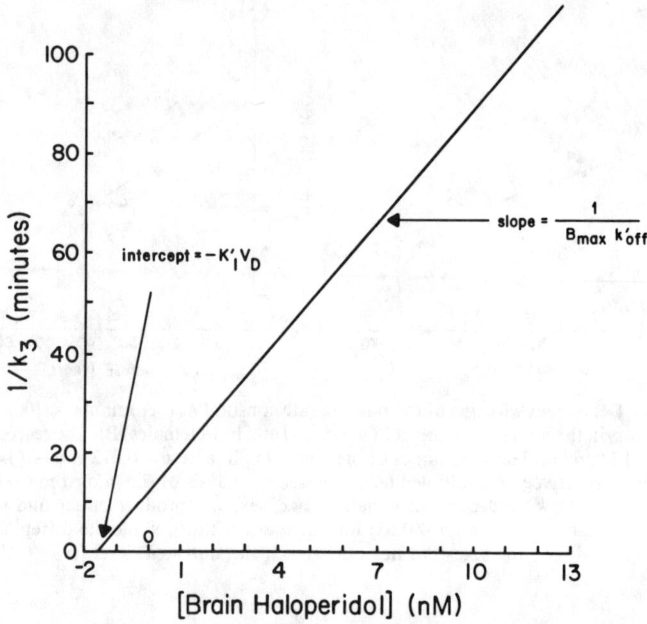

FIGURE 4. Schematical representation of the linear relationship between the reciprocal of the rate constant k_3 ($1/k_3$) and the tissue concentration of haloperidol. In our calculation of the absolute receptor density B_{max}, the brain haloperidol concentration was estimated from its serum values using the brain-to-plasma partition coefficient of haloperidol. The latter was determined both from average values of the K_1/k_2 ratios of [11C]NMSP for normal subjects and by *in vitro* experiments. These studies consisted of incubating [3H]haloperidol in human total plasma with minced prisms of rat cerebellum. The partition coefficient was obtained by measuring the loss of radioactive haloperidol from the plasma, as well as by measuring the uptake in brain on filters.

(41.7 $\pm$ 4.6 pmol/g) in the caudate nucleus of drug-naïve schizophrenic patients,[25] but are in agreement with our previous interpretation of the caudate/cerebellum ratio data.[17]

These preliminary results are in good agreement with those obtained from our simpler ratio approach. This decline has been observed also with *in vitro* experiments in both animals and humans.[6-14] Possible changes in cerebral blood flow that are associated with the aging process[26-30] cannot account for our measured decline in D_2 dopamine receptors with age because the model that we employed specifically measures a binding rate constant, k_3, that is independent of blood flow.

INFLUENCE OF THE MENSTRUAL CYCLE ON D_2 DOPAMINE RECEPTORS

In our original aging study,[17] we suggested that there was a sex difference in the distribution of the caudate/cerebellar ratio as a function of age. Some of these changes might be due in part to effects of male and female hormones. Current research demonstrates that gonadal steroid hormones, particularly estrogen, modulate some aspects of the function of the dopaminergic system.[31–34] In ovariectomized rats, striatal D_2 dopamine receptor density (B_{max}) is decreased; however, it is increased in nonovariectomized rats and in ovariectomized rats and male rats after long-term estrogen administration.[35–37]

To determine whether hormonal effects could be influencing the levels of cerebral dopamine receptors, we have recently been studying women at different stages of their menstrual cycle. Every woman received two PET scans, so each one served as their own control. Six women [mean age: 32.2 ± 4.9 (SD)] were selected from a group of gynecologically healthy young women who had regular uneventful mentrual cycles. None were taking exogenous estrogens or progesterones. The phase of the menstrual cycle was assessed by history, basal body temperature, and urine hormonal values. All of them had no more than one cycle between the two PET scans. In these six subjects, we computed the receptor binding using the full model. We noted that the binding rate constant (k_3) had a small, but definite trend (all in the same direction) between the different phases of the menstrual cycle (as illustrated in FIGURE 5). These results demonstrate that k_3 fluctuates during the normal menstrual cycle, with it tending to be lower in the follicular phase and higher in the periovulatory and luteal phases.

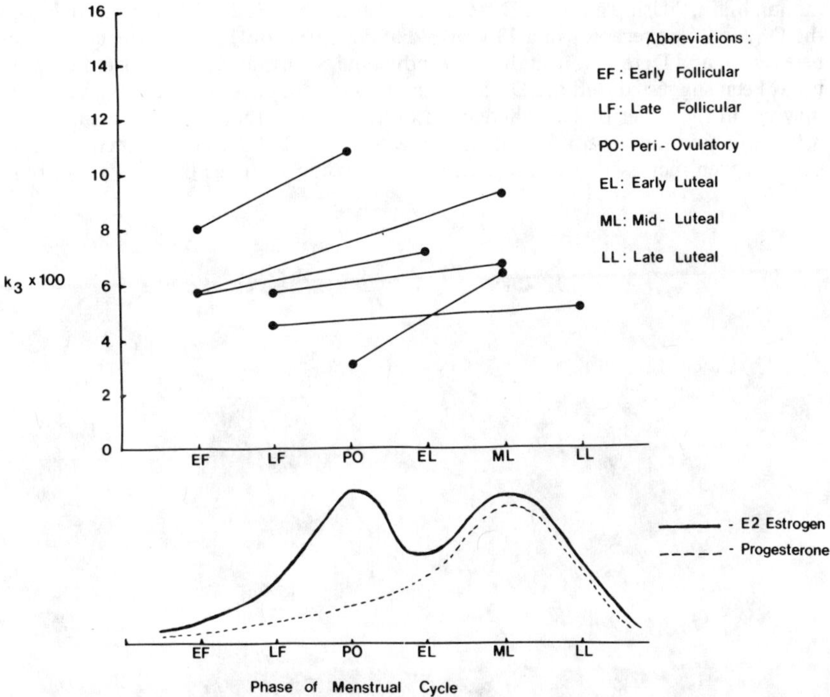

FIGURE 5. Fluctuations of the binding rate constant k_3 to the D_2 dopamine receptors in the caudate during the menstrual cycle in six healthy women. Each subject had two PET scans that were performed at different phases of the cycle. There was a trend to a slight increase of k_3 between the follicular and the luteal phase. Depicted in the lower graph is a schematic representation of variations in plasma estrogen and progesterone during a typical menstrual cycle.

Such a fluctuation of D_2 dopamine receptor density during the estrous cycle has been reported in rodent *in vitro* binding experiments, mainly in the anterior pituitary gland rather than in the striatum.[34,38,39] The pituitary-gonadal axis (possibly estrogens) may play an important role in the regulation of striatal D_2 dopamine receptors during the menstrual cycle and also with aging. Striatal dopaminergic function responds differently to estrogen in old animals as compared to younger animals.[40] Estrogens inhibit the dopaminergic supersensitivity induced by neuroleptics,[41] and estrogen therapy has been proposed to prevent or attenuate neuroleptic-induced tardive dyskinesia in older patients who are at greater risk for this severe secondary effect.[42]

In order to verify whether the presently observed fluctuations of the D_2 dopamine receptors in the striatum during the menstrual cycle are regulated by gonadal estrogens, further studies are being carried out to correlate these changes with hormone levels in serum. Also, other PET scans will be performed in postmenopausal women and in males in a similar manner.

IMAGING THE D_1 DOPAMINE RECEPTORS: PRELIMINARY STUDIES

Another recent development is the imaging of D_1 dopamine receptors in the living human brain.[43] Using a potent D_1 receptor ligand, [^{11}C]-SCH 23390, we have imaged the D_1 dopamine receptor in a 23-year-old and a 5-year-old subject. The comparison between D_1 and D_2 receptors in the same individual is illustrated in FIGURE 6. Recently,[44] it has been suggested that the D_1/D_2 ratio in young subjects at about 20 years of age may be on the order of 1:1, whereas, in older subjects, the ratio may be as high as 3:1. If this finding was confirmed, an explanation could be that the nonchanging (or perhaps even increased) value in D_1 receptor binding with age (as shown by human

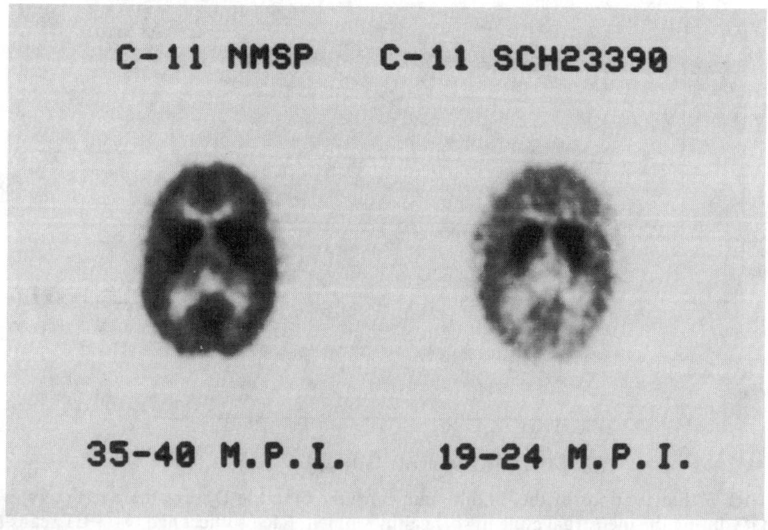

FIGURE 6. PET images in a 23-year-old subject passing through the caudate and putamen showing the uptake of [^{11}C]NMSP (35–40 min postinjection: MPI) and of [^{11}C]SCH 23390 (19–24 MPI). Both ligands show a high concentration in the basal ganglia.

autopsy studies)[45,46] added to a decline of D_2 dopamine receptors (as shown above). Although possible alterations of D_1 receptors with age are still a preliminary and controversial finding, our ability to measure [^{11}C]-SCH 23390 in human brain will allow imaging of the two dopamine receptor subtypes in the same subject (as a function of age) to determine possible D_1-D_2 receptor interaction. Breese *et al.*[47,48] proposed that the D_1 receptor function in severe neurodegenerative disorders such as Lesch-Nyhan syndrome could be modulated in part by D_2 receptors. Studies on D_1 and D_2 receptors in aging may provide further information about their interrelationship in normal physiological conditions.

CONCLUSIONS

The present data on the *in vivo* decline of the rate constant of binding of [^{11}C]NMSP to the D_2 dopamine receptors, k_3, as a function of age in men and women further reflect the likelihood that dopamine receptor densities in human caudate fall with age. Our preliminary data on receptor densities B_{max} in three old and nine young subjects also support this hypothesis. Future studies will involve calculation of receptor densities using varying levels of blocking doses of unlabeled neuroleptics for both D_1 and D_2 receptors.

The sex differences that are suggested from the menstrual cycle data introduce the novel studies that can be performed essentially by only *in vivo* techniques such as PET.

Thus, the promising investigations of normal physiological events as aging and sex differences in neuroreceptor systems will naturally lead to a better understanding of disease processes.

ACKNOWLEDGMENTS

We thank A. A. Wilson, H. T. Ravert, F. Gilbart, S. Herda, S. Bosley, D. Clough, M. Stumpf, H. Drew, B. Scheinin, C. Trauma, J. Schmidt, C. Schultz, M. Murrell, K. Prendergast, D. Starkey, K. Kofsky, and M. J. Kuhar for technical assistance and general discussion.

REFERENCES

1. HANDBOOK OF THE PSYCHOLOGY OF AGING. 1977. J. E. Birren & K. W. Shaie, Eds. Van Nostrand–Reinhold. Princeton, New Jersey.
2. PRADHAN, S.N. 1980. Central neurotransmitters and aging. Life Sci. **26:** 1643–1656.
3. ROTH, G. S. & G. D. HESS. 1982. Changes in the mechanisms of hormones and neurotransmitter action during aging: Current status of the role of receptor and post-receptor alterations. A review. Mech. Ageing Dev. **20:** 175–194.
4. SEVERSON, J. A. 1984. Neurotransmitter receptors and aging. J. Am. Geriatr. Soc. **32:** 24–27.
5. BURCHINSKY, S. G. 1984. Neurotransmitter receptors in the central nervous system in aging: Pharmacological aspect (review). Exp. Gerontol. **19:** 227–239.
6. MEMO, M., L. LUCCHI, P. F. SPANO & M. TRABUCCHI. 1980. Aging process affects a single class of dopamine receptors. Brain Res. **202:** 488–492.
7. MISRA, C. H., H. S. SHELAT & R. C. SMITH. 1980. Effect of age on estrogenic and dopaminergic receptor binding in rat brain. Life Sci. **27:** 521–526.
8. THAL, L. J., S. G. HOROWITZ, B. DVORKIN & M. H. MAKMAN. 1980. Evidence for loss of brain ^{3}H-spiroperidol and ^{3}H-ADTN binding sites in rabbit brain with aging. Brain Res. **192:** 185–194.

9. SEVERSON, J. A. & C. E. FINCH. 1980. Reduced dopaminergic binding during aging in the rodent striatum. Brain Res. **192:** 147–162.

10. JOSEPH, J. A., C. R. FILBURN & G. S. ROTH. 1981. Development of dopamine receptor denervation supersensitivity in the neostriatum of the senescent rat. Life Sci. **29:** 575–584.

11. SEVERSON, S. A., J. MARCUSSON, B. WINBLAD & C. E. FINCH. 1982. Age correlated loss of dopaminergic binding sites in human basal ganglia. J. Neurochem. **39:** 1623–1631.

12. SEVERSON, J. A. & P. K. RANDALL. 1985. D_2 dopamine receptors in aging mouse striatum: Determination of high- and low-affinity agonist binding sites. J.. Pharmacol. Exp. Ther. **233:** 361–368.

13. JOYCE, J. N., S. K. LOESCHEN, D. W. SAPP & J. F. MARSHALL. 1986. Age related regional loss of caudate-putamen dopamine receptors revealed by quantitative autoradiography. Brain Res. **378:** 158–163.

14. STAHL, S. M., S. THIEMANN, K. F. FAULL, J. D. BARCHAS & P. A. BERGER. 1986. Neurochemistry of dopamine in Huntington's dementia and normal aging. Arch. Gen. Psychiatry **43:** 161–164.

15. MORGAN, D. G. & C. E. FINCH. 1988. Dopaminergic changes in the basal ganglia: A generalized phenomenon of aging in mammals. This volume.

16. WAGNER, H. N., JR., H. D. BURNS, R. F. DANNALS, D. F. WONG, B. LANGSTROM, T. DUELFER, J. J. FROST, H. T. RAVERT, J. M. LINKS, S. B. ROSENBLOOM, S. E. LUKAS, A. V. KRAMER & M. J. KUHAR. 1983. Imaging dopamine receptors in the human brain by positron tomography. Science **221:** 1264–1266.

17. WONG, D. F., H. N. WAGNER, JR., R. F. DANNALS, J. M. LINKS, J. J. FROST, H. T. RAVERT, A. A. WILSON, A. E. ROSENBAUM, A. GJEDDE, K. H. DOUGLASS, J. D. PETRONIS, J. K. FOLSTEIN, J. K. T. TOUNG, H. D. BURNS & M. J. KUHAR. 1984. Effects of age on dopamine and serotonine receptors measured by positron emission tomography in the living human brain. Science **226:** 1393–1396.

18. BAUDRY, M., M. MARTRES & J. SCHWARTZ. 1977. *In vivo* binding of ^{3}H-pimozide in mouse striatum: effects of dopamine agonists and antagonists. Life Sci. **21:** 1163–1170.

19. HOLLT, V., A. CZLONKOWSKI & A. HERZ. 1977. The demonstration *in vivo* of specific binding sites for neuroleptic drugs in mouse brain. Brain Res. **177:** 176–183.

20. LADURON, P. M., P. F. M. JANSSEN & J. E. LEYSEN. 1978. Spiperone: A ligand of choice for neuroleptic receptors. 2. Regional distribution and *in vivo* displacement of neuroleptic drugs. Biochem. Pharmacol. **27:** 317–321.

21. KUHAR, M. J., L. C. MURRIN, A. T. MALOUF & N. KLEMM. 1978. Dopamine receptor binding *in vivo*: The feasibility of autoradiographic studies. Life Sci. **22:** 203–210.

22. WONG, D. F., A. GJEDDE & H. N. WAGNER, JR. 1986. Quantification of neuroreceptors in the living human brain. I. Irreversible binding of ligands. J. Cereb. Blood Flow Metab. **6:** 137–146.

23. WONG, D. F., A. GJEDDE, H. N. WAGNER, JR., R. F. DANNALS, K. H. DOUGLAS, J. M. LINKS & M. J. KUHAR. 1986. Quantification of neuroreceptors in the living human brain. II. Inhibition studies of receptor density and affinity. J. Cereb. Blood Flow Metab. **6:** 147–153.

24. WONG, D. F., H. N. WAGNER, JR., R. F. DANNALS, J. M. LINKS, M. J. KUHAR & A. GJEDDE. 1986. Human brain receptor distribution. (Letter.) Science **232:** 1270–1271.

25. WONG, D. F., H. N. WAGNER, JR., L. E. TUNE, R. F. DANNALS, G. D. PEARLSON, J. M. LINKS, C. A. TAMMINGA, E. P. BROUSSOLLE, H. T. RAVERT, A. A. WILSON, J. K. T. TOUNG, J. MALAT, J. A. WILLIAMS, L. A. O'TUAMA, S. H. SNYDER, M. J. KUHAR & A. GJEDDE. 1986. Positron emission tomography reveals elevated D_2 dopamine receptors in drug-naive schizophrenics. Science **234:** 1558–1563.

26. KETY, S. S. 1956. Human cerebral blood flow and oxygen consumption as related to aging. J. Chronic Dis. **3:** 478–486.

27. LASSEN, N. A., I. FEINBERG & M. H. LANE. 1960. Bilateral studies of cerebral oxygen uptake in young and aged normal subjects and in patients with organic dementia. J. Clin. Invest. **39:** 491–500.

28. OBRIST, W. D., L. SOKOLOFF, N. A. LASSEN, M. H. LANE, R. N. BUTLER & I. FEINBERG. 1963. Relation of EEG to cerebral blood flow and metabolism in old age. EEG Clin. Neurophysiol. **15:** 610–619.

29. MELAMED, E., S. LAVY, S. BENTIN, G. COOPER & Y. RINOT. 1980. Reduction in regional cerebral blood flow during normal aging in man. Stroke **11:** 31–35.

30. LONDON, E. D. 1984. Metabolism of the brain. A measure of cellular function in aging. *In* Aging and Cell Function. J. E. Johnson, Jr., Ed.: 187–210. Plenum. New York.

31. JOYCE, J. N., R. L. SMITH, C. VAN HARTESVELDT. 1982. Estradiol suppresses then enhances intracaudal dopamine-induced contralateral deviation. Eur. J. Pharmacol. **81:** 117–122.

32. GORDON, J. H. & K. O. PERRY. 1983. Pre- and postsynaptic neurochemical alterations following estrogen-induced striatal dopamine hypersensitivity. Brain Res. Bull. **10:** 425–428.

33. PICCARDI, P., F. BERNARDI, Z. ROSSETTI & G. CORSINI. 1983. Effect of estrogens on dopamine autoreceptors in male rats. Eur. J. Pharmacol. **91:** 1–9.

34. VAN HARTESVELDT, C. & J. N. JOYCE. 1986. Effects of estrogen on the basal ganglia. Neurosci. Biobehav. Rev. **10:** 1–14.

35. DIPAOLO, T., R. CARMICHAEL, F. LABRIE & J-P. RAYNAUD. 1979. Effects of estrogens on the characteristics of ^{3}H-spiroperidol and ^{3}H-RU 24213 binding in rat anterior pituitary gland and brain. Mol. Cell. Endocrinol. **16:** 99–112.

36. HRUSKA, R. E., L. M. LUDMER, K. T. PITMAN, M. DERYCK & K. SILBERGELD. 1982. Effects of estrogen on striatal dopamine receptor function in male and female rats. Pharmacol. Biochem. Behav. **16:** 285–291.

37. DIPAOLO, T., P. POYET & F. LABRIE. 1982. Prolactin and estradiol increase striatal dopamine receptor density in intact, castrated and hypophysectomized rats. Prog. Neuro-Psychopharmacol. Biol. Psychiatry **9:** 473–480.

38. HEIMAN, M. L. & N. BEN-JONATHAN. 1982. Dopaminergic receptors in the rat anterior pituitary change during the estrous cycle. Endocrinology **11:** 37–41.

39. DIPAOLO, T. & P. FALARDEAU. 1985. Modulation of brain and pituitary dopamine receptors by estrogens and prolactin. Prog. Neuro-Psychopharmacol. Biol. Psychiatry **9:** 473–480.

40. ROY, E. J., S. SHEINKOP & M. A. WILSON. 1982. Age alters dopaminergic responses to estradiol. Eur. J. Pharmacol. **82:** 74–75.

41. FIELDS, J. Z. & J. H. GORDON. 1981. Estrogen inhibits the dopaminergic supersensitivity induced by neuroleptics. Life Sci. **30:** 229–234.

42. GLAZER, W. M., F. NAFTOLIN, H. MORGENSTERN, E. R. BARNEA, N. J. MACLUSY & L. M. BRENNER. 1985. Estrogen replacement and tardive dyskinesia. Psychoneuroendocrinology **10:** 345–350.

43. WONG, D. F., C. BRAESTRUP, J. HARRIS, R. F. DANNALS, H. RAVERT, A. WILSON, J. WILLIAMS, J. LINKS, U. SCHEFFEL, L. O'TUAMA, G. FANARAS, H. MOSER, S. NAIDU, W. NYHAN, H. N. WAGNER, JR. & A. GJEDDE. 1986. Assessment of D_1 and D_2 dopamine receptors in Lesch-Nyhan syndrome by positron emission tomography. J. Nucl. Med. **27:** 1027 (abstract).

44. MORGAN, D. G., P. C. MAY & C. E. FINCH. 1986. Neurotransmitter receptors in normal human aging and Alzheimer's disease. *In* Receptors and Ligands in Psychiatry and Neurology. A. K. Sen & T. Y. Lee, Eds.

45. O'BOYLE, K. M. & J. L. WADDINGTON. 1984. Loss of striatal dopamine receptors with aging is selective for D_2 but not D_1 sites = association with increased non-specific binding of the D_1 ligand ^{3}H-piflutixol. Eur. J. Pharmacol. **105:** 171–174.

46. MORGAN, D. G., P. C. MAY & C. E. FINCH. 1986. Dopamine and serotonin systems in human and rodent brain: Effects of age and degenerative disease. J. Am. Geriatr. Soc. In press.

47. BREESE, G. R., A. A. BAUMEISTER, T. J. MCCROWN, S. G. EMERICK, G. D. FRYE & R. A. MUELLER. 1984. Neonatal 6-hydroxydopamine treatment: Model of susceptibility for self mutilation in the Lesch-Nyhan syndrome. Pharmacol. Biochem. Behav. **21:** 459–461.

48. BREESE, G. R., A. A. BAUMEISTER, T. C. NAPIER, G. D. FRYE & R. A. MUELLER. 1985. Evidence that D_1 dopamine receptors contribute to the supersensitive behavioral responses induced by L-dihydroxyphenylalanine in rats treated neonatally with 6-hydroxydopamine. J. Pharmacol. Exp. Ther. **235:** 287–295.

DISCUSSION OF THE PAPER

A. ALTAR (*CIBA–GEIGY Corporation, Summit, NY*): Are you able to detect D_1 binding in the substantia nigra? I noticed that the striatum was extremely high *C* labeled.

D. WONG (*The Johns Hopkins University School of Medicine, Baltimore, MD*): No; unfortunately, the current state of the art allows us only to make definitive comments about the caudata putamen because of the spatial resolution.

D. B. CALNE (*University of British Columbia, Vancouver, British Columbia, Canada*): Have you noticed any differences between caudate and putamen in your studies?

WONG: So far, we have not because it is very time-consuming to do all these fitting studies. I was principally looking at the caudate and, in our initial ratio studies, we did not see a difference between caudate and putamen. In general, the residue curves were almost completely superimposable. However, I do know that there have been some reported differences in the putamen and the caudate in different human and animal studies. I think that perhaps with better resolution elements — with better resolution PET scanners — it may be possible to pick those things up. In addition, we are going to try to refit all those putamens as well and I will have an answer for you in a few months.

J. TOBIN (*NIA, Bethesda, MD*): Just a technical question — do you give a PET scan and then a dose of prelabeling with pretreatment with haloperidol and then another PET scan?

WONG: That is correct.

TOBIN: Do you ever have a dose response of the pretreatment? Does it really fall on that slope if you use smaller doses for your pretreatment?

WONG: First, we do a control PET scan with the labeled compound. Then, four hours before the second PET scan, we give a dose of haloperidol in order to reduce the available number of receptors for the second PET scan. Thus, we have been able to show a dose response with different doses of haloperidol. Of course, we picked the dose that we have right now because that is the one that seems to be convenient and that tends to minimize acathexia.

D. INGRAM (*NIA, Baltimore, MD*): I know you used the Lesch-Nyhan data just for illustrative purposes, but why is there a higher D_1/D_2 ratio?

WONG: That is a good question. I am collaborating now with George Breese, who feels that there is a very strong D_1 behavioral response, but not necessarily D_1 receptor increases. However, other people have recently suggested D_1 elevations (perhaps in Parkinson's disease and other diseases). In addition, we know that the D_1 receptor is extremely important because if you use D_1 antagonists, you can block the self-injurious behavior in animal models; thus, it would not be inconceivable that the D_1 receptor would be relatively elevated to D_2.

Basal Ganglia Dopamine Receptor Autoradiography and Age-related Movement Disorders[a]

JOHN F. MARSHALL[b] AND JEFFREY N. JOYCE[c]

[b]Department of Psychobiology
University of California
Irvine, California 92717

[c]Department of Pharmacology
University of Pennsylvania
Philadelphia, Pennsylvania 19104

The existence of important regional differences in the structure and function of the striatum has become evident in recent years. Different regions of the striatum contribute to different behaviors; have a different mix of neurotransmitters, their synthetic enzymes, and their receptors; and receive information from widely differing sources. FIGURE 1 illustrates the regional specificity within the rat striatum by virtue of the topographic segregation of cortical inputs. Projections from motor cortex to the caudate-putamen (CP) of the rat are most dense in the dorsolateral sector at this relatively anterior level.[1,2] Projections from the somatic sensory cortex to the rat CP follow a similar pattern.[3] At more caudal levels, the densest projections of motor and somatosensory cortex are to the ventrolateral CP. In contrast, the more ventral and medial zone of the anterior striatum (i.e., the ventromedial CP, the nucleus accumbens septi [NAS], and the olfactory tubercle [OT]) receives few, if any, direct inputs from motor/somatosensory cortex. This ventromedial zone receives inputs principally from nonsensory, nonmotor regions of neocortex, the hippocampus, the entorhinal cortex, the amygdala, and related "limbic" structures.[4–6]

This description of corticostriatal neuroanatomy, although simplified, suggests two broad domains of information processing in the rodent striatum: one is related to somatic sensorimotor integration, while the other is not. Although the functions of the ventromedial striatum are poorly understood, the integration of information from cortical and subcortical limbic structures in this zone suggests a role in associative processes or spatial localization (two properties commonly attributed to limbic structures) or both. From this perspective, the reports of impaired egocentric localization[7] and of poor performance in tasks requiring spatial localization after CP lesions[8] are intriguing.

A corollary to this anatomy is that age-related striatal changes relevant to movement abnormalities are likely to occur in the dorsolateral sector of the anterior striatum (and in the ventrolateral posterior striatum). Although morphological and transmitter changes associated with the aging process may occur throughout the striatum,

[a] This research was supported by the following Public Health Service grants to J.F.M.: Nos. AG 00538, NS 20122, and NS 22698. J.N.J. was supported by Public Health Service Postdoctoral Fellowship No. IF 32 NS 07674.

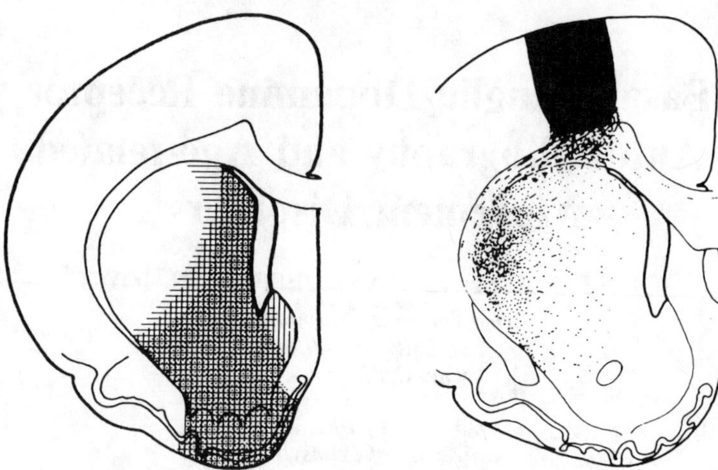

FIGURE 1. Left panel: projections to rat striatum from ventral tegmental area (vertical lines), amygdala (stipple), and prefrontal cortex (horizontal lines). Right panel: fiber labeling after injection of tritiated leucine and proline into the medial sensorimotor cortex of rat. (From reference 2.)

those occurring within the sensorimotor zone probably contribute most directly to the movement disturbances.

RELATIONSHIP OF DOPAMINERGIC SYNAPSES TO THE STRIATAL HETEROGENEITY

Much research concerning the role of the basal ganglia in age-related movement disorders has concentrated on the striatal dopaminergic synapses. The dopamine content of the striatum declines in the senescent rodent (reviewed in reference 9) and it declines progressively during the human life span.[10,11] In humans (but not in rats), the decline in caudate dopamine appears to be paralleled by a loss in the density of sites for dopamine uptake, which is a marker for dopamine nerve terminal density.[12,13] Accompanying these alterations in the striatal dopamine-containing elements are indications of lessened postsynaptic action of this transmitter. Decreases in striatal dopamine D_2 receptor binding are evident in the human and in rodents and are progressive during the adult life span.[14-16] A diminished capacity of dopamine to stimulate striatal adenylate cyclase activity has also been reported in the aged rodent,[17] which is a response to dopamine mediated through the D_1 receptor type.

The importance of these age-related alterations in striatal dopamine synapses for the movement limitations of senescence has been indicated by several experiments using rats. Specifically, some of the age-related impairments in the movements of aged rats can be reversed by (i) pharmacological treatment with L-dopa or directly acting dopamine agonists,[18] (ii) striatal transplants of fetal nigral dopamine-containing cells,[19] or (iii) manipulations that result in an increase in striatal D_2 receptors (dietary restriction or chronic treatment with dopamine receptor antagonists[20]).

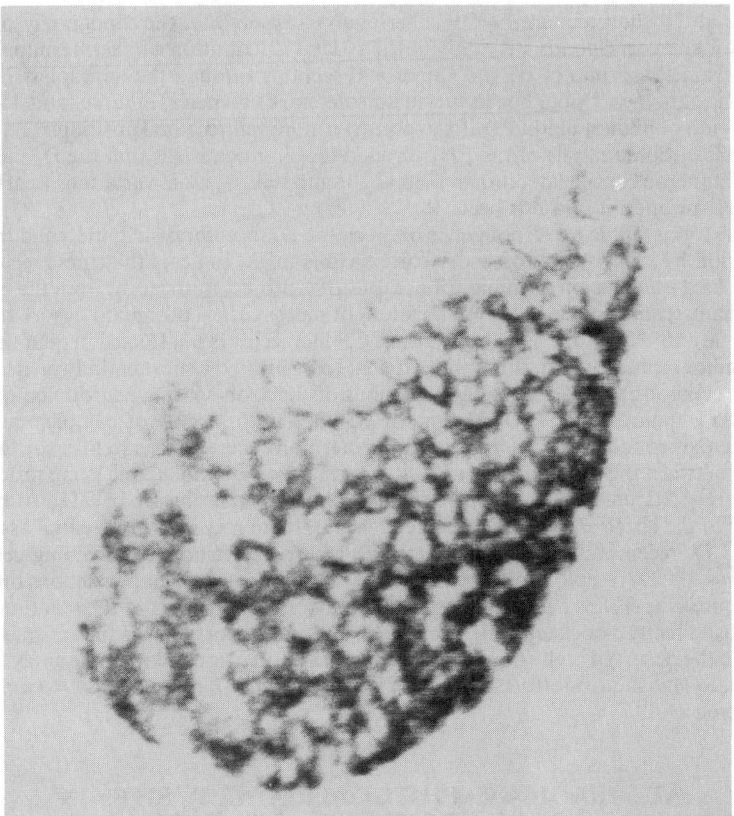

FIGURE 2. Image in horizontal plane of specific [³H]spiroperidol binding through the left striatum of a 5–6-month-old male F344 rat. Top is posterior; bottom is anterior. Medial is to left; lateral is to right.

In view of the importance of these dopaminergic synapses for movement, one might speculate that there are differences between the striatal dopaminergic input to the sensorimotor and limbic striatal zones previously described. However, the dopaminergic innervations of these zones of rodent CP appear very similar. For instance, the concentration of dopamine in the lateral CP is indistinguishable from that in the medial CP; neither do ventral versus dorsal differences in dopamine content exist.[21-23] A homogeneous distribution of the dopamine inputs along the dorsoventral and mediolateral CP axes has also been confirmed using semiquantitative fluorescence histochemistry of the striatal dopamine-containing nerve endings.[24]

However, the distribution of the D_2 class of dopamine receptor corresponds closely to the sensorimotor versus limbic domains. Using computer-assisted quantitative autoradiographic procedures to study the distribution of D_2 receptors in young adult rat striatum, we were struck by the marked regional variation in density of this site (FIGURE 2). The density of this site, labeled by [³H]spiroperidol, is severalfold higher in lateral CP than medially.[25,26] Further analysis shows that the topography of this receptor site corresponds strikingly to the striatal distribution of axon terminals derived from sensorimotor cortex. In coronal sections through the anterior striatum, the zone of highest D_2 binding occurs in dorsolateral CP, whereas at more caudal levels, this region of highest binding shifts to occupy a more ventrolateral position.[23] Equilibrium saturation analysis of the [3H]spiroperidol binding reveals that the D_2 sites are more numerous in the lateral than medial CP and that regional variations in affinity for [3H]spiroperidol do not occur.[23]

The topographic correspondence between the D_2 receptor distribution and the innervation by motor/somatosensory cortex axons might indicate that these receptors are located on the axon terminals of neurons that project to striatum from the motor or somatosensory cortex. However, ablations of motor cortex, of somatosensory cortex, or of the entire frontoparietal region leave CP D_2 receptors unaffected in quantitative autoradiographs. Instead, the D_2 sites appear to be located almost entirely on neurons whose cell bodies reside in the CP. Injections of the axon-sparing neurotoxin, quinolinic acid, reduces the CP D_2 binding by 90–95% in the region of complete neuron loss that surrounds the injection site.[27] Furthermore, there is a very close correspondence between the distribution of D_2 sites and indexes of cholinergic nerve processes in the rat striatum.[28] Because the striatal cholinergic neurons are believed to be intrinsic to the striatum (reviewed in reference 29), there may be a preferential association of D_2 receptors with the membranes of these acetylcholine-containing cells.

Thus, the D_2 receptor appears to mediate dopamine's postsynaptic actions on striatal neurons (perhaps cholinergic) preferentially in those regions of the striatum that are most directly associated with somatic sensory/motor cortex. This finding may help explain the observed high correlations between the potencies of dopamine antagonists in their *in vivo* motoric efforts and their affinities for the D_2 receptor *in vitro* (reviewed in reference 30).

AUTORADIOGRAPHY OF STRIATAL D_2 SITES IN YOUNG ADULT AND AGED RATS

In light of the marked striatal heterogeneity of D_2 receptors in young adult rats, we wished to determine whether the age-related decline in these receptors occurred uniformly throughout the CP. This issue was readily amenable to study using quantitative *in vitro* film autoradiography and image analysis.[31]

Horizontal sections were cut through the forebrain of senescent (26–28-month-old) and young adult (5–6-month-old) F344 male rats. Slide-mounted sections were incubated in [3H]spiroperidol (0.7 nM, 100 Ci/mmol; Amersham) for 60 min at 36 °C in 50 mM TRIS buffer plus ions. Ketanserin (40 nM) was included in the incubation medium to prevent [3H]spiroperidol binding to serotonin (S_2) sites. Alternate sections were incubated in a medium that also contained (+)-butaclamol (1 μM) to define the nonspecific binding of the radioligand. After exposure and development of the autoradiographic film ([3H]Ultrofilm, LKB Produkter), the autoradiographic images of the brain sections were digitized and linearized with the aid of a Spatial Data Systems Model 850 image analyzer. A calibration curve was generated using tritium-containing tissue standards, and the autoradiograph was transformed according to this curve (i.e., linearized) so that the grey values of each pixel were a linear function of the quantity of [3H]spiroperidol bound per mg protein. The linearized image of the nonspecific binding was subtracted from that of the total binding to obtain an image of the specific binding.

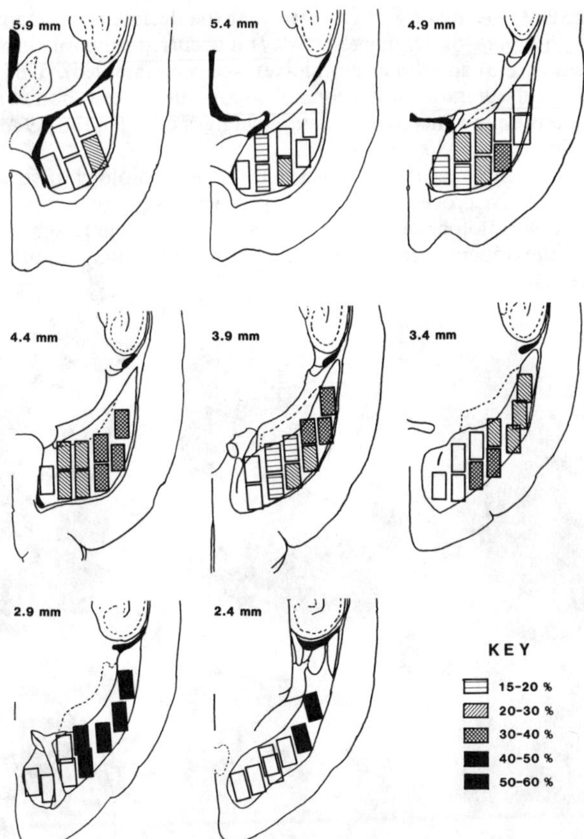

FIGURE 3. Diagram depicting the percentage reduction in specific [³H]spiroperidol binding in aged rats relative to young adult controls. Each frame depicts a different horizontal plane. Open rectangles demarcate zones in which no significant age differences were observed. The key indicates the percentile loss associated with the zones for which significant age differences were obtained. Orientation of striatum is the same as for FIGURE 2. (From reference 31.)

The aged rats showed an anatomically heterogeneous loss of D_2 sites. In general, the age-related decline in D_2 sites was most extensive in CP regions that showed the highest density of these receptors in young adult animals. As a result, the aged rats showed a greatly attenuated gradient of receptor binding. The zone of highest D_2 binding (which in young adult rats extends from the anterior dorsolateral CP through the posterior ventrolateral CP) is greatly diminished in the 26–28-month-old rats. FIGURE 3 depicts the age-related change in D_2 binding as the percentage decline relative to 5–6-month-old controls. Different regions of the striatum were quite differently affected. In many regions (open rectangles), no significant age differences were found. In others, the loss was as great as 60%. The regions in which substantial (30–60%) declines of D_2 binding were evident included the lateral, posterior, and ventral striatum.[31]

The finding that age-related synaptic changes in rat striatum can be regionally specific has precedent. Strong *et al.*[32] reported that the decline in dopamine content of the senescent (26-month-old) Sprague-Dawley rat occurred primarily in the caudal striatum (the mediolateral and dorsoventral axes were not sampled). This may relate to the morphological alterations in dopamine-containing cell bodies of the aged C57Bl/6NNia mouse in which the structural changes occur in the A9 and dorsal A10 cells, but not in ventral A10 neurons.[33]

Taken together, these results establish that the neurobiology of striatal aging can be a regionally selective process. Our results specifically suggest that the dopaminergic control of the sensorimotor domain of the striatum is more compromised in senescent rodents than is the dopaminergic influence over the limbic portion of this basal gangliar structure.

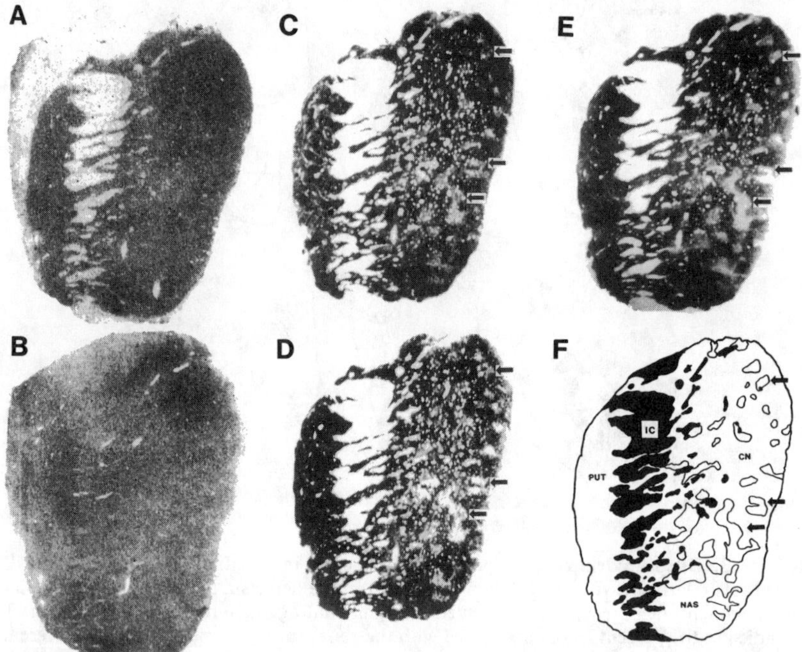

FIGURE 4. Effect of chloroform extraction of lipids on the nonspecific (A and B) and specific (C and D) binding of [³H]spiroperidol, and comparison with AChE staining (E and F) in an adjacent section of patient no. A-185-85. (A) Digitized image of an autoradiograph of nonspecific binding to a section not treated with chloroform. Note the apparent lower nonspecific binding of [³H]spiroperidol in white matter (e.g., the internal capsule). (B) Digitized image of an autoradiograph of nonspecific binding to the section adjacent to A, but treated with chloroform after incubation in [³H]spiroperidol. (C) Image of specific binding derived from a tissue section not treated with chloroform. (D) Image of specific binding derived from an adjacent section treated with chloroform after radioligand binding. (E) Photograph of an adjacent section that was stained for AChE. (F) Drawing (derived from E) showing the AChE-poor zones in outlines. Some AChE-poor zones are marked with arrows and they correspond to the D₂-poor zones that are marked in C and D. To assist in depicting the effect of chloroform extraction on the nonspecific binding, the photographic negatives of A and B were underexposed relative to the images of specific binding. IC = internal capsule; PUT = putamen; NAS = nucleus accumbens; CN = caudate nucleus. (From reference 36.)

DOPAMINE RECEPTOR TOPOGRAPHY IN HUMAN STRIATUM: NOVEL PRINCIPLES RELEVANT TO UNDERSTANDING BASAL GANGLIAR AGING

Human age-related changes in sensorimotor function believed to be due to the decline in basal ganglia dopamine transmission have long been recognized (e.g., see reference 34). More recent quantitative techniques support the view that slowing of movement with age may be secondary to the decline in dopamine's central action.[35] Recently, we have conducted studies to determine the distribution of dopamine D_2 receptors in caudate-putamen tissue sections derived from postmortem human brain.[36] Histochemical and immunocytochemical observations have provided convincing evidence for a complex compartmental organization of the striatum of carnivores and primates, including humans (reviewed in reference 29). The modular striatal chemoarchitecture, "striosomal",[37] appears to be obeyed by several transmitter-related compounds, as well as by afferent and efferent connections of the striatum.[29] A convenient histochemical marker for this striosomal organization is acetylcholinesterase (AChE) staining.[37]

Human brain material was obtained at autopsy from four patients (ages 34 to 68) after a postmortem interval of four hours. After sectioning and incubation in [³H]spiroperidol, sections were dried, fixed by exposure to paraformaldehyde vapors, and immersed briefly (2 min) in chloroform for extraction of lipids. This procedure avoids the difficulties otherwise associated with differential absorption of the beta emissions from tritium by white and gray matter.[38,39] Adjacent sections were not used for radioligand binding assays, but instead were stained for AChE.

The digitized, linearized images of [³H]spiroperidol binding revealed a striking pattern of high- and low-density patches in the caudate and putamen (FIGURE 4C,D). In coronal sections through the caudate and putamen of this individual (39 years old), the D_2-low patches form complexly shaped islands surrounded by a higher density matrix of D_2 binding. Quantification of this and the other cases revealed that the [³H]spiroperidol binding in the D_2-rich zones (420–450 fmol/mg protein) was approximately twice that of the D_2-poor zones (220–240 fmol/mg protein). The correspondence between the D_2 binding pattern (FIGURE 4C,D) and the AChE histochemistry on adjacent sections (FIGURE 4E,F) was quite close. Chloroform extraction of lipids from the tissue section improved the contrast between the D_2-rich and D_2-poor zones (compare FIGURE 4C with 4D), while it also elminated the differential absorption of tritium emissions (compare FIGURE 4A with 4B).

A comparison of the D_2 autoradiographs from each of the cases studied suggests that age may affect the patterning of the D_2 receptor. In each case, the density of D_2 binding within the D_2-rich regions was similar; however, the percentage of the striatal area containing D_2-rich area varied. Patient no. A-251-84 (age 68, FIGURE 5) had significantly less area of the caudate and putamen occupied by D_2-rich regions than did the younger patients (e.g., see FIGURE 4). For the older patient, the predominant patterning appears as circumscribed D_2-rich zones against a lighter background, yet circumscribed D_2-poor regions can also be identified. In all cases, it should be noted that the type of patterning evidenced by the D_2 receptor autoradiography closely matches that revealed in the AChE histochemistry.

These results on D_2 compartmentalization in human striatum have several implications. First, they suggest that D_2 receptors are strategically positioned to modulate dopamine's postsynaptic influence on a population of striatal outputs.[40,41] Second, they indicate that D_2 receptors are most dense in striatal regions that are high in acetylcholinesterase; this is consistent with previous studies from this laboratory indicating a close correspondence between D_2 receptor distribution in the rat striatum and markers

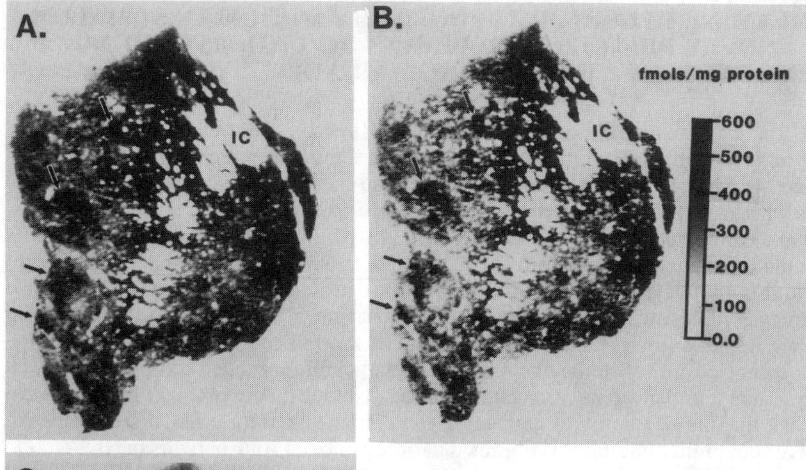
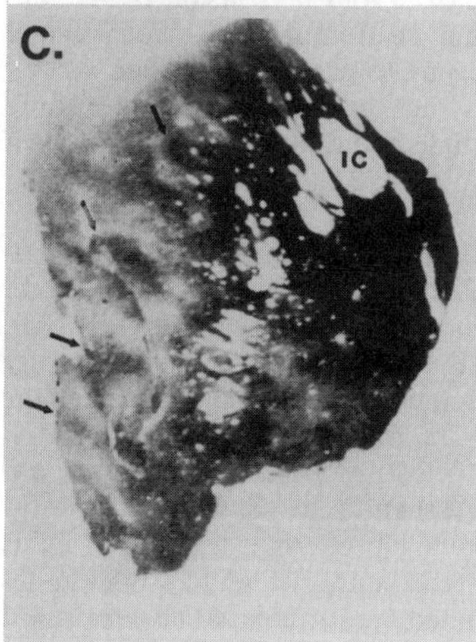

FIGURE 5. Comparison of D_2 receptor zones in the digitized image of the original autoradiograph (A) with the linearized version of the same image (B) and the adjacent section stained for AChE (C) in coronal sections of human striatum from the left hemisphere of patient no. A-251-84. (A) Digitized image of the autoradiograph of the total [³H]spiroperidol binding. Some of the D_2-rich zones in the nucleus accumbens septi and caudate nucleus are marked with arrows and they correspond to the D_2-rich zones in the linearized image and to the AChE-rich zones. (B) Same autoradiograph, but linearized to provide a quantitative representation of the amount of [³H]spiroperidol bound (fmol/mg protein). (C) Adjacent section, stained for AChE. Note that the AChE-poor zones (striosomes) and AChE-rich zones (arrows) correspond to D_2-poor and D_2-rich zones, respectively. IC = internal capsule. (From reference 36.)

for cholinergic neuron density.[28] Third, the results tentatively suggest that in the human striatum, as in the rodent, the age-related loss of D_2 receptors is anatomically distinct, thus affecting preferentially those zones rich in D_2 binding. The last of these conclusions will need to be tested further by analysis of additional striata derived from humans of different ages.

CONCLUDING COMMENTS

Studies concerning the neurobiology of basal ganglia in aging have largely focused on the development of neurochemical methods for assaying the presynaptic and postsynaptic changes that occur at dopaminergic, cholinergic, and other synapses during the life span. While these experiments have pointed out some reliable age changes in humans and rodents, there has been a tendency to treat the striatum as a structural unity. The deceptively homogeneous appearance of the caudate-putamen in Nissl-stained sections has undoubtedly reinforced this tendency. An appreciation of the domains, or compartments, of striatal information processing has developed only in the past few years because it has depended upon more recently devised anatomical/histochemical procedures such as immunocytochemistry, receptor autoradiography, and autoradiographic tracing of axonal projections. These and other techniques reveal a much richer and varied texture to the striatal neuropil than the Nissl stain suggests. The experiments described herein indicate that the aging process in rats, and perhaps in humans as well, respects the structural domains of the striatum. Thus, in order to understand fully the process of striatal aging, it will require an amalgamation of approaches — chemistry and morphology — so that we can address not only those classes of transmitters/receptor systems that are affected, but also the domains of striatal information processing that undergo synaptic alterations in the aging process.

ACKNOWLEDGMENTS

We thank Ronald C. Kim of the Long Beach Veterans Administration Hospital for assistance in obtaining human brain tissue at autopsy.

REFERENCES

1. COSPITO, J. A. & K. KULTAS-ILINSKY. 1981. Exp. Neurol. **72:** 257–266.
2. KELLEY, A. E., V. B. DOMESICK & W. J. H. NAUTA. 1982. Neuroscience **7:** 615–630.
3. WISE, S. P. & E. G. JONES. 1977. J. Comp. Neurol. **175:** 129–158.
4. BECKSTEAD, R. M. 1979. Neurosci. Lett. **12:** 59–64.
5. KELLEY, A. E. & V. B. DOMESICK. 1982. Neuroscience **7:** 2321–2335.
6. NEWMAN, R. & S. S. WINANS. 1980. J. Comp. Neurol. **191:** 167–192.
7. POTEGAL, M. 1972. Acta Neurobiol. Exp. **32:** 479–494.
8. DIVAC, I., H. J. MAKOWITSCH & M. PRITZEL. 1978. Brain Res. **151:** 523–532.
9. FINCH, C. E., P. RANDALL & J. F. MARSHALL. 1981. Annu. Rev. Gerontol. Geriatr. **2:** 49–87.
10. RIEDERER, P. & S. T. WUKETICH. 1976. J. Neural Transm. **38:** 277–301.
11. ADOLFSSON, R., C-G. GOTTFRIES, B-E. ROOS & B. WINBLAD. 1979. J. Neural Transm. **45:** 81–105.
12. ZELNICK, N., I. ANGEL, S. PAUL & J. E. KLEINMAN. 1986. Eur. J. Pharmacol. **126:** 175–176.
13. MARSHALL, J. F. & C. A. ALTAR. 1986. Brain Res. **379:** 112–117.
14. LEVIN, P., J. K. JANDA, J. A. JOSEPH, D. K. INGRAM & G. S. ROTH. 1981. Science **214:** 561–562.
15. SEVERSON, J. A. & C. E. FINCH. 1980. Brain Res. **192:** 147–162.
16. SEVERSON, J. A., J. MARCUSSON, B. WINBLAD & C. E. FINCH. 1982. J. Neurochem. **39:** 1623–1631.
17. PURI, S. K. & L. VOLICER. 1977. Mech. Ageing Dev. **6:** 53–58.
18. MARSHALL, J. F. & N. BERRIOS. 1979. Science **206:** 477–479.
19. GAGE, F. H., S. B. DUNNETT, U. STENEVI & A. BJORKLUND. 1983. Science **221:** 966–969.
20. JOSEPH, J. A., R. T. BARTUS, D. CLODY, D. MORGAN, C. FINCH, B. BEER & S. SESACK. 1983. Neurobiol. Aging **4:** 313–319.
21. DIPAOLO, T., M. DAIGLE & A. DUPONT. 1982. Can. J. Neurol. Sci. **9:** 421–427.
22. TASSIN, J. P., A. CHERAMY, G. BLANC, A. M. THIERRY & J. GLOWINSKI. 1976. Brain Res. **107:** 291–301.
23. JOYCE, J. N., S. K. LOESCHEN & J. F. MARSHALL. 1985. Brain Res. **338:** 209–218.
24. REDGRAVE, P. & I. MITCHELL. 1982. Neuroscience **7:** 871–883.
25. ALTAR, C. A., S. O'NEIL, R. J. WALTER, JR. & J. F. MARSHALL. 1985. Science **228:** 597–600.
26. ALTAR, C. A., R. J. WALTER, K. A. NEVE & J. F. MARSHALL. 1984. J. Neurosci. Methods **10:** 173–188.

27. JOYCE, J. N. & J. F. MARSHALL. 1986. Neuroscience **20**: 773–795.
28. JOYCE, J. N. & J. F. MARSHALL. 1985. Neurosci. Lett. **53**: 127–131.
29. GRAYBIEL, A. M. & C. W. RAGSDALE. 1983. *In* Chemical Neuroanatomy. P. C. Emson, Ed.: 427–504. Raven Press. New York.
30. SEEMAN, P. 1980. Pharmacol. Rev. **32**: 229–313.
31. JOYCE, J. N., S. K. LOESCHEN, D. W. SAPP & J. F. MARSHALL. 1986. Brain Res. **378**: 158–163.
32. STRONG, R., T. SAMORAJSKI & Z. GOTTESFELD. 1982. J. Neurochem. **39**: 831–836.
33. MCNEILL, T. H., L. L. KOEK & J. W. HAYCOCK. 1984. Mech. Ageing Dev. **24**: 293–307.
34. CRITCHLEY, M. 1956. J. Chronic Dis. **3**: 459–477.
35. MORTIMER, J. A. & D. D. WEBSTER. 1982. *In* The Aging Motor System. J. A. Mortimer, F. J. Pirozzolo & G. J. Maletta, Eds.: 217–241. Praeger. New York.
36. JOYCE, J. N., D. W. SAPP & J. F. MARSHALL. 1986. Proc. Natl. Acad. Sci. USA **83**: 8002–8006.
37. GRAYBIEL, A. M. & C. W. RAGSDALE. 1978. Proc. Natl. Acad. Sci. USA **75**: 5723–5726.
38. HERKENHAM, M. & L. SOKOLOFF. 1984. Brain Res. **321**: 363–368.
39. SAPP, D. W., J. N. JOYCE & J. F. MARSHALL. 1986. Neurosci. Abstr. **12**: 142.
40. GRAYBIEL, A. M., C. W. RAGSDALE & S. MOON-EDLEY. 1979. Exp. Brain Res. **34**: 189–195.
41. GERFEN, C. R. 1985. J. Comp. Neurol. **236**: 454–476.

DISCUSSION OF THE PAPER

G. S. ROTH (*NIA, Baltimore, MD*): A paper in the September 18th issue of *Nature* by Trugman *et al.* came to the same conclusion about the localization using cortical ablation, namely, that the D_2 receptors are on the cholinergic interneurons. However, I have a question with regard to your conclusion that this may be a cell loss phenomenon. I remember that Randy Strong presented data earlier showing no loss of the ChAT activity in the Fischer-344 rat. What do you think about that?

A. ALTAR (*CIBA–GEIGY Corporation, Summit, NJ*): That was a little puzzling to me. One would expect striatal cholinergic markers to decrease with D_2 receptor losses. Maybe Randy Strong has a better explanation for that.

R. STRONG (*Veterans Administration Medical Center, St. Louis, MO*): Thomas McNeill is going to present some data later showing morphological changes in what perhaps are cholinergic interneurons. His data suggest that there might be a loss of neurons, but then, in the ones remaining, there is an extensive dendritic arborization that is taking place. Therefore, maybe the storage sites for ChAT are not reduced, but the number of neurons may be reduced; this is evidenced by the decrease in high-affinity choline uptake.

ROTH: Are you then suggesting that perhaps the terminals are shrinking away and the cell bodies are more intact?

STRONG: Terminals are lost and some cells are lost, but the remaining cells are perhaps increasing in choline acetyltransferase (which is stored in other areas of the cell).

J. SEVERSON (*Amersham Corporation, Arlington Heights, IL*): I like the autoradiography concept. It is a good adjunct to what we have been doing with test tubes. One thing, though, that concerns me is the localization issue and the change with age. It is well known that the innervation of the striatum by the nigrostriatal pathway is highest in the head of the caudate and declines in the tail of the caudate. Therefore, are you saying that the major amount of decrease is in an area where dopamine innervation is least? What would be the functional significance of that?

ALTAR: The losses in striatal D_2 receptor binding of the aged rats were greatest in the caudal portions of the ventral striatum. However, the losses were expressed as percentile decreases from the specific D_2 binding of the young animals. The amounts of D_2 binding vary greatly through the striatum and are quite low in the caudal portions of the ventral striatum relative to the lateral striatum. Thus, the amounts of D_2 receptors lost may be similar in these regions. The functional significance of these D_2 losses can be better determined after a similar regional analysis is made for age-related decreases in striatal dopamine release.

Dopamine in the Extrapyramidal Motor Function

A Study Based upon the MPTP-Induced Primate Model of Parkinsonism[a]

C. C. CHIUEH

Clinical Brain Imaging Section
Laboratory of Cerebral Metabolism
National Institute of Mental Health
Bethesda, Maryland 20892-1000

INTRODUCTION

Since the discovery of dopamine in the central nervous system,[1] the extrapyramidal motor function of the nigrostriatal pathway has been studied extensively. Postmortem pathological and neurochemical studies of the parkinsonian brain have led to the introduction of L-dihydroxyphenylalanine (L-DOPA) for the treatment of Parkinson's disease.[2]

By using an intrastriatal or intranigral injection of a monoamine neurotoxin, 6-hydroxydopamine, Ungerstedt[3] has developed a rotational rodent model for studying postsynaptic supersensitivity of the nigrostriatal system. The contribution of this rotational animal model in developing D2 dopamine agonists for the treatment of Parkinson's disease has been well documented.

Through investigation of both the tragic consequences of several intravenous drug abusers[4-6] and industrial accidents that involved medicinal chemists, we have developed a primate model of parkinsonism[7] following intravenous administration of a nigrostriatal dopamine neurotoxin, 1-methyl-4-phenyl-1,2,3,6-tetrahydropyridine (MPTP). A primate model of hemiparkinsonism[8] was developed recently and was used for the study of postsynaptic supersensitivity. This discussion summarizes the use of this MPTP-induced primate model of parkinsonism for the reevaluation of the extrapyramidal motor function, for testing or screening of new antiparkinsonian agents, and for developing presynaptic and postsynaptic brain imaging ligands.

METHODS AND MATERIALS

Rhesus and cynomolgus monkeys (5–8 kg *Macaca mulatta*; 2–6 kg *Macaca fascicularis*) of both sexes, and female C57BL6 mice (National Institute on Aging, GRC

[a] This study was supported by the intramural research program of NIMH (Robert Cohen & Sanford Markey), NINCDS (Irwin J. Kopin), and NIA (Richard Greulich, GRC aging colony of C57BL6 mice).

colony; age 2, 12, and 24 months) were used in this study. MPTP free base (caution: sublimes at room temperature) was dissolved in saline solution containing 10% alcohol, and MPTP·HCl salt (RBI, Wayland, Massachusetts) was dissolved in saline for either intravenous administration to conscious monkeys[7] or infusion into the internal carotid artery of the anesthetized monkeys[8] (7 mg/kg ketamine with 0.7 mg/kg xylazine). MPTP solution was injected intraperitoneally to mice (15–30 mg/kg) every 12 hours for three times. Behavioral observations were performed either by direct observation or by videotaping as described previously.[7,8]

Sinemet (100 mg L-DOPA with 10 mg carbidopa) was suspended in juice and given orally. Apomorphine and LY 171555 (Quinperol) were dissolved in saline and injected subcutaneously (0.1–2 mg/kg for monkeys; 5–20 mg/kg for mice).

An HPLC procedure[9] was used to measure dopamine, L-DOPA, 6-F-L-DOPA, and their metabolites in the CSF and brain samples.

The *in vivo* imaging of the CNS dopaminergic system was performed in small animals[3] by using autoradiographic procedures following intravenous injection of 1-^{14}C-L-DOPA (Amersham) or ^{125}I-IBZM [S-3-iodo-N-{(1-ethyl-2pyrrolidinyl)}methyl-2-hydroxy-6-methoxybenzamide] synthesized by Kung *et al.*[10] The positron emission tomography (PET) of the brain dopamine procedure of Garnett *et al.*[11] was used to monitor brain damage in parkinsonian monkeys.

RESULTS

MPTP-Induced Primate Model of Parkinsonism and Hemiparkinsonism

Serotonin syndrome, mydriasis, sympathetic discharge, dystonia (discharge of striatal dopamine), and gastrointestinal bleeding (ulcer) were observed during acute phase after administration of MPTP. Not all of the MPTP-treated monkeys developed parkinsonism, though. The major clinical signs of the extrapyramidal motor dysfunction appeared only in monkeys with a more than 80% reduction in striatal dopamine. Full parkinsonism was observed in 4–8-kg monkeys two to three weeks following intravenous administration of MPTP free base (0.35 mg/kg, daily for five days)[7] or after administration of 1.5–2.5 mg/kg of MPTP·HCl salt. The high dose regimen often caused not only depletion of brain catecholamines, but also other side effects such as ulcer and aphagia or sudden death. In addition to an acute serotonin syndrome, MPTP (1.5–2.5 mg/kg, i.v.) caused a selective lesion of the neuromelanin-containing A9 substantia nigral compacta neurons and spared the ventrotegmental A10 neurons (TABLE 1). The symptoms and signs produced by MPTP in monkeys were similar to those produced in man. These extrapyramidal signs manifested within two to three weeks, which included flexed posture, drooling, freezing, rigidity, akinesia, eyelid closure, and decrease in vocalization (FIGURE 1). The only noticeable difference was the type of tremor; MPTP produced mostly postural tremor rather than resting tremor in "rhesus monkeys". MPTP also produced severe depletion of striatal dopamine in small experimental animals, but failed to induce extrapyramidal motor dysfunction in these animals (i.e., mice, rats, cats, and dogs).

Full parkinsonian monkeys required L-DOPA therapy in order to maintain life (FIGURE 1). The therapeutic effects of L-DOPA were significantly smaller in the severely lesioned monkeys (with a greater than 98% decrease in striatal dopamine). These monkeys required tube feeding and intensive care.

A primate model of hemiparkinsonism was produced in cynomolgus and rhesus monkeys following a slow infusion of MPTP·HCl (0.2–0.4 mg/kg) into the right in-

TABLE 1. MPTP Induced a Selective Depletion of Dopamine in the Putamen and Caudate Nucleus, but Not in the Nucleus Accumbens of Rhesus Monkeys

	Dopamine		
	Putamen	Caudate Nucleus	Nucleus Accumbens
		(pg/µg protein)	
Control	135.4 ± 9.6 (7)	152.6 ± 6.0 (7)	59.5 ± 10.2 (2)
MPTP[a]	6.4 ± 2.4[b] (5)	13.4 ± 5.3[b] (5)	66.5 ± 24.6 (4)

[a] MPTP (3.3 mg/kg, i.v., daily for five days; sacrificed one to two months later).
[b] $p < 0.05$.

ternal carotid artery. This procedure produced a greater than 95% depletion of dopamine in the caudate nucleus and putamen ipsilateral to the side of infusion of MPTP. These unilaterally lesioned monkeys exhibited a spontaneous circling behavior toward the side of lesion, while dystonia, bradykinesia, or rigidity (or any combination of these three) of the contralateral limbs appeared within two weeks. These symptoms were alleviated after treatment with L-DOPA or D2 agonists (apomorphine and LY 171555).[8] L-DOPA and apomorphine also caused a contralateral rotational behavior (TABLE 2) in some of these hemiparkinsonian monkeys. These results indicate that a postsynaptic D2 dopamine receptor supersensitivity develops following a selective lesion of the nigrostriatal dopaminergic neurons by MPTP. The receptor supersensitivity produced by MPTP in these hemiparkinsonian monkeys (TABLE 2) is similar to that reported in Ungerstedt's rotational rodent model following an intranigral injec-

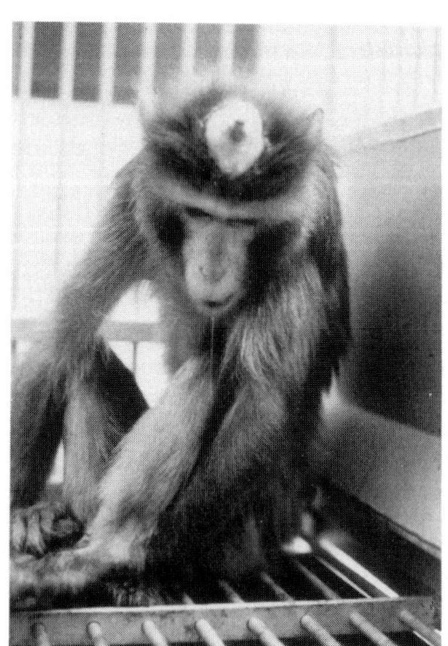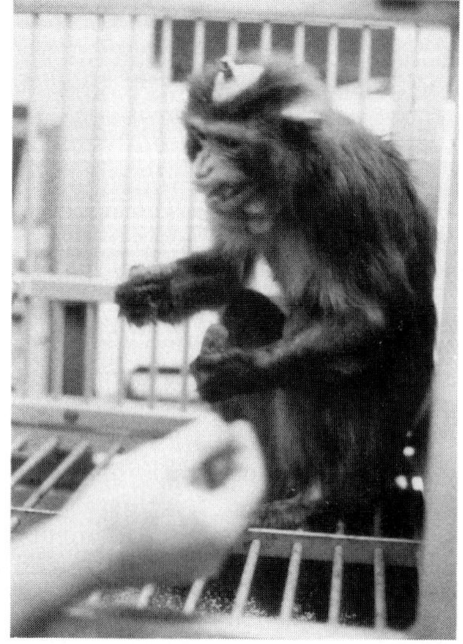

FIGURE 1. MPTP-induced primate model of parkinsonism: (A) before and (B) after treatment with L-DOPA (Sinemet 100/10).

TABLE 2. Rotational Behavior in MPTP-Induced Hemiparkinsonian Monkeys

| | Rotation (turns/20 min) | |
Treatment	Ipsilateral[a]	Contralateral
Spontaneous (saline; $N = 4$)	33 ± 14	—
Apomorphine (0.15 mg/kg, i.m., $N = 6$)	—	53 ± 17[b]
L-DOPA (Sinemet 100/10, p.o., $N = 4$)	—	15 ± 3[b]

[a] The dopamine content of the ipsilateral basal ganglia (control putamen 153 ± 19; control caudate nucleus 141 ± 27 pg/μg protein) decreased to about 2% of control after an infusion of MPTP into the internal carotid artery of anesthetized cynomolgus monkeys.
[b] $p < 0.05$.

tion of 6-hydroxydopamine. These hemiparkinsonian monkeys were able to eat and drink, and thus no daily medication was needed to maintain their lives. No progressiveness into full parkinsonism was observed. Some of these hemiparkinsonian monkeys showed a reduced visual recognition or interpretation in the contralateral eye field (Bankiewicz *et al.*, personal communication).

In northern California, a very few percent of MPTP users have developed irreversible parkinsonism.[4] Again, the sensitivity of an individual monkey to MPTP's neurotoxic insult was found to be variable and might be related to the age of the animal. Aged monkeys were consistently found to develop parkinsonism after administration of low dose MPTP. The greater sensitivity of aged animals is supported by the fact that MPTP produced a greater depletion of striatal dopamine in one- to two-year-old groups than in the two-month-old group (TABLE 3) of C57BL6 mice. This was observed although the MPTP's effects in rodents were reversible (see reference 17).

Comparison of the Major Clinical Signs of Idiopathic and MPTP-Induced Parkinsonism

There were several major differences in the pathogenesis or etiology (or both) of idiopathic and MPTP-induced parkinsonism (TABLE 4). The manifestation of parkinsonian signs in the MPTP-treated monkeys was over within 2–3 weeks. There was no

TABLE 3. Effects of Age on the Dopamine Depletion Effect of MPTP in C57BL6 Mice[a]

| | Striatal Dopamine | | |
Age (months)	2	12	24
	(ng/mg net wt)		
Control	18.5 ± 1.2	23.6 ± 1.7	21.2 ± 0.6
MPTP (mg/kg)			
15 × 3	13.9 ± 2.1	7.9 ± 0.9	8.2 ± 0.4
30 × 3	5.4 ± 0.4	—	1.2 ± 0.4

[a] $N = 4$–6, sacrificed three days after the last dose of MPTP.

TABLE 4. Comparison of the Idiopathic and MPTP-Induced Parkinsonism

Parkinsonism	Idiopathic	MPTP-Induced
(1) Pathological findings:		
(a) cell loss in substantia nigra	+	+
(b) depigmentation	+	+
(c) lipid pigmentation	?	+
(d) Lewy bodies[a]	+	−
(e) cell loss in monoaminergic group	+	±
(2) Neurochemical changes:		
(a) decrease in striatal dopamine	+	+
(b) decrease in other monoamines	+	±
(3) Treatments:		
(a) L-DOPA	+	+
(b) D2 dopamine receptor agonists	+	+
(4) Clinical signs:		
(a) extrapyramidal motor dysfunction	+	+
(b) tremor[a]	resting	postural
(c) progressiveness[a]	+	−
(d) spontaneous recovery[a]	−	+
(5) Sensory neglect in hemiparkinsonism	±	contralateral

[a] Major differences observed in MPTP-treated rhesus monkeys.

progressiveness or spray of the hemiparkinsonian symptoms into other limbs. Furthermore, spontaneous recovery was observed in some of the mildly affected parkinsonian monkeys. The CSF content of homovanillic acid (HVA) was found decreased by about 70% at one to two months after MPTP, which then showed a trend of recovery thereafter. The recovery of CSF content of MHPG and 5-HIAA was more rapid and complete.[7] In idiopathic parkinsonism, the CSF levels of these monoamine metabolites remain depressed.[6] Thus, compensation or sprouting (or both) of surviving nigral A9 neurons may occur in the MPTP-induced parkinsonian monkeys, but not in idiopathic Parkinson's patients. The ability of the nigral dopaminergic neurons of monkeys to repair the MPTP's damage and to sprout may play a role in the recovery of mildly affected parkinsonian monkeys. A selective lesion of the nigrostriatal dopaminergic neurons is sufficient to produce the extrapyramidal syndrome in monkeys following intravenous administration of below 2.5 mg/kg of MPTP. MPTP's neurotoxic damages may also involve noradrenergic systems or the mesolimbic system (or both) when higher doses of MPTP (e.g., more than 2.5 mg/kg) are given to aged monkeys. Finally, no Lewy bodies were found in remaining substantia nigral neurons of the NIMH MPTP patient[4] or of MPTP-induced parkinsonian monkeys.

TABLE 5. Effects of MPTP[a] on the Dopamine Content in the Zona Compacta Area of the Substantia Nigra of Rhesus Monkeys

Area	Time after MPTP (weeks)		
	0	1	4
	Dopamine (pg/µg protein)		
Zona compacta	47.43	22.74	33.11
Area above zona compacta	8.93	18.83	31.60

[a] MPTP: 1.5 mg/kg, i.v.

Compensation of Remaining Nigrostriatal Neurons
in MPTP-Induced Parkinsonian Monkeys

The tyrosine hydroxylase containing substantia nigra compacta neurons decreased by more than 80% in all parkinsonian monkeys. However, the dopamine content in the compacta area decreased by only 40–50%, whereas a threefold increase in dopamine was observed in the area above the substantia nigra (TABLE 5). The notion of sprouting from the remaining nigral neurons was confirmed by an immunohistochemical procedure. As mentioned above, this phenomenon of sprouting in nigral neurons is unique to the MPTP-induced parkinsonism and results in spontaneous recovery of extrapyramidal motor dysfunction.

A compensatory increase of the ratio of homovanillic acid to dopamine (HVA/DA) in the caudate nucleus and putamen was observed in MPTP-induced parkinsonian monkeys (TABLE 6). The HVA/DA ratio or the dopamine content of the nucleus accumbens—which receives most of its innervation from the ventrotegmental A10 neurons—was not altered. This result supports the pathological finding that the A10 neurons in the ventrotegmental area were not damaged by MPTP. Thus, the dopamine turnover in the remaining nigrostriatal neurons was increased after MPTP in order to compensate for the loss of striatal dopamine.

The denervation-induced postsynaptic supersensitivity of the striatal dopamine receptors has been demonstrated previously in Ungerstedt's rotational rodent model. L-DOPA and apomorphine produced contralateral circling behavior in the MPTP-induced hemiparkinsonian monkeys (TABLE 2) that was similar to that observed in Ungerstedt's rodent model. A unilateral increase in D2 dopamine receptors of the denervated striatum might be responsible for the D2 agonists inducing contralateral rotational behavior (Bruecke *et al.*, unpublished observation).

Application of MPTP-Induced Primate Model of Parkinsonism in Developing Presynaptic and Postsynaptic Imaging Ligands for Brain Dopaminergic Systems in Vivo

This primate model of parkinsonism is employed not only for reevaluation of the role of the nigrostriatal dopaminergic system in the extrapyramidal motor function, but also for developing and testing presynaptic and postsynaptic imaging ligands of brain dopaminergic systems. We have previously identified 6-F-L-DOPA as a potential presynaptic imaging ligand for brain dopaminergic systems.[9] In collaboration with the PET team of the McMaster University Medical Centre, we have synthesized 6-^{18}F-L-DOPA[17,18] and have used it to image the damage of striatal dopamine in the living

TABLE 6. The Ratio of HVA/DA in the Brain of Monkeys Following MPTP-Induced 80–95% Cell Loss in the Substantia Nigra

MPTP	Substantia Nigra	Putamen	Caudate Nucleus	Nucleus Accumbens
Before	1.95 ± 0.30	1.30 ± 0.22	0.75 ± 0.13	1.62 ± 0.19
1–5 Days after MPTP	1.53 ± 0.13	0.34 ± 0.08[b]	0.26 ± 0.04[b]	0.50; 0.75
1–2 Months after MPTP[a]	1.93 ± 0.27	8.34 ± 1.62[b]	3.48 ± 1.25[b]	1.21 ± 0.21

[a] Dopamine content decreased by more than 90% (control putamen 135 ± 10; control caudate nucleus 153 ± 6 pg/µg protein) at 1–2 months after MPTP (0.33 mg/kg, i.v., daily for five days); N = 4–7.
[b] $p < 0.05$.

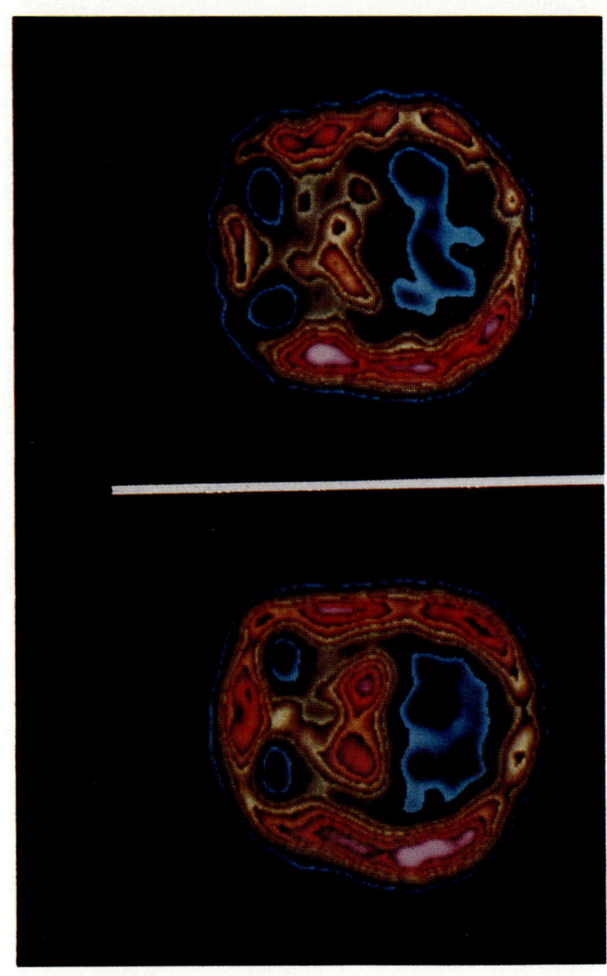

FIGURE 2. 6-^{18}F-L-DOPA/Positron Emission Tomographic imaging of striatal dopamine in MPTP-induced parkinsonian monkeys: (A) partially lesioned (left panel); (B) severely lesioned (right panel).

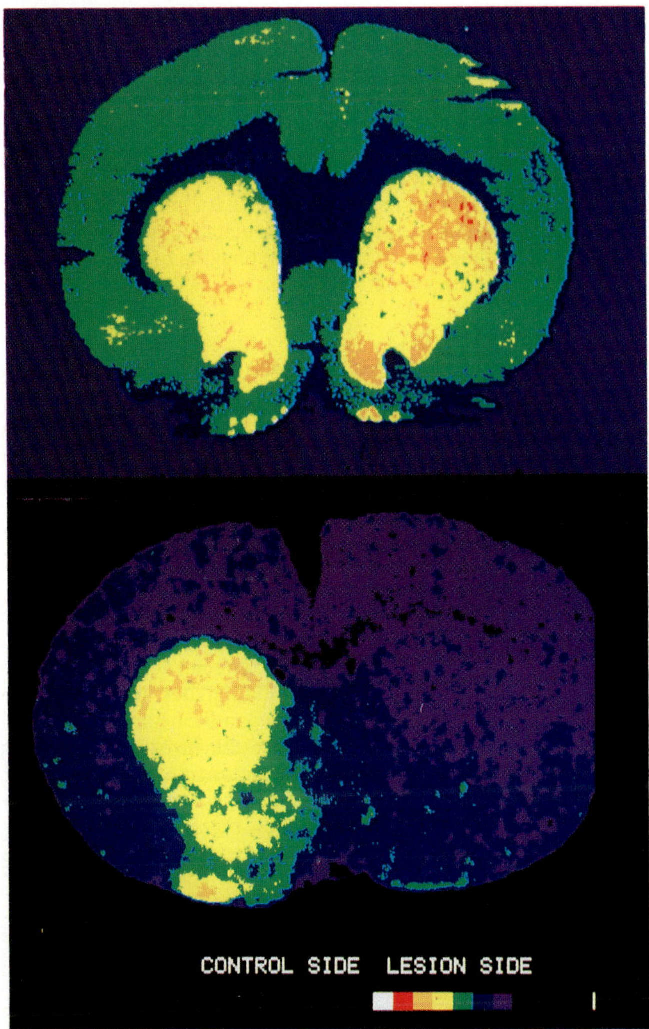

FIGURE 3. ^{125}I-IBZM *in vivo* binding and *ex vivo* autoradiographic imaging of supersensitive D2 dopamine receptors and ^{14}C-L-DOPA imaging of dopaminergic terminals following unilateral lesioning of the medial forebrain bundle by intracerebral injection of MPP[+] (8 μg). (A) Post-synaptic imaging of D2 dopamine receptors by ^{125}I-IBZM (upper panel), which shows 10–50% increase in D2 receptor density in the lesioned side. (B) Presynaptic imaging of dopamine terminals by ^{14}C-L-DOPA (lower panel), which shows disappearance of dopamine in the caudate nucleus, nucleus accumbens, and olfactory tubercle ipsilateral to the side of lesion (unpublished observation of Kung, Singhaniyom, Bruecke, Tsai, Namura, and Chiueh).

MPTP-treated monkeys with various degrees of parkinsonism (FIGURE 2). The results indicate that depletion of brain dopamine in Parkinson's patients can be semiquantified by this 6-^{18}F-L-DOPA/PET imaging procedure.[11,19]

We have also employed Ungerstedt's rotational rodent model[3] in screening of an *in vivo* imaging ligand for D2 dopamine receptors. In the present preliminary study, a newly developed ligand ^{125}I-IBZM of Kung *et al.*[10] was used to study *in vivo* binding of D2 receptors. The results showed that ^{125}I-IBZM recognized D2 receptors in the caudate nucleus, nucleus accumbens, olfactory tubercle, olfactory bulb, adrenal gland, kidney, etc. This *in vivo* binding of ^{125}I-IBZM was blocked by pretreatment of animals with D2 agonist (LY 171555) and antagonist (YM 09151-2). Furthermore, the *in vivo* binding sites of ^{125}I-IBZM increased by 10–50% in the denervated caudate nucleus (FIGURE 3, unpublished observation of Kung, Singhaniyom, Tsai, Bruecke, Namura, and Chiueh). Thus, ^{125}I-IBZM appears to meet criteria for an ideal *in vivo* postsynaptic imaging ligand for D2 dopamine receptors. It is speculated that this ligand after labeling with ^{123}I may be useful for single photon (SPECT) imaging of the up and down regulation of D2 receptors in the Parkinson's patients.

DISCUSSION

MPTP is a selective nigrostriatal dopaminergic neurotoxin that causes a severe cell loss in the pigmented substantia nigra compacta A9 neurons, but spares the nonpigmented A10 mesolimbic neurons following systemic administration.[7,12] Despite MPTP-induced depletion of striatal dopamine in several animal species (TABLE 7), a parkinsonian syndrome appears "only" in subhuman primates and humans.[20] MPTP must also cause more than 80% depletion of the striatal dopamine before parkinsonian symptoms are seen.[12] In a proper dose regimen, MPTP's effects on the mesolimbic system and other monoaminergic systems were found to be short-lasting and insignificant.

An age-dependent increase in the dopamine-depleting effect of MPTP is observed in C57BL6 mice and possibly in monkeys. A spontaneous age-dependent decrease in dopamine content, decrease in D2 antagonist binding sites, increase in monoamine oxidase activity, and increase in accumulation of dopamine neuromelanin and/or dopamine toxic metabolites (e.g., dopamine aldehyde, 5,6-dihydroxyindoline, and quinones) in the substantia nigra may have exaggerated or augmented MPTP's neurotoxic effects. MPTP's effects on the nigrostriatal system appear to shorten, from years into weeks, the slow age-dependent degeneration of these nigral dopamine neurons (FIGURE 4). It is interesting to note that deprenyl, an inhibitor of type B monoamine oxidase,

TABLE 7. MPTP Produced Various Effects in Different Animal Species

	Man	Monkey	Dog	Rat	Mice
(1) Dopamine neuromelanin in substantia nigra	+	+	±	−	−
(2) Cumulative dose (mg/kg)	?	2.5	2.5	150	300
(3) Depletion of striatal dopamine	+ + (irreversible)	+ +	+ +	− (reversible)	±
(4) Cell loss in substantia nigra compacta A9 area	+ + +	+ + +	+ + +	−	±
(5) Serotonin syndrome	+	+	+	+	+
(6) Parkinsonian syndrome	+ + +	+ + +	−	−	−

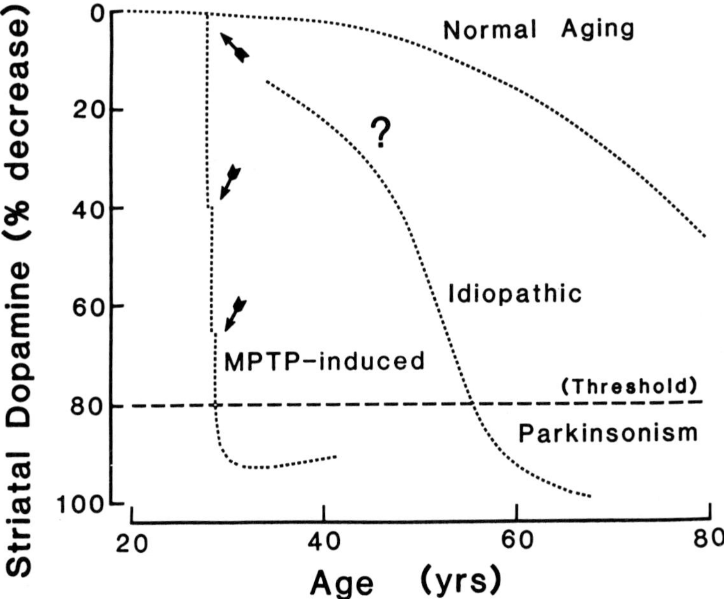

FIGURE 4. Time course of decline of striatal dopamine in the brain of MPTP-induced parkinsonism, idiopathic parkinsonism, and normal aging control (arrows indicate repeat exposures to MPTP).

retards the progressiveness of idiopathic parkinsonism and blocks MPTP's neurotoxicity in monkeys.[13] Therefore, environment toxins might enter the central nervous system and trigger or accelerate (or both) an age-dependent decline of the extrapyramidal motor function of the nigrostriatal dopaminergic pathway.

The exact mechanism by which MPTP selectively destroys the nigrostriatal neurons but spares other dopaminergic systems is not clear. It has been demonstrated that MPTP has to be oxidized to 1-methyl-4-phenylpyridine (MPP^+) in order to express its neurotoxic action.[14] It is postulated that MPP^+ inside the nigrostriatal neurons produces a chain of events, that is, inhibition of ATP formation, accumulation of intracellular Ca^{++}, accumulation of toxic metabolites of dopamine, depletion of glutathione, and dissolution of cell membranes or neuromelanin (or both). Lack of adequate compensation or ability to repair injured nigrostriatal neurons might also contribute to the selective cell death of the A9 neurons caused by MPTP. MPP^+ is known to cause nonspecific cytoplasmic damage to monoamine neurons,[15] hepatic cells, and spinal neurons, in addition to causing cataracts and lesions of the lung and gastrointestinal tract.

One of the major differences between idiopathic and MPTP-induced parkinsonism is the progressiveness of the extrapyramidal symptoms in idiopathic Parkinson's disease. Parkinsonian signs usually begin from one limb and spray to all four limbs with no sign of spontaneous recovery. On the other hand, though, there is spontaneous recovery of the extrapyramidal signs and CSF HVA in some mildly affected parkinsonian monkeys. There is no progress of the hemiparkinsonian monkeys into full parkinsonism in the MPTP-treated monkeys.

Sensory neglects have been reported in rodents following unilateral lesioning of

TABLE 8. Compensations[a] of the Nigrostriatal System to MPTP-Induced Selective Cell Loss in the Substantia Nigra Compacta

(1) Increase in HVA/DA ratio of the caudate nucleus and putamen, but not in the nucleus accumbens.
(2) Increase in either dopamine receptor numbers or sensitivity to D2 agonists (or both).
(3) Increase in dopamine content or sprouting of remaining substantia nigra dopaminergic neurons (or both).
(4) Increase in enzymatic activities of tyrosine hydroxylase and L-aromatic amino acid decarboxylase in basal ganglia.

[a] These compensations may not be observed in severely lesioned monkeys.

the nigrostriatal pathway[3] and have been confirmed by observation in the MPTP-induced hemiparkinsonian monkeys. The significance and consequence of this sensory neglect phenomenon in the idiopathic Parkinson's patients remains to be investigated.

Most of the compensation of the remaining nigrostriatal dopaminergic neurons (i.e., increase in striatal HVA/DA turnover ratio, increase in biosynthetic enzymes, increase in D2 antagonist binding sites and/or postsynaptic supersensitivity) are observed in both idiopathic[16] or MPTP-induced parkinsonism (TABLE 8). Nevertheless, increases in sprouting or regeneration activities have only been observed in MPTP-treated monkeys and other lower animals.[17] Thus, either the lack of ability of the survived nigral neurons to sprout or repair damaged terminals or a continuous presence of endogenous neurotoxins (e.g., toxic dopamine metabolites) of the idiopathic Parkinson's patients may account for the progressive deterioration of extrapyramidal motor function.

The monkeys with hemiparkinsonism were able to feed themselves and were able to maintain good health without daily medication or intensive care despite contralateral motor and sensory impairments. We have used Ungerstedt's rodent model and the MPTP-induced monkey model in screening and testing of both PET ligands for dopaminergic neurons (6-^{18}F-L-DOPA; synthesized by G. Firnau)[18] and of Single Photon Emission Computerized Tomography (SPECT) imaging ligands for D2 dopamine receptors (^{123}I-IBZM; synthesized by H. Kung).[10] The preliminary results show that these imaging ligands recognize specifically the dopaminergic systems in the brain following intravenous administration (FIGURE 3). The effects of MPP$^+$ lesion on the medial forebrain bundle (i.e., decrease in dopamine and increase of D2 dopamine receptor) are visualized in the rat brain. Furthermore, the depletion of striatal dopamine in parkinsonian monkeys was semiquantified by the 6-^{18}F-L-DOPA/PET procedure.[19] The ^{123}I-IBZM/SPECT procedure after testing in the hemiparkinsonian monkeys may prove to be useful in imaging of postsynaptic supersensitivity or of up and down regulation (or both) of D2 dopamine receptors in Parkinson and neuropsychiatric research.

In conclusion, the MPTP-induced primate model of parkinsonism not only provides an excellent animal model for investigating the function of the nigrostriatal dopaminergic system, for screening of new antiparkinsonian agents, and for developing agents that retard the progress of Parkinson's disease, but it also provides for studying transplantation of dopamine-producing cells and for preclinical trials of *in vivo* imaging procedures (i.e., PET or SPECT) using presynaptic or postsynaptic ligands of brain dopaminergic systems.

ACKNOWLEDGMENTS

The author wishes to thank collaborations of R. Stanley Burns and Irwin J. Kopin (primate model of parkinsonism), Gunter Firnau (6-F-DOPA/PET imaging of brain dopamine), and Hank Kung (IBZM binding of D2 dopamine receptor).

REFERENCES

1. CARLSSON, A., M. LINDQVIST, T. MAGNUSSON & B. WALDECK. 1958. Science **127:** 471.
2. BIRKMAYER, W. & O. HORNYKIEWICZ. 1961. Wien. Klin. Wochenschr. **73:** 787–788.
3. UNGERSTEDT, U. 1971. *In* 6-Hydroxydopamine and Catecholamine Neurons. T. Malmfors & H. Thoenen, Eds.: 315–322. North-Holland. Amsterdam.
4. DAVIS, G. C., A. C. WILLIAMS, S. P. MARKEY, M. H. EBERT, E. D. CALNE, C. M. REICHERT & I. J. KOPIN. 1979. Psychiatry Res. **1:** 249–254.
5. LANGSTON, J. W., P. BALLARD, J. W. TETRUD & I. IRWIN. 1983. Science **219:** 979–980.
6. BURNS, R. S., P. A. LEWITT, M. H. EBERT, H. PAKKENBERG & I. J. KOPIN. 1985. N. Engl. J. Med. **312:** 1418–1421.
7. BURNS, R. S., C. C. CHIUEH, S. P. MARKEY, M. H. EBERT, D. M. JACOBOWITZ & I. J. KOPIN. 1983. Proc. Natl. Acad. Sci. **80:** 4546–4550.
8. BANKIEWICZ, K. S., E. H. OLDFIELD, C. C. CHIUEH, J. L. DOPPMAN, D. M. JACOBOWITZ & I. J. KOPIN. 1986. Life Sci. **39:** 7–16.
9. CHIUEH, C. C., Z. ZUKOWSKA-GROJEC, K. L. KIRK & I. J. KOPIN. 1983. J. Pharmacol. Exp. Ther. **225:** 529–533.
10. KUNG, H. F., J. J. BILLINGS, Y. Z. GUO & X. XU. 1987. Int. J. Nucl. Med. Biol. In press.
11. GARNETT, E. S., G. FIRNAU & C. NAHMIAS. 1983. Nature **305:** 137–138.
12. CHIUEH, C. C., R. S. BURNS, S. P. MARKEY, D. M. JACOBOWITZ & I. J. KOPIN. 1985. Life Sci. **36:** 213–218.
13. COHEN, G., P. PASIK, B. COHEN, A. LEIST, C. MYTILINEOU & M. YAHR. 1984. Eur. J. Pharmacol. **106:** 209–210.
14. MARKEY, S. P., J. N. JOHANNESSEN, C. C. CHIUEH, R. S. BURNS & M. A. HERKENHAM. 1984. Nature **311:** 464–467.
15. NAMURA, I., P. DOUILLET, C. J. SUN, A. PERT, R. M. COHEN & C. C. CHIUEH. 1987. Eur. J. Pharmacol. **136:** 31–37.
16. HORNYKIEWICZ, O. 1982. *In* Movement Disorders. C. D. Marsden & S. Fahn, Eds.: 41–58. Butterworths. London.
17. CHIUEH, C. C., J. N. JOHANNESSEN, J. L. SUN, J. P. BACON & S. P. MARKEY. 1986. *In* MPTP: A Neurotoxin Producing a Parkinsonian Syndrome. S. P. Markey, N. Castagnoli, A. J. Trevor & I. J. Kopin, Eds.: 473–480. Academic Press. New York.
18. FIRNAU, G., R. CHIRAKAL & E. S. GARNETT. 1984. J. Nucl. Med. **25:** 1228–1233.
19. CHIUEH, C. C., R. S. BURNS, I. J. KOPIN, K. L. KIRK, G. FIRNAU, C. NAHMIAS, R. CHIRAKAL & E. S. GARNETT. 1986. *In* MPTP: A Neurotoxin Producing a Parkinsonian Syndrome. S. P. Markey, N. Castagnoli, A. J. Trevor & I. J. Kopin, Eds.: 327–338. Academic Press. New York.
20. CHIUEH, C. C., S. P. MARKEY, R. S. BURNS, J. N. JOHANNESSEN, D. M. JACOBOWITZ & I. J. KOPIN. 1984. Psychopharmacol. Bull. **20:** 548–553.

DISCUSSION OF THE PAPER

D. WONG (*The Johns Hopkins University School of Medicine, Baltimore, MD*): Can you comment on the advantage of I-123 over C-11 for the benzamide compound for external imaging?

C. CHIUEH (*National Institute of Mental Health, Bethesda, MD*): The advantage of an iodine-labeled IBZM is that we can make it as specific as possible. We can make it around 2000 curies per millimole. Moreover, because this ligand is partially reversible, it can be displaced by both D2 agonists and D2 antagonists *in vivo*. Therefore, now in my laboratory, we are trying to see endogenous dopamine-displaced binding of these iodocompounds. I-123-Labeled compounds are designed for SPECT imaging.

WONG: I think that C-11 and N-methylspiperone, as well as C-11-raclopride in Sweden, have specific activities of at least 2000 curies. In fact, it is more like 3000 curies per millimole with C-11. Therefore, I disagree quite strongly with your comment.

CHIUEH: No, I just said specific binding; we can clear out nonspecific binding *in vivo* within 30 minutes.

WONG: However, I meant that the specific activity of C-11 compounds is generally much higher than iodinated compounds.

CHIUEH: The half-life, though, is only 20 minutes, so the half-life of these I-123-labeled compounds is about 13 hours.

WONG: Is the technique of producing the hemiparkinsonian syndrome with intracarotid MPTP a matter of dosage? Why does the toxin circulate and reach other parts of the brain?

CHIUEH: We put the angiocatheter through the femoral artery and it travels through the aorta up to the carotid artery. We then bend the catheter into the internal carotid artery (we use a fluoroscope to guide the catheter into the internal carotid artery). After that, we use a slow infusion of MPTP solution because MPTP is a lipid soluble compound; it can be taken up by the brain through the blood-brain barrier by the one-pass uptake procedure. The other side of brain only sees about one-tenth of that MPTP dose as compared to the infusion site. Hence, by using this procedure, we can really create specific hemiparkinsonism.

Age-related Changes in the Nigrostriatal System[a]

THOMAS H. McNEILL,[b] LAURIE L. KOEK,[c] SALLY A. BROWN,[c]
AND JOSE A. RAFOLS[d]

[b]Departments of Neurology, Neurobiology, and Anatomy
and of Oncology in the Cancer Center
[c]Department of Neurology
University of Rochester Medical Center
Rochester, New York 14642

[d]Department of Anatomy
Wayne State University
Detroit, Michigan 48201

INTRODUCTION

Age-related changes in the neural circuitry of the basal ganglia have been postulated to contribute to a disruption of motor function and balance associated with advancing age.[1] Previous biochemical studies in rodent and human brain have reported age-related declines in a number of neurotransmitter systems in the striatum and the substantia nigra,[2] as well as decreases in the number of dopaminergic[3,4] and cholinergic binding sites[5] in the caudate nuclei and putamen. Morphological studies have reported age-correlated declines in the number of cells in both the striatum[6,7] and the substantia nigra[8] of rat and human brain. In addition, a previous report from our laboratory has shown age-correlated morphological changes in A-9, but not all A-10 dopaminergic neurons of the midbrain in the C57BL/6N mouse.[9] Because it is known that both medium spiny (medium spiny I)[10–13] and aspiny (aspiny I and II)[14] neurons of the striatum may be target populations for afferent nigrostriatal dopamine fibers,[15–19] we undertook a study to examine the question as to whether striatal target neurons undergo compensatory dendritic growth or regression with age in response to possible degeneration of neighboring and/or afferent projecting neurons.

METHODS AND MATERIALS

Five age groups (6, 10, 20, 25, and 30 months) of C57BL/6N mice were used for this study and mice were obtained through the National Institute on Aging (NIA). Mice were sacrificed by decapitation under light anesthesia in random order and were prepared by the Golgi Cox method according to the procedure of Van der Loos.[20] Tissue

[a] Thomas H. McNeill is the recipient of a Research Career Development Award from the National Institute on Aging (AG00300). The studies were supported by PHS Grant Nos. AG05445 and AG03254.

sections containing the striatum were cut in a coronal plane at 200 microns and slides were coded so that it would be unknown during data gathering which slide came from which age group. A sample of 20–30 neurons (based on a predetermined 95% confidence interval) was randomly chosen from each mouse at both a rostral and caudal level of the striatum from among all well-impregnated cells. Only cells with their soma in the center one-third of the section and whose dendrites were unobscured by overlying glia, blood vessels, other neurons, and nonspecific deposits of stain were examined. Based on previous observations, terminal dendritic segments were required to be tapered at their tips and were found to lack spines, thus indicating the complete impregnation of the dendrite. For our study, medium spiny (medium spiny I) and two types of aspiny neurons (aspiny I and II) were analyzed (classification after DiFiglia[14]). Profiles of the cell soma and dendrites were traced using a $40\times$ or $100\times$ objective lens and a camera lucida drawing tube. Cells were entered into an IBM microcomputer system using a digitizing tablet and DAN software.[21] Analysis of dendritic parameters of medium spiny I and aspiny I and II neurons included total and terminal segment lengths, as well as the number of dendritic segments per neuron. The motor performance of the animal was then tested by recording coordination and balance using the rotorod and balance beam.[22]

RESULTS

Qualitative examination of the striatum showed that medium spiny I (MS) neurons were characterized by round, ovoid, fusiform, or triangular cell bodies. Moreover, they represented over 95% of all impregnated neurons. MS neurons had four to eight primary dendrites that emerged from the cell soma and each gave rise to several branches that radiated in all directions. Primary dendrites and the initial segments of the secondary branches were spine-free; however, the rest of the branches were covered with numerous spines of heterogeneous shapes and sizes. In general, MS neurons at the caudal level of the striatum had more robust dendritic arbors than MS neurons at the more rostral level of the striatum.

For all age groups examined, we identified three populations of MS neurons based on their total and terminal dendritic lengths (FIGURE 1). The first population was a group of cells with short dendrites that had a total dendritic length of less than 600 microns. The second size population represented a majority of the impregnated MS neurons of the striatum and had a total dendritic length ranging from 600–1200 microns per neuron. The third population comprised neurons with total dendritic lengths longer than 1200 microns. Our analysis of the five age groups based on the total or terminal dendritic lengths of all of the MS neurons drawn without significant motor impairment revealed a significant increase in the total dendritic length between 6 and 30 months of age in the caudal striatum (FIGURE 2). However, while there was a significant increase in total dendritic length between young and aged mice without motor impairment, there was a substantial decrease in dendritic length in MS neurons of the striatum in aged mice that were motor impaired based on the rotorod and balance-beam tests. A correlation analysis between dendritic parameters and functional scoring revealed that mice that tested poorly on the balance beam and rotorod showed an overall loss of total and terminal dendritic length of MS neurons and an increased number of cells with small shrunken dendrites (FIGURE 3). Conversely, 30-month-old mice that showed no functional impairment likewise showed no statistical deficits in dendritic parameters when compared to young mice.

Because almost all synaptic input into MS neurons is axospinous, we are also in-

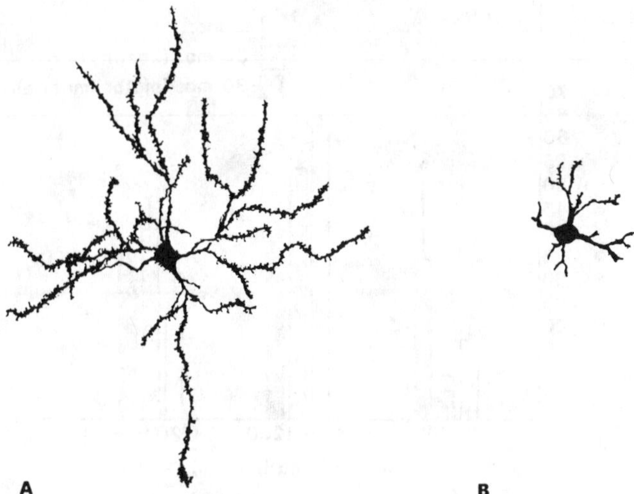

FIGURE 1. Camera lucida drawings of two MS neurons of the striatum with a total dendritic length of (A) 1200 μm and (B) <600 μm. The neuron with short dendritic branches may be indicative of atrophic changes that ultimately lead to cell death.

terested in examining age-related changes in the linear density of dendritic spines in young and aged mice. As shown in FIGURE 4, the linear density of dendritic spines was calculated in 20-μm intervals centripetally from the cell body to the tip of the terminal segment. The highest density of dendritic spines was found on the 41–60-μm

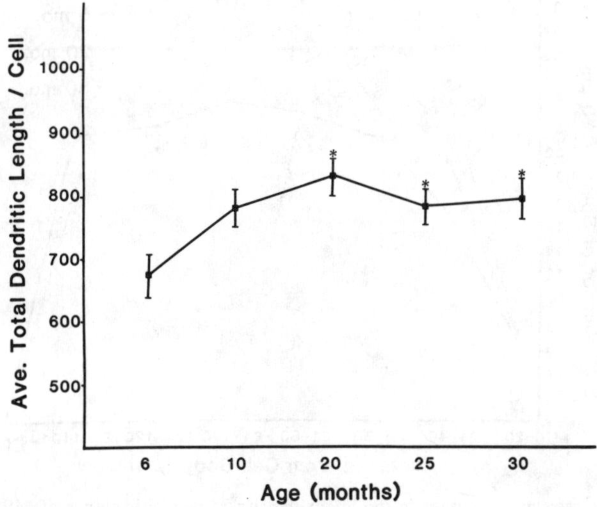

FIGURE 2. Age changes in the total dendritic length of MS neurons at a caudal level of the striatum. Each data point represents the mean total dendritic length of 30 cells drawn from each of five mice ± SEM.

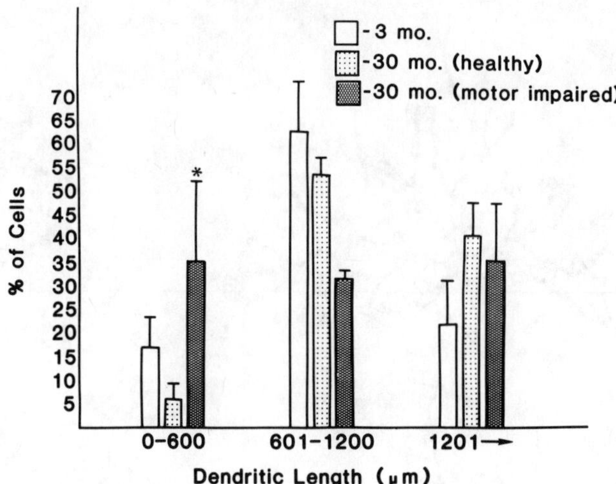

FIGURE 3. Frequency analysis of the number of large-sized (>1200 μm), medium-sized (600–1200 μm), and small-sized (<600 μm) neurons in 3-month and 30-month motor impaired and unimpaired mice. The 30-month-old motor impaired mice showed a significant increase in the number of cells with short dendrites.

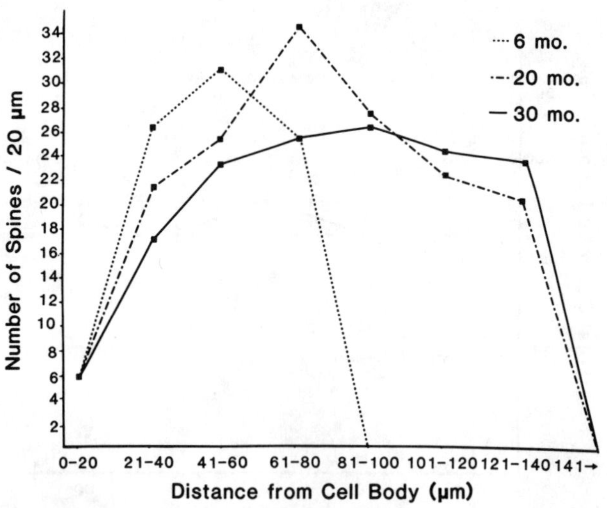

FIGURE 4. Age-related changes in the linear density of dendritic spines of MS neurons. The linear density of dendritic spines was calculated in 20-μm intervals centripetally from the cell body to the tip of the terminal segment. Each data point represents the mean number of dendritic spines of 20 cells from each of five mice.

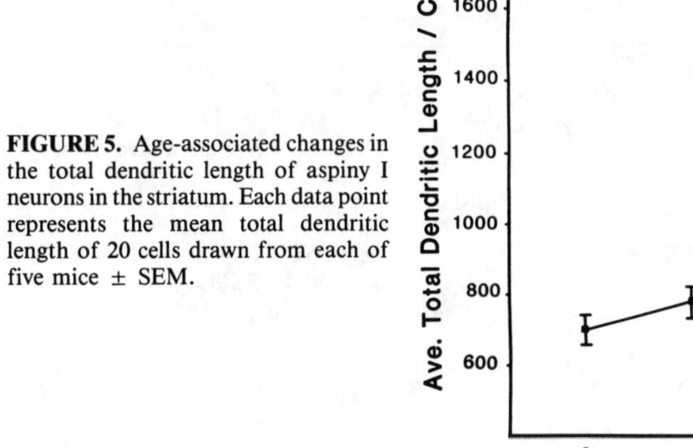
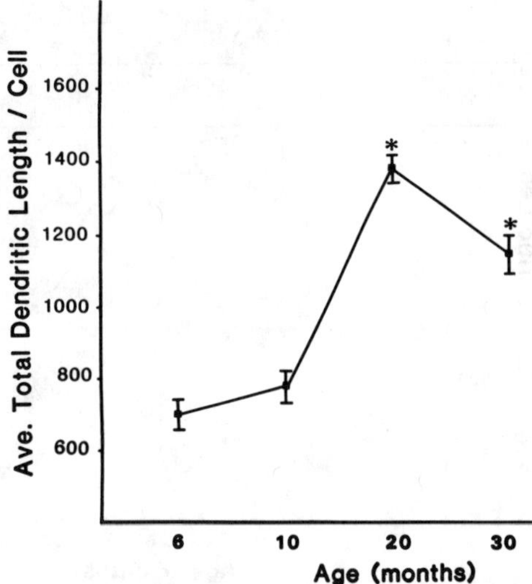

FIGURE 5. Age-associated changes in the total dendritic length of aspiny I neurons in the striatum. Each data point represents the mean total dendritic length of 20 cells drawn from each of five mice ± SEM.

interval at 6 months of age and between 61–80 µm at 20 months of age. However, at 30 months of age, there was significant loss of dendritic spines at the 60–80-µm interval as compared to that at 20 months of age.

Qualitative examination of aspiny (AS) neurons of the striatum showed two different patterns of dendritic growth. Aspiny I neurons were the second most frequently found cell type in the striatum and were characterized by medium-sized cell bodies with thin varicose dendrites. In the normally aging mouse, the dendritic tree was relatively simple at 6 months of age, but became increasingly more complex with advancing age. Our

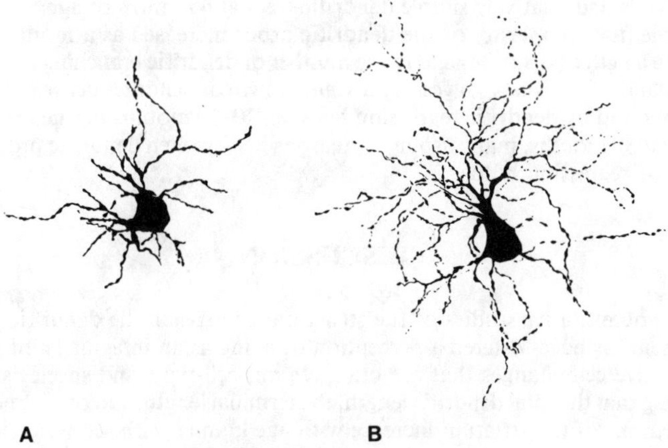

FIGURE 6. Camera lucida drawings of aspiny II neurons of the striatum in (A) 6-month-old and (B) 25-month-old mice. The complexity of the dendritic arbor increases with advancing age as a result of increases in both the length of the dendrites and in the number of branching points.

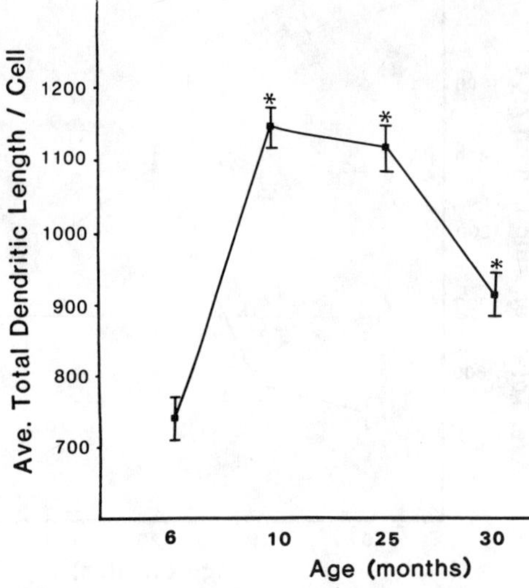

FIGURE 7. Age-associated changes in the total dendritic length of aspiny II neurons in the striatum. Each data point represents the mean total dendritic length of 20 cells drawn from each of five mice ± SEM.

quantitative data suggest that a continuous growth of aspiny I dendrites occurred well into middle age (20 months), with the most significant growth between 10–20 months (FIGURE 5). In contrast, dendritic regression was found between 20–30 months of age; however, the average total dendritic length per aspiny I cell was still greater than that measured at 6 months of age. Overall, this cell type seems to have the greatest capacity of growth in normal aging.

On the other hand, aspiny II neurons were the largest neurons found within the striatum and were found distributed homogeneously throughout the extent of the nuclei. These cells were characterized by large, bulbous somata, thick dendritic trunks, and thin varicose dendrites with few spines and appendages. As with the aspiny I cells, aspiny II cells had relatively simple dendritic trees at 6 months of age; then, with advancing age, the complexity of the dendritic arbor increased as a result of increases in both the length of dendrites and in the number of dendritic branching points (FIGURE 6). Our quantitative figures suggest significant growth of dendrites between 6–10 months of age, followed by dendritic regression between 10–30 months of age (FIGURE 7). In addition, at 30 months, many aspiny II neurons had swollen dendritic processes characteristic of regression bulbs.

DISCUSSION

Recent quantitative studies of the structural changes in the dendritic parameters of aged neurons have fostered a perception of aging as an integration of progressive and regressive cell changes that are brain-region, cell-type, and species specific.[23-28] Our finding that the total dendritic length, the terminal length, and the segment number of MS neurons of the striatum increase with age in mice without motor impairment supports this view and adds another brain region to the list of structures that show a significant degree of growth and plasticity with advancing age. In addition, the presence of three populations of MS neurons based on the sizes of their dendritic arbors at each of the five age groups reinforces the idea that aging is a continuing process made up of both regressing and growing cells.[23,24] The regressing population, characterized by shrinking dendritic branches, may be indicative of atrophic changes that ultimately lead to cell death, while the surviving population shows continued growth. Therefore, in aged C57BL/6N mice without motor impairment, our data suggest that the balance between the growing population and the regressing population rests in favor of the surviving cells such that the total dendritic length of MS neurons increases with age. However, later in life, the process begins to reverse and the dendritic growth of the surviving cells is not sufficient to offset the increase in regressive cell changes. This results in a net dendritic loss by 30 months of age in regions of the striatum. The question of whether or not the dendritic regression — seen at 25 and 30 months of age in MS neurons of the striatum — continues on into very old age (i.e., greater than 40 months) is not known. However, concurrent cell counts and Golgi studies are presently under way in 45-month-old mice to determine if dendritic regression as a result of age-related neuronal loss is characteristic of advancing age in this brain region.

The finding that there is a significant increase in the dendritic length of MS neurons between 6 and 30 months of age does not necessarily lead to the conclusion that the functional integrity of the receptive fields of MS neurons remains uncompromised. In fact, preliminary data from our study collected at three ages suggest that there is a significant loss of dendritic spines in old mice. Previous biochemical studies using kainate acid have shown medium-sized striatal neurons to be associated with dopamine receptors,[29,30] and studies by Severson and co-workers[3,4] have reported a decrease in the number of dopaminergic binding sites in the striatum associated with advancing age. Because it is known that almost all afferent inputs to MS cells are axospinous, it may be suggested that a reduction in the linear density of dendritic spines along with dendrites of MS neurons in the aged mice provides a morphological basis for the reduction of dopaminergic postsynaptic binding sites in the striatum, as well as changes in motor function associated with advancing age. Whether the loss of dendritic spines in the aged mouse along selected segments of the dendritic shaft reflects a topography of different synaptic inputs is not known and is thus currently under investigation.

Another finding of ours suggests that there is a positive correlation between structure and function in the striatum. Specifically, this finding is that in aged mice that show significant motor impairment, there is a significant decrease in the dendritic extent of MS neurons. Furthermore, this suggests that while dendritic regression of MS neurons is not correlated with chronological age, there is a close association between functional deficits and the number of MS neurons with very small dendritic arbors. In addition, the correlation between structure and function — but not with age — within the striatum points towards a reality that has been recapitulated by clinical scientists for years (personal communication, T. Franklin Williams, NIA): namely, that not all old individuals present clinically with motor impairment and not all elderly can be stereotyped as parkinsonian. Thus, although striatal motor deficits may be associated with old age, they should not be considered synonymous with old age. On the contrary, in normal aging without disease, our data suggest that there is considerable potential for growth and plasticity in the aged striatum. Hence, it is only through studies that correlate structure, function, and chronological age that we may assess true aging from other age-associated functional deficits.

Our finding of a difference in the temporal patterns of dendritic growth between the three types of striatal neurons suggests that advancing age may have a differential effect on selected populations of striated cells based on differences in their neurotransmitter content and afferent inputs. Previous studies by Freund *et al.*[16] have shown that

MS neurons of the striatum represent the principal target neuron population for dopaminergic fibers of the substantia nigra. Moreover, they have shown that dopamine plays an inhibitory role through its modulation of afferent inputs of other intrinsic neurons of the striatum or afferent projecting neurons from the cortex and thalamus. In addition, it is thought that some MS neurons contain the neurotransmitter GABA and form a reciprocal descending projection pathway to the substantia nigra.[31,32] In contrast, afferent inputs to large aspiny II and aspiny I cells — the principal intrinsic cholinergic (aspiny II) and somatostatin-like (aspiny I) containing populations of the striatum[31] — are mainly axodendritic with few dopaminergic synapses. Previous studies in rodents have shown an age-related decline in striatal dopamine[33-35] (but not in glutamic acid decarboxylase[36]) between 24–30 months of age, and histological examination of the aged striatum has shown marked declines in the number of medium and small neurons.[6] Whether the differences in dendritic growth between MS and AS neurons represent different compensatory growth responses to death of neighboring striatal neurons or whether they may be related to the loss of selected afferent neuronal inputs to the striatum is not known. Studies directed at addressing this question are currently under way by using anatomical and biochemical lesions of afferent inputs to the striatum (including the substantia nigra, thalamus, and cortex) and cell counts of striatal neurons in aged mice.

SUMMARY

These data support the view that the rate at which an organism ages is a summation of factors throughout life. While some cells seem to remain stable or even grow with age, others show significant regression. In this regard, different populations of striatal neurons show unique and different patterns of growth and development with advancing age. While aspiny II neurons show peak growth by 10 months of age, aspiny I and medium spiny I cells do not reach a growth peak until much later in life. In addition, our data support the notion that the occurrence and severity of structural changes in the aged brain are not distributed homogeneously and that many of the so-called "age-related" changes that were once generalized to the entire brain are brain-region, cell-type, and species specific. Furthermore, our data reinforces the concept that the correlation of structure and function is central to the analysis of an aging population because considerable differences may be found in data based on functionally impaired and unimpaired groups.

REFERENCES

1. HODKINSON, H. M. 1980. *In* Common Symptoms of Disease in the Elderly. Second Edition. Blackwell. Oxford.
2. FINCH, C. E., P. E. RANDALL & J. F. MARSHALL. 1981. Aging and basal gangliar functions. *In* Annual Review of Gerontology and Geriatrics. Volume 2. C. Eisdorfer, Ed.: 48–86. Springer Pub. New York.
3. SEVERSON, J. A. & C. E. FINCH. 1980. Reduced dopaminergic binding during aging in the rodent striatum. Brain Res. **192:** 147–162.
4. SEVERSON, J. A., J. MAECUSSON, B. WINBLAD & C. E. FINCH. 1982. Age-correlated loss of dopaminergic binding sites in human basal ganglia. J. Neurochem. **39:** 1623–1631.
5. STRONG, R., P. HICKS, L. HSU, R. T. BARTUS & S. J. ENNA. 1980. Age-related alterations in the rodent brain cholinergic system and behavior. Neurobiol. Aging **1:** 59–63.
6. MENSAH, P. L. 1979. The effects of aging on neuron "cell islands" in the mouse neostriatum. Soc. Neurosci. Abstr. **5:** 250.18.

7. BUGIANI, O., S. SLAVARANI, F. PERDELLI, G. L. MANCARDI & A. LEONARDI. 1978. Nerve cell loss with aging in the putamen. Eur. Neurol. **17:** 286–291.

8. McGEER, P. L., E. G. McGEER & J. S. SUZUKI. 1977. Aging and extrapyramidal function. Arch. Neurol. **34:** 33–35.

9. McNEILL, T. H., L. L. KOEK & J. W. HAYCOCK. 1984. Age-correlated changes in dopaminergic nigrostriatal perikarya of the C57BL/6NNia mouse. Mech. Ageing Dev. **24:** 293–320.

10. DIMOVA, R., J. VUILLET & R. SEITE. 1980. Study of the rat neostriatum using a combined Golgi-electron microscope technique and serial sections. Neuroscience **5:** 1581–1596.

11. KEMP, J. M. & T. P. S. POWELL. 1971. The structure of the caudate nucleus of the cat: Light and electron microscopy. Philos. Trans. R. Soc. London Ser. **B262:** 383–401.

12. FOX, C. A., A. N. ANDRADE, D. E. HILLMAN & R. C. SCHWIN. 1971. The spiny neurons in the primate striatum: A Golgi and electron microscopic study. J. Hirnforsch. **13:** 181–201.

13. RAFOLS, J. A. & C. A. FOX. 1979. Fine structure of the primate striatum. Appl. Neurophysiol. **42:** 13–16.

14. DiFIGLIA, M., P. PASIK & T. PASIK. 1976. A Golgi study of neuronal types in the neostriatum of monkeys. Brain Res. **114:** 245–256.

15. CHANG, H. T. & S. T. KITAI. 1982. Large neostriatal neurons in the rat: An electron microscope study of gold-toned, Golgi-stained cells. Brain Res. Bull. **8:** 631–643.

16. FREUND, T. F., J. F. POWELL & A. D. SMITH. 1984. Tyrosine hydroxylase-immunoreactive boutons in synaptic contact with identified striatonigral neurons, with particular reference to dendritic spines. Neuroscience **13**(4): 1189–1215.

17. GROVES, P. M. 1980. Synaptic endings and their postsynaptic targets in neostriatum: synaptic specializations revealed from analysis of serial sections. Proc. Natl. Acad. Sci. USA **77:** 6926–6929.

18. LEHMAN, J. & S. Z. LANGER. 1983. The striatal cholinergic interneuron: Synaptic target of dopaminergic terminals? Neuroscience **10**(4): 1105–1120.

19. WILSON, C. J. & P. M. GROVES. 1980. Fine structure and synaptic connections of the common spiny neuron of the rat neostriatum: A study employing intracellular injection of horseradish peroxidase. J. Comp. Neurol. **194:** 599–615.

20. VAN DER LOOS, H. 1956. Une combinaison de deux vieilles methodes histologiques pour le systeme nerveux central. Monatsschr. Psychiatr. Neurol. **132:** 330–334.

21. MOYER, A., V. MOYER & P. D. COLEMAN. 1985. An inexpensive PC based system for quantification of neuronal processes. Soc. Neurosci. **11:** 261.18.

22. INGRAM, D. K., E. L. LONDON, M. A. REYNOLDS, S. B. WALLER & C. L. GOODRICK. 1981. Differential effects of age on motor performance in two mouse strains. Neurobiol. Aging **2:** 221–227.

23. BUELL, S. J. & P. D. COLEMAN. 1979. Dendritic growth in the aged human brain and failure of growth in senile dementia. Science **206:** 854–856.

24. BUELL, S. J. & P. D. COLEMAN. 1981. Quantitative evidence for selective dendritic growth in normal human aging but not in senile dementia. Brain Res. **214:** 23–41.

25. CONNOR, J. R., M. C. DIAMOND & R. E. JOHNSON. 1980. Occipital cortical morphology of the rat: alterations with age and environment. Exp. Neurol. **68:** 158–170.

26. FLOOD, D. G., S. J. BUELL, C. H. DEFIORE, G. J. HORWITZ & P. D. COLEMAN. 1985. Age-related dendritic growth in dentate gyrus of human brain is followed by regression in the "oldest old". Brain Res. **345:** 366–368.

27. HINDS, J. W. & N. A. McNELLY. 1977. Aging of the rat olfactory bulb: Growth and atrophy of constituent layers and changes in size and number of mitral cells. J. Comp. Neurol. **171:** 345–368.

28. HINDS, J. W. & N. A. McNELLY. 1981. Aging in the rat olfactory system: Correlation of changes in the olfactory epithelium and olfactory bulb. J. Comp. Neurol. **203:** 341–342.

29. McGEER, E. G. & P. L. McGEER. 1976. Duplication of biochemical changes of Huntington's chorea by intrastriatal injections of glutamic and kainic acids. Nature **263:** 517–519.

30. SCHWARCZ, R., I. CREESE, J. T. COYLE & S. H. SNYDER. 1978. Dopamine receptors localized on cerebral cortical afferents to rat corpus striatum. Nature **271:** 766–768.

31. GRAYBIEL, A. M. & C. W. RAGSDALE. 1983. Biochemical anatomy of the striatum. *In* Chemical Neuroanatomy. P. C. Emson, Ed.: 317–504. Raven Press. New York.

32. PRESTON, R. J., G. A. BISHOP & S. T. KITAI. 1980. Medium spiny neuron projection from
     the rat striatum: An intracellular horseradish peroxidase study. Brain Res. **183:** 253–263.
33. FINCH, C. E. 1973. Catecholamine metabolism in the brains of aging male mice. Brain Res.
     52: 261–276.
34. JOSEPH, J. A., R. E. BERGER, B. T. ENGLE & G. S. ROTH. 1978. Age-related changes in
     the neostriatum: A behavioral and biochemical analysis. J. Gerontol. **33:** 643–649.
35. OSTERBERG, H. H., H. G. DONAHUE, J. A. SEVERSON & C. E. FINCH. 1981. Catecholamine
     level and turnover during aging in brain regions of male C57BL/6J mice. Brain Res. **234:**
     337–352.
36. MCGEER, E. G., H. C. FIBIGER, P. L. MCGEER & V. WICKSON. 1971. V. Aging and brain
     enzymes. Exp. Gerontol. **6:** 391–396.

DISCUSSION OF THE PAPER

M. S. LEVINE (*University of California, Los Angeles, CA*): We have similar data
for the cat and I will discuss some of that later. However, now I want to reiterate a
point that you made because I think it is very true of both species. The point is that
there is a lot of heterogeneity in the neurons that you looked at. You even mentioned
individual neurons being different. In support of this, I will show some pictures on
the same neuron having one dendrite looking almost perfectly normal (just like very
young animals) and then, on the same neuron, another dendrite almost denuded of
spines at its end, which is a very abnormal looking spine.

General Discussion of Part III

D. B. CALNE

Division of Neurology
Department of Medicine
University of British Columbia
Health Sciences Centre Hospital
Vancouver, British Columbia, Canada V6T 1W5

REVIEW

In this session, we heard David Morgan report on the effect of aging on the nigrostriatal dopamine system. The 50% loss of dopamine in a normal human life span was matched by a somewhat lesser fall in rats and mice. The D2 receptors fell by 25–50%. The D1 receptor density increased with human aging, so there was a 2–3-fold rise in the D1-to-D2 ratio.

Randy Strong then reported on the heterogeneous changes in the various transmitters of the striatum. James Severson discussed high-affinity D2 binding sites in mice and described a 25% decline between the ages of 3 and 12 months, followed by stabilization. In contrast, the total D2 receptor population fell progressively from 3 to 24 months. Gary Freeman presented evidence that elderly mice were more sensitive to metabolic disturbances (such as those induced by thiamin deficiency).

Dean Wong introduced the topic of PET scanning. He reviewed the evidence for age-related loss of D2 receptors in human subjects and described the mathematical modeling employed to derive quantitative information. Anthony Altar (who presented John Marshall's paper) then described autoradiographic studies on the uniform distribution of dopamine receptors in the striatum of rats. The D2 binding was highest in the lateral striatum. The 30–60% loss of D2 binding with aging was most marked in the lateral and caudal regions. In human subjects, the D2 binding was patchy, which corresponded to the acetylcholinesterase-rich pattern in the striosome-matrix organization. The D1 binding was more uniform.

C. C. Chiueh discussed PET scanning with fluorodopa in monkeys, along with application of a unilateral MPTP model induced by injecting this toxin into one carotid. Finally, Thomas McNeill provided morphological evidence of diverse reactions of striatal neurons to aging. While the dendritic arbor of some neurons regressed, others enlarged.

COMMENT

We have heard an excellent range of reports concerning the consequences of aging on the nigrostriatal pathway. I have a comment on where, perhaps, we might hope to see this work evolving over the next few years. It would be of value to obtain more morphometric observations because alterations in neuronal numbers need not correlate directly with changes in transmitters, receptors, or dendrites. Quantitative information on neuronal loss is important because, ultimately, the crucial questions are when, why, and where do neurons die in the aging process. Only answers to these questions will allow a rational strategy to be developed towards attaining methods to modify the onset and progress of age-related neurological problems. Excellent pioneering cell countings have been undertaken, but the reports are few in number; in fact, in most cases, only a small group of subjects was studied. These results need to be confirmed and extended; furthermore, there is only one really satisfactory species for these studies, *Homo sapiens.*

THE RELATIONSHIP BETWEEN AGING AND DEGENERATIVE NEUROLOGICAL DISEASE OF THE ELDERLY

From the practical viewpoint, society needs some explanation of the relationship between normal aging and neurological disorders of senescence such as Alzheimer's disease, Parkinson's disease, and motoneuron disease. I believe the most viable hypothesis at present is that these disorders result from environmentally induced subclinical damage to the nervous system, which is followed over several decades by age-related attrition of neurons. This eventually leads to the emergence and progression of symptoms. Recent evidence in support of this concept comes from studies on the ALS-PD complex of Guam.

This disease comprises any combination of parkinsonism, dementia, or a motoneuron disease resembling ALS. The disorder is clearly environmental because it is disappearing as Guam is westernized. Some Guamanians who emigrated from the island have been found to present with symptoms over 30 years after leaving. This, of course, is an observation in accord with the hypothesis of subclinical damage followed by age-related attrition. We are currently collaborating with Peter Spencer and John Steele in studying Guamanians by PET in an attempt to demonstrate subclinical neurochemical changes (just as conventional neuropathology has revealed excessive neurofibrillary tangles in clinically normal Guamanians).

The Neurobiology of Cerebellar Senescence

JOSEPH ROGERS

Institute for Biogerontology Research
Sun Health Corporation
Sun City, Arizona 85372

Mechanisms of neural senescence have been intensely pursued, but any kind of fundamental understanding remains elusive.[1] The difficulty is not in finding significant effects of age in the nervous system, but rather arises from the fact that aging is as ubiquitous in brain as it is in phylogeny: age changes can be detected at practically any level of analysis, from the molecular biology of ribosomes to the neuropsychology of cognition.[2] Faced with this plethora of effects, perhaps the most difficult challenge facing those who study neural aging is the determination of which phenomena are primary, which are secondary, which are important, and which are only trivial epiphenomena.

Because the cerebellum is one of the most extensively studied, best understood, and accessible structures in brain,[3-10] our laboratory has used it as a model system in which to characterize age changes in brain microanatomy,[11-16] physiology,[11-15] and function.[17] Based on these results, a primary cytoarchitectural mechanism — the differential loss of specific terminal areas on the dendrite arbor of large output neurons, and the relative preservation of other terminal areas on these neurons — is hypothesized to account for many of the physiologic and functional alterations that characterize the senescent cerebellum. A hypothesis such as this may generalize to other structures that, like the cerebellum, depend on highly arborized, long projecting, large diameter neurons for the final output of information processing.

THE CEREBELLUM AS A MODEL SYSTEM FOR
NEUROGERONTOLOGIC RESEARCH

Over a century of investigation, researchers (see references 3–10) have established ultrastructural, cytoarchitectural, biochemical, and physiological properties that characterize the normal cerebellum of a young or mature animal. Because of this extensive data base, cerebellar preparations have been frequently and advantageously employed to assay a wide variety of phenomena,[18-25] including the role and mechanisms of action of most of the major neurotransmitters.[26-31]

For the same reasons that the cerebellum has historically been such a useful model for studying the effects of various agents and processes on brain function generally, so also it recently has proven to be an excellent substrate for investigating mechanisms of brain senescence.[11-17,32-46] There is now extensive ultrastructural,[16,36,47] morphological,[11-16,37,38] biochemical,[11,35,39-42,45] physiological,[11-16,33,34] and behavioral[17,43-46] evidence of significant cerebellar alterations with age. These findings about aging follow directly from the proposition that by understanding (as one can with the cerebellum) what constitutes normality in young subjects, it becomes possible quickly to appreciate and effectively to study what has changed about old subjects. Such advantages for aging research are not so clearly afforded by other models and brain structures (including cortex and striatum), where many rudimentary elements of synaptic circuitry remain a very important target for basic research, but not for aging research.

RECENT RESEARCH ON CEREBELLAR AGING

Over several years, our laboratory has carried out electrophysiologic, light and electron microscopic, biochemical, and behavioral research on age changes in the rat cerebellum.[11-17] The experimental results can generally be divided into studies of afferents, studies of the Purkinje cell target, studies of efferents, and studies of cerebellum-related behaviors.

Age Changes in Cerebellar Afferents

Four afferent systems converge on the dominant element of cerebellar information processing, the Purkinje cell. Mossy fiber afferents to the cerebellum arise from diverse structures, including the labyrinth (through primary vestibular root fibers and

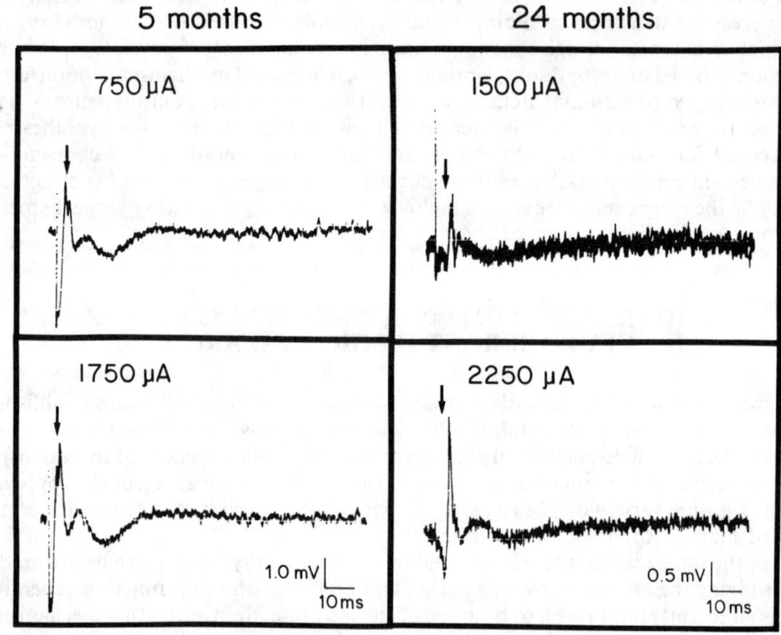

FIGURE 1. Sample parallel fiber volley records obtained from a 5-month-old rat (left) and a 24-month-old rat (right). The baseline-to-peak volley amplitudes are as much as four times greater in the younger rat. Note that the calibration references show twice as much amplification of signal for records of the old rat and that the stimulation currents are greater. Arrows in these traces are at 3 ms poststimulus onset to help indicate the typical slower conduction velocity of the parallel fiber volley in the old rats.[13]

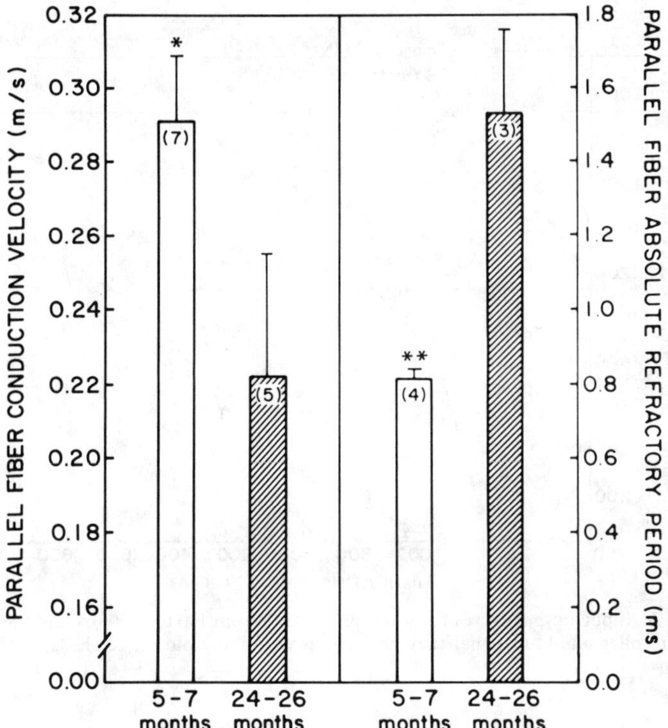

FIGURE 2. Mean parallel fiber conduction velocity (m/s) and mean parallel fiber absolute refractory period (ms) in young and old rats (* = $p < 0.05$; ** = $p < 0.01$).[13]

efferents of the medial and descending vestibular nuclei), skin and muscle receptors (through the spinocerebellar tracts), and pontine nuclei (through the pontocerebellar tracts). These afferents typically enter by way of the inferior and middle cerebellar peduncles and then synapse in characteristic rosettes with granule cell dendrites and cerebellar Golgi cell axons. In turn, granule cell axons, parallel fibers, rise up through the cerebellar molecular layer, bifurcate, and course laterally in separate beams parallel to the long axis of Purkinje cell folia. Our studies show significant age changes in parallel fiber afferents: conduction velocity decreases (FIGURE 1),[13,14] refractory period increases (FIGURE 2),[13,14] and there is both electron microscopic[16] and physiologic (FIGURES 1 and 3)[13,14] evidence of decline in the number of parallel fibers. The ability to drive Purkinje unit firing via this pathway is also significantly impaired in old rats (FIGURES 4A and 4B).[13,14]

Parallel fibers also innervate cerebellar interneurons (e.g., basket cells), providing a disynaptic, inhibitory, parallel fiber–interneuron–Purkinje cell circuit. Electrophysiologic evidence suggests additional senescent decline in this pathway (FIGURE 5).[13]

Climbing fiber afferents to the cerebellum originate in the (usually contralateral) inferior olivary nucleus. Virtually every olivary neuron projects to the cerebellum, with each Purkinje cell receiving a single climbing fiber.[4,5] Climbing fiber input to the cere-

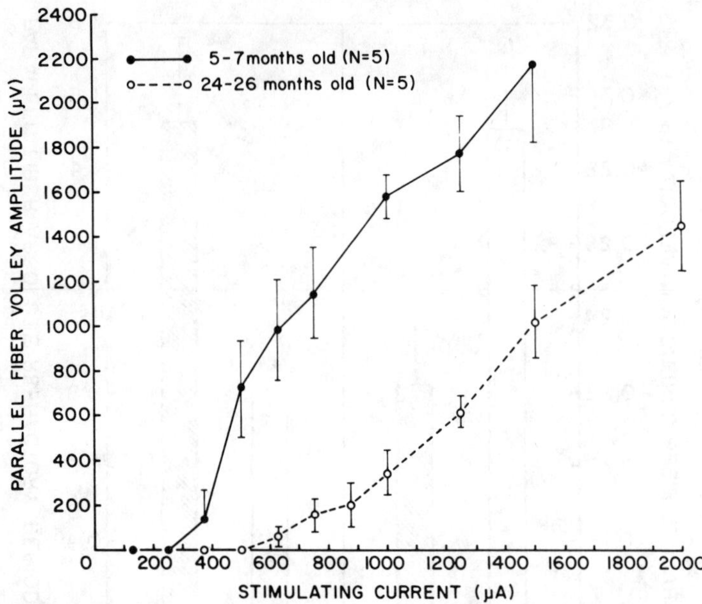

FIGURE 3. Input/output curves for stimulus currents from 100 to 2000 μA and the mean parallel fiber volley amplitudes that they produce in young and old rat cerebella.[13]

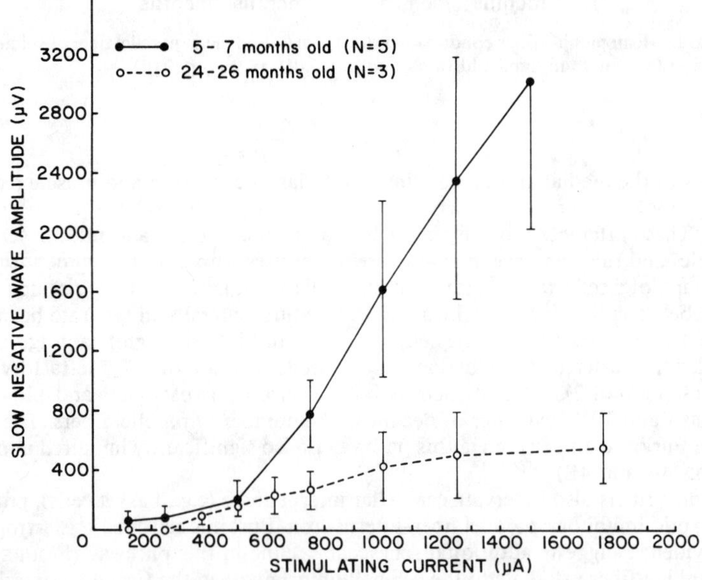

FIGURE 4A. Slow negative wave amplitude (a summed potential evoked in Purkinje cells by parallel fiber stimulation) in young and old rats at stimulus currents from 125 to 1750 μA.

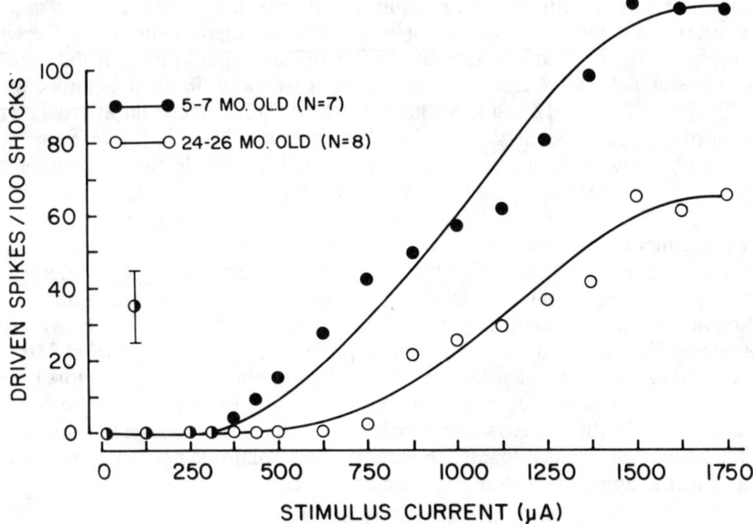

FIGURE 4B. Excitatory responses of single Purkinje units to parallel fiber stimulation at currents from 0 to 1750 µA. The number of driven spikes is summed over 100 stimulus trials.[13]

bellum is easily identified by the characteristic burst of spikes it generates in Purkinje cells.[4] Our studies to date do not show any evidence of senescent change in climbing fiber–mediated firing of Purkinje cells.[11,12] However, it should be pointed out that because Purkinje cells are identified electrophysiologically on the basis of their climbing fiber response, the above data are possibly somewhat biased (i.e., a Purkinje unit that

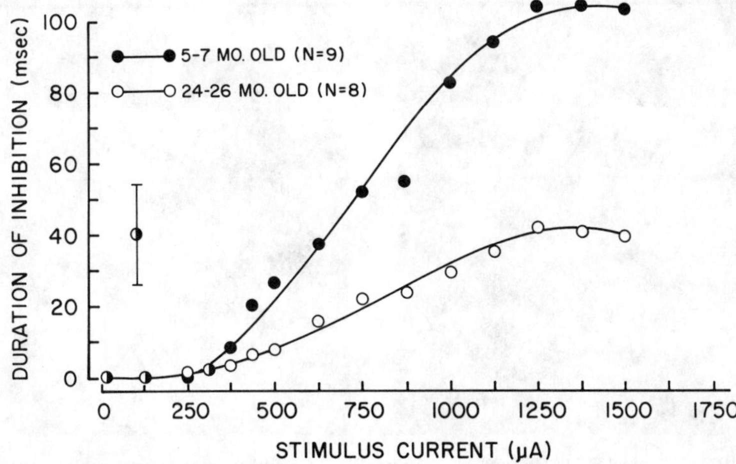

FIGURE 5. Inhibitory responses of single Purkinje units to molecular layer stimulation at currents from 0 to 1750 µA. This inhibition is mediated primarily by interneurons on adjacent parallel fiber beams.[13]

had completely lost its climbing fiber input would probably be misidentified as a cerebellar interneuron and thus would not have been included in the data). Cerebellar climbing fiber field potentials generated after olivary stimulation will be necessary to confirm the lack of age change in this afferent pathway. To do so is important because of cytoarchitectural considerations (i.e., why do some cerebellar afferents remain viable in old age, while others do not?) (see below) and because the inferior olivary nucleus reportedly accumulates more intraneuronal lipofuscin than any other brain structure.[48-50] Whether liposfuscin ("aging pigment") deposition is pathologic,[51] inconsequential,[11,12] or even beneficial[52] has been debated for nearly two decades. More direct experiments could help settle the argument: if lipofuscin-filled olivary cells still fire normally, then it will be difficult to maintain that lipofuscin accumulation with age is more than an epiphenomenon (rather than a cause) of neural aging.

Fine varicose norephinephrine (NE) fibers originating in the nucleus locus ceruleus terminate on Purkinje cells, particularly, secondary and tertiary dendrites,[53] in characteristic small granular vesicle boutons.[54] Neither we nor other investigators have observed any age-dependent alteration in cerebellar NE content[11,32] or catecholamine fluorescence[11,12] in the rat. However, Hoffer and colleagues (reviewed in this volume) have identified numerous dynamic changes in catecholamine neurotransmission and function in the aging cerebellum and locus ceruleus.

Aging Studies of the Purkinje Cell Target

At the level of the Purkinje cell, the essential target for cerebellar afferents, a number of age changes have been demonstrated by our laboratory.[11-16] Ethanolic phosphotungstic acid–(EPTA)–stained synaptic profiles in the upper molecular layer of old and young rat cerebella show a significant decline in number with age (FIGURE 6).[16]

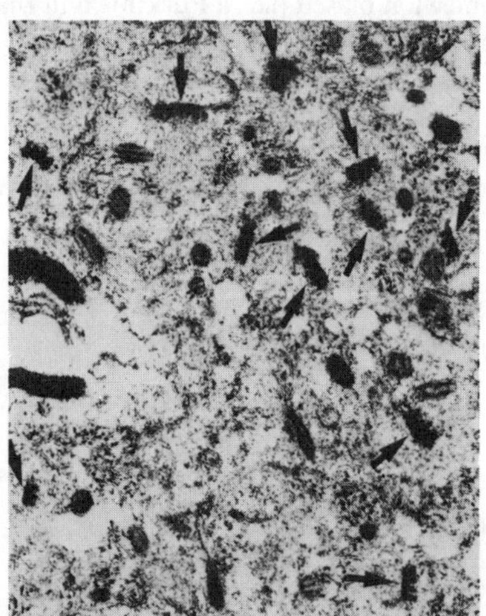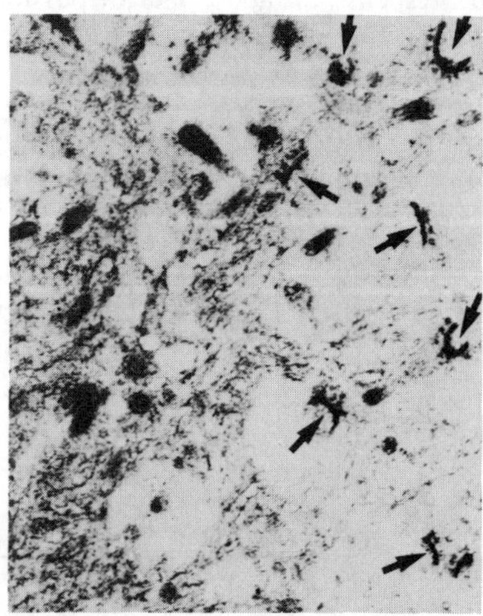

FIGURE 6. Typical EPTA-stained synaptic profiles (arrows) from the upper molecular layer of 6-month-old (left) and 26-month-old (right) rats. Young rats averaged 150,485 ± 3641 synapses/mm², which was significantly more than the 125,000 ± 4849 synapses/mm² average for old rats.[17]

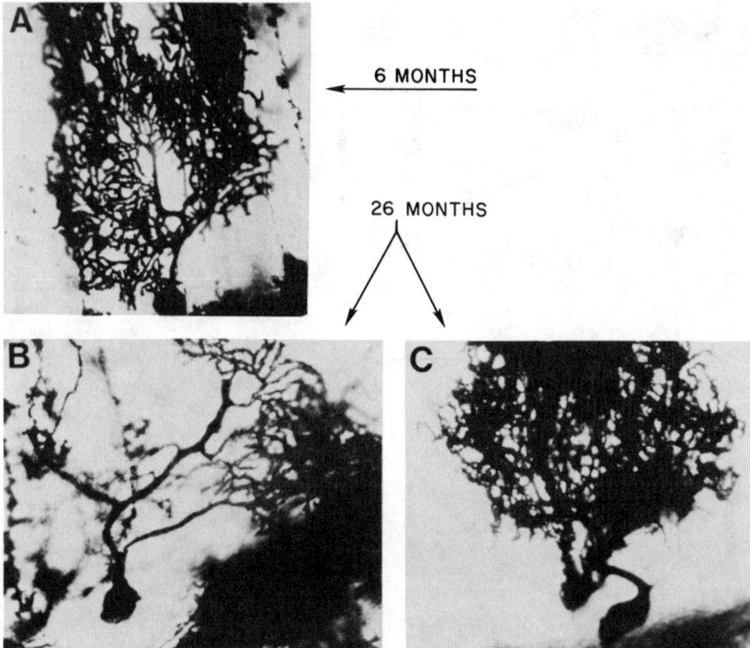

FIGURE 7. Typical Golgi-impregnated Purkinje neurons from 6-month-old (A) and 26-month-old (B,C) rats.[17]

Golgi sections have provided a light microscopic correlate to these ultrastructural findings (FIGURE 7).[16] FIGURE 7A, for example, illustrates the beautiful, full dendrite arbor of the young rat Purkinje cell. Although many relatively normal looking Purkinje neurons are also evident in old rats (FIGURE 7B), atrophic, severely defoliated Purkinje cells (FIGURE 7C) begin to appear in significant numbers.[16] Whether these are cells in the process of dying remains to be determined. However, using both cresyl violet and hematoxylin and eosin stains, we have demonstrated significant loss of Purkinje neurons in old rats.[11,16] Indeed, senescent loss of Purkinje cells is one of the oldest findings in aging research.[55] Given these results on atrophy and death of old Purkinje cells, perhaps it is not surprising that their spontaneous firing patterns are significantly altered (FIGURE 8)[11] nor that reactive gliosis can be demonstrated in the cerebellar white matter (FIGURE 9).[16]

Behavioral Correlates

Although it is axiomatic that correlations cannot establish causation, our recent experiments[17] have shown relationships between aspects of cerebellar morphologic change and locomotor performance. For example, there is a 0.84 correlation, within subjects, between EPTA synaptic density and rotorod performance of young and old rats (FIGURE 10).[17] Similar correlations are found on comparison of Purkinje cell counts and rotorod performance.[17] Balance beam performance is also impaired with age in our studies.[17]

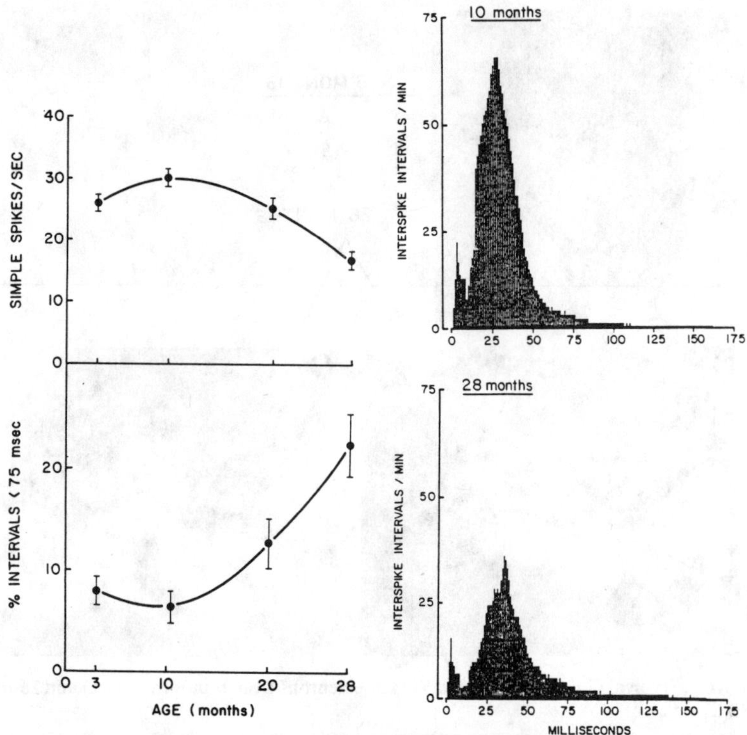

FIGURE 8. Age-dependent changes in rat Purkinje cell electrical activity. (Top left) Simple spike rate declines significantly from 3–28 months of age. (Bottom left) Percentage of long (>75 ms) interspike intervals increases significantly from 3–28 months of age. This suggests that the slowing of firing rate with age is not so much due to a general lengthening of the intervals between all spikes; instead, it is better explained by erratic long pauses between a few spikes. (Top right) Computer average of interspike interval histograms from the 48 cells recorded in four 10-month-old rats. (Bottom right) Computer average of interspike interval histograms from the 50 cells recorded in four 28-month-old rats. Note that the modal interspike interval has shifted very little with age: even the slow-firing cells of very old rats retain a strong tendency to fire at normal (25–30 ms) interspike intervals.[11]

OTHER STUDIES OF CEREBELLAR AGING

Much of the above work from our laboratory has been confirmed and extended by other investigators. For example, the massive lipofuscin deposition that we have observed in old rat cerebellar Purkinje cells[11,12] has been described recently in old monkeys.[51] Nosal[36] has performed ultrastructural studies in which extensive disruption of the granular endoplasmic reticulum is seen in old Purkinje cells. This provides an electron microscopic correlate to our work with Nissl stains.[11,12] Numerous studies, dating as far back as 1920,[56] have reported senescent losses of Purkinje neurons that are in general agreement with our data.[11,16] Scheibel and Scheibel's early Golgi studies on the aging cortex[57] and brain stem[58] bear clear parallels to our morphologic work on the aging cerebellum.[16] Although there has been one report, using Golgi techniques,

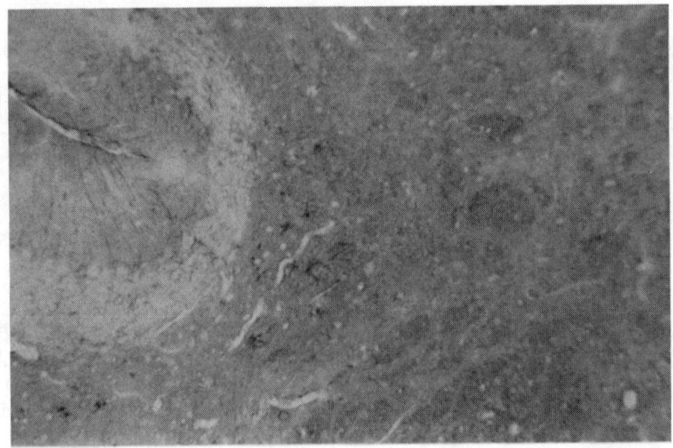

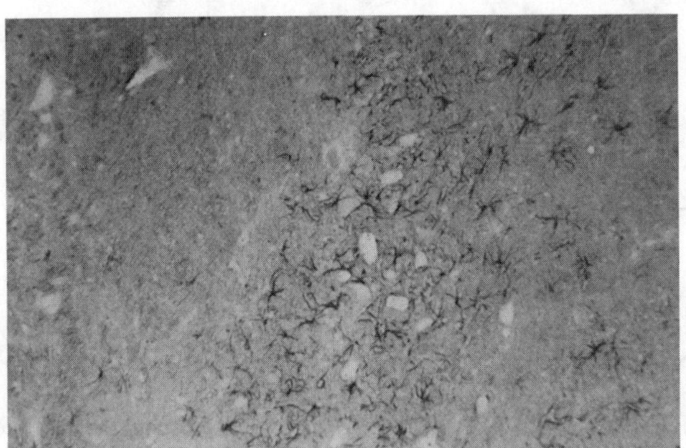

FIGURE 9.   Reactive gliosis (glial fibrillary acidic protein stain) in comparable cerebellar white matter sections from 5-month-old (top) and 24-month-old (bottom) rats.[17]

suggesting a lack of age change in Purkinje neurons,[59] that report appeared in abstract form and, to our knowledge, has never been formally published. An earlier paper by Bondareff,[47] who employed glutaraldehyde-osmium fixation, describes an age-dependent decline in cerebellar synaptic density that is similar to our results based on EPTA staining.[16]

Several pharmacological studies on aging of the cerebellum are also relevant to our work. Plaitakis *et al.*[45] have shown impaired cerebellar glutamate catabolism in adult onset olivopontocerebellar degeneration. Glutamate reuptake is known to be impaired in striata of old rats,[60] and glutamate/quinolinic acid neurotoxicity has become an increasingly plausible mechanism for progressive destruction of specific afferent target systems both in neural aging and in Huntington's disease. The excitatory par-

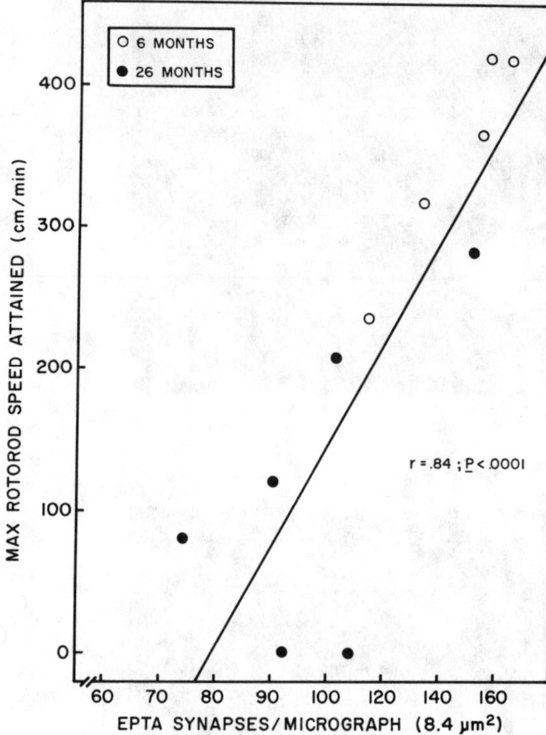

FIGURE 10. EPTA synapses versus rotorod performance in the same young and old rats as in FIGURE 9. Note that the best old rat overlaps the worst young one.[15]

allel fiber–Purkinje cell neurotransmitter is almost certain to be glutamate (cf. reference 27).

Coleman and Goldman[61] report no age change in rat locus ceruleus cell number, and we have been unable to detect a senescent decline in cerebellar catecholamine fluorescence.[11,12] Other experimenters[32,62] have replicated our finding[11,12] that cerebellar NE concentrations are not significantly lower in old animals. However, Hoffer and his colleagues have observed significant diminution in the response of old Purkinje units to iontophoretic and pressure-ejected NE and cAMP,[33,34] and Schmidt reports diminished adenylate cyclase activity after incubation of cerebellar slices from old rats with NE agonists.[35] Thus, presynaptic measures of NE afferents consistently fail to find evidence of senescent change (cf. references 11, 12, 32, 61, and 62), whereas postsynaptic measures almost invariably do (cf. references 33–35). Iontophoretic response to GABA, the inhibitory neurotransmitter probably used by basket cells and Purkinje-cell recurrent collaterals, is unaltered with age in the cerebellum.[33]

A HYPOTHESIS OF SENESCENT CEREBELLAR CHANGE

It is our belief that much of the data so far reported on cerebellar aging, including superficially contradictory findings, can be made coherent if one starts with specific cytoarchitectural degeneration of Purkinje cells. That this could be a primary mechanism is suggested by both the dominant role and the vulnerability of Purkinje cells in cerebellar function: Purkinje neurons are the essential target of all cerebellar afferents, the dominant element of cerebellar information processing, and the final output neuron (excluding the deep nuclei) of the olivocerebellar system. Moreover, they are one of the most exquisitely sensitive neuron types in brain to vascular, hyperthermic, and other insults,[63–67] and the evidence for their loss with age is, without doubt, the strongest in the nervous system (reviewed in reference 68).

Purkinje cells are very large and must support a densely arborized dendritic field and a lengthy, highly ramified axonal projection. Their metabolic requirements exceed that of all other neurons in the brain except cortical pyramidal cells.[69] Like cortical pyramidal cells,[57] their most vulnerable anatomic locus appears to be the most distal and fine elements of the dendrite field, the synaptic thorns and spiny branchlets. These are, especially in the upper molecular layer of the cerebellum, almost exclusively the site for glutamatergic parallel fiber–Purkinje cell contacts. Their loss with age, as demonstrated in both EPTA[16] and glutaraldehyde-osmium[47] preparations, thus provides at least a partial cytoarchitectural basis for the decreased ability to drive old Purkinje units via parallel fiber stimulation.[13]

The next most distal and fine elements of the dendritic arbor are secondary and tertiary dendrites, which provide a terminal projection area for catecholamine fibers[53] among others. Golgi sections[16] reveal these dendrites, especially the tertiary dendrites, to be nearly as vulnerable as the spiny branchlets. Hence, loss of the former provides a cytoarchitectural explanation for why presynaptic measures of cerebellar NE input (e.g., NE concentrations, catecholamine fluorescence, locus ceruleus cell counts)[11,32,61] fail to detect an aging change, whereas postsynaptic measures (e.g., response to iontophoretic NE, adenylate cyclase activation)[33–35] do detect an aging change.

Still further down the dendrite arbor are the Purkinje cell's large primary dendrites and trunk. These terminal projection areas for olivary climbing fibers appear to be relatively well preserved even in the oldest, most severely defoliated Purkinje cells.[16] This preservation provides a cytoarchitectural basis for our physiological finding that climbing fiber responses are unaltered in old Purkinje neurons,[11] as well as for Bondareff's ultrastructural finding that synapses characteristic of parallel fiber contacts are lost with age, whereas synapses characteristic of climbing fiber contacts are not.[47]

FIGURE 11 pictorially summarizes many of the arguments for a cytoarchitectural hypothesis of senescent cerebellar dysfunction. In an early publication,[11] we noted that about 60–70% of old rat Purkinje cells fired quite normally (as in FIGURE 11A). However, in the same electrode penetration, occasional, quite abnormally firing Purkinje units could also be found (FIGURE 11B, taken from the same 28-month-old rat as FIGURE 11A). These abnormally firing units, the number of which increases significantly to around 30% in old age,[11] are identifiable as Purkinje cells because of their normal and characteristic climbing fiber response (the leftmost peak of intervals in the histograms). It is their simple spike firing (reflected in the modal, rightmost peak of intervals) that shows pathologic slowing. In a more recent study,[16] we found that about 60–70% of old, Golgi-impregnated Purkinje cells appeared morphologically normal (as in FIGURE 11C). In the same sections, however, other morphologically abnormal Purkinje neurons could also be found (FIGURE 11D). These abnormal cells, the number of which is significantly increased in old rats, show defoliation precisely at the site most influencing Purkinje unit modal, simple spike firing, the fine distal branchlets where parallel fibers synapse. There is relative preservation at the site for climbing fiber input, namely, the large primary dendrites and trunk.

Whether Purkinje neuron defoliation is the first stage of a process leading to cell death or is concurrent with it cannot yet be stated; however, the two processes are significantly correlated.[16] Moreover, the reactive gliosis that can be detected in the white

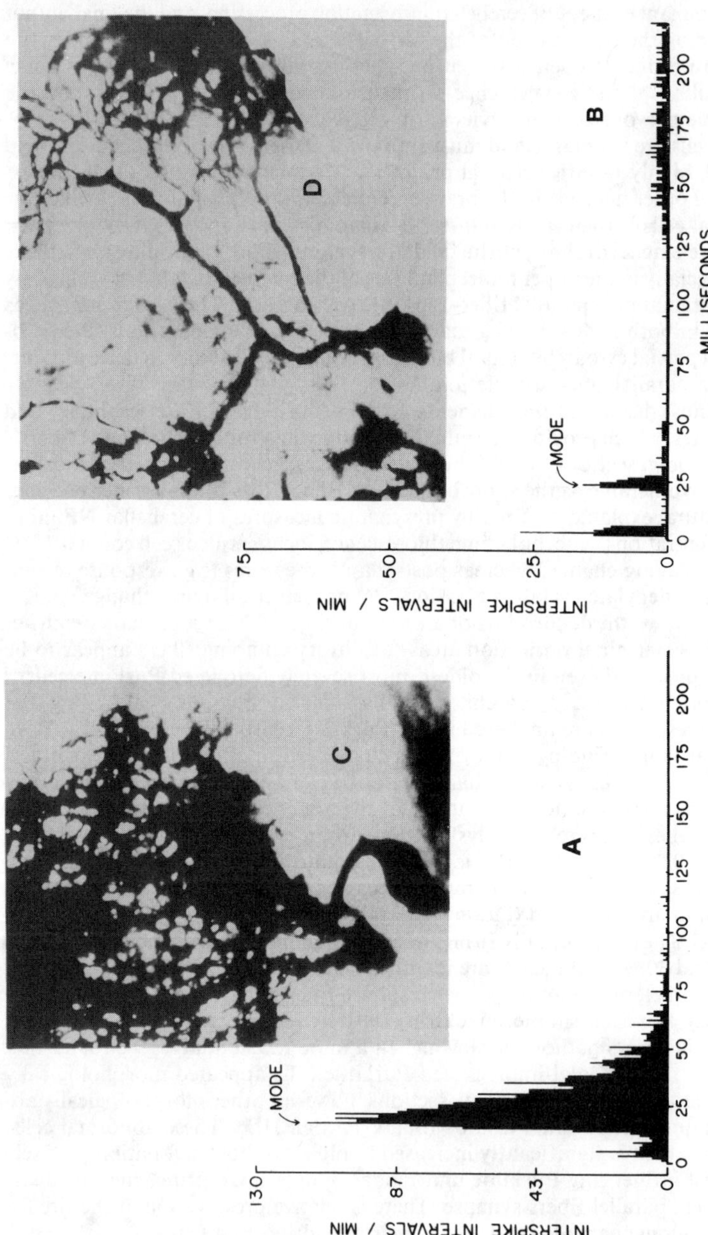

FIGURE 11. (Bottom graphs) Interspike interval histograms of single Purkinje units from a 28-month-old rat.[11] (Top photographs) Golgi-impregnated Purkinje neurons from the same 28-month-old rat.[17] The histogram and morphology seen in the left panels are normal and are observed in 60–70% of old rat Purkinje cells. About 30–40% of old Purkinje cells in the same rat fire abnormally and appear defoliated (right panels).[11,17]

matter of old rat cerebella[16] seems likely to be related to Purkinje neuron atrophy[16] and death.[11,16]

Several issues will have to be addressed by a cytoarchitectural hypothesis of senescent cerebellar change. These include the role of concurrent afferent degeneration and the consideration of why some areas of the Purkinje cell dendritic arbor should be more vulnerable than others. One possible answer for the latter is that the farther one gets from somatic metabolic reserves (as in distal dendrite spines), the more precarious survival becomes (an argument advanced by Scheibel and Scheibel).[57] A second possibility is that the bigger a neurite is, the more of it there is to lose and the longer it will take to do so (i.e., primary dendrites could be degenerating along with more distal elements, but the latter, being smaller, would disappear first). A third possibility concerns the role of afferents. Our work,[13-16] in addition to that of others,[70] suggests senescent deterioration of parallel fibers, and this deafferentation could exacerbate the loss of Purkinje unit spiny branchlets. An intriguing alternative is that glutamate/quinolinic acid toxicity from parallel fiber input could cause the loss of Purkinje cell spiny branchlets. Olney[60] and others[45,71] have put forward the notion that if glutamate reuptake or catabolism fails as a means for glutamate synaptic inactivation, then a kainitelike lesion of terminals might result. Striatal glutamate reuptake has already been shown to be impaired in old rats[60] and a defect in glutamate catabolism is now known to exist in adult onset olivopontocerebellar degeneration.[66]

In light of our hypothesis of cerebellar aging, the work of Coleman and his associates[72] must also be considered. Morphologic research by this group (in contrast to our results and those of Mervis,[37,73] Scheibel and Scheibel,[57,58,74] and others) is widely perceived as demonstrating age-related dendritic growth rather than atrophy. It is seldom appreciated that Coleman and his co-workers actually showed both dendritic growth and dendritic atrophy during senescence, leading them to conclude: "When considered together, data from qualitative and quantitative studies of Golgi material suggest that there are two populations of neurons in the aging mammalian brain. One is undergoing dendritic atrophy, probably as a prelude to neuronal loss through cell death. The other is undergoing dendritic growth."[75] In an exhaustive review of this issue, Mervis[76] comes to a nearly identical conclusion.

POTENTIAL APPLICATIONS OF CEREBELLAR AGING RESEARCH

Heretofore, the technique of intracellularly staining a recorded neuron has been used primarily to determine what kind of cell was recorded. However, because the characteristic firing patterns of Purkinje units uniquely identify them at the time of recording and their morphology has already been described in great detail, it becomes possible in the cerebellum to extend intracellular staining techniques to a more specific task—the correlation of neuronal cytoarchitecture with neuronal electrical activity. Llinas and his colleagues, among others, have already begun such investigations. Such an approach could have wide basic science significance because central nervous system cytoarchitectural alterations are not limited to senescence: they may occur in learning and memory,[77,78] in recovery from central nervous system injury,[79,80] and in other phenomena.[55,81-83] Walker and his colleagues,[84,85] for example, present Golgi sections of Purkinje cells from ethanol-naive and chronic-ethanol mice that are virtually indistinguishable from those obtained in our studies of old rats.[16] Interestingly, in two alcohol-related studies in our laboratory,[11,18] electrophysiological changes in Purkinje cells after chronic-ethanol treatment[18] also bear clear parallels to those seen in aging.[11]

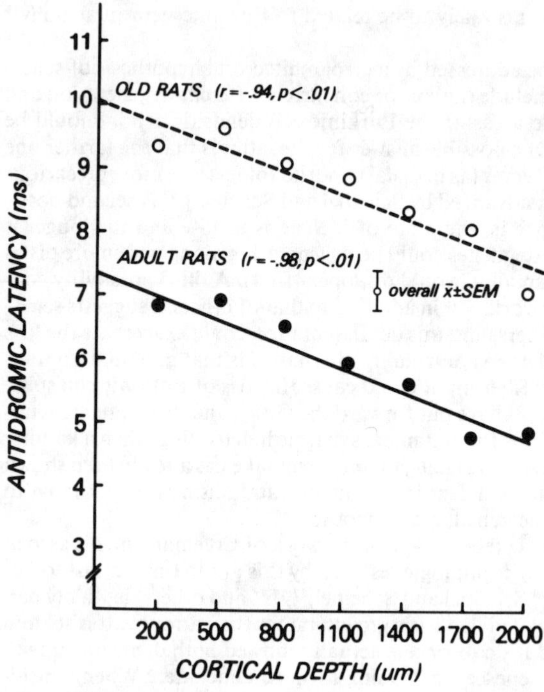

FIGURE 12. Mean antidromic conduction latency for nucleus basalis neurons in adult and aged rats. The recording electrode placement was in the nucleus basalis. The stimulation of nucleus basalis axons projecting to the cortex was accomplished using a cortical electrode that could be moved to progressively lower cortical depths. Note that the slopes of the curves are identical, although the conduction latencies are consistently longer at all depths for aged rats. Thus, intracortical conduction velocities of basalis axons are unaltered with age; the significant senescent decline in impulse conduction is wholly due to changes that occur in the white matter.[86]

The senescent cytoarchitectural changes that we have hypothesized to be a primary determinant of cerebellar aging are, moreover, not limited to cerebellar Purkinje cells. Indeed, cortical pyramidal cells[57] and hippocampal pyramidal cells[74] exhibit very similar changes, including a particular vulnerability of dendrite spines. These and other shared features of Purkinje and pyramidal cells (e.g., large size; lengthy axon; highly arborized dendrites; use of spines or thorns for certain synaptic contacts; exquisite sensitivity to hypoxic, hyperthermic, and other insults; highest metabolic requirements in brain)[63–67] may provide insights for a common cytoarchitectural basis of senescent neuronal dysfunction. Lessons learned about mechanisms of senescence in the more easily studied and better characterized cerebellum are likely to prove extendable to aging processes in other brain structures underlying other geriatric disorders (e.g., the cortex and dementia). For example, our laboratory, in collaboration with that of Gary Aston-Jones, has recently demonstrated changes in conduction properties of cholinergic afferents from the nucleus basalis to cortex (FIGURE 12) that are reminiscent of cerebellar parallel fiber alterations.[86]

Because the cerebellum lends itself so well to systems analysis, it could also have utility for the evaluation of aging therapies. Presently, there are no useful, comprehensive protocols for screening putative "antigeriatric" compounds. Several such compounds (e.g., Hydergine) are now being marketed despite a paucity of information about their mechanism of action or their efficacy in treating neurologic problems of the elderly.[87] Centrophenoxine, for instance, reportedly reduces CNS lipofuscin in guinea pigs,[88] but it remains unclear whether such an action is therapeutic or worthless.[52,89,90] Similar statements could probably be made about all of the present antigeriatric compounds because clear cellular endpoints do not presently exist against which they can be tested. With further refinement, the cerebellum could become a practical model with both cellular and behavioral endpoints for testing or screening so-called "anti-aging" compounds.

Finally, cerebellar senescence is not without clinical correlates.[43-46,91-94] As Bondareff has put it: "It is tempting to speculate that abnormalities of coordination and gait, well known in older persons, might relate to a similar loss of cerebellar circuitry."[47] Infirmities of gait and station are, in fact, one of the most common repercussions of cerebellar lesions;[8,46] they are estimated to occur to a disabling extent in at least 15% of the aged population, even in the absence of Parkinson's disease.[91]

In addition to the direct clinical correlates of cerebellar senescence, indirect relationships with disorders of other motor centers may exist. For example, adult onset olivopontocerebellar degeneration was originally discovered serendipitously in patients initially examined because of progressive extrapyramidal syndromes.[92] Klawans[93] has pointed out that "supranuclear palsy and olivopontocerebellar degeneration frequently include among their manifestations signs and symptoms which are considered to be part of the usual spectrum of Parkinsonism." Moreover, in their olivopontocerebellar cases, Critchley and Greenfield[94] have noted a "tendency towards degeneration of other nuclei and fibre tracts subserving movement, but not directly concerned with the cerebellum."

Abnormalities of cognition, especially those related to senescence, also appear to co-occur with adult onset olivopontocerebellar disorders. For example, Hutton *et al.*[44] observe a highly significant correlation between visual tracking disability (a cerebellar test) and the severity of cognitive dysfunction in Alzheimer's disease. According to a survey by Heshe,[95] 65% of patients suffering spinocerebellar and "pure" cerebellar degeneration are also diagnosed as demented. Both a clinical study using CT scans[96] and a morphological survey of the Yakolev Collection[97] report a surprising but significant incidence of cerebellar vermis atrophy in previously diagnosed schizophrenics. Although it is true that the cerebellar vermis is linked automatically and physiologically with areas of the limbic forebrain previously implicated in cognitive disorders,[98-100] few would take seriously a direct role of the cerebellum in such diseases (however, see reference 101). What these data do reasonably and importantly suggest is that mechanisms of brain senescence and dysfunction may not always be restricted to just one neural circuit nor even to one brain region. Thus, cerebellar aging studies may provide information relevant not only to specific geriatric motor infirmities, but also to mechanisms of senescence in other senile disorders, particularly Parkinson's disease and senile dementia.

With regard to age-related motor dysfunction, it cannot be emphasized enough that efferents from the cerebellum provide highly processed information both to the motor cortex and to the basal ganglia.[3-6,8,102] Thus, even if cerebellar changes do not play a primary role in senescent motor dysfunction, they are in a position to exacerbate age-related disorders of pyramidal and extrapyramidal centers.

REFERENCES

1. ROCKSTEIN, M. 1974. Theoretical Aspects of Aging. Academic Press. New York.
2. BIRREN, J. 1980. Handbook of Mental Health and Aging. Prentice–Hall. Englewood Cliffs, New Jersey.
3. ECCLES, J., M. ITO & J. SZENTAGOTHAI. 1967. The Cerebellum as a Neuronal Machine. Springer Pub. New York.
4. LLINAS, R. 1969. Neurobiology of Cerebellar Evolution and Development. AMA-ERF Institute for Biomedical Research. Chicago.

5. PALAY, S. & V. CHAN-PALAY. 1974. Cerebellar Cortex. Springer Pub. New York.
6. CHAN-PALAY, V. 1977. Cerebellar Dentate Nucleus. Springer Pub. New York.
7. RAMON Y CAJAL, S. 1894. Proc. R. Soc. London 7: 12–30.
8. GILMAN, S., J. R. BLOEDEL & R. LECHTENBERG. 1981. Disorders of the Cerebellum. Davis. Philadelphia.
9. DOW, R. S. & G. MORUZZI. 1958. The Physiology and Pathology of the Cerebellum. University of Minnesota Press. Minneapolis.
10. HOFFER, B. J., G. R. SIGGINS, D. J. WOODWARD & F. E. BLOOM. 1971. Brain Res. 30: 425–430.
11. ROGERS, J., M. A. SILVER, W. J. SHOEMAKER & F. E. BLOOM. 1980. Neurobiol. Aging 1: 3–11.
12. ROGERS, J., M. SILVER & F. BLOOM. 1979. Soc. Neurosci. Abstr. 5: 10.
13. ROGERS, J., S. ZORNETZER & F. BLOOM. 1981. Neurobiol. Aging 2: 15–25.
14. ROGERS, J. 1981. In Brain Neurotransmitters and Receptors in Aging and Age-Related Disorders. Raven Press. New York.
15. ROGERS, J. & S. ZORNETZER. 1984. In Assessment in Geriatric Psychopharmacology. Raven Press. New York.
16. ZORNETZER, S., F. BLOOM, R. MERVIS & J. ROGERS. 1981. Soc. Neurosci. Abstr. 7: 690.
17. ROGERS, J., S. F. ZORNETZER, F. E. BLOOM & R. E. MERVIS. 1984. Senescent microstructural changes in rat cerebellum. Brain Res. 292: 23–32.
18. ROGERS, J., G. SIGGINS, J. SCHULMAN & F. BLOOM. 1980. Brain Res. 196: 183–198.
19. LAMARRE, Y., C. DE MONTIGNY, M. DUMONT & M. WEISS. 1971. Brain Res. 32: 246–250.
20. LLINAS, R. & R. VOLKIND. 1973. Exp. Brain Res. 18: 69–78.
21. PURO, D. & D. WOODWARD. 1977. Brain Res. 129: 141–146.
22. GRUNER, J. A., J. ALTMAN & N. SPIVACK. 1980. Exp. Brain Res. 40: 361–373.
23. LLINAS, R. & M. SUGIMORI. 1980. J. Physiol. 305: 171–213.
24. LANDIS, S. 1973. J. Cell Biol. 57: 782–797.
25. SIGGINS, G. R. & J. E. SCHULTZ. 1979. Proc. Natl. Acad. Sci. USA 76: 5987–5991.
26. FREEDMAN, R., B. J. HOFFER, D. J. WOODWARD & D. PURO. 1977. Exp. Neurol. 55: 269–288.
27. WIKLUND, L., G. TOGGENBURGER & M. CUENOD. 1982. Science 216: 78–79.
28. BLOEDEL, J. R. & J. COURVILLE. 1981. In Handbook of Physiology. Amer. Physiol. Soc. Washington, D.C.
29. SHINNAR, S., R. MACIEWICZ & R. SHOFER. 1975. Brain Res. 97: 139–145.
30. ROBERTS, E. & K. KURIYAMA. 1968. Brian Res. 8: 1–35.
31. SALMOIRAGHI, G. & F. H. STEINER. 1963. J. Neurophysiol. 26: 581–597.
32. OSTERBERG, H., H. DONAHUE, I. SEVERSON & C. E. FINCH. 1981. Brain Res. 224: 337–352.
33. MARWAHA, J., B. HOFFER, R. PITTMAN & R. FREEDMAN. 1980. Brain Res. 201: 85–97.
34. MARWAHA, J., B. HOFFER & R. FREEDMAN. 1981. Neurobiol. Aging 2: 95–98.
35. SCHMIDT, M. J. & J. F. THORNBERRY. 1978. Brain Res. 139: 159–177.
36. NOSAL, G. 1979. Mech. Ageing Dev. 10: 295–314.
37. MERVIS, R. F. 1979. Gerontol. Soc. Abstr. 19: 119.
38. MEHRAEIN, P., M. YAMADA & E. TARNOWSKA-DZIDUSKO. 1975. In Advances in Neurology, Vol. 12. Raven Press. New York.
39. MORIN, A. M. & C. G. WASTERLAIN. 1980. Neurochem. Res. 5: 301–308.
40. SPOKES, G. S. 1979. Brain 102: 333–346.
41. UNSWORTH, B. R., L. H. FLEMING & P. C. CARON. 1980. Mech. Ageing Dev. 134: 205–217.
42. ENNA, S. J. & R. STRONG. 1981. In Brain Neurotransmitters and Receptors in Aging and Age-Related Disorders. Raven Press. New York.
43. SPOONER, J. W., S. M. SAKALA & R. W. BALCH. 1980. Arch. Neurol. 37: 575–576.
44. HUTTON, J. T., I. SHAPIRO, R. B. LOEWENSON, B. L. CHRISTIANS & J. A. NAGEL. 1982. Abstr. Am. Neurol. Assoc., p. 102.
45. PLAITAKIS, A., S. BERL & M. D. YAHR. 1982. Science 216: 194–196.
46. ADAMS, R. D. & M. VICTOR. 1981. Principles of Neurology, p. 418–426. McGraw-Hill. New York.
47. GLICK, R. & W. BONDAREFF. 1979. J. Gerontol. 34: 818–822.
48. BRODY, H. 1976. In Neurobiology of Aging, Vol. 5. Raven Press. New York.

49. MONAGLE, R. & H. BRODY. 1974. J. Comp. Neurol. **155**: 61–66.
50. BRIZZEE, K., J. HARKIN, J. ORDY & B. KAACK. 1975. *In* Aging, Vol. 1. Raven Press. New York.
51. NANDY, K. 1981. Neurobiol. Aging **2**: 61–64.
52. KARNAUKNOW, V. N. 1973. Tsitologya **15**: 538–542.
53. KIMOTO, Y., M. TOHYAMA, K. SATOH, T. SAKUMOTO, Y. TAKAHASHI & N. SHIMIZU. 1981. Neuroscience **6**: 47–58.
54. MOORE, R. Y. & F. E. BLOOM. 1979. Annu. Rev. Neurosci. **2**: 113–168.
55. PYSH, J. J. & G. M. WEISS. 1979. Science **206**: 230–232.
56. ELLIS, R. S. 1920. J. Comp. Neurol. **32**: 1–32.
57. SCHEIBEL, M. E. & A. B. SCHEIBEL. 1975. *In* Aging, Vol. 1. Raven Press. New York.
58. MACHADO-SALAS, J. P., M. E. SCHEIBEL & A. B. SCHEIBEL. 1977. Exp. Neurol. **54**: 504–512.
59. PYSH, J. J. & M. D. BENSON. 1980. Soc. Neurosci. Abstr. **6**: 281.
60. PRICE, M. T., J. W. OLNEY & R. HAFT. 1981. Life Sci. **28**: 1365–1370.
61. GOLDMAN, G. & P. D. COLEMAN. 1981. Neurobiol. Aging **2**: 33–36.
62. FINCH, C. E. 1973. Brain Res. **52**: 261–276.
63. EADIE, M. J., J. H. TYRER & J. R. KUKUMS. 1971. Brain **94**: 647–660.
64. SCHADE, J. P. & W. H. MCMENEMY. 1963. Selective Vulnerability of the Brain in Hypoxaemia. Oxford University Press. London/New York.
65. GREENFIELD, J., W. BLACKWOOD, W. MCMENEMY, A. MEYER & R. NORMAN. 1958. Neuropathology. Arnold. London.
66. SNIDER, R. S., W. THOMAS & S. R. SNIDER. 1978. Experientia **34**: 479–489.
67. MARGERISON, J. H. & J. A. N. CORSELLIS. 1966. Brain **89**: 499–509.
68. CORSELLIS, J. A. N. 1976. *In* Aging, Vol. 3. Raven Press. New York.
69. EPSTEIN, M. H. & P. R. THORNE. 1970. Exp. Neurol. **26**: 586–594.
70. OGRA, M., R. YATES & C. KNOX. 1980. Proceedings of the American Aging Association. Houston, Texas.
71. COYLE, J. T., E. MCGEER, P. L. MCGEER & R. SCHWARCZ. 1978. *In* Kainic Acid as a Tool in Neurobiology. Raven Press. New York.
72. BUELL, S. J. & P. D. COLEMAN. 1979. Science **206**: 854–856m.
73. MERVIS, R. & R. BARTUS. 1981. J. Neuropathol. Exp. Neurol. **40**: 313–322.
74. MACHADO-SALAS, J. P. & A. B. SCHEIBEL. 1979. Exp. Neurol. **63**: 347–355.
75. COLEMAN, P. D. & D. G. FLOOD. 1986. Prog. Brain Res. **70**: 227–237.
76. MERVIS, R. 1981. *In* Aging and Cell Structure. Plenum. New York.
77. VAN HARREVELD, A. & E. FIFKOVA. 1974. Brain Res. **81**: 455–467.
78. FIFKOVA, E. & A. VAN HARREVELD. 1977. J. Neuropsychol. **6**: 211–230.
79. LYNCH, G., S. MOSKO, T. PARKS & C. COTMAN. 1973. Brain Res. **50**: 174–178.
80. LYNCH, G., S. DEADWYLER & C. COTMAN. 1973. Science **180**: 1364–1366.
81. FLOETER, M. K. & W. T. GREENOUGH. 1979. Science **206**: 227–229.
82. FIALA, B., J. JOYCE & W. GREENOUGH. 1978. Exp. Neurol. **59**: 372–382.
83. VALVERDE, F. 1971. Brain Res. **33**: 1–10.
84. RILEY, J. N. & D. W. WALKER. 1978. Science **201**: 646–648.
85. RILEY, J. N. 1977. Doctoral dissertation. Department of Neuroscience, College of Medicine, University of Florida, Gainesville.
86. ASTON-JONES, G., J. ROGERS, R. D. SHAVER, D. G. DINAN & D. E. MOSS. 1985. Nature **318**: 462–464.
87. BANN, T. 1980. Psychopharmacology for the Aged. Karger. Basel.
88. NANDY, K. 1968. J. Gerontol. **23**: 82–92.
89. ZEMAN, W. 1974. J. Neuropathol. Exp. Neurol. **33**: 1–12.
90. HASAN, M. & P. GLEES. 1972. Gerontologia **18**: 217–236.
91. DRACHMAN, D. A. 1980. *In* Handbook of Mental Health and Aging. Prentice-Hall. Englewood Cliffs, New Jersey.
92. ADAMS, R. D., L. VAN BOGAERT & H. VANDER EECKEN. 1964. J. Neuropathol. Exp. Neurol. **23**: 584–608.
93. KLAWANS, H. L. 1973. The Pharmacology of Extrapyramidal Movement Disorders. Karger. Basel.
94. CRITCHLEY, M. & J. G. GREENFIELD. 1948. Brain **71**: 343–363.

95. HESHE, J. 1970. Acta Neurol. Scand. **46**(suppl. 43): 83–85.
96. WEINBERGER, D. R., E. F. TORREY & R. J. WYATT. 1979. Lancet **i:** 718–719.
97. WEINBERGER, D. R., J. E. KLEINMAN, D. J. LUCHINS, E. B. BIGELOW & R. J. WYATT. 1980. Am. J. Psychiatry **137:** 359–361.
98. HEATH, R. G., C. W. DEMPSEY & C. J. FONTANA. 1978. Biol. Psychiatry **13:** 501–529.
99. SNIDER, R. S., A. MAITI & S. R. SNIDER. 1976. Exp. Neurol. **53:** 714–728.
100. SNIDER, S. R. & R. S. SNIDER. 1977. J. Neurol. Trans. **40:** 115–128.
101. HEATH, R. G. 1977. J. Nerv. Ment. Disorders **165:** 300–305.
102. MASSION, J. & K. SASAKI. 1979. Cerebro-Cerebellar Interactions. Elsevier. Amsterdam/New York.

Age-related Changes in Cerebellar Noradrenergic Function[a]

BARRY J. HOFFER,[b] GREG ROSE,[b,c] KAREN PARFITT,[b]
ROBERT FREEDMAN,[b,c,d] AND PAULA C. BICKFORD-WIMER[b,c]

[b]Department of Pharmacology
University of Colorado Health Sciences Center
Denver, Colorado 80262

[c]Veterans Administration Hospital
Denver, Colorado 80220

[d]Department of Psychiatry
University of Colorado Health Sciences Center
Denver, Colorado 80262

INTRODUCTION

The elucidation of age-related alterations in central nervous system function is a necessary prerequisite to understanding the causes of behavioral deficits in the elderly. A good strategy for identifying such changes, as well as their functional consequences, is to look for them in specific, well-characterized neuronal systems. It is well known that central catecholamine pathways are altered during aging. Several areas of the central nervous system (CNS) demonstrate decreases in catecholamine turnover[1] and tyrosine hydroxylase activity in aging.[2] Reductions in beta-adrenergic receptor numbers have been described.[3,4] Moreover, decreases in catecholamine-stimulated adenylate cyclase[5,6] and cyclic nucleotide accumulation[7] in old animals have been reported.

We have examined the functional consequences of alteration in the central noradrenergic system during aging using the cerebellum as a model.[8,9] The inhibitory noradrenergic input from the locus coeruleus to the cerebellum has been extensively studied in terms of its anatomy, physiology, and pharmacology.[10,11] Noradrenergic fibers arising from the pontine nucleus locus coeruleus (LC) ascend through the superior cerebellar peduncle to synapse on cerebellar Purkinje neurons. Activation of this input inhibits spontaneous discharge of the cerebellar Purkinje neurons via a cyclic-AMP–dependent process.[10]

The interaction of norepinephrine (NE) with cerebellar neuronal circuitry has been shown to be more complex than a simple effect on spontaneous discharge.[12,13] NE is thought to have neuromodulatory actions because it preferentially decreases spontaneous discharge while leaving evoked activity relatively intact. Cerebellar Purkinje neurons receive two major afferent connections, in addition to a smaller noradrenergic input from the LC. The first one is the excitatory climbing fiber input from the inferior olive; this produces characteristic complex discharges in Purkinje neurons.[11] The

[a] This work was supported by USPHS Grant Nos. AG-04418 and NS-09199 and by the Veterans Administration Medical Research Service.

269

mossy fiber input (via a granule cell interneuron) provides the other major excitatory afferent; it produces only simple spike discharges in Purkinje neurons.[11] The granule cell parallel fibers synapse on basket and stellate cells in addition to the Purkinje cells. Activation of this intrinsic pathway inhibits Purkinje cell discharge in a row or beam adjacent to the Purkinje cell that is being excited by the parallel fiber.

The effect of NE on Purkinje cell responses to electrical activation of these connections has been studied in our laboratory using computer-generated peristimulus time histograms (PSTHs) of evoked neuronal discharge. Local application of NE in young animals preferentially inhibits spontaneous activity over simple or complex spike excitations induced by stimulation of mossy or climbing fiber afferents. Moreover, NE augments evoked inhibition to a greater extent than it inhibits spontaneous activity. These differential effects of NE on spontaneous and evoked activity—either excitatory or inhibitory—suggest a significant functional role for NE in the operation of cerebellar circuitries. A large body of evidence links cerebellar function with motor coordination and motor learning. More recently, a specific involvement of cerebellar NE in motor learning has been described.

The central noradrenergic system is also thought to be involved in the mechanism of action of some tricyclic antidepressant drugs (such as desipramine). Depression is a major problem among the aged population and it affects approximately 13 million elderly individuals. Although the cerebellar cortex may not be a critical area for the action of antidepressant drugs, it provides a good system in which to investigate the possibility of altered noradrenergic function as the basis for age-related differences in the efficacy of antidepressant agents.

METHODS

Young (3–6 month) and old (18–26 month) male Fischer 344 rats were obtained from the National Institute on Aging contract colonies maintained by Charles River or Harlan Laboratories. In addition, 18- to 26-month-old Sprague-Dawley rats were obtained from Zivic-Miller.

Rats were anesthetized with urethane (0.75–1.5 g/kg), intubated, and allowed to breathe spontaneously. Body temperature was maintained at 37 °C with a heating pad. The animal was placed in a stereotaxic frame and the skin and muscle over the posterior cerebellar vermis were excised. After cisternal drainage, the skull and dura over this region were removed; then, the brain surface was covered with warm 2% agar in saline. Recordings were made from Purkinje cells in the vermis, lobule VI, and lobule VII. Cells were identified by anatomical location and by their characteristic discharge of simple and complex spikes.[11]

The activity of single Purkinje neurons were recorded using glass micropipettes filled with 5 M NaCl (resistance of 1–3 megohms). Action potentials were displayed on an oscilloscope and were separated from background activity using a window discriminator. The output of the discriminator was integrated over one-second intervals and was displayed as a firing rate using a chart recorder. The output of the window discriminator was also led to a microcomputer for construction of peristimulus time histograms or interspike interval histograms.

For all experiments in which spontaneous firing rates were determined, single-barrel glass electrodes were used for recording. The mean firing rate of 10 cells was determined from their interspike interval histograms. In some cases, propranolol was administered intraperitoneally (5 mg/kg), and 30 minutes later, another 10 Purkinje neurons were sampled.

Norepinephrine (2×10^{-2} M) was locally applied from one barrel of a multibarreled micropipette using pressure microejection. The pressure applications, ranging from 1 to 35 pounds per square inch (psi), were controlled by a Medical Systems Corporation pneumatic pump that regulated the magnitude of pressure delivered and the timing of the pressure pulse. Pressure ejection from glass micropipettes has been reported to release the drug in an amount linearly related to pressure and time.[14] For each cell, the drug was tested at least twice at each dose with consistent effects required. Data from cells that showed a decrease in the action potential amplitude during drug response or that did not show recovery after cessation of drug application were discarded. A schematic of the recording setup is illustrated in FIGURE 1.

Changes in spontaneous and evoked activity were determined by comparing identical portions of histograms computed during control and drug periods. Cell discharge rate was computed for each evoked and spontaneous period by dividing the number of spikes within the period by the number of sweeps multiplied by the length of that period. The difference in firing rate between control and drug periods was expressed as a percentage inhibition or excitation.[12,13]

Afferents to the Purkinje cells were electrically activated using monophasic 0.05-ms to 0.1-ms square wave pulses of 1 to 80 V. The sensorimotor cortex was stimulated

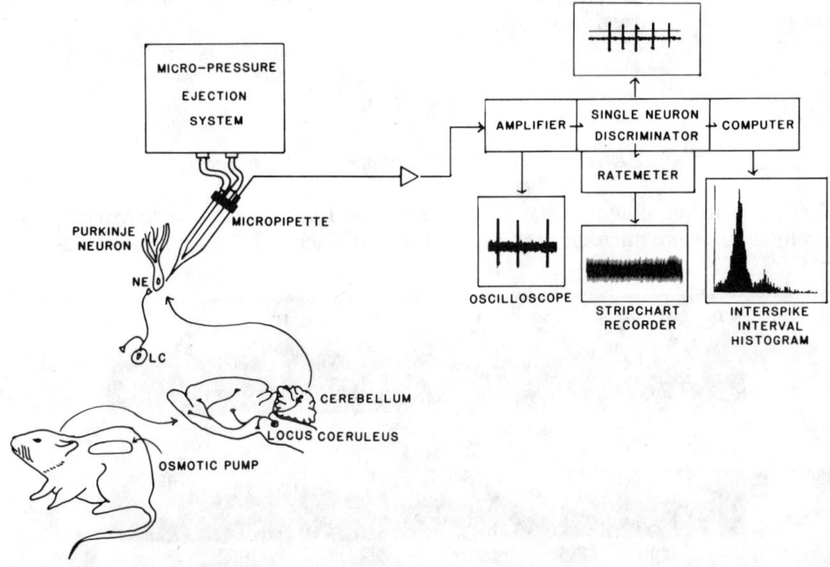

FIGURE 1. Diagrammatic representation of the recording facility used for the experiments reported here. Rats were prepared for electrophysiological recording of cerebellar Purkinje neurons. Depicted in the diagram of the rat brain is the noradrenergic innervation to the cerebellum from the nucleus locus coeruleus; note that this nucleus is the source of noradrenergic innervation for most of the neuraxis. A glass micropipette was used to record the extracellular action potentials of cerebellar Purkinje neurons, as well as to apply drugs locally by pressure microejection. The signal recorded via the electrode was amplified and viewed on an oscilloscope. Single neurons were discriminated from background as shown on the top right side of the figure. Any action potential passing above the line was converted to a five-volt pulse and then led either to a ratemeter for illustration as a strip-chart recording or to a computer for compilation of interspike interval histograms, or peristimulus time histograms.

using an array of concentric bipolar electrodes. Parallel fibers were stimulated using bipolar electrodes—made from two twisted wires with a tip separation of 0.1 mm—placed on the surface of the cerebellum. The inferior olive was stimulated with a single concentric bipolar electrode placed contralateral to the recording site. All stimulating electrode placements were verified histologically.

Desipramine hydrochloride (10 mg/kg/day) was administered via subcutaneous Alzet osmotic pumps (model 2ML4) for a period of three weeks. At the end of the experiment, the cerebellum was rapidly removed and frozen at −70 °C for analysis of desipramine.[15] After addition of a known amount of imipramine, which was used as an internal standard, brain samples were sonicated. Then, the homogenate was made basic with NaOH and extracted three times with hexane. The hexane was evaporated under a stream of nitrogen and the residue was resuspended in 0.1 N HCl. Levels of desipramine and imipramine were finally determined by the National Psychopharmacological Laboratory (Knoxville, Tennessee) using gas chromatography with electron capture detection.

A group of rats also received intracisternal 6-hydroxydopamine (6-OHDA, 200 μg in 50 μL saline with 1 mg/mL ascorbate, repeated after 48 hours) one week prior to implantation of the osmotic pump containing desipramine. Six 3-month-old rats were treated with DSP4 [N-(2-chloroethyl)-N-ethyl-2-bromobenzylamine; 50 mg/kg, i.p.] to deplete the central stores of NE.[16,17] Animals were used for experimentation one to two weeks after treatment.

RESULTS

Effects of NE on Spontaneous Discharge

The electrophysiological response of cerebellar Purkinje neurons to drugs applied locally by pressure microejection was assessed in Fischer 344 rats at 3–6, 18–20, and

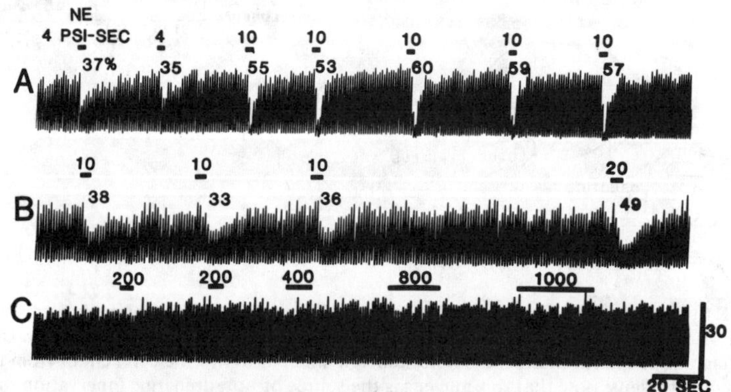

FIGURE 2. Ratemeter recordings showing three cerebellar Purkinje neuron responses to local application of NE. Several doses of drug were tested to determine a dose that produced a 50% decrease in Purkinje cell firing rate. In some cases, Purkinje neurons from old animals did not respond to locally applied drugs, even at doses as high as 1000 psi-seconds (C). Purkinje neurons illustrated are from Fischer 344 rats: (A) 3 months old; (B) and (C) 18 months old. Bars above the trace indicate the dose of drug in psi-seconds; the number below the bar indicates the percent depression of firing rate. Calibration bars: vertical = 30 spikes/second; horizontal = 20 seconds.

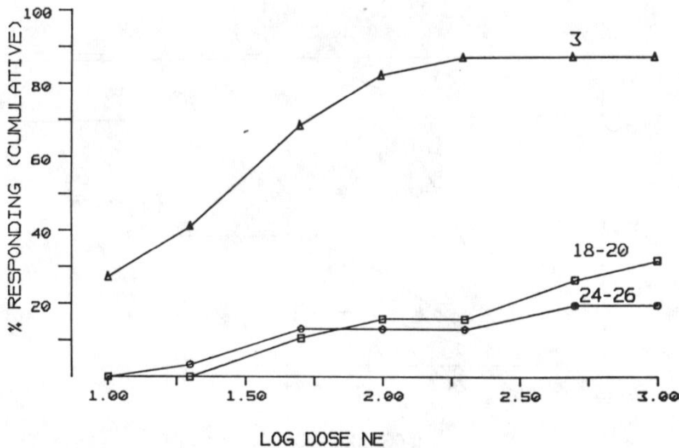

FIGURE 3. Cumulative dose response curves of cerebellar Purkinje cell responses to local application of NE in Fischer 344 rats. Dose response curves from 18–20- and 24–26-month-old rats differed significantly from the 3-month-old rats ($p < 0.02$; Kolmogorov-Smirnov statistic). The number of cells represented is $N = 20$ (3 month), $N = 21$ (18–20 month), and $N = 31$ (24–26 month).

24–26 months of age. Local application of NE to the Purkinje cells resulted in a depression of the spontaneous discharge rate. For each neuron tested, the dose of NE (in psi-seconds) that produced an approximately 50% inhibition in discharge rate was determined (see FIGURE 2). These values were used to construct a cumulative dose response curve for the entire population of cells.

The cumulative dose response curve to NE in 3-month-old Fischer 344 rats shows the majority of Purkinje cells responding to low doses of NE between 1 and 20 psi-seconds (FIGURE 3). In contrast, a much smaller percentage of cells in 18–20- and 24–26-month-old F344 rats responded to low doses of NE. Higher doses were needed to produce a response in the 18–20- and 24–26-month-old rats; in these animals, approximately 70% of Purkinje cells did not respond to NE at doses up to 1000 psi-seconds (FIGURE 3). Mean firing rates of Purkinje neurons from F344 rats of different ages, determined using single-barrel electrodes, were as follows: 27.24 ± 1.7 ($N = 16$, 3 month), 26.11 ± 2.2 ($N = 16$, 18–20 month), and 20.76 ± 2.1 ($N = 16$, 24–26 month). Similar results were observed in rats of the Sprague-Dawley strain; for these animals, Purkinje cell spontaneous discharge rates were: 26.7 ± 1.0 ($N = 30$, 3 month), 29.16 ± 1.3 ($N = 35$, 18–20 month), and 20.65 ± 1.1 spikes/second ($N = 27$, 24–26 month). These results are consistent with previous works.[18,19] The 24–26-month-old groups had significantly lower firing rates than the 3-month-old groups in both rat strains ($p < 0.01$; two-tailed Student's t test).

The responsiveness of Purkinje cells to phencyclidine (PCP), an indirect noradrenergic agonist, was also tested in F344 rats (FIGURE 4). As was seen with NE, higher doses of PCP were necessary to elicit a response in the older age groups; in addition, more neurons remained unresponsive even at high ejection pressures.

The responsiveness to locally applied norepinephrine and PCP was also tested in Sprague-Dawley rats of different ages. As was seen with the F344 strain, the responsiveness to both NE and PCP was significantly diminished in the 18–20- and 24–26-month-old animals.

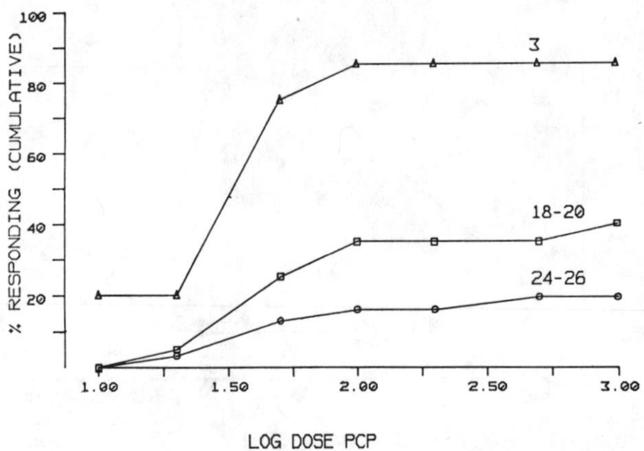

FIGURE 4. Cumulative dose response curves of cerebellar Purkinje neuron responses to local application of PCP in Fischer 344 rats. Dose response curves from older groups differed from the 3-month-old animals ($p < 0.01$; Kolmogorov-Smirnov statistic). The number of cells represented is $N = 23$ (3 month), $N = 19$ (18–20 month), and $N = 31$ (24–26 month).

Effects of NE on Evoked Activity

The modulatory effects of NE on primary cerebellar afferent pathways were investigated in young (3–6 month) and old (18–20 month) Fischer 344 rats. For these experiments, NE was applied continuously during the collection of data for the drug PSTHs.

Inhibition

Basket-stellate cell inhibitions of Purkinje cell activity, elicited by stimulation of parallel fibers, were studied in the two age groups. The inhibitory pause elicited by parallel fiber stimulation was similar: 24.2 ± 2.7 versus 22.4 ± 2.0 ms for the 3- and 18–20-month-old rats, respectively. However, the stimulation voltage necessary to elicit an inhibition of similar magnitude was significantly greater in old animals (37.7 ± 3.6 versus 50.6 ± 3.9 V, $p < 0.02$, two-tailed Student's t test). Similar changes are seen in young adult rats that have been treated with DSP4 to deplete central noradrenergic stores. In DSP4-treated animals, a stimulation voltage of 50.6 ± 4.9 V was needed to elicit inhibitory pauses of similar magnitude and duration.

The modulatory actions of NE on evoked inhibitions in 3–6-month-old rats is illustrated in FIGURE 5. In FIGURE 5A, during NE application, it can be seen that the evoked inhibition (solid bar underneath the histogram) is greatly enhanced. The spontaneous activity at this same time (broken bar beneath the histogram) is decreased by only 11%. Therefore, the evoked inhibition is augmented with respect to the spontaneous discharge of the Purkinje cell. In FIGURE 5B, the results from all the cells tested in young animals are shown. An NE-induced increment in evoked inhibition versus spontaneous activity is clearly seen insofar as all points but one fall above the 45° line.

In sharp contrast, the administration of NE to Purkinje cells from 18–20-month-old rats elicited a greater effect on spontaneous firing than on evoked inhibition. As shown in FIGURE 6, the majority of cells fall below the 45° line, thus indicating that

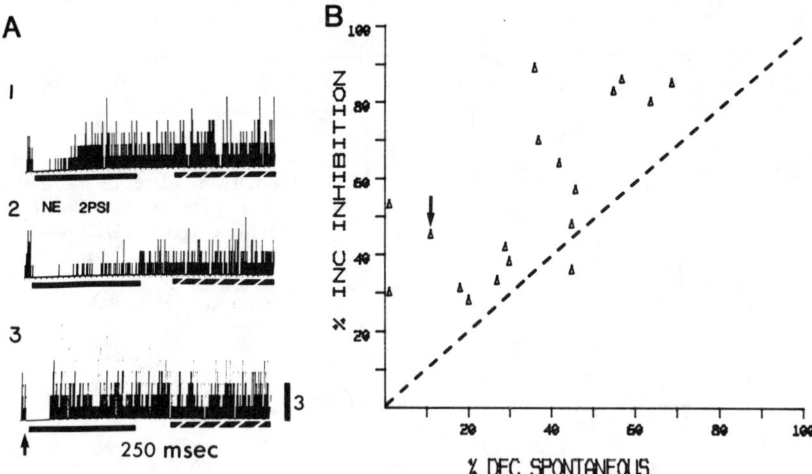

FIGURE 5. Effect of NE on basket-stellate cell inhibitions on Purkinje cells from 3-month-old rats. (A) PSTHs from a single cerebellar Purkinje cell (1) before, (2) during, and (3) after local application of NE. In this and all subsequent histograms, the period of evoked activity is indicated by the solid bar underneath the histogram; the period of spontaneous activity used for analysis is indicated by the broken bar under the histogram. These periods of activity were used to calculate the percent changes in evoked versus spontaneous activity during NE application. The stimulus was observed at the point indicated by the arrow on lowest PSTH. (B) Each point on the graph indicates a single neuron. The neuron in (A) is indicated by an arrow. The x-axis represents the percent decrease (DEC) in spontaneous activity induced by NE. The y-axis represents the percent augmentation (INC) by NE of the evoked inhibition.

the NE decreased spontaneous activity to a greater extent than it augmented the evoked inhibition in the old rats. The two age groups were significantly different with respect to the effects of NE on evoked inhibitions versus spontaneous activity ($p < 0.01$; Mann-Whitney U test).

Excitation

Simple and complex spike excitations were elicited by stimulation of either the parallel fiber or climbing fiber afferents to the Purkinje neurons. A difference between the old and young animals was observed in the percentage of neurons in which evoked climbing fiber excitation was found. In the young rats, all of the neurons examined responded to inferior olivary stimulation; in contrast, only 54% (14 of 26) of the Purkinje neurons demonstrated an evoked complex spike after olivary stimulation in the 18–20-month-old rats.

The effect of NE on simple and complex spike excitations was studied in 3–6- and 18–20-month-old F344 rats. The cell illustrated in FIGURE 7A was driven by parallel fiber stimulation in a young F344 rat. When NE was applied locally from the micropipette throughout the stimulation period, the spontaneous activity, as measured from the latter part of the PSTH (dashed line under the histogram), was decreased by 53%. At the same time, the evoked excitation (indicated by the solid bar under the histo-

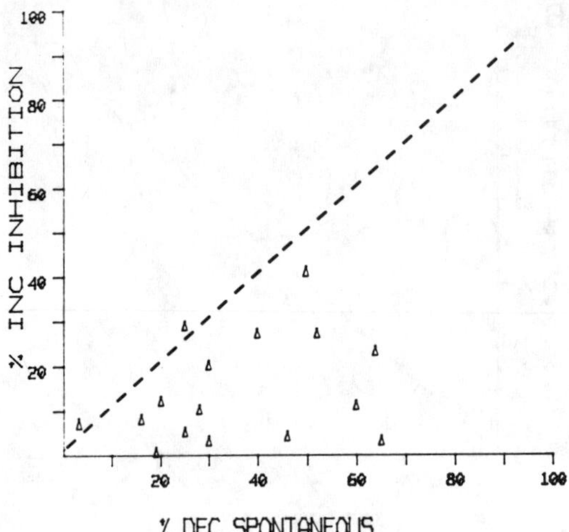

FIGURE 6. Effect of NE basket-stellate cell inhibitions of cerebellar Purkinje cells from 18–20-month-old rats. Each point on the graph represents a single neuron. The axes are marked as in FIGURE 5.

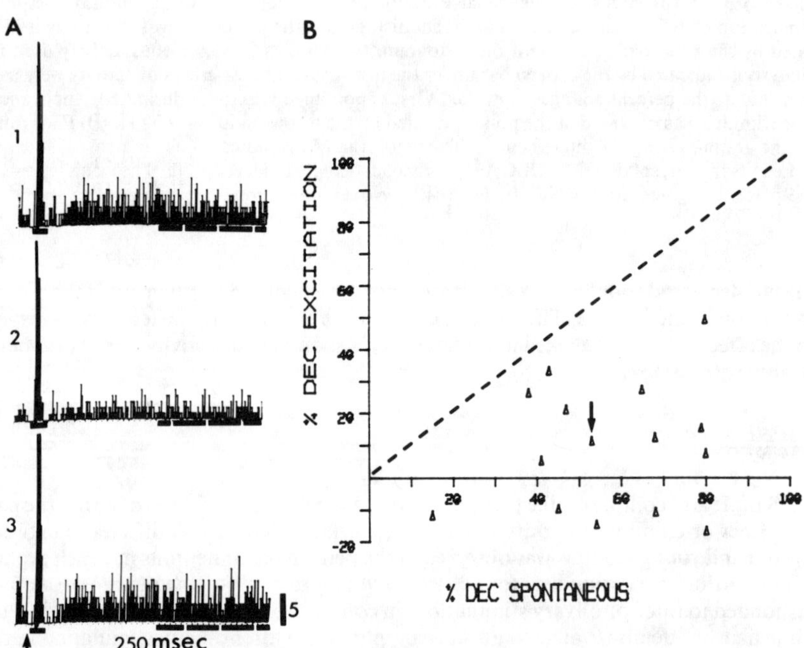

FIGURE 7. Effect of NE on afferent excitations of cerebellar Purkinje neurons from 3-month-old rats. (A) Peristimulus time histograms (1) before, (2) during, and (3) after local application of NE to a single cerebellar Purkinje cell. (B) Each point on the graph represents a single Purkinje neuron. The point indicated by the arrow is the Purkinje cell illustrated in (A). The x-axis represents the percent decrease (DEC) in spontaneous activity during NE application and the y-axis represents the percent decrease (DEC) in excitations evoked by climbing fibers, mossy fibers via granule cells, or parallel fibers.

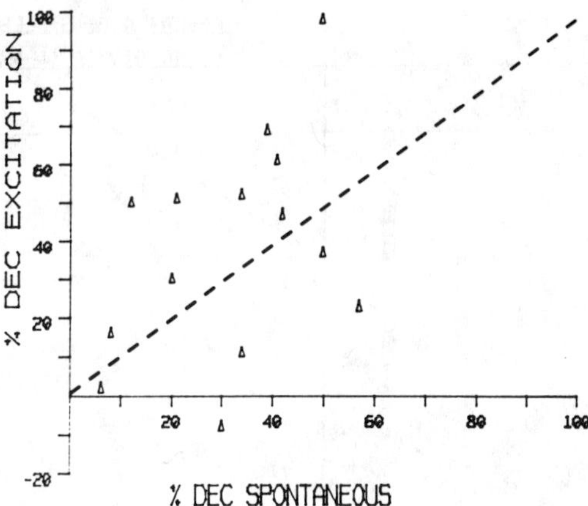

FIGURE 8. Effect of NE on evoked excitations of cerebellar Purkinje neurons from 18–20-month-old rats. Each point on the graph indicates a single neuron. The axes are labeled as in FIGURE 7.

gram) in this cell was decreased by only 11%. Hence, there was a differential effect of NE on spontaneous versus evoked Purkinje cell firing. As shown in FIGURE 7B, all cells from the 3–6-month-old animals were below the 45° line. Thus, they manifested a greater NE-induced depression in spontaneous activity versus evoked excitations. In fact, in 30% of the neurons, there was an absolute augmentation of the evoked excitation during an application of NE that decreased spontaneous activity.

In contrast, the 18–20-month-old rats did not manifest the same differential effect on evoked versus spontaneous activity as was observed in the 3-month-old animals. In fact, there was a tendency towards the opposite effect, that is, a greater effect of NE on the evoked excitations rather than spontaneous activity (FIGURE 8). When comparing the noradrenergic modulation of these responses in the two age groups, a significant difference was observed ($p < 0.01$; Mann-Whitney U test).

The ability of NE to modulate climbing fiber afferent excitation evoked by stimulation of the inferior olive in young F344 rats is summarized in FIGURE 9A; in this figure, the percent inhibition of spontaneous discharge rate during NE application is plotted with respect to the percent change in the evoked excitation induced by this agent. The solid line indicates the hypothetical distribution if each parameter would be equally affected by NE. Twelve of the 13 cells lie below the line, thereby indicating a differential effect. In fact, 5 of the 13 neurons lie below the abscissa, thus showing an absolute augmentation of the excitatory response during an application of NE that decreased spontaneous activity. Therefore, in young animals, NE clearly increased the evoked climbing fiber response with respect to the background spontaneous activity.

The actions of NE on climbing fiber excitations are also altered in senescent F344 rats. The results for all neurons tested are summarized in FIGURE 10A. Four of the 14 cells lie above the solid line. An additional 6 Purkinje neurons fall below, but they are actually very close to this line, thus suggesting a modest modulatory action at best. In only one case was the excitation unequivocally augmented in the senescent rats. The difference between young and old rats was significant ($p < 0.01$; Mann-Whitney U test).

A striking feature of the interaction of NE with evoked climbing fiber excitations in young rats is the observation of an increased tendency for the complex spike to include more full-sized action potentials during drug application. FIGURE 9B illustrates that the probability of observing a complex spike in the control condition with only

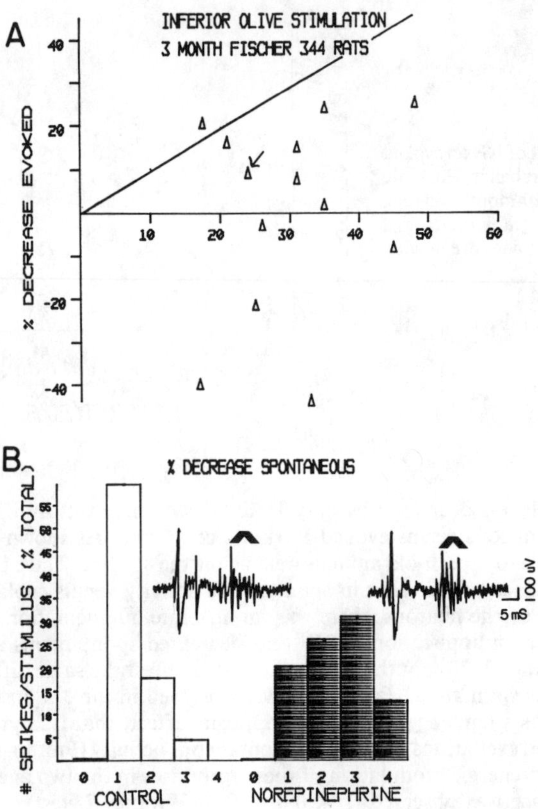

FIGURE 9. Effect of NE on climbing fiber evoked excitations of cerebellar Purkinje neurons from 3–6-month-old rats. (A) Each point on the graph indicates one Purkinje neuron. The x-axis represents the percent decrease in spontaneous discharge during NE application with respect to a control period prior to NE application. The y-axis represents the percent decrease in the climbing fiber evoked excitations during NE application; negative numbers represent an absolute augmentation of the response during NE application. Data from five rats are shown. (B) A bar graph demonstrating the number of full-sized action potentials occurring in climbing fiber bursts as a result of inferior olive stimulation. Each individual evoked response was evaluated for the number of full-sized action potentials elicited per stimulus. The data are represented as the percent of the total number of stimulation trials for the individual cell during the control period and during local application of NE. Examples of individual responses are inset above the bar graph; brackets above the trace indicate the climbing fiber complex spike. Before NE application, the evoked response consists of a single full-sized spike followed by action potentials of reduced amplitude; during NE application, the response shifts to full-sized action potentials. The data represent four cells from one rat.

a single full-sized action potential is much greater than the chance of seeing complex spikes with either two or three full-sized action potentials. None of the control cells, though, demonstrated four full-sized action potentials. However, during local application of NE, the probability of a complex spike containing multiple full-sized spikes increased. In fact, about 15% of the evoked climbing fiber discharges consisted of

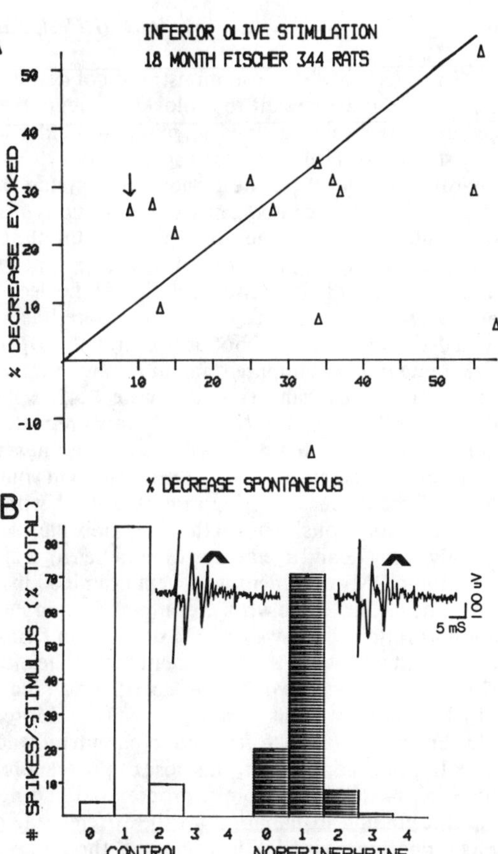

FIGURE 10. (A) Effect of NE on climbing fiber evoked excitations of cerebellar Purkinje neurons recorded from five 18–20-month-old F344 rats. Each point on the graph indicates a single Purkinje neuron. The axes are similar to those in FIGURE 9. (B) A bar graph demonstrating the number of full-sized action potentials occurring as a result of inferior olive stimulation in 18–20-month-old rats. The data are represented as in FIGURE 9. Even during NE application, the oscilloscope tracing insets show that the climbing fiber response (below the bracket) tended towards only one full-sized spike followed by reduced amplitude spikes. The data represent 10 neurons.

four full-sized spikes. The oscilloscope tracing inserts in FIGURE 9B illustrate this finding. The tracing before norepinephrine shows a typical complex spike with one full-sized action potential that is followed by a series of action potentials with decreasing amplitude. When NE is locally applied to this same neuron, the evoked complex spike consisted of four full-sized spikes. The neuron then recovered to control values after the application of NE was terminated.

The number of full-sized action potentials per stimulus (with and without NE) was also altered in the old rats when compared to the young rats (FIGURE 10B). In control recordings prior to NE, there was a 10% chance of zero spikes and none of the cells examined fired as many as three full-sized spikes; however, in the young animals, 5% of the evoked complex spikes contained three full-sized action potentials (this difference was significant at $p < 0.05$ using a chi-square analysis). Furthermore, a significant difference was noted in the effect of local application of NE on the number of full-sized spikes. Compared to young rats, there was an increase in the probability of zero evoked activity and there was no significant tendency towards complex spikes with more full-sized spikes ($p < 0.001$, chi-square analysis). This phenomenon is also illustrated by the oscilloscope tracing insert in FIGURE 10B; during application of NE, the complex spike is basically unaltered from that seen in the control period.

Actions of Desipramine

The effects of chronic administration of desipramine (DMI; 10 mg/kg for 21 days), a tricyclic antidepressant that blocks the reuptake of NE, on spontaneous Purkinje cell discharge was examined in young and old F344 rats. In young rats, chronic administration of DMI decreased spontaneous discharge rates (FIGURE 11). Pharmacological manipulation of the noradrenergic system of young rats was used in an attempt to assess the relative importance of endogenous NE in the mechanism of DMI's action on spontaneous discharge. After propranolol (the beta-adrenergic antagonist) was administered (5 mg/kg, i.p.), the firing rate returned to control level, thereby suggesting an involvement of NE in the mediation of the decreased firing rate. In addition, young animals were treated with 6-OHDA, a noradrenergic neurotoxin, prior to treatment with desipramine and did not demonstrate the DMI-induced reduction in spontaneous firing rate that was apparent in animals with intact noradrenergic innervation of the cerebellum. The mean firing rates were 31.42 ± 0.8 ($N = 20$) in 6-OHDA pretreated rats versus 30.83 ± 0.8 ($N = 40$) in rats pretreated with 6-OHDA followed by DMI administration. Taken together, these experiments establish that the presence of an intact noradrenergic input to the cerebellum in young rats is necessary for the development of the decreased firing rate associated with chronic DMI treatment.

We had previously shown that the cerebellar cortex of old rats demonstrated a subsensitivity to NE and a reduction of noradrenergic modulatory effects. The consequences of chronic DMI treatment were next examined in 18–20- and 26–28-month-old F344 rats. The results of the work are summarized in FIGURE 11. Following 21 days of DMI administration, there was a 22% decrease in firing rate of Purkinje cells in the 3–6-month-old rats. After the same treatment in the old rats, no change in the spontaneous firing rate was observed. This effect of age on the response to chronic administration of DMI was significant ($p < 0.05$; ANOVA). Moreover, the 18–20- and 26–28-month-old control rats failed to respond to parenterally administered propranolol (5 mg/kg, i.p.). In young control rats, this dose of propranolol increased cell firing rates by 15%; however, in the older groups, propranolol had no effect (TABLE 1).

One possible explanation for the difference in effects of DMI in young versus old rats is pharmacokinetic. In young rats, though, cerebellar DMI levels were measured to be 3.61 ± 1.0 ng/mg ($N = 5$), whereas concentrations of 5.56 ± 1.4 ng/mg (N

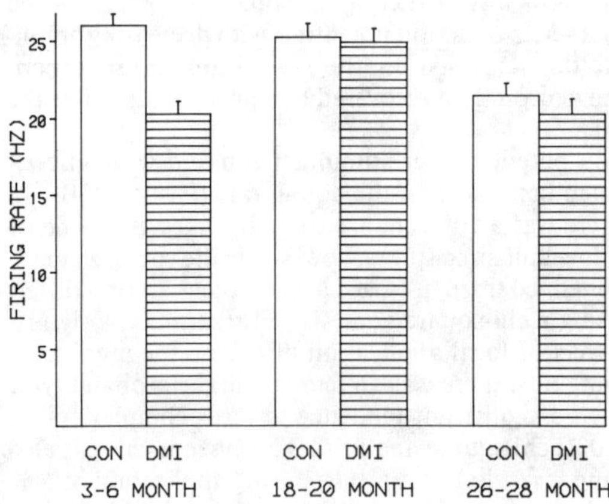

FIGURE 11. Effect of age on response to desipramine. The bar graph demonstrates the lack of effect of 21 days of treatment with DMI (10 mg/kg/day) via Alzet osmotic pumps in rats of 18–20 and 26–28 months of age. The effect of DMI treatment was significant only for the 3–6-month age group ($p < 0.05$). The control discharge rate was also significantly lower in the 24–26-month-old animals versus the 3–6-month-old group. The vertical axis indicates the firing rate in spikes per second. The N's for the groups, in the order presented in the figure from left to right, are 30, 26, 41, 50, 41, and 30.

TABLE 1. Effect of Propranolol on Cerebellar Purkinje Neuron Spontaneous Discharge

Age	Control Mean $\pm$ SEM (N)	After Propranolol Mean $\pm$ SEM (N)
3–6	26.03 $\pm$ 0.8 (30)	29.8 $\pm$ 1.3 (31)[a]
18–20	25.3 $\pm$ 0.9 (41)	26.0 $\pm$ 0.9 (40)
24–26	21.5 $\pm$ 0.8 (41)	21.5 $\pm$ 1.0 (37)

[a] $p < 0.01$.

= 7) DMI were measurable in the old rats. Thus, DMI levels were actually greater in older animals despite the reduced effect of this drug on Purkinje cell discharge rate.

DISCUSSION

These experiments have demonstrated an age-associated decrease in the postsynaptic sensitivity of cerebellar Purkinje neurons to NE. The age-related noradrenergic subsensitivity was apparent using drugs that either modulated the extracellular cells of endogenous NE or that directly activated the postsynaptic receptor: PCP and NE, respectively. When the responses to these two drugs were examined within a strain, no differences could be seen. This decreased postsynaptic sensitivity of neurons to NE is probably a meaningful physiological change and it accounts for markedly decreased adrenergic neurotransmission in older animals.

The electrophysiological experiments described here do not delineate a specific mechanism of postsynaptic subsensitivity, such as a change in receptor type or number, or an alteration in transduction. Indeed, transduction mechanisms such as the activation of adenylate cyclase or the cyclic-AMP induction of protein kinase are known to be altered in the aged animal.[5,7] Moreover, the above experiments do not exclude possible changes in presynaptic function; further investigation is needed to assess the integrity of the noradrenergic afferents to the cerebellum.

The study of inbred rat strains is helpful when comparing responses in different age groups because it reduces one possible source of error, namely, genetic variability. The use of inbred strains, though, may also bias one's findings because the inbreeding process may select for a trait not commonly seen in a genetically heterogeneous population. Thus, two strains of rats were used here. Because similar findings of decreased responsiveness to NE are observed in both the Sprague-Dawley and the Fischer 344 rats, we believe that it is unlikely to be a unique phenomenon resulting from the selective breeding process. Rather, we believe that it is a generalized property of aging in these animals.

A second aspect of age-related changes in noradrenergic function addressed here was the interaction of NE with noncatecholaminergic afferents to the Purkinje cells. In young animals, NE enhances excitatory or inhibitory evoked responses of Purkinje cells to a greater extent than it decreases spontaneous activity. Therefore, the action of NE is more complex than a simple depression of spontaneous activity. In the older F344 animals, this more complex modulatory action of NE was markedly reduced. The observed changes in the interaction of NE with other cerebellar inputs may also be of functional importance. It has been postulated that this differential effect of NE increases the bias for evoked activity to be translated into a functional output of the cerebellar cortex.[12,13] A change in this bias could have an effect on cerebellar information processing and on subsequent motor regulation.

Age-related changes in cerebellar anatomy and physiology are well documented in the literature. There is a loss in the number of cerebellar Purkinje neuron dendrites and parallel fiber synapses.[19,20] Threshold currents needed to evoke parallel fiber volleys and to drive single spikes in 24–26-month-old rats are significantly higher than for 5–7-month-old rats.[21] In light of these changes, it is of interest that higher stimulation voltages were necessary to induce similar parallel fiber basket-stellate cell–mediated inhibitions in the older rats studied here. Rogers[21] has correlated changes in parallel fiber synapses with the loss of Purkinje cell tertiary dendritic branches in a population of slow, aberrantly firing Purkinje cells in 24–26-month-old rats. The present work, however, was performed in 18–20-month-old rats. At this age, the firing rates of Purkinje neurons are normal, thus suggesting that this degeneration of parallel fiber synapses has not occurred to a significant extent.

In the senescent rats studied here, there was only a 54% probability that a given Purkinje neuron would demonstrate a climbing fiber evoked excitation after stimulation of the inferior olive. In contrast, 100% of the neurons from young rats demonstrated such evoked activity. Moreover, even those neurons from senescent rats showing climbing fiber responses manifested a 10% probability of response failure after a given stimulus. Because Glick and Bondareff[22] have shown that the number of synapses associated with Purkinje cell apical dendrite proximal shafts does not change in 26-month-old F344 rats, one would predict that the number of climbing fiber contacts remains intact. Thus, an alteration in Purkinje cell responsiveness to olivary excitation needs to be explained by a mechanism other than a simple loss of anatomical connections. Another explanation for the decreased ability to evoke Purkinje cell parallel and climbing fiber responses in 18–20-month-old animals is that the decreased modulatory efficacy of endogenous noradrenergic inputs from locus coeruleus leads to a condition in which it is more difficult to elicit an evoked response. In young animals depleted of central NE stores with DSP4, it was also more difficult to elicit parallel fiber responses.

The age-dependent decrease in the modulatory effect of NE that we have observed may lead to changes in cerebellar information processing by decreasing the bias for afferent inputs to be translated into a functional output. The cerebellum has been implicated in the regulation of posture and movement,[23] and in motor learning.[24,25] Using 6-OHDA-induced depletions, cerebellar NE has been shown to be important for learning a novel locomotor task in rats.[25] In addition, there is evidence from electrophysiological recordings in monkeys that an increased inferior olive-induced complex spike frequency is associated with an acquisition of new motor tasks.[24] It has been shown that elderly humans are impaired in the ability to acquire a novel motor task.[26] Although one cannot causally relate changes in cerebellar function (as those observed here) to behavioral changes, it is of interest that several correlational studies have supported such a relationship.[20] However, one must also keep in mind that other CNS areas and monoamines have been implicated in age-related movement disorders. For instance, psychomotor performance is improved in aged rats pretreated with haloperidol to up-regulate striatal dopamine receptors,[27] while swimming behavior in aged rats is improved following administration of apomorphine or L-dopa.[28]

Another facet of cerebellar pharmacology that was examined here was the ability of the tricyclic antidepressant, desipramine, to functionally alter noradrenergic transmission in this structure. Chronic administration of DMI decreased the mean firing rate of cerebellar Purkinje neurons in young animals. In contrast, there was no effect of chronic administration of DMI in senescent rats. The level of DMI in the cerebella of the older rats was significantly higher than that in the younger rats, which was consistent with previous findings.[29] In all probability, though, the increased level in old rats does not underlie the loss of efficacy of this drug. Administration of 20 mg/kg/day DMI to young rats will produce an equivalent decrease in discharge rate,[30] presumably with a commensurately higher level of cerebellar DMI.

There is additional evidence for deficiencies in noradrenergic neurotransmission with age. Other work has shown that the disruption of noradrenergic input to the cerebellar Purkinje neuron with reserpine or 6-OHDA does not alter the spontaneous discharge rate in 15–24-month-old rats.[18] In addition, intraperitoneal administration of indirect NE agonists and antagonists fails to have the same effect on spontaneous Purkinje cell firing in 12- to 20-month-old Sprague-Dawley rats as that observed in younger animals.[18] We have also demonstrated here that propranolol had no effect on the spontaneous discharge rate in the older control rats. It appears that Purkinje neurons of senescent rats are insensitive to a number of different pharmacological manipulations of noradrenergic transmission. Given this marked insensitivity, it appears that even if DMI treatment was effective in the older rats at the presynaptic level, no postsynaptic changes would be observed.

In conclusion, the data reported here demonstrate a significant effect of age on the postsynaptic efficacy of NE on Purkinje cell discharge and on the ability of NE to modulate afferent inputs to the cerebellum. Additionally, the action of the tricyclic antidepressant, desipramine, was reduced in senescent rats. The alterations demonstrated here could, in part, underlie changes in drug efficacy and motor programming seen in senescence.

REFERENCES

1. OSTERBURG, H. H., H. G. DONAHUE, J. A. SEVERSON & C. E. FINCH. 1981. Catecholamine levels and turnover during aging in brain regions of male C57BL/6J mice. Brain Res. **224:** 337–352.
2. MCGEER, E. G., H. C. FIBIGER, P. L. MCGEER & V. WICKSON. 1971. Aging and brain enzymes. Exp. Gerontol. **6:** 391–396.
3. MISRA, C. H., H. S. SHELAT & R. C. SMITH. 1980. Effect of age on adrenergic binding in rat brain. Life Sci. **27:** 521–526.
4. PITTMAN, R. W., K. P. MINNEMAN & P. B. MOLINOFF. 1980. Alteration in b*1*- and b*2*-adrenergic receptor density in the cerebellum of aging rats. J. Neurochem. **35:** 273–275.
5. MAKMAN, M. H., H. S. AHN, L. J. THAL, N. S. SHARPLESS, B. DVORKIN, S. G. HOROWITZ & M. ROSENFELD. 1980. Evidence for selective loss of brain dopamine- and histamine-stimulated adenylate cyclase activities in rabbits with aging. Brain Res. **192:** 177–183.
6. WALKER, J.B. & J. P. WALKER. 1973. Properties of adenylate cyclase from senescent rat brain. Brain Res. **54:** 391–396.
7. SCHMIDT, M.J. & J. F. THORNBERRY. 1978. Cyclic AMP and cyclic GMP accumulation *in vitro* in brain regions of young, old and aged rats. Brain Res. **139:** 169–177.
8. BICKFORD, P. C. 1983. Age-related alterations in noradrenergic neurotransmission in Sprague-Dawley and Fischer 344 rat strains. Age **6:** 100–105.
9. BICKFORD, P. C., B. J. HOFFER & R. FREEDMAN. 1985. Interaction of norepinephrine with Purkinje cell responses to cerebellar afferent inputs in aged rats. Neurobiol. Aging **6:** 89–94.
10. BLOOM, F. E., B. J. HOFFER & G. R. SIGGINS. 1979. Norepinephrine mediated cerebellar synapses: A model for neuropsychopharmacology. Biol. Psychiatry **4:** 157–178.
11. ECCLES, J. C., M. ITO & J. SZENTAGOTHAI. 1967. The cerebellum as a neuronal machine. Springer Pub. New York.
12. FREEDMAN, R., B. HOFFER, D. WOODWARD & D. PURO. 1977. Interaction of norepinephrine with cerebellar activity evoked by mossy and climbing fibers. Exp. Neurol. **55:** 269–288.
13. MOISES, H. C., D. J. WOODWARD, B. J. HOFFER & R. FREEDMAN. 1979. Interactions of norepinephrine with Purkinje cell responses to putative amino acid neurotransmitters applied locally by microiontophoresis. Exp. Neurol. **64:** 493–515.
14. PALMER, M. R., S. M. WUERTHELE & B. J. HOFFER. 1980. Physical and physiological char-

acteristics of micropressure ejection of drugs from multibarreled pipettes. Neuropharmacology **19:** 931–938.

15. RIVA, R., P. D. HRDINA & P. MORSELLI. 1975. Measurement of desipramine in brain tissue
by a radioisotope derivative technique. J. Pharm. Pharmacol. **27:** 797–799.

16. JONSSON, G., H. HALLMAN, F. PONZIO & S. ROSS. 1981. DSP4 (N-(2-chloroethyl)-N-ethyl-
2-bromobenzylamine), a useful denervation tool for central and peripheral noradrenergic
neurons. Eur. J. Pharmacol. **72:** 173–188.

17. BICKFORD, P. C., W. F. MOSIMAN, B. J. HOFFER & R. FREEDMAN. 1984. Effects of the
selective noradrenergic neurotoxin DSP4 on cerebellar Purkinje neuron electrophysiology.
Life Sci. **34:** 731–741.

18. MARWAHA, J., B. J. HOFFER & R. FREEDMAN. 1981. Changes in noradrenergic neurotransmission in rat cerebellum during aging. Neurobiol. Aging **2:** 95–98.

19. ROGERS, J., M. A. SIVER, W. J. SHOEMAKER & F. E. BLOOM. 1980. Senescent changes in
a neurobiological model system: cerebellar Purkinje cell electrophysiology and correlative anatomy. Neurobiol. Aging **2:** 15–25.

20. ZORNTZER, S., F. BLOOM, R. MERVIS & J. ROGERS. 1981. Senescent changes in balance,
coordination, and cerebellar microanatomy. Soc. Neurosci. Abstr. **7:** 187.

21. ROGERS, J., S. F. ZORNETZER & F. E. BLOOM. 1981. Senescent pathology of cerebellum:
Purkinje neurons and their parallel fiber afferents. Neurobiol. Aging **2:** 15–25.

22. GLICK, R. & W. BONDAREFF. 1979. Loss of synapses in the cerebellar cortex of the senescent rat. J. Gerontol. **34:** 818–822.

23. BROOKS, V. B. 1984. Cerebellar functions in motor control. Hum. Neurobiol. **2:** 251–260.

24. GILBERT, P. F. C. & W. T. THACH. 1977. Purkinje cell activity during motor learning.
Brain Res. **128:** 309–328.

25. WATSON, M. & J. G. MCGELLIGOTT. 1984. Cerebellar norepinephrine depletion and impaired acquisition of specific locomotor tasks in rats. Brain Res. **296:** 129–138.

26. WRIGHT, B. M. & R. B. PAYNE. 1985. Effects of aging on sex differences in psychomotor
reminiscence and tracking proficiency. J. Gerontol. **40:** 179–184.

27. JOSEPH, J. A., R. T. BARTUS, D. CLODY, D. MORGAN, C. FINCH, B. BEER & S. SESACK.
1983. Psychomotor performance in the senescent rodent: Reduction of deficits via striatal dopamine receptor up-regulation. Neurobiol. Aging **4:** 313–319.

28. MARSHALL, J. F. & N. BERRIOS. 1979. Movement disorders of aged rats: Reversal by dopamine receptor stimulation. Science **206:** 477–479.

29. GREENBERG, L. H. & B. WEISS. 1979. Ability of aged rats to alter beta adrenergic receptors
of brain in response to repeated administration of reserpine and desmethylimipramine.
J. Pharmacol. Exp. Ther. **211:** 309–316.

30. YEH, H. H. & D. J. WOODWARD. 1983. Alterations in beta adrenergic physiological response characteristics after long-term treatment with desmethylimipramine: interaction
between norepinephrine and gamma-aminobutryic acid in rat cerebellum. J. Pharmacol.
Exp. Ther. **226:** 126–134.

DISCUSSION OF THE PAPER

J. ROGERS (*Sun Health Corporation, Sun City, AZ*): You talked mainly about postsynaptic phenomena here and I think that there are a lot of investigations that suggest
that the noradrenergic content of cerebellum does not change with age in rodent models.
Are those fibers relevant in old age once you get to the point where the postsynaptic
mechanisms are simply not responding? If so, why do the fibers not just go away?

B. HOFFER (*University of Colorado Health Sciences Center, Denver, CO*): Let me
provide several answers to that. First of all, I would not dare say that any sort of catecholamine presynaptic afferent mechanism is irrelevant. I might think that, but I would
not say it. Secondly, it is true that the levels of norepinephrine do not change and
this is something that we have confirmed in our own models. Therefore, my hypothesis
is that the lion's share of the kinds of changes we see are indeed postsynaptic. How-

ever, this is something that is probably somewhat species-specific because certain mouse species lose locus coeruleus neurons, while certain rodent species do not. I might add that in terms of this postsynaptic sensitivity, we have seen this in more than one species — we have seen it in Sprague-Dawleys and in Fischers — but Sprague-Dawleys and Fischers have very different age-related presynaptic noradrenergic changes.

G. KING: In your experiments, have you looked at the sort of dose response relationship of the anesthetic that you used on the noradrenergic response in your young animals? Moreover, can that be involved in the age difference that you see?

HOFFER: To begin with, let me indicate that we are basically using animals for most of these studies in the 18- to 20-month-old range. These are considerably younger than the 24- to 26-month-old ones that J. Rogers uses. Furthermore, on the cells that most of our data comes from, we do not see the cell population of slowly firing cells. We do not have this phenomena that is seen in older animals that are exquisitely sensitive to anesthetics. You have to give things in quarter doses and just hope that the bottom does not fall out. Over a fairly wide range of anesthetic agents and anesthetic levels, the noradrenergic suppression in young animals is fairly uniform. However, in old animals, there is a good bit of variability. In general, though, our animals are at the same levels in terms of superficial signs of anesthesia, corneal reflex, pupil constriction, etc. Therefore, I do not think that this would contribute much to the subsensitivity.

D. B. CALNE (*University of British Columbia, Vancouver, British Columbia, Canada*): I would like to ask a question about the clinical correlation of your findings. For the other systems that either have been or will be discussed, we have well defined clinical problems for striatal disease, we have Alzheimer's disease for cortical and basal forebrain lesions, and we have motor neuron disease for the upper and lower motor neuron. However, for the cerebellum, we do not really have a common disease of late life that is particularly separated from the specific genetic disorders of cerebellar function of focal lesions such as tumors. It seems that there are two possible explanations, but I would like to know whether you feel either of these is more likely than another. One is that these findings are all above a threshold to produce neurological deficits within a normal life span. The second one is that the neurologists are not good enough at looking at cerebellar deficits and their neurological examinations fail to reveal any cerebellar deficits. Is it just that we do not know how to examine?

ROGERS: Some of the latter things that you said are somewhat true. In particular, it has been established in everything from honey bees to human beings that the most reliable loss of neurons in brain with age is in the cerebellum; yet, when deficits are seen in balance and coordination that are well known to occur with age, we still do not have any cerebellar correlates of these motor dysfunctions. However, I know that we have had them. What happens, though, is that we tend to want to make the cerebellar physical dysfunction out to be the same as the effect of the cerebellar stroke, which does not necessarily need to be.

CALNE: However, even if you have an analogy of a more widespread degenerative disease or a hereditary cerebellar degeneration, there are other signs that go with that and yet we do not see them in the majority of old people.

ROGERS: There have been several clinical reports of deficits in eye tracking, for example, with age. There is one specific cerebellar circuit that is just devoted to that and we also have to remember that the cerebellum provides highly processed information to the motor cortex and to the basal ganglia. Therefore, the well-known deficits that occur with age in the cerebellum could in fact be manifest as motor cortex or striatal deficits because the striatum is not doing as well (this could be because it is missing information that it should be getting from the cerebellum).

LAPP: Maybe the aging group is not the best group to look at the threshold effect in cerebellar disease. There have been a number of studies looking at cerebellar atrophy with falls and gait abnormalities that have not been able to show a deficit. However, in a number of studies looking at atrophic cerebellar diseases (comparing cerebellar atrophy on CT scan with clinical findings), there is a suggestion that the greater the atrophy, the more developed the clinical syndrome.

P. LEWITT (*Lafayette Clinic, Detroit, MI*): I think there have been some children born as cerebellar deficits who are coordinated, so that is another side issue. However, let me ask this question. The Purkinje cell is among the most sensitive to oxygen deprivation and it is one of the first systems to actually go. The hippocampus is about the same order as that with memory as another vulnerable activity. Have you seen any parallels or have you studied hypoxia as a way to create the equivalent or nonequivalent of aging in the Purkinje cell?

ROGERS: I suggested that in a grant proposal once and it was not too popular. Therefore, I concluded that there was not.

HOFFER: The problem, though, with that kind of an experiment is really a technical one. Indeed, the Purkinje cells are so sensitive to hypoxia that if you make the animal hypoxic at some point during the preparative procedure, you then get this very bizarre abnormal firing. Thus, it becomes extremely difficult to test inputs because the cells have this sort of cyclical waxing and waning of excitability that appears to be totally indifferent to any inputs that you can muster. You really then cannot study cells after they are significantly hypoxic because of this technical problem.

ROGERS: I was thinking more of chronic exposure, and I think that any tissue that undergoes as much change with aging as the cerebellum does and is so vulnerable might be telling us a clue there.

LIPSITZ: I find this reduced sensitivity to norepinephrine quite interesting particularly because it seems to be more systemic than just in the cerebellum—especially in older humans, where there is a reduced sensitivity to norepinephrine in the heart and in the vasculature. That may be due to some postreceptor defect and I wondered whether the receptors in the Purkinje cells are looked at as we have looked at receptors elsewhere. Could there be some uniformity of receptor problem or postreceptor problem that ties all of this together?

P. BICKFORD-WIMER (*University of Colorado Health Sciences Center, Denver, CO*): People actually have looked at receptor numbers in the cerebellum. What is interesting is that the absolute number of beta-receptors goes down, but the subtype that is thought to be neuronal goes up. Maybe some type of intracellular mechanism is defective that does not affect the actual receptor number, but maybe there is also another type of mechanism that is defective that actually increases the number in a sort of compensatory fashion.

ROGERS: You mean upregulation. There might be upregulating in a place where there is no noradrenergic axon to terminate there. Still, for me, the bottom line is that if you lose the dendrites where noradrenergic axons should terminate, then you will lose the noradrenergic receptors there. You may get some compensation at another point in the neuron, but it is not going to do you any good if it is way down where the fibers do not normally go.

D. INGRAM (*NIA, Baltimore, MD*): I was intrigued by the correlations between the individual performances and the cell counts. The data you showed were for rotorod performance and your fine slides were on balance beam performance. Did you see the same sort of correlations for the balance beam performance?

ROGERS: Yes, we did.

Parkinsonian Symptomatology

An Anatomical and Physiological Analysis[a]

WILLIAM C. MILLER AND

MAHLON R. DeLONG

Departments of Neurology and Neuroscience
The Johns Hopkins University School of Medicine
Baltimore, Maryland 21205

INTRODUCTION

The parkinsonian syndrome includes disturbances of motor function such as akinesia, bradykinesia, tremor and rigidity, disturbances of eye movements, and cognitive impairment. It is difficult to understand how a relatively small and specific lesion of midbrain dopamine neurons could produce such a diverse syndrome. Two recent developments permit a reexamination of this question: (1) the increased understanding of the anatomical relations between the basal ganglia and the cerebral cortex, and (2) the development of a suitable primate model of parkinsonism using the neurotoxin MPTP. In recent years, a system of functionally segregated parallel basal ganglia–thalamocortical circuits has been proposed.[1] In this scheme, the basal ganglia and the related portions of the thalamus are viewed as components of larger cortico-subcortical circuits whose ultimate influences are directed upon specific cortical areas. It therefore follows that the functional contributions of the basal ganglia must be considered in terms of their influences on these cortical areas. Moreover, disturbances in basal ganglia function, as occur in neurological diseases such as Parkinson's disease, must result in part from abnormal cortical output. The recent development of the MPTP model of Parkinson's disease has provided the opportunity to study the changes in neuronal activity within the basal ganglia and to delineate further the pathophysiologic basis of this disorder. In the following discussion, we will consider the impairments in Parkinson's disease in light of this newly acquired data.

CIRCUITS

General Model

In the past, it generally was believed that the basal ganglia integrated inputs from widespread cortical areas and funneled this information to the motor cortex via the ventrolateral thalamus.[2] In particular, the basal ganglia were believed to integrate input from association cortices and derive a signal responsible for movement initiation that was then directed to the motor cortex. Recent anatomical and physiological data have

[a] This work was supported by grants from the U.S.P.H.S. (NIH NS15417 and NS20471, and NRSA 5-F32-NS-08130) and by donations from the E. K. Dunn family.

necessitated a revision of this scheme.[1,3] These data have suggested that the inputs to the basal ganglia from the sensorimotor and association areas tend to remain anatomically and functionally segregated throughout the basal ganglia–thalamocortical circuitry. Five distinct basal ganglia–thalamocortical circuits have been proposed: the motor, oculomotor, dorsolateral prefrontal, orbitofrontal, and anterior cingulate circuits, as shown schematically in FIGURE 1. The specific details of each of these circuits will be discussed briefly in the sections below. The anatomical and physiological evidence for these circuits has been reviewed in detail previously.[1]

Each of the specific circuits appears to be organized in a similar fashion. In each, the striatum receives multiple, overlapping inputs from several cortical areas. Striatal projections are directed toward the internal pallidal segment (GPi) and the substantia nigra pars reticulata (SNr), which project to a restricted portion of the thalamus. Each circuit is partially closed by thalamic projections to one of the original cortical areas supplying the striatal input. In a sense, the concept of funneling is retained because a single cortical area receives information derived from the processing of inputs from several cortical areas by the basal ganglia. The important difference, however, is that the processing of sensorimotor, oculomotor, "association", and "limbic" inputs remains segregated throughout the basal ganglia.

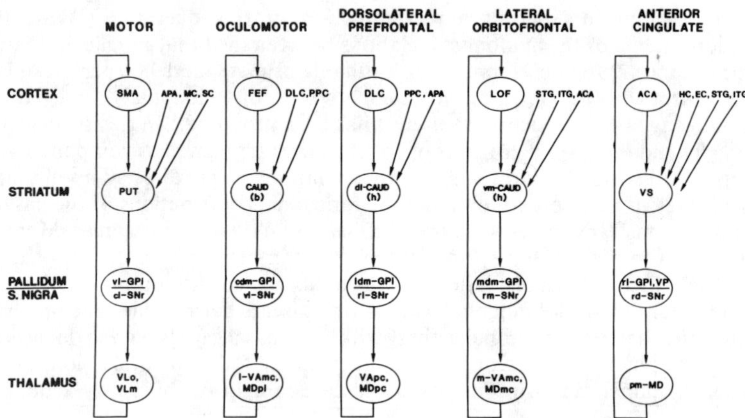

FIGURE 1. Proposed basal ganglia–thalamocortical circuits. Parallel organization of the five basal ganglia–thalamocortical circuits. Each circuit engages specific regions of the cerebral cortex, striatum, pallidum, substantia nigra, and thalamus. Abbreviations are as follows—ACA: anterior cingulate area; APA: arcuate premotor area; CAUD: caudate—(b) body, (h) head; DLC: dorsolateral prefrontal cortex; EC: entorhinal cortex; FEF: frontal eye fields; GPi: internal segment of globus pallidus; HC: hippocampal cortex; ITG: inferior temporal gyrus; LOF: lateral orbitofrontal cortex; MC: motor cortex; MDpl: medialis dorsalis pars paralamellaris; MDmc: medialis dorsalis pars magnocellularis; MDpc: medialis dorsalis pars parvocellularis; PPC: posterior parietal cortex; PUT: putamen; SC: somatosensory cortex; SMA: supplementary motor area; SNr: substantia nigra pars reticulata; STG: superior temporal gyrus; VAmc: ventralis anterior pars magnocellularis; VApc: ventralis anterior pars parvocellularis; VLm: ventralis lateralis pars medialis; VLo: ventralis lateralis pars oralis; VP: ventral pallidum; VS: ventral striatum; cl: caudolateral; cdm: caudal dorsomedial; dl: dorsolateral; l: lateral; ldm: lateral dorsomedial; m: medial; mdm: medial dorsomedial; pm: posteromedial; rd: rostrodorsal; rl: rostrolateral; rm: rostromedial; vm: ventromedial; and vl: ventrolateral.

Motor Circuit

The cortical areas from which the motor circuit originates include the motor, premotor, supplementary motor, and somatosensory areas, as well as the superior parietal lobule. Each cortical area projects upon the putamen, which is the principal striatal component of the motor circuit. The portions of the putamen that receive these sensorimotor inputs project to specific portions of the external (GPe) and internal pallidal segments. The GPi efferents terminate primarily in the pars oralis portion of the ventrolateral thalamus (VLo), which has been shown recently to project to the supplementary motor area (SMA). By virtue of direct projections to the motor cortex and the spinal cord, the SMA provides two parallel routes whereby the basal ganglia can influence the segmental motor apparatus.

The motor circuit is somatotopically organized throughout due to topographically organized projections linking the different structures, as shown in FIGURE 2. Corticostriatal fibers originating from cortical "leg" areas terminate in a dorsolateral portion of the putamen, fibers from the "face" areas terminate in a ventromedial sector, and fibers from "arm" areas terminate in a region that is in between. The somatotopic organization of the putamen and pallidum has been confirmed in neurophysiological studies.[4-6]

Neurophysiologic studies of the basal ganglia have demonstrated that neurons within the motor circuit are related to active or passive movements (or both) of specific body parts.[7-10] Parametric studies of active movements have revealed relations to movement

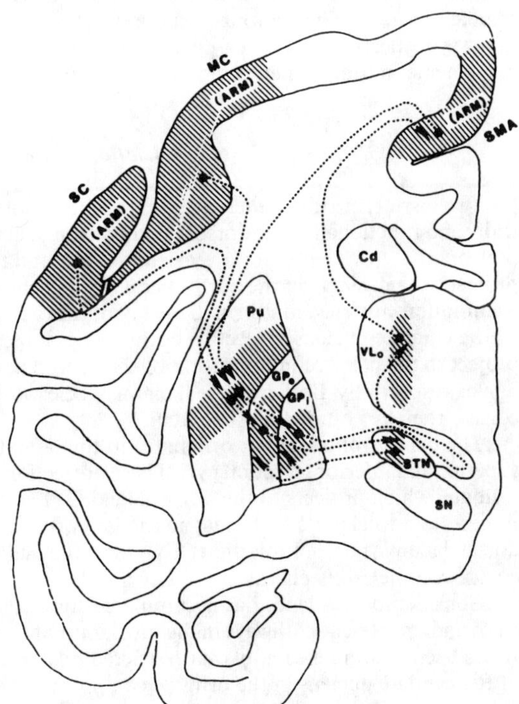

FIGURE 2. Somatotopic organization of the "motor" circuit showing the maintained somatotopy throughout this pathway: Cd = caudate; Pu = putamen.

direction, amplitude/velocity, and load. The directional component appears relatively independent of the pattern of muscle activity. Neurons within the motor circuit have also been shown to be involved in the preparation for movement.[11-13] Neurons in the putamen, globus pallidus, and SMA demonstrate instruction-dependent activity during the period before a movement is made, thus suggesting that this may be an important aspect of the functions of the motor circuit.

Oculomotor Circuit

Cortical inputs to the oculomoter circuit originate from the frontal eye fields (FEF), the dorsolateral prefrontal cortex, and the posterior parietal cortex. Each of these cortical areas projects to the central portion of the body of the caudate nucleus. This portion of the caudate projects to a caudal, dorsomedial portion of the GPi and to the ventrolateral SNr. The magnocellular portion of the ventral anterior thalamus and the paralamellar portion of the mediodorsal nucleus receive the output from this portion of the SNr, and both thalamic areas project back to the FEF. In addition to the cortical output of the oculomotor circuit, the SNr projects to the superior colliculus. Hence, the oculomotor circuit may influence oculomotor functions through both cortical and collicular mechanisms.

Neurons within the caudate and SNr have been shown to respond to visual stimuli, particularly in relation to saccade generation.[14,15] Caudate and nigral neurons also demonstrate responses preceding saccade generation.[14,15] In addition, nigral neurons demonstrate memory-contingent saccade responses prior to saccades to a previously instructed area.[14,16] The neuronal responses in the oculomotor circuit appear analogous in many respects to the activity within the motor circuit related to passive and active movements and movement preparation.

"Association" Circuits

Two distinct circuits centered in the prefrontal cortex can be distinguished anatomically and functionally. The dorsolateral prefrontal circuit originates in the dorsolateral prefrontal cortex, the posterior parietal cortex, and the arcuate premotor area. These projections terminate in the dorsolateral head of the caudate nucleus and throughout a continuous rostrocaudal strip to the tail of the caudate. Rostral dorsolateral portions of the caudate nucleus project to both the dorsomedial GPi and rostral SNr, which project to the parvocellular portion of the ventral anterior and mediodorsal thalamic nuclei, respectively. Both of these thalamic nuclei project to the dorsolateral prefrontal cortex, thereby completing the circuit.

The orbitofrontal circuit originates in the lateral orbitofrontal cortex and in the superior and inferior temporal gyri. These projections are received in the ventromedial caudate, which projects to the dorsomedial GPi and the rostromedial SNr. The SNr projects to medial parts of the magnocellular portions of the ventral anterior and mediodorsal thalamic nuclei. Projections from these thalamic nuclei to the lateral orbitofrontal cortex complete this circuit.

Considerable evidence has accumulated for a role of portions of the caudate nucleus and its efferent pathways in the mediation of behaviors other than simple motor. It has been shown repeatedly that restricted bilateral lesions of the appropriate areas of the caudate nucleus in the primate can produce an impairment of performance in behavioral tasks (e.g., delayed response, delayed alternation, and object-reversal tasks) similar to deficits seen after restricted lesions of corresponding regions of the frontal cortex. The most distinct impairments have been observed in performance on delayed alternation tasks after lesions of the dorsolateral prefrontal cortex or its projection area in the head of the caudate nucleus (the anterodorsal portion) and in performance on object-reversal tasks after lesions of the orbitofrontal cortex or the ventrolateral portion of the caudate nucleus. These studies support the distinction of two separate association circuits.

Anterior Cingulate Circuit

The ventral striatum (the striatal component of the cingulate circuit) receives inputs from a number of "limbic" structures including the hippocampus, amygdala, and entorhinal and perirhinal cortices. In addition to these structures, the anterior cingulate cortex, the temporal lobe, and the medial orbitofrontal cortex also contribute to the circuit. The ventral striatum projects to the rostrodorsal SNr, the ventral pallidum, and the rostrodorsal GPi. Projections of the SNr and GPi to posterior and medial portions of the mediodorsal thalamic nucleus and thalamocortical projections to the anterior cingulate area complete the circuit.

The functions of the anterior cingulate circuit remain highly speculative. The input from "limbic" areas may favor a possible role in aspects of motivation and drive. One issue of interest is how these "limbic" areas can influence the motor areas of the brain. The suggested parallel circuits provide no clear mechanism. This topic has been addressed by others[17] and will not be discussed further here.

APPLICATIONS TO PARKINSON'S DISEASE

In the following discussion, we will review the actions of dopamine within the striatum and briefly discuss recent findings in the primate MPTP model of parkinsonism. We will then discuss possible relationships of the proposed circuits to some of the signs and symptoms of parkinsonism.

Actions of Dopamine

In recent years, the majority of studies (using both intracellular and extracellular recordings) are consistent with the view that dopamine exerts a modulatory effect by reducing the tonic activity of striatal neurons and decreasing the response of striatal neurons to cortical stimulation, peripheral stimulation, or glutamate administration.[18-21] Intracellular recordings suggest that dopamine acts to reduce the amplitude of both excitatory and inhibitory postsynaptic potentials produced by cortical stimulation or iontophoresis of glutamate and GABA.[21] Loss of the net inhibitory action of dopamine should produce an increase in the tonic activity of striatal neurons and enhance responsiveness to extrinsic inputs. These effects have been observed in several studies.[18-20] In addition, recordings from the globus pallidus, which receives the major output from the striatum, have suggested that the striatal activity changes are transmitted into the basal ganglia circuitry as pallidal activity is also altered under these conditions.[22,23] These findings suggest that damage to the nigrostriatal dopamine system, as occurs in Parkinson's disease, may lead to altered tonic and phasic neuronal activity within the striatum and pallidum and that these changes are transmitted to the cerebral cortex through the basal ganglia–thalamocortical circuitry.

Recent studies in the primate MPTP model of parkinsonism support this hypothesis. Thus far, neurophysiological recording studies in these animals have focused on the globus pallidus, which is the source of the major output from the basal ganglia. In monkeys rendered parkinsonian with MPTP, altered tonic and phasic activities have been observed.[24-27] In GPe, tonic activity is decreased as determined by a shift in the mean discharge rate of GPe neurons. By contrast, in GPi, mean tonic activity is increased as shown in FIGURE 3. The pattern of neuronal discharge is also altered with a tendency for pronounced bursting, especially within GPi. In some GPi neurons, a regular, repetitive bursting pattern at about 12–15 Hz has been observed. Similar changes in discharge pattern were previously observed in animals with electrolytic lesions of the substantia nigra.[28]

Phasic activity has been examined in MPTP-treated animals primarily in response to passive manipulations of the limbs. These studies indicate that phasic responses of pallidal neurons to natural stimuli are enhanced.[25,27] With perturbation of the limb by a torque pulse, it can be demonstrated that the pallidal responses are increased in

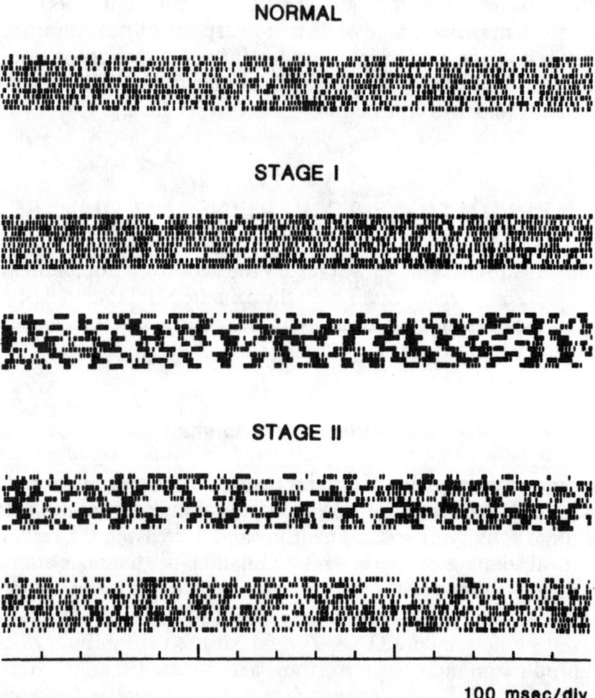

FIGURE 3. Tonic activity of representative GPi neurons. The upper raster is the activity of a normal GPi neuron, while the lower four rasters show examples of neuronal activity following MPTP treatment. Stage I is a period of severe impairment, whereas stage II represents gradual behavioral improvement and milder impairment. Note the increased discharge rate and the pronounced bursting observed following MPTP treatment. The second stage-I neuron demonstrates the dramatic regular bursting observed in some cells.

magnitude and duration in the parkinsonian monkey.[27] Responses to displacement of the limb are also detectable in a larger percentage of pallidal neurons. Although phasic activity during movement or in more complex tasks has not yet been studied in detail, it seems likely that the responses of GP neurons during these tasks would also be enhanced. Together, these data suggest that there is increased tonic output from the basal ganglia (GPi) in animals rendered parkinsonian with MPTP and that phasic signals throughout the circuit have increased gain and decreased selectivity.

When considered in the context of the segregated circuit model, it is apparent that these changes in neuronal activity within the basal ganglia might produce behavioral effects through a number of mechanisms. First, the increase in tonic output from GPi might result in corresponding changes in the tonic activity of the specific target nuclei in the thalamus and cortex. Such changes in tonic activity at the cortical level might directly produce behavioral changes. Altered tonic output from GPi might also disrupt cortical processing by altering the responsiveness of the cortical target areas. This could occur even if the level of tonic activity of these areas was not obviously altered. Altered phasic signals within the basal ganglia might disturb the normal processing and integration of signals within the basal ganglia. The information conveyed by these signals to the thalamus and cortex would be incorrect, thereby contributing to the production of the abnormal behaviors.

It is conceivable that altered output from the basal ganglia may have effects on cortical function and behavior that are largely independent of the normal functions of the basal ganglia. Even the abnormal behaviors associated with abnormal phasic activity in the basal ganglia may reflect the utilization and integration of the abnormal output by the cortex. Although Parkinson's disease has generally been considered prototypical of basal ganglia dysfunction, these factors emphasize the point that the behavioral deficits observed in this disorder must largely reflect abnormal cortical function. As a result, it is difficult to infer basal ganglia functions solely on the basis of observations of parkinsonian patients.

The segregated circuit model predicts that the behavioral deficits of Parkinson's disease should reflect abnormal processes in the SMA for the motor circuit, in the frontal eye fields for the oculomotor circuit, and in the prefrontal cortex for the association circuits. The variety of signs and symptoms of Parkinson's disease becomes more easily understood when considered with this circuit model in mind. Motor symptoms, such as rigidity and bradykinesia, and perhaps akinesia, reflect disruption of the motor circuit and the SMA. Similarly, oculomotor deficits reflect the oculomotor circuit and FEF, and cognitive deficits reflect the association circuits and the prefrontal cortex. Deficits referable to dysfunction of the anterior cingulate circuit are less certain. In the following discussion, we will briefly examine several signs and symptoms of Parkinson's disease and relate these problems to possible dysfunction within specific segregated circuits.

Motor Symptoms

Rigidity

In Parkinson's disease, there are two related but dissociable disorders of muscle activity. First, there is an increase in the resting level of EMG activity with a corresponding difficulty in achieving complete muscle relaxation. Second, there is increased resistance to passive stretch of the muscle; this is clinically defined as rigidity. In recent years, several studies have demonstrated abnormal long latency reflexes (LLR) in parkinsonian patients and this abnormality appears to contribute to rigidity.[29-31] The LLR occurs approximately 40–100 ms following the passive stretch of a muscle and is distinguishable from the shorter latency spinal reflex. In normal individuals, the magnitude of the LLR is dependent upon several factors, including instructions to respond to the perturbation, stretch velocity, magnitude, and duration.[32] However, in parkinsonian subjects, the LLR appears relatively independent of instruction and is nearly maximal at relatively small stretch parameters; hence, this indicates that the gain is relatively fixed and abnormally high.[32]

It is not known with certainty whether the basal ganglia or the SMA normally contribute to the production of long latency reflexes. Indeed, the transcortical nature of the LLR remains an issue of some controversy. However, it has been shown that motor cortical projection neurons respond appropriately to contribute to the production of the LLR[33] and that stimulation of the SMA can modulate the responses of motor cortex neurons.[34]

The demonstration of enhanced responses to passive stretch in pallidal neurons in the MPTP model of parkinsonism suggests several possible relations to LLR production. It is possible that the abnormal phasic responses generated within the basal ganglia are responsible for the LLR production through the motor circuit projection to the SMA. An alternative possibility is that the enhanced responses reflect abnormally large inputs to the striatum from the motor or somatosensory cortices that are engaged in the LLR production. In such a case, the abnormal responses may be due, in part, to altered responsiveness at the cortical level resulting from the increased tonic output from GPi.

It is possible that the increase in resting EMG activity may be due to the increased tonic output from GPi; this presumably occurs by altering tonic activity in the thalamus and SMA. Altered tonic activity in the SMA might produce the resting muscle activity directly through its corticospinal projections or through projections to the motor cortex. It is of interest that tonic EMG activity can be produced in rats by the injection of GABA agonists into the thalamus,[35] which is a finding consistent with increased tonic activity in the GABAergic output neurons in GPi. It is well recognized that lesions of GPi or its thalamic projections in humans can abolish rigidity, as predicted by these findings.

Rest Tremor

Although tremor in Parkinson's disease has been the subject of numerous investigations, the mechanism for its generation is not well understood. There remains some controversy as to whether the tremor results solely from a central oscillation generator. Some recent evidence suggests that peripheral feedback may act upon a centrally generated oscillatory output.[36]

In the past, the thalamus has been considered to be the principal candidate for tremor generation. This has been derived from the observation that surgical lesions in the thalamus [principally, the Ventralis intermedius (Vim) nucleus] abolish the tremor of Parkinson's disease. Furthermore, recordings of the neuronal activity in the thalamus during these operations have revealed oscillatory bursting in Vim that is consistent with tremor generation. However, it is important to note that the Vim portion of the thalamus does not receive direct projections from GPi and is not a component of the motor circuit.[37] Rather, the Vim appears to receive principally cerebellar input.

Because the site for surgical treatment of parkinsonian tremor is outside the motor circuit, it is of interest that in animal models of tremor and parkinsonism, lesions of the dopaminergic neurons of the substantia nigra alone do not produce tremor.[38] Additional lesions involving the cerebellum or its connections have usually been required to produce tremor. In the MPTP model of parkinsonism, the majority of nonhuman primate species tested thus far do not exhibit a rest tremor; rather, they exhibit an action tremor or postural tremor (or both) and this is typically the least consistent feature of the syndrome.[39] However, in at least one monkey species and in some of the human cases of MPTP-induced parkinsonism, a clear rest tremor has been observed.[40] The development of tremor in the MPTP model may be related to damage of other catecholaminergic nuclei, such as the locus ceruleus that projects heavily to the cerebellum. Loss of this projection to the cerebellum may produce changes in cerebellar activity to such an extent that they establish the oscillatory bursting observed in the Vim. The possibility remains, though, that the tremor may be at least partially related to abnormal activity in the basal ganglia resulting from nigral destruction. Three possible mechanisms are suggested. First, some neurons within the globus pallidus exhibit a characteristic oscillatory bursting pattern following MPTP treatment or electrolytic lesion of the substantia nigra that may contribute to the generation of tremor. Alternatively, the abnormal tonic output from GPi may establish a level of tonic activity or responsiveness within the SMA that is conducive to the development of the oscillation within the reciprocal thalamocortical circuits involving Vim and the motor cortex. Finally, the apparent increase in the gain of the motor circuit in relation to passive limb perturbations may also contribute to the development of oscillation. Clearly, the role of the motor circuit and the basal ganglia in the production of tremor remains poorly understood.

Bradykinesia

In recent years, several studies of parkinsonian subjects have examined the basis for bradykinesia at the muscular level. In normal individuals, rapid limb movements are performed with a triphasic pattern of muscle activity involving an initial agonist burst, an antagonist burst, and a second agonist burst.[41] As movement amplitude is increased, movement velocity is also increased. The increase in movement velocity is produced by generating a greater initial agonist burst. In parkinsonian subjects, the normal amplitude-velocity relation is disturbed and the large amplitude movements are performed at abnormally low velocities.[42] The abnormal velocities are due to a failure of these subjects to generate adequate initial agonist bursts.[43] The resultant movement appears discontinuous with several segmented, small-amplitude movements apparent in the velocity tracing.

It has been suggested that the basal ganglia motor circuit may play a role in the scaling of movement amplitude. This hypothesis was based upon several factors, including the abnormal amplitude/velocity relations in Parkinson's disease, the effects of GP lesions and stimulation in trained animals,[44,45] and the linearly graded discharge of pallidal neurons with increasing amplitudes of movement.[7] According to the scaling hypothesis, it would be predicted that during movement, neurons in the globus pallidus of a parkinsonian animal would discharge proportionately less during a large amplitude movement, thus corresponding to the decrease in movement velocity. Although active movements have not as yet been studied in detail in the MPTP model, the enhanced responses observed during passive movements suggest the possibility that responses during active movement may actually be enhanced rather than be diminished. It would also be predicted that the response magnitude would be relatively unmodifiable.

Altered activity in the basal ganglia during movement could account for bradykinesia in several different ways. First, there may be relatively less grading of the responses during attempted movements of different amplitudes. This would diminish the range of velocities produced by the basal ganglia output. Alternatively, it may be that the linearly graded responses observed in normal animals are not directly related to the scaling of movement amplitude and velocity. Instead, such responses could reflect the feed-forward of motor commands from the motor cortex and SMA, and the basal ganglia could be involved in a complex monitoring or comparator function. Abnormally large phasic output from the basal ganglia in the parkinsonian condition might lead to misinterpretation of the command within the SMA and to reduced output to the agonist musculature. This type of feed-forward system would be particularly important in movements performed without visual feedback, which are precisely the types of movements most dramatically impaired in parkinsonian subjects. Unfortunately, parametric studies of the motor functions of the SMA have not been performed and it is not known how the SMA utilizes the information it receives from the basal ganglia. Abnormal tonic output could also contribute to bradykinesia by altering the tonic activity or by reducing the responsiveness of the SMA (as discussed above for rigidity).

Akinesia

Akinesia may be simply defined as an impairment in movement initiation that results in a paucity of movement. In parkinsonian patients, the absence of movement is particularly prominent for movements that are internally generated. External stimuli often facilitate movement initiation. In addition to the deficit in movement initiation, parkinsonian subjects have difficulty performing complex motor acts, such as simultaneous and sequential movements.

Ideally, akinesia should be studied in patients performing internally generated movements because these are the types of movement most severely impaired. However, in such movements, the cue for movement is internal and, unlike a light or a tone, it cannot be accessed by the experimenter for determination of the process of movement initiation. Therefore, most attempts to assess movement initiation in parkinsonian patients have focused on reaction-time tasks in which a stimulus is presented and the patient must respond. In the majority of these studies, the principal finding is that reaction time in these subjects is highly variable with a slight tendency for prolongation.[46] However, in some studies where the EMG reaction time (i.e., the time from stimulus to EMG onset) has been monitored, the EMG reaction times were within normal limits.[47] This suggests that the observation of prolonged reaction times in stimulus-triggered movements is chiefly due to the inappropriate magnitude of the initial agonist burst and reflects the slowing of movements rather than a deficit in the command for movement initiation.

Recent studies of complex movements in parkinsonian subjects have revealed deficits that cannot be accounted for simply on the basis of slowed movements alone. In normal individuals, the simultaneous or sequential performance of two simple motor acts does not significantly affect the movement time of each act. In parkinsonian subjects, however, movement times are prolonged to a greater extent when simple movements are performed sequentially or simultaneously than when performed alone.[48,49] In sequential movements, the deficit arises from both a prolongation of the individual movement times and an abnormal delay between the movements.

Neurophysiological recording studies in the SMA of primates may provide some additional insight into akinesia. In animals performing self-paced movements without trigger stimuli, the discharge of SMA neurons appears coupled to the onset of the movement.[50] Other studies suggest that the SMA and the motor circuit may be involved in movement preparation, as discussed earlier. In parkinsonism, inappropriate activity in these classes of SMA neurons may interfere with the initiation of movement, thereby producing akinesia.

Dysfunction of the motor circuit and the SMA appears to be the most likely source for the production of akinesia. Destruction of the SMA and adjacent areas in humans may produce akinesia,[51,52] although effects of SMA lesions in monkeys are relatively mild.[53] Deficits in the preparatory motor functions of the motor circuit are supported by the observation of reduced readiness potentials in parkinsonian patients prior to movement[54] (these are normally maximal over the mesial cortex). In addition, the SMA has been implicated in the performance of complex movements on the basis of cerebral blood flow studies.[55]

Although it is suggested that akinesia results from dysfunction of the motor circuit, the nature of the disorder makes it plausible that dysfunction of the association or limbic circuits may also be important. In rats, involvement of the limbic circuit is suggested by the development of akinesia following dopamine depletion of the nucleus accumbens (see reference 3).

Oculomotor Symptoms

There are several oculomotor deficits that have been observed in Parkinson's disease and the correspondence of these symptoms to some of the motor symptoms is striking. In studies of saccadic eye movements, parkinsonian subjects demonstrate abnormally low peak velocities.[56] This deficit appears to be exaggerated during saccades of larger amplitudes, thus suggesting a disruption of normal amplitude-velocity relationships. Parkinsonian subjects also tend to make hypometric saccades, and large amplitude eye movements are produced by several small saccadic steps.[57] These findings appear analogous to the observations in bradykinetic parkinsonian patients where mean movement velocity is decreased, particularly with larger movements that are accomplished by several step movements. Parkinsonian subjects demonstrate some difficulty in initiating saccadic eye movements. Saccadic reaction times to external trigger stimuli are prolonged. When saccades are made between two stationary targets, the period of fixation between saccades is prolonged in parkinsonian subjects.[57] Moreover, patients with Parkinson's disease tend to make fewer spontaneous saccades. Therefore, these deficits in saccade initiation appear to reflect a "saccadic akinesia".

Presumably, the mechanisms underlying the oculomotor deficits of Parkinson's disease are similar to those of voluntary movements. The inappropriate tonic and phasic activities described above as possible mechanisms for motor dysfunction may be applicable to the oculomotor circuit as well. A critical difference, though, between the motor and oculomotor circuits is in the projection of the SNr to the superior colliculus, which creates a direct subcortical outlet for oculomotor processing from the basal ganglia. Thus, abnormal activity within the oculomotor circuit may produce the deficits either by acting directly on the superior colliculus or through the thalamocortical projection to the frontal eye fields.

In addition to these deficits, parkinsonian subjects appear to have altered smooth pursuit and vestibulo-ocular reflexes (VOR).[56,58] In both cases, the gains of the responses are diminished. Visual suppression, voluntary facilitation, and voluntary suppression of the VOR were also impaired in these subjects. The changes in the gain and control of the VOR highlight a point made previously, that is, the possible dissociation of parkinsonian deficits and normal functions of the basal ganglia. It is known that the VOR is controlled by a short three-neuron reflex arc within the brain stem. Clearly, the basal ganglia do not contribute phasically to this system. Whether or not the basal ganglia contribute normally to the gain control of this system is unknown. However, it is clear that abnormal output, presumably tonic output, from the basal ganglia may produce deficits in gain control of the VOR in parkinsonian subjects. Such an effect could be mediated by either collicular or cortical pathways.

Cognitive Symptoms

The precise role of the basal ganglia in disturbances of higher functions in humans is controversial because of the associated neuropathological changes occurring in other structures. As discussed earlier, data from experimental animals leave little doubt as to a role of the basal ganglia in cognitive functions (as suggested by the anatomical relations between the prefrontal cortex and the basal ganglia). Cognitive impairment frequently has been reported in Parkinson's disease. The degree of reported impairment has ranged from minimal impairment to global dementia. The relationship of Parkinson's disease and dementia, though, is controversial and beyond the scope of this paper. Instead, we will focus on some recent studies that have identified several specific impairments in parkinsonian patients without global dementia and that appear to be consistent with frontal lobe dysfunction.

One of the most consistent cognitive deficits observed in parkinsonian subjects is a failure to perform card sorting tasks, such as the Wisconsin Card Sorting Task (WCST), normally.[59-62] This task requires the subject to select an object on each card presented on the basis of a particular characteristic of the object such as color or shape. After a certain number of correct responses, the correct category of classification is altered (i.e., from color to shape) and the subject must utilize error feedback to determine the new category. Parkinsonian subjects are impaired on these tasks, reflecting a deficit in the manipulation of mental sets. Unfortunately, because of the modifications and differences in the presentation of the task, the conclusions of different authors regarding the specific nature of the impairment have differed; abnormal initiation, switching, and maintenance of sets have all been offered as explanations.[60-62] These differences in interpretation have largely been derived from the modifications of the tasks used and the error analyses used. Future studies of this kind should include complete analysis and description of both the number and specific nature of the errors made by the subjects. Perhaps, this would provide a clearer interpretation of the principal deficit in the manipulation of mental sets.

The deficits observed in the sorting tasks described above are similar to those in patients with frontal lobe lesions and several authors have suggested that the deficits reflect frontal lobe dysfunction.[59,60] In a recent study, the hypothesis that the cognitive impairments of Parkinson's disease were related to dysfunction of the frontal cortex (as suggested by the segregated circuit model) was examined.[60] A battery of neuropsychological tests was administered and it was determined that the deficits of the parkinsonian subjects were restricted to a limited number of tests specifically related to frontal dysfunction. The argument was strengthened by the lack of deficits on tests related to other cortical areas, such as recognition memory and most visuospatial tasks. Other studies have also reported minimal deficits on these tasks,[63,64] although visuospatial deficits have at times been reported.[65]

The presence of frontal lobe–related deficits could be related to abnormal activity within the association circuits of the basal ganglia. Indeed, the authors of the extensive neuropsychological study described above[60] suggested that the dorsolateral prefrontal circuit is the principal circuit involved. Altered tonic and phasic activity within this circuit (or the orbitofrontal circuit) could produce these deficits through any of the basic mechanisms previously elucidated, such as changes in frontal cortex responsiveness or altered processing within the caudate or pallidum.

CONCLUSIONS

In this brief paper, we have reviewed selective data from parkinsonian patients and the MPTP model of parkinsonism in light of the recently proposed scheme of segregated basal ganglia–thalamocortical circuits. It has been emphasized that the signs and symptoms of Parkinson's disease, although resulting from the loss of dopamine-containing midbrain neurons, must, ultimately, be the result of altered cortical activity. The basal ganglia are viewed as components of larger circuits that influence the activity of selective frontal areas. Clearly, the basal ganglia must play an important role in the normal functions of these cortical areas and, in disorders such as Parkinson's disease, they can produce disturbances of motor and cognitive function that depend on altered cortical output.

REFERENCES

1. ALEXANDER, G. E., M. R. DeLONG & P. L. STRICK. 1986. Parallel organization of functionally segregated circuits linking basal ganglia and cortex. Annu. Rev. Neurosci. **9:** 357–381.
2. KEMP, J. M. & T. P. S. POWELL. 1971. The connections of the striatum and globus pallidus: synthesis and speculation. Philos. Trans. R. Soc. London **B262:** 441–457.
3. DeLONG, M. R. & A. P. GEORGOPOULOS. 1981. Motor functions of the basal ganglia. *In* Handbook of Physiology, The Nervous System. J. M. Brookhart, V. B. Mountcastle, & V. B. Brooks, Eds.: 1017–1061. Amer. Physiol. Soc. Bethesda, Maryland.
4. ALEXANDER, G. E. & M. R. DeLONG. 1985. Microstimulation of the primate neostriatum: II. Somatotopic organization of striatal microexcitable zones and their relation to neuronal response properties. J. Neurophysiol. **53:** 1417–1430.
5. CRUTCHER, M. D. & M. R. DeLONG. 1984. Single cell studies of the primate putamen. I. Functional organization. Exp. Brain Res. **53:** 233–243.
6. DeLONG, M. R., M. D. CRUTCHER & A. P. GEORGOPOULOS. 1985. Primate globus pallidus and subthalamic nucleus: functional organization. J. Neurophysiol. **53:** 530–543.
7. GEORGOPOULOS, A. P., M. R. DeLONG & M. D. CRUTCHER. 1983. Relations between parameters of step-tracking movements and single cell discharge in the globus pallidus and subthalamic nucleus of the behaving monkey. J. Neurosci. **3:** 1586–1598.
8. CRUTCHER, M. D. & M. R. DeLONG. 1984. Single cell studies of the primate putamen. II. Relations to direction of movement and pattern of muscular activity. Exp. Brain Res. **53:** 244–258.
9. LILES, S. L. 1985. Activity of neurons in putamen during active and passive movements of wrist. J. Neurophysiol. **53:** 217–236.
10. MITCHELL, S. J., R. T. RICHARDSON, F. H. BAKER & M. R. DeLONG. 1987. The primate globus pallidus: neuronal activity related to direction of movement. Exp. Brain Res. In press.
11. ALEXANDER, G. E. 1987. Selected neuronal discharge in monkey putamen reflects intended direction of planned limbic movements. Exp. Brain Res. **67:** 623–634.
12. MILLER, W. C., S. J. MITCHELL & M. R. DeLONG. 1986. Instruction-dependent changes in neuronal activity in the primate globus pallidus. Soc. Neurosci. Abstr. **12:** 207.
13. TANJI, J., K. TANIGUCHI & T. SAGA. 1980. Supplementary motor area: neuronal response to motor instructions. J. Neurophysiol. **43:** 60–68.

14. HIKOSAKA, O. & M. SAKAMOTO. 1986. Cell activity in monkey caudate nucleus preceding saccadic eye movements. Exp. Brain Res. **63:** 659–662.

15. HIKOSAKA, O. & R. H. WURTZ. 1983. Visual and oculomotor functions of monkey substantia nigra pars reticulata. I. Relation of visual and auditory responses to saccades. J. Neurophysiol. **49:** 1230–1253.

16. HIKOSAKA, O. & H. WURTZ. 1983. Visual and oculomotor functions of monkey substantia nigra pars reticulata. III. Memory-contingent visual and saccade responses. J. Neurophysiol. **49:** 1268–1284.

17. NAUTA, H. J. W. 1986. The relationship of the basal ganglia to the limbic system. *In* Handbook of Clinical Neurology. Volume 5. H. L. Klawans, Ed.: 19–31. Elsevier. Amsterdam/New York.

18. ABERCROMBIE, E. D. & B. L. JACOBS. 1985. Dopaminergic modulation of sensory responses of striatal neurons: single unit studies. Brain Res. **358:** 27–33.

19. HIRATA, K., C. Y. YIM & G. J. MOGENSON. 1984. Excitatory input from sensory motor cortex to neostriatum and its modification by continuing stimulation of the substantia nigra. Brain Res. **321:** 1–8.

20. JOHNSON, S. W., M. R. PALMER & R. FREEDMAN. 1983. Effects of dopamine on spontaneous and evoked activity of caudate neurons. Neuropharmacology **22:** 843–851.

21. MERCURI, N., G. BERNARDI, P. CALABRESI, A. COTUGNO, G. LEVI & P. STANZIONE. 1985. Dopamine decreases cell excitability in rat striatal neurons by pre- and postsynaptic mechanisms. Brain Res. **358:** 110–121.

22. TOAN, D. L. & W. SCHULTZ. 1985. Responses of rat pallidum cells to cortex stimulation and effects of altered dopaminergic activity. Neuroscience **15:** 683–694.

23. HIRATA, K. & J. MOGENSON. 1984. Inhibitory response of pallidal neurons to cortical stimulation and the influence of conditioning stimulation of substantia nigra. Brain Res. **321:** 9–19.

24. FILION, M., R. BOUCHER & P. BEDARD. 1985. Globus pallidus unit activity in the monkey during the induction of parkinsonism by 1-methyl-4-phenyl-1,2,3,6-tetrahydropyridine (MPTP). Soc. Neurosci. Abstr. **11:** 1160.

25. FILION, M., L. TREMBLAY & P. J. BEDARD. 1986. Responses of globus pallidus neurons to electrical stimulation of striatum and to passive joint rotation in MPTP treated monkeys. Soc. Neurosci. Abstr. **12:** 208.

26. MILLER, W. C. & M. R. DELONG. 1987. Altered tonic activity of neurons in the globus pallidus and subthalamic nucleus in the primate MPTP model of parkinsonism. *In* Basal Ganglia: Structure and Function II. M. Carpenter, Ed. Plenum. New York. In press.

27. MILLER, W. & M. DELONG. 1987. Altered responses of pallidal neurons to limb perturbations following MPTP treatment in the monkey. In preparation.

28. FILION, M. 1979. Effects of interruption of the nigrostriatal pathway and of dopaminergic agents on the spontaneous activity of globus pallidus neurons in the awake monkey. Brain Res. **178:** 425–441.

29. TATTON, W. G. & R. G. LEE. 1975. Evidence for abnormal long-loop reflexes in rigid parkinsonian patients. Brain Res. **100:** 671–676.

30. BERARDELLI, A., A. SABRA & M. HALLETT. 1983. Physiological mechanisms of rigidity in Parkinson's disease. J. Neurol. Neurosurg. Psychiatry **46:** 45–53.

31. ROTHWELL, J. C., J. A. OBESO, M. M. TRAUB & C. D. MARSDEN. 1983. The behaviour of the long-latency stretch reflex in patients with Parkinson's disease. J. Neurol. Neurosurg. Psychiatry **46:** 35–44.

32. LEE, R. G., J. T. MURPHY & W. G. TATTON. 1983. Long-latency myotatic reflexes in man: mechanisms, functional significance, and changes in patients with Parkinson's disease or hemiplegia. *In* Motor Control Mechanisms in Health and Disease. J. E. Desmedt, Ed.: 489–507. Raven Press. New York.

33. CHENEY, P. D. & E. E. FETZ. 1984. Corticomotoneuronal cells contribute to long-latency stretch reflexes in the rhesus monkey. J. Physiol. **349:** 249–272.

34. HUMMELSHEIM, H., M. WEISENDANGER & M. BIANCHETTI. 1986. The supplementary motor area modulates perturbation-evoked discharges of neurons in the precentral motor cortex. Neurosci. Lett. **67:** 119–122.

35. KLOCKGETHER, T., M. SCHWARZ, L. TURSKI, S. WOLFARTH & K. H. SONTAG. 1985. Ri-

gidity and catalepsy after injections of muscimol into the ventromedial thalamic nucleus: an electromyographic study in the rat. Exp. Brain Res. **58:** 559–569.

36. RACK, P. M. H. & H. F. ROSS. 1986. The role of reflexes in the resting tremor of Parkinson's disease. Brain **109:** 115–141.

37. SCHELL, G. R. & P. L. STRICK. 1984. The origin of thalamic inputs to the arcuate premotor and supplementary motor areas. J. Neurosci. **4:** 539–560.

38. POIRIER, L. J., J. C. PECHADRE, C. LAROCHELLE, J. DANKOVA & R. BOUCHER. 1975. Stereotaxic lesions and movement disorders in monkeys. Adv. Neurol. **10:** 5–22.

39. BURNS, R. S., C. C. CHIUEH, S. P. MARKEY, M. H. EBERT, D. M. JACOBOWITZ & I. J. KOPIN. 1983. A primate model of parkinsonism: Selective destruction of dopaminergic neurons in the pars compacta of the substantia nigra by N-methyl-4-phenyl-1,2,3,6-tetrahydropyridine. Proc. Natl. Acad. Sci. USA **80:** 4546–4550.

40. BALLARD, P. A., J. W. TETRUD & J. W. LANGSTON. 1985. Permanent human parkinsonism due to 1-methyl-4-phenyl-1,2,3,6-tetrahydropyridine (MPTP): seven cases. Neurology **35:** 949–956.

41. HALLETT, M. & C. D. MARSDEN. 1979. Ballistic flexion movements of the human thumb. J. Physiol. **294:** 33–50.

42. DRAPER, I. T. & R. J. JOHNS. 1964. The disordered movement in parkinsonism and the effect of drug treatment. Bull. Johns Hopkins Hosp. **115:** 465–480.

43. HALLETT, M. & S. KHOSHBIN. 1980. A physiological mechanism of bradykinesia. Brain **103:** 301–314.

44. HORAK, F. V. & M. E. ANDERSON. 1984. Influence of globus pallidus on arm movements in monkeys. I. Effects of kainic acid–induced lesions. J. Neurophysiol. **52:** 290–304.

45. HORAK, F. V. & M. E. ANDERSON. 1984. Influence of globus pallidus on arm movements in monkeys. II. Effects of stimulation. J. Neurophysiol. **52:** 305–322.

46. EVARTS, E. V., H. TERAVAINEN & D. CALNE. 1981. Reaction time in Parkinson's disease. Brain **104:** 167–186.

47. WIESENDANGER, M., P. SCHNEIDER & J-P. VILLOZ. 1969. Electromyographic analysis of a rapid volitional movement. Am. J. Phys. Med. **48:** 17–24.

48. BENECKE, R., J. C. ROTHWELL, J. P. R. DICK, B. L. DAY & C. D. MARSDEN. 1987. Simple and complex movements off and on treatment in patients with Parkinson's disease. J. Neurol. Neurosurg. Psychiatry **50:** 296–303.

49. BENECKE, R., J. C. ROTHWELL, J. P. R. DICK, B. L. DAY & C. D. MARSDEN. 1986. Performance of simultaneous movements in patients with Parkinson's disease. Brain **109:** 739–757.

50. BRINKMAN, C. & R. PORTER. 1979. Supplementary motor area in the monkey: activity of neurons during performance of a learned motor task. J. Neurophysiol. **42:** 681–709.

51. DAMASIO, A. R. & G. W. VAN HOESEN. 1980. Structure and function of the supplementary motor area. Neurology **30:** 359.

52. LAPLANE, D., J. TALAIRACH, V. MEININGER, J. BANCAUD & J. M. ORGOGOZO. 1977. Clinical consequences of corticectomies involving the supplementary motor area in man. J. Neurol. Sci. **34:** 301–314.

53. BRINKMAN, C. 1984. Supplementary motor area of the monkey's cerebral cortex: short- and long-term deficits after unilateral ablation and the effects of subsequent callosal section. J. Neurosci. **4:** 918–929.

54. NIIJIMA, K. & M. YOSHIDA. 1983. Clinical neurophysiological study of akinesia in patients with disorders of the extrapyramidal system. Clin. Neurol. **23:** 288–293.

55. ROLAND, P. E., B. LARSEN, N. A. LASSEN & E. SKINHOJ. 1980. Supplementary motor area and other cortical areas in organization of voluntary movements in man. J. Neurophysiol. **43:** 118–136.

56. WHITE, O. B., J. A. SAINT-CYR, R. D. TOMLINSON & J. A. SHARPE. 1983. Ocular motor deficits in Parkinson's disease II. Control of the saccadic and smooth pursuit systems. Brain **106:** 571–587.

57. DEJONG, J. D. & G. M. JONES. 1971. Akinesia, hypokinesia, and bradykinesia in the oculomotor system of patients with Parkinson's disease. Exp. Neurol. **32:** 58–68.

58. WHITE, O. B., J. A. SAINT-CYR & J. A. SHARPE. 1983. Ocular motor deficits in Parkinson's disease I. The horizontal vestibulo-ocular reflex and its regulation. Brain **106:** 555–570.

59. LEES, J. & E. SMITH. 1983. Cognitive deficits in the early stages of Parkinson's disease. Brain **106**: 257–270.

60. TAYLOR, A. E., J. A. SAINT-CYR & A. E. LANG. 1986. Frontal lobe dysfunction in Parkinson's disease. Brain **109**: 845–883.

61. COOLS, A. R., J. H. L. VAN DEN BERCKEN, M. W. I. HORSTINK, K. P. M. VAN SPAENDONCK & H. J. C. BERGER. 1984. Cognitive and motor shifting aptitude disorder in Parkinson's disease. J. Neurol. Neurosurg. Psychiatry **47**: 443–453.

62. FLOWERS, K. A. & C. ROBERTSON. 1985. The effect of Parkinson's disease on the ability to maintain a mental set. J. Neurol. Neurosurg. Psychiatry **48**: 517–529.

63. BROWN, R. G. & C. D. MARSDEN. 1986. Visuospatial function in Parkinson's disease. Brain **109**: 987–1002.

64. FLOWERS, K. A., I. PEARCE & J. M. S. PEARCE. 1984. Recognition memory in Parkinson's disease. J. Neurol. Neurosurg. Psychiatry **47**: 1174–1181.

65. BOLLER, F., D. PASSAFIUME, N. C. KEEFE, K. ROGERS, L. MORROW & Y. KIM. 1984. Visuospatial impairment in Parkinson's disease. Arch. Neurol. **41**: 485–490.

DISCUSSION OF THE PAPER

J. SLADEK (*University of Rochester Medical School, Rochester, NY*): In one of your very nice flow diagrams, the caudate nucleus was conspicuously absent. We also heard a great deal about D2 receptors in different parts of the striatum. Therefore, I was quite interested in the human work presented in the dorsal-medial distribution in caudate nucleus. Could you comment on what role the caudate may or may not play?

M. DELONG (*The Johns Hopkins Medical School, Baltimore, MD*): The main thing about the caudate is that it receives input from the sensory motor areas. The caudate is intimately linked with the functions of the prefrontal cortex in general. In fact, in the primate, this has been studied extensively and it has been found that if you bilaterally lesion the areas that receive their input from that dorsal-lateral prefrontal cortex, you produce exactly the same impairment that you do from lesioning the cortical areas. This subcortical system thus seems to be as important in mediating that behavior as does the cortex itself. Therefore, the functions of prefrontal cortex are dependent on processing within specific regions of the caudate. However, to disrupt that function (just as for the cortex), you would have to make bilateral lesions. If you take out half or one side of the predorsal-lateral prefrontal, the animal does fine and does not have any trouble performing the complex task. Moreover, there are no motor impairments. Damage to the caudate has absolutely no effect on movement.

Effects of Age on the Motor Unit

A Study on Single Motor Units in the Rat[a]

LARS LARSSON AND TOR ANSVED

Departments of Clinical Neurophysiology and Neurology
Karolinska Hospital
S-104 01 Stockholm, Sweden

INTRODUCTION

In the process of aging, profound alterations take place in the neuromuscular system in most mammals. By far, senile muscle atrophy is the most commonly encountered kind of muscle atrophy in man. In spite of this, the influence of age-related muscle atrophy on muscle function and the mechanisms underlying senile atrophy have so far received relatively little scientific attention. This is probably due, at least in part, to the large number of methodological problems encountered in aging studies. In addition, this is coupled with the very complex pathogenesis of senile muscle atrophy, which involves different levels of nervous and endocrine systems (see reference 1). The most significant methodological problems, and those that are most difficult to handle in old age, are the secondary influences on muscle tissue of disuse, malnutrition, and degenerative lesions due to diseases of the cardiovascular, nervous, or locomotor systems (see reference 1). The impact of these conditions is of considerable importance for the overall aging process; however, they should be separated by studying populations that are homogeneous in these respects in order to increase the knowledge about "primary" aging mechanisms.

In a previous series of studies, we attempted to shed some light on the mechanisms underlying the impaired muscle function in old age in man.[2-8] Investigations of enzyme-histochemical, biochemical, and morphological properties of the quadriceps muscle were made concomitantly with functional measurements in the knee-extensor muscles in sedentary men of ages between 22 and 65 years. The subjects were carefully selected as having equivalent physical activity levels both occupationally and during leisure. The quadriceps muscle was studied because proximal lower limb muscles have been reported to be especially affected by impaired function in old age in man (see reference 1). In this series of investigations, significant age-related alterations were observed in torque outputs during maximum voluntary knee extensions of various speeds of movement, and in the maximum speed of movement, fiber-type proportions, fiber size, and mitochondrial volumes. However, activities of different enzymes that were representative of major pathways of muscle energy metabolism did not change during this age span. A number of statistically significant correlations were found between muscle function and the various enzyme-histochemical, biochemical, and morphological muscle

[a] This study was supported by grants from the Swedish Medical Research Council (Project No. B86-12X-03875-14A), the Swedish Society of Medical Sciences, the Karolinska Institute, and the Swedish Sports Research Council.

properties, with the most pertinent being a relation between the reduced muscle force (both isometric and dynamic) and the fiber atrophy, which preferentially affected the fast-twitch (type II) fibers in old age. The reduced maximum speed of movement in old age correlated with an age-related change in fiber-type proportions, that is, a decline in the proportion of type II fibers.

From the results of these experiments, though, it cannot be determined whether these correlations reflect causal relations or not. Furthermore, it is not known if the maximum capacity for the generation of force by material that is maintained in a contractile state is impaired or not in old age. It has been proposed, on the one hand, that the age-related decrease in muscle force is caused exclusively by a loss of contractile material, that is, by a decrease in the number and size of fibers.[9,10] On the other hand, some authors have emphasized the importance of qualitative changes in the contractile machinery in old age as the factor in impairing the capacity for force generation.[11,12] Moreover, the cause of the reduced speed of contraction in old age is not known, but it has been suggested that it may be related to a selective fallout of fast-twitch units or a change in contractile properties within remaining motor units (or both).[13]

Hence, in view of the fact that many of the age-related effects on striated muscle are still poorly understood and cannot be explained in human studies with presently available techniques, we have undertaken a series of animal experiments with the aim of elucidating the mechanisms underlying the age-related declines in force and speed of contraction and also the differential effects of aging on fast- and slow-twitch muscles and single motor units. In studies of the final functional unit in the motor system (i.e., the motor unit),[14] the technique of glycogen depletion was used as a marker of previous muscle contraction[15-17] in order to permit direct examination of the morphological-physiological correlations. Part of this work has been published elsewhere.[18-21]

MATERIALS AND METHODS

Male albino rats of the same strain (Wistar) — fed *ad libitum* with standard laboratory food and tap water — were studied in all experiments. The animals were divided into a young adult (3–6 months) and an old (20–24 months) group. In some preliminary experiments, animals of 7–8 months and 16–18 months of age were also studied. Animals that were sick, moribund, or that showed gross pathological organ changes were excluded from the study. Rats of the Wistar strain have a mean life duration of 24 months and may live for approximately 36 months.[22] In order to avoid unpredictable influences (such as extreme obesity, disease, and disuse) on skeletal muscle in very old age, we chose to study rats that had not reached an advanced age.

Physiological Technique

The animals were anesthetized with pentobarbital administered intraperitoneally. The ventral roots — L4 to the tibial anterior (TA) and L5 to the soleus (S) muscle — were exposed by laminectomy. The skin over the lower part of the left hind limb was removed, and the tendon from TA or S was cut distally and attached to a strain gauge (UC 2, Statham Instruments, Oxnard, California). A load cell accessory (UL 4–10, Statham Instruments) was attached to the strain gauge when whole muscle responses were recorded. The mechanical responses were amplified (AD 6, Medelec, Old Woking, Surrey, United Kingdom), displayed on an oscilloscope (M-scope, Medelec), and recorded on Kodak Linagraph direct print paper (Eastman Kodak, Rochester, New York). The surrounding muscles were denervated or tenotomized. The left popliteal artery was exposed and a fine thread was placed loosely around the artery to make it easily accessible.

The animal was placed in a prone position and the limb was put into a bath circulated with mineral oil maintained at 36 °C. The limb was fixed rigidly in the bath with a steel drill through the tibia close to the knee joint and with a clamp on the foot. Single motor units in TA and S were functionally isolated by microdissection of the L4 and L5 ventral roots, respectively (FIGURE 1). The criterion was an all-or-none twitch response to finely graded current pulses of 0.2 ms duration. Supramaximal stimulation was used in all experiments. Contractions were recorded with the muscle set at an optimum length as determined from the maximum isometric twitch force. The isometric twitch contraction time was measured from the beginning of contraction to the peak force, and the half-relaxation time was measured from the peak force to the time when the force had fallen by 50%. Mechanical properties of single motor units were recorded during repetitive stimulation. Stimulation trains with frequencies of 10, 46, and 196 Hz and with a duration of 7 s were used. In some experiments,

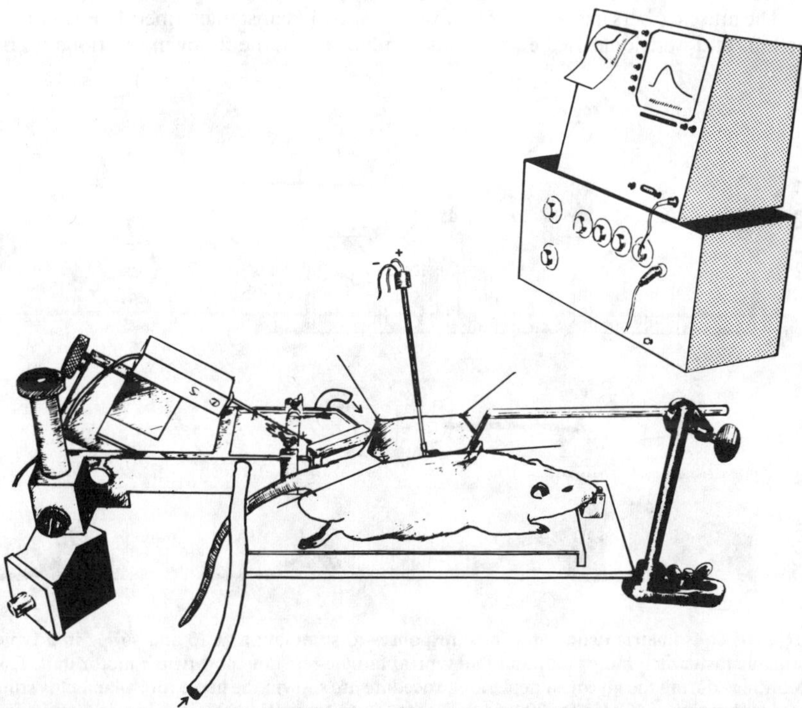

FIGURE 1. Schematic illustration of the experimental setup. The rat is placed in the prone position on a steel plate (which is heated to maintain body temperature). The left hind limb is rigidly fixed in a bath circulated with mineral oil maintained at 36 °C. The tendon of the muscle is oriented along its natural pull and aligned with a strain gauge. The ventral root is exposed by laminectomy. Single motor units are functionally isolated by microdissection and the contractile properties of the motor unit are recorded.

the muscle length was increased in steps of 1 mm to study the influence of muscle length on twitch and tetanus force.

The muscle fibers of the unit were depleted of glycogen by stimulation with trains of 20 impulses with a frequency of 100 Hz. This was repeated once a second until the tetanic force had dropped to nearly zero. The stimulation was then terminated and the unit was stimulated with one impulse train every 10 s until the force had almost recovered. This sequence was repeated 3–5 times (FIGURE 2). Fatigue-resistant units in TA and all units in S were stimulated during ischemia, which was produced by clamping of the popliteal artery with a small clip. The clip was removed during the recovery periods (for detailed information, see references 15, 17, 18, 23, and 24).

Histological Technique

After each experiment, the muscle was gently dissected free from surrounding tissue and clamped at the approximate *in situ* length. The muscle was weighed, frozen in freon chilled with liquid nitrogen, and stored at $-80\,°C$ until processed further, which is when it was cut perpendicular to its longitudinal axis into serial 10-μm-thin cross sections with a cryotome ($-20\,°C$) at the motor point (S) or at the greatest girth (TA).

The muscle fibers in the motor unit were mapped as unstained fibers in PAS-stained sections and were identified enzyme-histochemically in the following sections stained

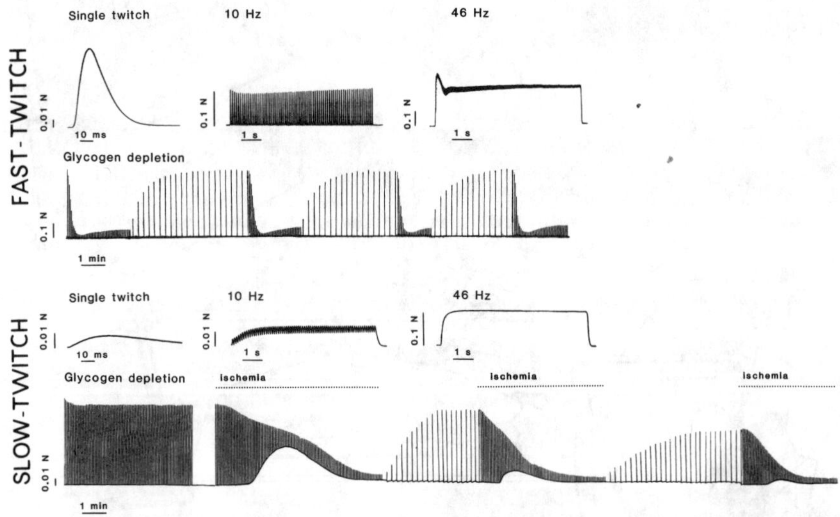

FIGURE 2. Isometric twitch and force responses to stimulation at 10 and 46 Hz in a typical fatigable fast-twitch motor unit and in a typical fatigue-resistant slow-twitch motor unit. Force recordings during the glycogen depletion procedure are shown; the nerve root filament is stimulated with trains of 100 Hz for 200 ms each second until a considerable decrease in tetanus force is recorded. Stimulation is then terminated and the filament is stimulated with one impulse train every 10 s until the tetanus force has almost recovered. This sequence is repeated 3–5 times. In fatigue-resistant units, the tetanus force does not decrease until ischemia is produced by clamping the popliteal artery with a small spring clip. The clip is removed during recovery periods. The clamping of the artery is indicated as a dotted line in the figure. The force recordings during the glycogen depletion are retouched for greater contrast.

for myofibrillar ATPase. They were classified into types I, IIA, IIB, and IIC on the basis of the ATPase stainings (for detailed information, see references 17–19, 23, and 24).

A special model was designed to assess the randomness of muscle fibers in the unit. With this model, the motor unit territory was divided into eight sectors. The angle between the two radii of the sectors was 45°, the center of the sectors was at the midportion of the axis between the two most distant muscle fibers in the unit, and the border of the motor unit territory was the base of each sector. The average differences in the predicted and measured numbers of muscle fibers in the sectors were corrected for differences in innervation ratios. These were then used as an index of the randomness of the fiber arrangement in the motor unit (for detailed information, see reference 18).

RESULTS AND DISCUSSION

In conformity with findings in various albino rat strains (e.g., reference 25), the body weight increased from young age (3–6 months, 441 ± 51 g, $n = 69$) to old age (20–24 months, 605 ± 87 g, $n = 67$). In contrast, though, the weight of the fast-twitch TA (931 ± 104 mg versus 1078 ± 265 mg) and the slow-twitch S (214 ± 49 mg versus 240 ± 89 mg) did not change significantly from young to old age. The increased body weight in old age appeared to be due mainly to a greater amount of subcutaneous adipose tissue (often noticed during dissections) rather than to increased muscle weight.[19]

Number of Muscle Fibers and Proportions of Fiber Types in Fast- and Slow-Twitch Muscles

In the fast-twitch TA, the proportions and sizes of muscle fibers of different types did not differ between adult (6 months) and old (20–24 months) animals. The proportions of type I, IIA, and IIB fibers were 3 ± 1%, 19 ± 2%, and 78 ± 1% in the adult and 4 ± 2%, 15 ± 4%, and 80 ± 3% in the old animals, respectively.[19] The total number of fibers counted from one single cross-sectional cut at the greatest girth of the muscle was 13,303 ± 1032 in the adult and 13,691 ± 1333 in the old animals, thus indicating that there was no major change in this number with age. However, these figures have to be treated with caution because all fibers probably do not pass through the greatest girth of TA (see reference 19).

On the other hand, in the slow-twitch S muscles, all fibers pass the motor point. Therefore, accurate measurements of the total number of fibers can accordingly be made in this muscle from single cross-sectional cuts (see reference 19). This total number decreased ($p < 0.001$) by approximately 13% from the young adult age to old age, whereas there was no significant change in the number of type I fibers. This resulted in an increase ($p < 0.001$) in the proportion of type I fibers from 88 ± 5% to 99 ± 3%.[19] The cross-sectional area of the muscle fibers decreased in parallel with the age-related decrease in the number of muscle fibers, with fibers of type I and II being 23% and 55% smaller ($p < 0.05$–0.01), respectively, in old age (FIGURES 3 and 4).[19] In spite of the age-related decrease in the number and size of muscle fibers in S, the muscle weight was not significantly affected during aging; this indicates that contractile material was gradually replaced by fat and connective tissue (cf. reference 2).

The most probable mechanism underlying the age-related alterations in the number and size of S fibers appears to be either a selective fallout and degeneration of type II fibers or a transformation of type II to type I followed by fiber loss and atrophy

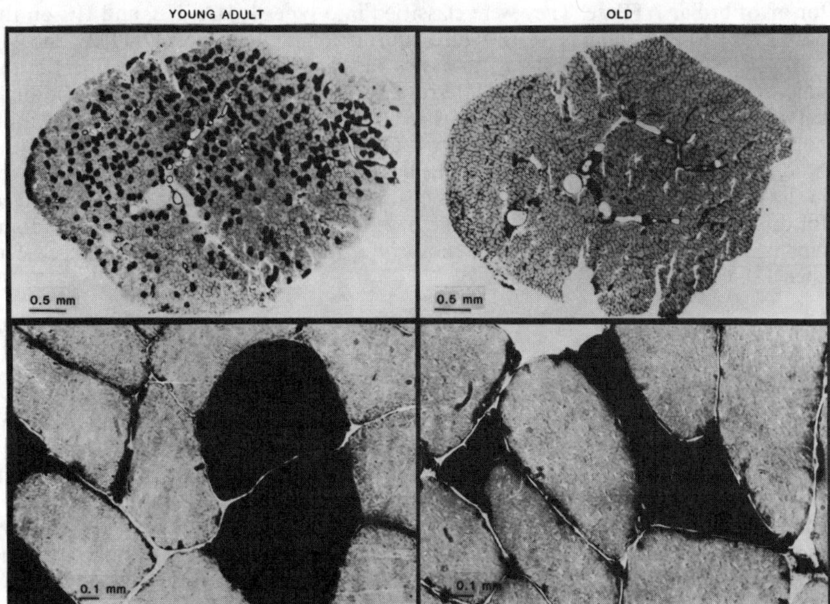

FIGURE 3. Transverse sections of a young and an old rat soleus muscle. The sections are stained for myofibrillar ATPase at pH 9.4 after formaldehyde fixation. Type I fibers show low activity. Type II fibers show strong and several shades of intermediate activities.

irrespective of the enzyme-histochemical type. Severe muscle fiber atrophy (cross-sectional areas less than 1000 μm) was predominantly seen in type II fibers, particularly in animals in which the total number of type II fibers was below the average innervation ratio.[19] These atrophic fibers often had an angular appearance (FIGURE 3), thus suggesting previous denervation. These findings indirectly point to a selective fallout of fast-twitch motor units in old age. However, preliminary results from rats of ages between 6 and 20 months indicate that there is a continuation in adult and middle-aged animals of the process of transformation of type II to type I fibers seen during early development.[24] There would seem to be an unselected fallout of motor units. Therefore, the atrophic and angular type II fibers seen in old age may in fact be type I fibers that, by loss of neuronal control, have been transformed to type II. Supporting this possibility is the observation that fast myosin is preferentially synthesized in slow muscles after denervation (see reference 26). The transformation process in the adult and middle-aged rats presumably reflects the same mechanism as has been proposed for developing rat muscle,[24] that is, transformation of type II fibers to type I as a result of a change in motoneuron properties related to altered functional demands in connection with the increased body weight.

Morphometrical Properties of Fast- and Slow-Twitch Single Motor Units

The fast-twitch motor units in TA covered 18 ± 8% and 22 ± 15% of muscle

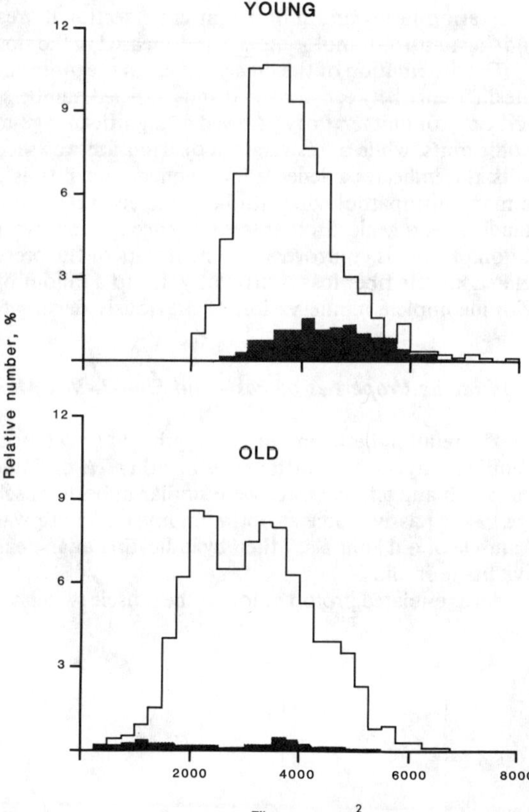

FIGURE 4. The distribution of the average cross-sectional areas of soleus muscle fibers of type I (unfilled histogram) and type II (filled histogram) in rats 3–6 (n = 5) and 20–24 (n = 5) months of age.

cross sections, comprised 148 ± 59 and 162 ± 59 muscle fibers, and had a total area of 0.05 ± 0.32 mm² and 0.44 ± 0.22 mm² in the young adult (3–6 months) and old (20–24 months) animals, respectively. Hence, neither the motor unit territory, the innervation ratio, nor the motor unit area changed with age in the fast-twitch units.[18] The total number of motor units was not calculated in TA because the total number of muscle fibers could not be determined accurately from single cross-sectional cuts in this muscle (see above).

The slow-twitch motor units in S covered 53 ± 10% and 74 ± 11% of muscle cross sections (p = n.s.), comprised 55 ± 9 and 83 ± 12 muscle fibers ($p < 0.01$), and had a total area of 0.14 ± 0.02 mm² and 0.22 ± 0.06 mm² ($p < 0.01$) in the young adult (3–6 months) and old (20–24 months) animals, respectively. The total number of motor units (calculated under the assumption that the mapped motor unit was representative of the rest of the units in the muscle) decreased ($p < 0.01$) from 49 ± 10 in the young adult animals to 29 ± 10 in the old ones. Similar numerical decreases in motor units were observed when the number of isolated single motor units was counted during whole ventral root microdissection and when the average single motor unit twitch force was related to the twitch force evoked by whole ventral root stimulation.[18] Thus, the innervation ratios and motor unit cross-sectional areas were significantly increased and the number of motor units was decreased in the slow-twitch units of old animals.[18]

The distribution of the muscle fibers in the motor unit (assessed as the mean absolute difference between measured and predicted numbers of muscle fibers in eight sectors of the motor unit territory) showed no significant age-related change in the fast-twitch motor units, while a less random distribution was seen in the old slow-twitch motor units; this indicates a denervation-reinnervation process. It also conforms with findings in many histopathological studies of aged skeletal muscle showing signs of a long-standing neurogenic disorder (see reference 1). However, the site of the age-related denervation process is controversial. The results of the present study suggest that the age-related muscle fiber loss is primarily due to a fallout of whole motor units combined with incomplete reinnervation of previously denervated fibers.

Contractile Properties of Fast- and Slow-Twitch Muscles and Single Motor Units

The relation between muscle length and twitch or tetanus force did not show any significant age-related differences in either TA or S and the optimum muscle lengths for twitch and tetanus force were similar in both muscles, irrespective of the animal's age.[19] The passive force at optimum muscle length was significantly increased in the S muscle of old animals,[19] thereby indicating an increased relative amount of connective tissue in old S.

An age-related prolongation of the muscle twitch was noted both in the fast-twitch

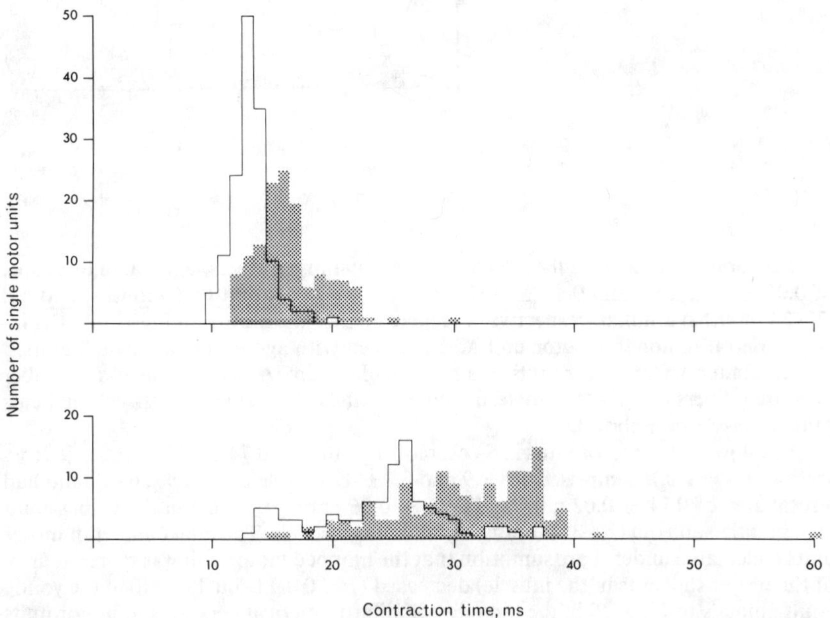

FIGURE 5. Contraction times in 274 tibial anterior (the upper figure) and 236 soleus (the lower figure) single motor units in young (3–6 months, unfilled histograms) and old rats (20–24 months, filled histograms).

TA and in the slow-twitch S. The contraction time increased from 17 ± 2 ms to 21 ± 3 ms ($p < 0.001$) in TA and from 25 ± 4 ms to 34 ± 12 ms ($p < 0.01$) in S from young adult age (6 months) to old age (20–24 months).[19] A corresponding increase in twitch duration was recorded from single motor units of both the fast- and slow-twitch type (FIGURE 5). It is thus concluded that the reduced speed of contraction in old age is due to altered contractile properties in remaining motor units in both the fast- and slow-twitch muscles, along with a decreased number of fast-twitch muscle fibers in the slow-twitch S.[18] A series of events in the excitation-contraction coupling determines the time course of the contractile response. The key factors that decide the contraction time of the muscle twitch are (1) the capacity of the sarcoplasmic reticulum for calcium release and recapture and (2) the composition of fast and slow isoforms of the myofibrillar proteins (see reference 19). The very coordinated appearance of sarcoplasmic reticulum proteins and myofibrillar proteins in fast- and slow-twitch muscle fibers in young adults, presumably triggered by motoneuron discharge properties, is reported to be partially lost in old age.[27] In addition, the surface and volume densities of the T-tubular and sarcoplasmic reticulum are claimed to be decreased.[28] Therefore, these complex age-related alterations may have obvious effects on the excitation-contraction coupling and may underlie the reduced speed of contraction seen in both fast- and slow-twitch motor units in this study.

The effects of age on the twitch and tetanus force differed significantly between fast- and slow-twitch muscles. In the fast-twitch TA, the twitch force increased ($p < 0.05$) in old age, while the tetanus force showed no age-associated change. This resulted in an increased ($p < 0.01$) twitch:tetanus ratio. Similar results were obtained at the single motor unit level.[18] In S, both the twitch and tetanus force decreased ($p < 0.05$) in old age and the twitch:tetanus ratio therefore remained unaltered. The tetanus tension (i.e., tetanus force per total muscle fiber cross-sectional area) did not differ between adult and old muscles of either the fast- or slow-twitch type; this thus indicates that the force-generating capacity of the contractile material is maintained in old age.[19]

In conclusion, the present results demonstrate that aging affects muscle tissue in both quantitative and qualitative terms and that these age-related alterations affect fast- and slow-twitch muscles and motor units in different ways. It is shown that the decrease in muscle force in old age is due to a reduction in the number and size of muscle fibers, whereas the capacity of maintained contractile material to generate force is intact. The loss of contractile material in old age is mainly due to a fallout of whole motor units and an incomplete reinnervation of previously denervated muscle fibers. The age-related reduction in the speed of contraction is primarily due to altered contractile properties (irrespective of the motor unit type) and a decreased number of fast-twitch (type II) muscle fibers in the slow-twitch muscle.

ACKNOWLEDGMENTS

We wish to thank Birgitta Lindegren and Birgitta Hedberg for excellent laboratory assistance.

REFERENCES

1. LARSSON, L. 1982. Aging in mammalian skeletal muscle. *In* The Aging Motor System. F. J. Pirozzolo & G. J. Maletta, Eds.: 60–98. Praeger. New York.
2. LARSSON, L. 1978. Morphological and functional characteristics of the ageing skeletal muscle in man. A cross-sectional study. Acta Physiol. Scand. Suppl. **457**: 1–36.

3. LARSSON, L. 1982. Physical training effects on muscle morphology in sedentary males. Med. Sci. Sports **14:** 203–206.

4. LARSSON, L. 1983. Histochemical characteristics of human skeletal muscle during aging. Acta Physiol. Scand. **117:** 469–471.

5. LARSSON, L. & J. KARLSSON. 1978. Isometric and dynamic endurance as a function of age and skeletal muscle characteristics. Acta Physiol. Scand. **104:** 129–136.

6. LARSSON, L., B. SJÖDIN & J. KARLSSON. 1978. Histochemical and biochemical changes in human skeletal muscle with age in sedentary males, age 22–65 years. Acta Physiol. Scand. **103:** 31–39.

7. LARSSON, L., G. GRIMBY & J. KARLSSON. 1979. Muscle strength and speed of movement in relation to age and muscle morphology. J. Appl. Physiol. **46:** 451–456.

8. ÖRLANDER, J., K-H. KIESSLING, L. LARSSON, J. KARLSSON & A. ANIANSSON. 1978. Skeletal muscle metabolism and ultrastructure in relation to age in sedentary men. Acta Physiol. Scand. **104:** 249–261.

9. ERMINI, M. 1976. Ageing changes in mammalian skeletal muscle. Biochemical studies. Gerontology **22:** 301–316.

10. MCCARTER, A. J. 1978. Effects of age on contraction of mammalian skeletal muscle. *In* Aging in Muscle. Vol. 6. G. Kaldor & W. J. D. Battista, Eds.: 1–21. Raven Press. New York.

11. GUTMANN, E. & V. HANZLIKOVA. 1972. Age changes in the neuromuscular system. Scientechnica (Bristol).

12. MATSUKI, H., Y. TAKEDA & Y. TONOMURA. 1966. Changes in biochemical properties of isolated human skeletal myofibrils with age and in myasthenia gravis. J. Biochem. **59:** 122–125.

13. CAMPBELL, M. J., A. J. MCCOMAS & F. PETITO. 1973. Physiological changes in ageing muscles. J. Neurol. Neurosurg. Psychiatry **36:** 174–182.

14. SHERRINGTON, C. S. 1929. Some functional problems attaching to convergence. Ferrier Lecture. Proc. R. Soc. London **105:** 332–362.

15. EDSTRÖM, L. & E. KUGELBERG. 1968. Histochemical composition, distribution and fatiguability of single motor units. Anterior tibial muscle of the rat. J. Neurol. Neurosurg. Psychiatry **31:** 424–433.

16. KUGELBERG, E. & L. EDSTRÖM. 1968. Differential histochemical effects of muscle contraction on phosphorylase and glycogen in various types of fibres: relation to fatigue. J. Neurol. Neurosurg. Psychiatry **31:** 415–423.

17. KUGELBERG, E. & B. LINDEGREN. 1979. Transmission and contraction fatigue of rat motor units in relation to succinate dehydrogenase activity of motor unit fibres. J. Physiol. (London) **288:** 285–300.

18. EDSTRÖM, L. & L. LARSSON. 1986. Effects of age on contractile, enzyme-histochemical and morphometrical properties of fast- and slow-twitch single motor units in the rat. J. Physiol. (London) **392:** 129–145.

19. LARSSON, L. & L. EDSTRÖM. 1986. Effects of age on enzyme-histochemical fibre spectra and contractile properties of fast- and slow-twitch skeletal muscles in the rat. J. Neurol. Sci. **76:** 69–89.

20. LARSSON, L. & L. EDSTRÖM. 1986. Effects of aging on enzyme-histochemical and contractile properties of fast- and slow-twitch skeletal muscles and single motor units in the rat. Muscle Nerve **9:** 169.

21. LARSSON L. & L. EDSTRÖM. 1986. Effects of aging on enzyme-histochemical and contractile properties of fast- and slow-twitch single motor units in the rat. Proc. Int. Union Physiol. Sci. XXXth Congr. (Vancouver) **XVI:** 273.

22. ILAR (INSTITUTE FOR LABORATORY ANIMAL RESEARCH). 1981. Mammalian Models for Research on Aging, p. 75–132. Nat. Acad. Press. Washington, D.C.

23. KUGELBERG, E. 1973. Histochemical composition, contraction speed and fatiguability of rat slow motor units. J. Neurol. Sci. **20:** 177–198.

24. KUGELBERG, E. 1976. Adaptive transformation of rat soleus motor units during growth. J. Neurol. Sci. **27:** 269–289.

25. FUJISAWA, K. 1974. Some observations on the skeletal musculature of aged rats. Histological aspects. J. Neurol. Sci. **22:** 353–366.

26. JENNY, E., H. WEBER, H. LUTZ & R. BILLETER. 1980. Fibre populations in rabbit skeletal muscles from birth to old age. *In* Plasticity of Muscle. D. Pette, Ed.: 97–109. de Gruyter. Berlin.

27. SALVIATI, G., R. BETTO, D. DANIELI BETTO & M. ZEVIANI. 1983. Myofibrillar-protein isoforms and sarcoplasmic-reticulum Ca^{2+}-transport activity of single human fibers. Biochem. J. **224:** 215–225.

28. DeCOSTER, W., J. DeREUCK, G. SIEBEN & H. VANDER EECKEN. 1981. Early ultrastructural changes in aging rat gastrocnemius muscle. A stereologic study. Muscle Nerve **4:** 111–116.

DISCUSSION OF THE PAPER

A. ALTAR (*CIBA–GEIGY Corporation, Summit, NJ*): Does the denervation occurring as a function of old age occur before the fallout of entire motor units? If so, is there any evidence for upregulation of nicotinic receptors that could compensate for this loss of innervation?

L. LARSSON (*Karolinska Hospital, Stockholm, Sweden*): The fall of the motor unit, of course, is the denervation. However, the reinnervation is incomplete and, thus, there is a loss of muscle cells during aging. The change in fiber-type proportion, though, precedes the loss in muscle cells. After that, there is an unselected loss of motor units irrespective of type (phasic or tonic).

ALTAR: Therefore, is it more likely that you would see some upregulation of nicotinic receptors?

LARSSON: We have not looked into that particularly.

D. B. CALNE (*University of British Columbia, Vancouver, British Columbia, Canada*): That seems to be a rather characteristic feature of the aging process; that is, that the normal regulatory mechanisms do not take place. For example, from D. Wong's data on the aging loss of dopamine receptors, we know that nigral cells are dying. Are then the dopamine receptors going up? No, they are going down, which is exactly analogous to the situation here.

G. KAMEN (*Indiana University, Bloomington, IN*): Is it that there is no upregulation?

CALNE: No. I do not know about the muscle situation, but during an actively progressive loss of motor neurons (as in motor neuron disease), you get a spreading of fibers and a hypertrophy of some of the remaining fibers. I do not know, though, specifically about the receptor data.

KAMEN: Can you tell us something about how these animals were housed? To what extent were these changes due to aging and to what extent were they due to a lifetime of reduced physical activity?

LARSSON: They were all caged under the same conditions. There were about three to four animals per cage (which was about half a meter wide) and they were fed the same diets. Most of these rats were physically inactive. However, I do not think that the observed changes were due to inactivity because the fast-twitch muscles (which are most prone to show signs of inactivity) showed no signs of fiber atrophy. This was true for the fast-twitch tibular anterior muscle and the fast-twitch EDL muscle. Thus, I do not think that an inactivity effect is at work here—perhaps in man, but not in the rat.

M. YAHR (*Mount Sinai School of Medicine, New York, NY*): Is there a difference between small and large muscles?

LARSSON: Yes, in man, it is claimed that there is a difference—that is, that the large muscles are more affected by age than the small muscles.

Neurophysiological and Morphological Alterations in Caudate Neurons in Aged Cats[a]

MICHAEL S. LEVINE

Mental Retardation Research Center
University of California at Los Angeles
Los Angeles, California 90024

Our laboratory has been studying the changes that occur in the basal ganglia of cats as they age from young adults through middle age to senescence. We have identified a series of morphological and neurophysiological alterations that occur both in middle-aged and older cats. The purpose of this paper is to briefly describe this work and to show that the results of this research provide a standardized set of neurophysiological and morphological measures for qualitative and quantitative determination of changes due to aging. These findings indicate that the basal ganglia can provide a useful and important model system for both the determination of the mechanisms involved in aging and for the development of strategies that can restore neuronal communication, alleviate deficiencies, and prevent additional changes due to the aging process from occurring.

There is pharmacological, neurochemical, and morphological evidence indicating that marked alterations in neuronal function occur in the basal ganglia in aged humans and animals.[1-4] A large portion of this research concerns the neostriatum [caudate nucleus (Cd) and putamen], which is a major component of the basal ganglia. In contrast, there is relatively little information on the neurophysiological changes that occur as a consequence of the aging process or how these changes relate to morphological and pharmacological indices. The present research was thus designed to assess the neurophysiological and morphological changes that occur in Cd neurons in aged cats.[5,6] Extracellular recordings were used to determine the electrophysiological alterations in Cd neurons. In parallel experiments, morphological changes that occur in Cd medium-sized spiny neurons stained by the rapid Golgi technique were assessed. In the mature cat, these neurons are distributed throughout the Cd nucleus and appear to constitute a very high proportion of all Cd cells.[7,8]

METHODS

Neurophysiology

Extracellular single unit recordings were obtained from neurons in the Cd of 14 cats. Seven mature adult cats of 1–3 years of age and two cats of 6–7 years of age were obtained from the Mental Retardation Research Center (MRRC) cat breeding

[a] This work was supported by USPHS Grant Nos. AG 01558 and HD 05958.

colony at the University of California at Los Angeles (UCLA). Five cats of 11–14 years of age were obtained from two sources: retired breeders from the UCLA colony (n = 2) and the Starkist Cat Food Company (n = 3). The animals were divided into three age groups (1–3, 6–7, and 11–14 years) (TABLE 1).

Surgical procedures for acute electrophysiological preparations and computer-assisted data analysis have been detailed elsewhere.[9–11] Briefly, all animals were anesthetized initially with sodium brevital (a short-acting barbiturate). Throughout the experiment, anesthesia was maintained by continuous administration of respiratory mixtures of halothane, nitrous oxide, and oxygen. Stimulating electrodes were placed in the precruciate cortex (CX) and in the substantia nigra (SN) ipsilateral to the recorded Cd; these structures provide two major inputs to the Cd.[8] When a neuron was isolated, spontaneous activity was recorded and then the ability of the neuron to respond to electrical stimulation of each site was tested. The following measurements were obtained: type of response (excitation, inhibition, excitation-inhibition sequence), response threshold (minimum current necessary to produce the response), response latency (for initially excitatory responses), response duration (for inhibitory responses), and ability to follow pairs of stimuli (for initially excitatory responses). For each evoked neuronal response, thresholds were determined by decreasing the stimulation current until a response was no longer evident on the oscilloscopic monitor. Response type, response latency, and responses to paired pulses were tested at 1.5 times the threshold current. At this intensity, the type of response and its latency were stable for each neuron.

Morphology

Eleven cats were used as subjects in the morphological experiments. Five mature adult cats of 1–3 years of age were obtained from the MRRC colony. Six cats of 13–18 years of age were obtained from three different sources: retired breeders from the UCLA colony (n = 1), the Starkist Cat Food Company (n = 3), and the brains of two cats were obtained from local veterinarians. The animals were divided into four age groups (1–3, 13, 15, and 18 years) (TABLE 1).

Animals were sacrificed by vascular perfusion with 10% neutral buffered formalin. Brains obtained from the veterinarians were not perfused, but they had been immersed in 10% buffered formalin within one hour of death. The time interval between death and tissue immersion was well within the limits to avoid postmortem artifact.[12] Tissue blocks were dissected from the Cd and processed by the rapid Golgi method. Only

TABLE 1. Age Groups and Number of Neurons Examined

Age (years)	Number of Cats	Gender		Total Neurons Examined
		Males	Females	
Neurophysiology				
1–3	7	1	6	111
6–7	2	0	2	36
11–14	5	0	5	85
Morphology				
1–3	5	2	3	75
13	2	1	1	30
15	2	0	2	29
18	2	1	1	30

well-impregnated tissue that satisfied all the criteria for quantitative analyses was included in this study.[12] These criteria were: (1) good impregnation of all dendrites with continuous staining throughout their lengths; (2) neuron soma located in the middle of each section and all (or nearly all) of the dendritic field confined to the section; (3) "medium-spiny" neurons as defined by the presence of dendritic spines and by soma diameters not larger than about 25 µm; and (4) neurons selected from the head of the Cd nucleus.

Details of computer-assisted techniques for three-dimensional reconstruction of neurons have been published.[13] For each cell, the following parameters were determined: number of dendrites, average dendritic field radius, average dendritic length, average number of branches per dendrite, average branch length, and total dendritic length. The total dendritic length represented the summed distance of all branches of all dendrites of a single neuron. The dendritic field radius was calculated by taking the dis-

TABLE 2. Response Type and Threshold

Age (years)	Neurons Tested	Number Responding	Initial Excitation	Initial Inhibition	Average Latency to Excitation (ms)
			Cortex		
1–3	100	89 (89%)[a]	67 (75%)	22 (25%)	15.2 ± 0.95^b
6–7	33	30 (91%)	16 (53%)[c]	14 (47%)	11.3 ± 0.85
11–14	80	65 (81%)	40 (62%)[c]	25 (38%)	12.1 ± 0.87^d
			Substantia Nigra		
1–3	81	64 (79%)	44 (69%)	20 (31%)	18.4 ± 1.11
6–7	28	15 (54%)	3 (20%)[c]	12 (80%)	13.3 ± 1.2
11–14	68	46 (68%)	16 (35%)[c]	30 (65%)	17.5 ± 2.02

	Response Threshold (mA)		
	Excitation	Inhibition	% Increase (Excitation/Inhibition)
		Cortex	
1–3	1.27 ± 0.13	1.13 ± 0.17	12%
6–7	2.42 ± 0.30	1.35 ± 0.25	79%
11–14	1.37 ± 0.12	0.95 ± 0.11	$44\%^e$
		Substantia Nigra	
1–3	0.62 ± 0.05	0.57 ± 0.11	9%
6–7	0.68 ± 0.09	0.49 ± 0.09	39%
11–14	0.76 ± 0.12	0.54 ± 0.11	$41\%^e$

[a] Percentage of total.

[b] Mean ± SE.

[c] Decrease in excitation statistically significant: $\chi^2 = 3.91$, df = 1, $p < 0.04$ for cortex; $\chi^2 = 23.15$, df = 1, $p < 0.003$ for substantia nigra.

[d] Decrease in latency statistically significant: $t = 2.20$, df = 105, $p < 0.025$.

[e] Increase in threshold statistically significant: $t = 5.16$, df = 4, $p < 0.01$ for cortex; $t = 2.70$, df = 4, $p < 0.05$ for substantia nigra.

tance from the soma origin to the distalmost branch point or to the free end of each dendrite and then determining that mean value for each neuron. The values for these parameters for all cells in a given age group were averaged. Spines were counted along the longest terminal branch of the longest dendrite of a population of neurons in each age group. The criteria for selection of dendritic spines were similar to those used in recent reports.[7,13]

RESULTS

Neurophysiology

Extracellular single unit recordings were obtained from 232 neurons located in the head of the Cd nucleus (TABLES 1 and 2). Histological reconstruction of the recording sites indicated that the same region of the head of the Cd was sampled in each age group. There were no consistent differences among the three age groups in the duration of action potentials, their amplitude, or waveform (FIGURE 1).

The proportion of Cd neurons responding to stimulation of CX was similar in the 1–3- and 6–7-year-old groups. However, there was a slight decrease in this value in the 11–14-year-old animals (TABLE 2). When SN was stimulated, decreases in the proportion of responsive neurons occurred in both groups of aged cats (TABLE 2). A major finding was that there was a significant change in the proportion of occurrence of different types of evoked neuronal responses in both groups of aged cats as compared to the 1–3-year-old cats (TABLE 2). The types of responses that were evoked in each age group consisted of either excitation (increase in the frequency of occurrence

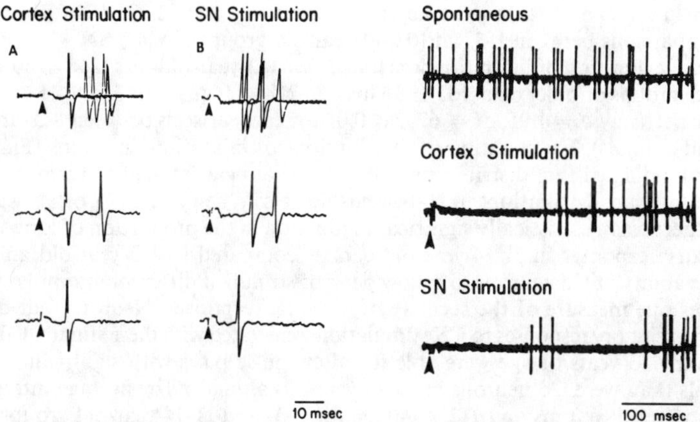

FIGURE 1. Examples of excitatory and inhibitory responses to activation of CX and SN in Cd neurons from a 14-year-old cat. (A) CX stimulation. Top: Four superimposed traces. The two traces below are single responses. There is a fixed latency excitatory response at about 7 ms that is followed by a variable latency second response. (B) SN stimulation. Top: Four superimposed traces. The two traces below are single responses. There is a variable latency excitatory response between 7–15 ms. Right panel: Examples of inhibitory responses to activation of CX and SN. Each trace is 10 superimposed responses. Top: Spontaneous activity. The inhibitory response in this neuron was 160 ms in duration after CX stimulation (middle) and 125 ms in duration after SN stimulation (bottom). In all traces, stimulation occurs at the arrows.

of action potentials), inhibition (decrease in frequency of action potentials), or a sequence of excitation followed by inhibition (FIGURE 1). For purposes of this analysis, responses were considered as being either initially excitatory or initially inhibitory. Sequences of excitation followed by inhibition were considered to be initially excitatory responses. The decreases in the frequency of occurrence of initially excitatory responses in Cd neurons in aged cats when either CX or SN was stimulated were statistically significant (TABLE 2). When CX was stimulated, the proportion of initially excitatory responses decreased by 13–25%, while when SN was stimulated, the decrease in the frequency of occurrence of initially excitatory responses was greater (35–49%).

There was a statistically significant increase in threshold current for evoking excitatory responses in Cd neurons of aged cats (TABLE 2). This increase occurred in both the 6–7- and 11–14-year-old groups. In cats of 1–3 years of age, the thresholds for evoking either initially excitatory or initially inhibitory responses were approximately equal for stimulation of either CX or SN. In 6–7- and 11–14-year-old cats, there were 79% and 44% increases in threshold for evoking excitatory responses when CX was stimulated and 39% and 41% increases when SN was stimulated, respectively.

The average latencies to orthodromically evoked action potentials in Cd neurons decreased in both groups of aged cats as compared to animals in the 1–3-year-old group. The decrease in average latency when CX was stimulated was statistically significant for comparisons between 1–3- and 11–14-year-old animals (TABLE 2). Distributions of latencies of excitatory responses evoked by CX or SN stimulation in aged cats were significantly different from those of 1–3-year-old animals (FIGURES 2A and 2C). Examination of the differences among the distributions indicated that the decrease in latency was due to a loss of longer latency responses.

The duration of inhibition decreased in both groups of aged cats regardless of which input was stimulated. The average duration of inhibition for CX stimulation in 1–3-year-old cats decreased from 333 ± 37 ms (mean $\pm$ SE) to 259 ± 26 ms and 244 ± 15 ms in 6–7- and 11–14-year-old cats, respectively ($t = 2.09$, df $= 85$, $p < 0.025$ for comparisons between 1–3- and 11–14-year-old groups). When SN was stimulated, the average duration of inhibition was longer for 1–3-year-old cats (248 ± 19 ms) than for both groups of older cats (162 ± 16 ms and 211 ± 16 ms in 6–7- and 11–14-year-old cats, respectively; $t = 1.95$, df $= 67$, $p < 0.05$ for comparisons between 1–3- and 11–14-year-old animals). Examination of distributions of inhibition durations (FIGURES 2B and 2D) indicated that distributions in 1–3-year-old cats tended to be more variable and flatter than distributions in 11–14-year-old cats. When either CX or SN was stimulated, there was a statistically significant reduction in the proportion of long-duration inhibitory responses in 11–14-year-old cats as compared to 1–3-year-old animals.

The ability of Cd neurons to follow pairs of stimuli at different interpulse intervals provides one measure of the security of synaptic responses. Neurons that displayed initially excitatory responses to CX stimulation were tested with these stimuli. Cd neurons in cats of 1–3 years of age were able to follow pulse pairs with significantly shorter intervals than were Cd neurons in 11–14-year-old animals. The average interpulse intervals were 45 ± 7 ms and 112 ± 40 ms for 1–3- and 11–14-year-old groups, respectively ($t = 2.19$, df $= 81$, $p < 0.05$). The differences between distributions of these measures were also statistically significant (FIGURE 2E). Although neurons were encountered in both age groups that could follow pulse pairs at relatively short intervals (10–50 ms), there was a marked increase in the aged animals in the proportion of neurons that followed at extremely long intervals (>200 ms).

There also was a decrease in the spontaneous firing rates of Cd neurons recorded from the 11–14-year-old group as compared to the 1–3-year-old group. The distributions of mean interspike intervals for all neurons in each age group were significantly

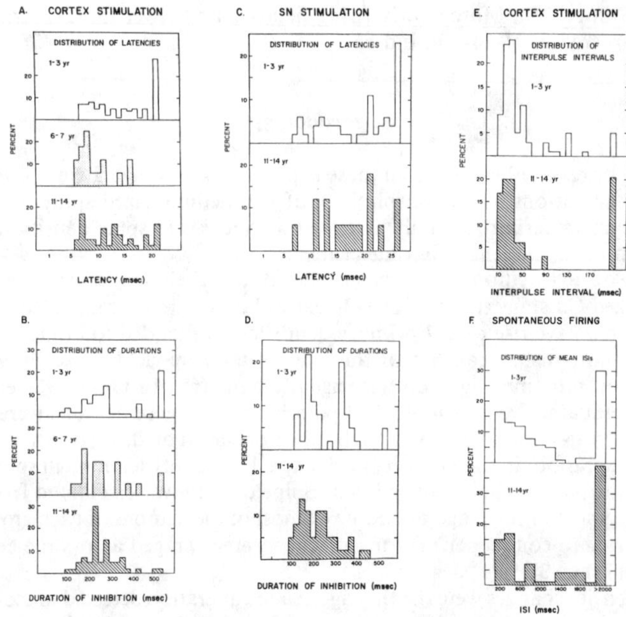

FIGURE 2. Frequency distributions for neurophysiological measures. In this figure, the last bin of each distribution is an overflow bin and contains all values equal to or greater than the value indicated on the abscissa. (A) Frequency distributions of latencies of excitatory responses evoked by CX stimulation. Note the decrease in longer latency responses (>20 ms) in 6–7- and 11–14-year-old groups. Distributions from 1–3- and 11–14-year-old groups were significantly different ($\chi^2 = 31.6$, df = 15, $p < 0.0079$). The bin size is 1 ms. All responses greater than 20 ms in latency are contained in the overflow bin. (B) Frequency distributions of durations of inhibitory responses evoked by CX stimulation. Note the reduction in the proportion of long-duration inhibitory responses in 6–7- and 11–14-year-old groups. Distributions from 1–3- and 11–14-year-old groups were significantly different ($\chi^2 = 42.8$, df = 17, $p < 0.0005$). Bin size is 25 ms. All responses greater than 500 ms are contained in the overflow bin. (C) Frequency distributions of latencies of excitatory responses evoked by SN stimulation. There is a decrease in longer latency responses (>25 ms) in 11–14-year-old cats. Distributions from 1–3- and 11–14-year-old groups were significantly different ($\chi^2 = 59.8$, df = 18, $p < 0.00025$). Bin size is 1 ms. All responses greater than 25 ms are contained in the overflow bin. Data from 6–7-year-old cats are not plotted because only a small number of excitatory responses occurred. (D) Frequency distributions of durations of inhibitory responses evoked by SN stimulation. Note the decrease in frequency of long-duration responses and the flattening of the distribution in the 11–14-year-old group. Distributions from 1–3- and 11–14-year-old groups were significantly different ($\chi^2 = 66.9$, df = 15, $p < 0.0002$). Bin size is 25 ms. All responses >500 ms are contained in the overflow bin. (E) Frequency distribution of minimum interpulse intervals. Overall, there was a reduction in the proportion of shorter minimum intervals in 11–14-year-old cats and an increase in the proportion of longer intervals. Distributions from 1–3- and 11–14-year-old groups were significantly different ($\chi^2 = 21.9$, df = 11, $p < 0.025$). Bin size is 10 ms. All responses >200 ms are contained in the overflow bin. Data from SN stimulation are not plotted because only a small number of neurons were tested. (F) Frequency distributions of mean interspike intervals (ISIs) for Cd neurons. Distributions from 1–3- and 11–14-year-old groups were significantly different ($\chi^2 = 24.1$, df = 10, $p < 0.0079$). There was an increase in the proportion of occurrence of slowly firing neurons in 11–14-year-old cats. Only data obtained from 1–3- and 11–14-year-old groups are plotted. Bin size is 200 ms. All mean ISIs >2000 ms are contained in the overflow bin.

different (FIGURE 2F). More slowly firing neurons and fewer rapidly firing neurons were encountered in 11–14-year-old cats.

Morphology

The major result obtained from these experiments was that there is a sequence of age-related alterations in the morphology of Cd medium-sized spiny neurons. This sequence is characterized, initially, in time by decreases in spine density followed by decreases in dendritic length in older cats.

A total of 164 neurons were reconstructed and their processes were measured. Medium-sized Cd spiny neurons in 1–3-year-old cats were characterized by round to oval soma that gave rise to 3–7 primary dendrites that tended to branch close to the soma. The more distal branches of these dendrites were richly covered with spines, while the most proximal segments were usually spine-free. In 15- and 18-year-old cats, many of the qualitative morphological parameters for these neurons were similar to those of 1–3-year-old animals. Although spines occurred on distal dendritic segments, there were alterations in their density and shape. For quantification, all spine-like profiles on dendritic branches were counted. Spine density was calculated from the longest distal segment of the longest dendrite of most of the neurons of each group. Counts were converted to counts per micron and they were averaged across the cells in each age group (TABLE 3).

Spine density changes were the first age-related alteration detected in these neurons. There was a statistically significant decrease in spine density in all older groups as compared to 1–3-year-old animals ($F = 21.3$, df $= 3/90$, $p < 0.05$). Spines were categorized into four groups according to shape: stalks with heads, heads with no stalks,

TABLE 3. Morphological Parameters

Age (years)	Total Length (μm)	Dendrite Length (μm)	Branch Length (μm)	Field Radius (μm)	Length Closed Ends (μm)	Length Free Ends (μm)
1–3	4202 ± 154^a	836 ± 75	89 ± 3	206 ± 5	29 ± 0.8	122 ± 4
13	3900 ± 142 $(-7\%)^b$	813 ± 30 (-3%)	86 ± 3 (-3%)	197 ± 8 (-4%)	28 ± 1.1 (-3%)	121 ± 4 (-1%)
15	2553 ± 142^c (-39%)	590 ± 29^c (-29%)	58 ± 3^c (-35%)	140 ± 6^c (-32%)	25 ± 0.7 (-14%)	82 ± 4^c (-33%)
18	2458 ± 185^c (-42%)	563 ± 30^c (-33%)	56 ± 2^c (-37%)	140 ± 6^c (-32%)	27 ± 1.5 (-7%)	76 ± 4^c (-37%)

Age	Number Dendrites	Branches/Dendrite	Spine Density (Spines/μm)
1–3	5.28 ± 0.14	9.9 ± 0.3	0.953 ± 0.039
13	5.18 ± 0.23 (-2%)	10.0 ± 0.6 $(+1\%)$	0.799 ± 0.054^c (-16%)
15	4.62 ± 0.26 (-12%)	10.3 ± 0.6 $(+4\%)$	0.488 ± 0.044^c (-49%)
18	4.67 ± 0.26 (-12%)	10.1 ± 0.7 $(+2\%)$	0.572 ± 0.052^c (-40%)

[a] Mean ± SE of mean.
[b] Percentage change from the 1–3-year-old group.
[c] Statistically significant difference from the 1–3-year-old group.

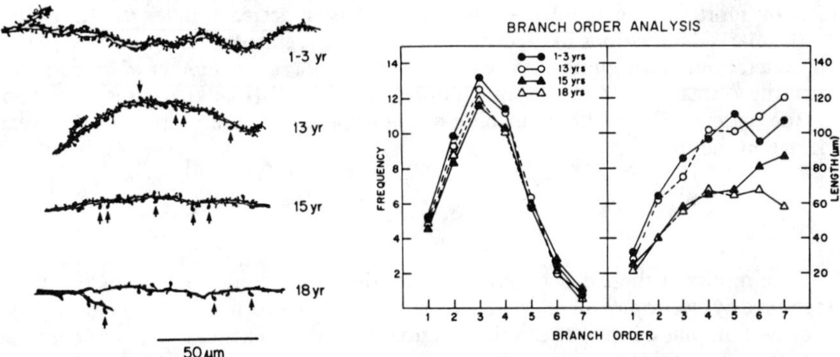

FIGURE 3. Left panel: Camera lucida drawings of distal dendritic segments of medium-sized spiny Cd neurons from 1–3-, 13-, 15-, and 18-year-old cats. Dendritic diameters are noticeably thinner and spine density is reduced in the 15- and 18-year-old dendrites. The arrows show some enlarged spine heads. Right panel: Branch order analysis. The left side of the drawing shows the average frequency per neuron of the number of branches at each order. The right side shows the average length per neuron of each branch order. Order 7 is an overflow category that contains data from all orders greater than 6.

pins (thin stalk with small heads), and enlarged heads. The frequency of occurrence of each of these categories was determined for each age group. In all aged animals, a population of spines with enlarged heads was observed (20–30%) (FIGURE 3). Such spines rarely occurred in cats of 1–3 years of age (less than 5%). In addition, a decrease in the thickness of distal segments was observed in some dendritic branches in aged cats (FIGURE 3). These thinner dendritic segments usually had few spines (FIGURE 3). While it was apparent that many distal dendritic segments displayed decreases in spine density, there was also a high degree of variation on different dendritic segments, even on the same neuron.[5]

There were marked statistically significant decreases in virtually all measures of dendritic length in aged cats (TABLE 3). These included the total length of all dendrites (−40%), the average dendrite length (−30%), the average branch length (−35%), and the radius of the dendritic field (−30%). The results of these analyses indicated that the major length decreases were occurring after 13 years of age. In order to determine if all dendritic branches were contributing to these decreases, the branch lengths for branches with free ends (terminal branches) and with closed ends were compared (TABLE 3). There were no decreases in the length of branches with closed ends. In contrast, the terminal branch length decreased significantly in cats over 13 years of age (−35%).

To further assess the contribution of different types of dendritic branches to this pattern of length decrease, an analysis of branch length by branch order was performed. Branch order for all branches on each dendrite was calculated by having the computer assign the order number 1 to the initial branch emanating from the soma. The numbering continued sequentially to the distal dendritic branches, with the number being raised by one beyond each branch point. Branch lengths were sorted into categories by order (FIGURE 3). The branch length changed significantly as a function of both age ($F = 6.3$, df $= 3/160$, $p < 0.01$) and order ($F = 17$, df $= 18/960$, $p < 0.01$). Statistically significant decreases in length occurred in both 15- and 18-year-old groups at all orders except the first. These decreases became more marked at the higher orders, with the more peripheral branches showing the largest decreases in length. In contrast to the marked alterations in the length of dendritic segments, there were few systematic alterations in the number of dendrites per neuron, in the number of branches per dendrite (TABLE 3), and in the branch order in aged cats (FIGURE 3). Reorganization of the pattern of dendritic branching did not appear to occur between 13–18 years of age in the cat.

DISCUSSION

The results of these experiments indicate that functional changes in Cd neurons measured by electrophysiological activity appear to be correlated morphologically with decreases in spine density. The major electrophysiological changes consist of decreases in the proportion of excitatory responses that can be evoked by activation of Cd inputs; increases in the threshold current necessary to evoke these excitatory responses; decreases in the ability of Cd neurons to follow temporally, closely spaced stimuli; reductions in the duration of inhibitory responses; and decreases in spontaneous activity. The first morphological alteration that occurs in Cd medium spiny neurons is a decrease in spine density on distal dendritic segments. In older animals, these decreases are followed by a loss of parts of distal dendritic segments. No significant changes appear in the organization of individual dendrites, in the number of dendrites per neuron, nor in the number of branches per dendrite in cats of 13–18 years of age.

The present evidence suggests that there are changes in excitatory activity in Cd neurons in aged cats. The most prominent change is a decrease in the proportion of initially excitatory responses that occurs when Cd inputs are activated. This decrease is largest when afferents from SN are stimulated, but it is also apparent when CX is stimulated. Reduced excitability is also reflected by decreases in spontaneous firing and increases in response threshold. Furthermore, intracellular recording experiments indicate that most Cd neurons respond to activation of their monosynaptic inputs with an initially excitatory postsynaptic potential (EPSP).[14-16] This response is usually followed by an inhibitory postsynaptic potential (IPSP).[14-16] This IPSP is thought to be generated, at least in part, by mutual inhibition from neighboring Cd neurons.[11,14,15] Frequently, the amplitude of the EPSP does not reach threshold for producing an action potential.[14-16] If extracellular recordings are made (as in the present experiment), an EPSP without an evoked action potential would be classified as an initially inhibitory response. From the present data, it cannot be ascertained whether there are proportionately fewer EPSPs or whether the EPSPs occur but are subthreshold for generation of action potentials in aged cats. The major morphological alteration occurring in 11–14-year-old cats is a decrease in spine density. Because most inputs to the Cd synapse on the spines[8] and produce initially excitatory effects, the loss of spines provides an anatomical substrate for the decrease in excitation in Cd neurons.

Although many Cd neurons in aged cats can follow paired pulses at short interpulse intervals, a population of cells in this group could only follow paired pulses at long interpulse intervals. This population is infrequent in 1–3-year-old cats. The fact, though, that this latter population exists in the aged cat indicates that the short-interval following failed in these neurons. Because of the long time period over which pairs of pulses could be separated (2–500 ms), several phenomena may contribute to the differences among the age groups. These include changes in inhibitory events in the Cd as well as changes in excitatory and inhibitory events outside the Cd, decreases in spine or synaptic density (see below),[17] decreases in the amount of transmitter released from Cd afferents, and increases in refractory periods of CX input fibers.

The frequency of occurrence of inhibitory responses in Cd neurons in aged cats increases. However, their duration decreases. The increase in frequency of inhibition is probably a result of the decrease in excitation. As indicated above, either fewer EPSPs or smaller amplitude EPSPs occur in a population of neurons in the Cd of the aged cat. Action potentials are evoked less frequently in this population of neurons. Consequently, these neurons do not produce as much lateral inhibition of neighboring cells via their local axon collaterals.[11,14,15] As our data indicate, all neurons are not equally affected by the aging process. Another population of neurons displays action potentials (and presumably undiminished EPSPs) when their inputs are activated. This population is capable of inhibiting neighboring cells. Thus, in the aged cat, neurons can display fewer excitatory responses, but they still can maintain inhibitory responses because they receive inhibitory inputs from neighboring neurons less affected by the aging process. When these events are observed with extracellular recordings in which EPSPs subthreshold for spike generation cannot be detected, the result is an increase in the proportion of inhibitory responses. Because fewer neurons display excitatory responses in aged cats, the lateral inhibition is reduced and the IPSPs should be of lower amplitude and of shorter duration. Although amplitude could not be measured in the present experiment, the duration of inhibition is reduced in aged cats. FIGURE 4 illustrates diagrammatically how the loss of excitatory inputs in Cd neurons in aged cats produces changes in inhibition.

A significant decrease in the average latency of responses evoked by CX stimulation was also observed in aged cats. This was an entirely unexpected finding because previous neurophysiological experiments have indicated that decreases in conduction velocity and hence increases in the latency of responses occur in aged animals.[18-20] Examination of distributions did not indicate that shorter latency responses occurred; instead, there was a loss of longer latency responses in aged animals. In fact, it has been demonstrated that some of these longer latency responses in the Cd are probably not monosynaptic; rather, they are due to indirect activation of Cd neurons.[21] In the aged cats, it is probably these multisynaptic responses that decrease in frequency of occurrence. Indirect polysynaptic responses would be more affected by decrements in both excitation and in synaptic security. Altered timing of these long-latency inputs in reaching Cd target neurons could result in less efficient spatial and temporal summation.

The present study is the first demonstration of regressive changes in the morphology of Cd neurons in aged cats. In many respects, these observations are similar to those reported for other areas of the brain.[22,23] A series of studies has provided evidence that there is also plasticity and growth in both human and rodent brains well past the period normally defined as the developmental phase.[24-26] For example, dendrites of mature neurons have been shown to expand in response to environmental manipulation, electrical stimulation, and experimental lesions.[27,28] In well-controlled quantitative studies, Buell and Coleman[29] reported that the dendrites of neurons in human parahippocampal gyrus continued to expand throughout the eighth decade of life. In a more recent study, it was shown that regressive changes occurred in the oldest cases examined.[30] In the age groups examined in the present experiments, though, there was no evidence of expansion in any of the parameters.

However, in recently completed unpublished studies, we have found that there is a significant increase in the number of branches per dendrite on Cd spiny neurons from 6–9 years of age in the cat.[17] These data provide evidence that dendritic growth continues past maturity at 1–3 years of age in the cat. The present findings, though, indicate that functional decrements begin to appear in Cd neurons of cats during this age period. There are proportionately fewer excitatory responses, the thresholds for

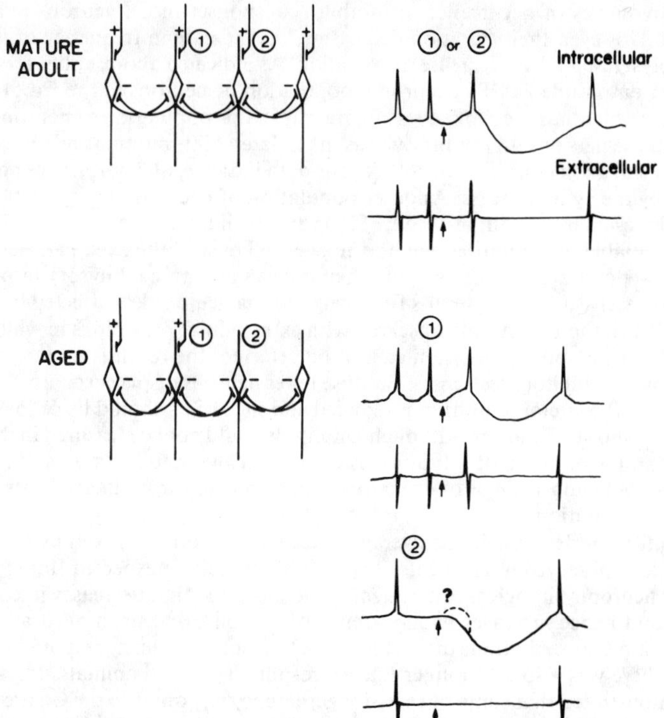

FIGURE 4. A diagram illustrating the hypothesis of how the loss of excitatory inputs of Cd neurons during aging alters duration and frequency of inhibitory responses. In the "mature" adult (top), excitatory inputs to the Cd synapse on neurons that mutually inhibit each other. Recording from any neuron (case no. 1 or 2) yields similar electrophysiological activity when inputs are activated. When such recordings are performed intracellularly and inputs are stimulated (at the arrow), the result is an evoked EPSP followed by an IPSP.[14-16] When extracellular recordings are performed (as in the present experiment), an evoked action potential is followed by a period of inhibition. In the aged animal (bottom), it is hypothesized that some neurons still receive excitatory inputs (the left two neurons), while others display a reduction in such inputs (the right two neurons). It is also hypothesized that neurons are still mutually inhibitory. If recordings are made from neurons that receive normal excitatory inputs (case no. 1), then the initial excitation will occur; however, the inhibition will be of smaller amplitude and duration because some of the surrounding neurons are not activated and hence cannot inhibit their neighbors. When extracellular recordings are made, shorter duration inhibitory responses should occur, as in the present experiments. When recordings are made from neurons that display reductions in excitation, only inhibitory responses are observed in extracellular records (case no. 2). This is because evoked EPSPs are either of insufficient magnitude to evoke action potentials or they do not occur (the question mark in the recording of case no. 2). Because intracellular recording experiments have not yet been performed in the Cd in aged animals, it has not been determined whether EPSPs are of smaller amplitude or are absent completely. However, the neuron illustrated in case no. 2 still receives inhibitory inputs. The extracellular recordings will show only the inhibitory responses. The duration of inhibition, though, will tend to be shorter because some of the surrounding neurons are also not activated.

evoking excitatory responses are higher, and the inhibitory responses are of shorter duration. Our unpublished studies also indicate that there are other morphological changes in 6–9-year-old cats that suggest that the newly formed branches may not become functional. The density of synapses in the neuropil and the density of dendritic spines are decreased and the new branches are significantly shorter.[17] Finally, behavioral alterations that may reflect impaired information processing in Cd neurons begin to occur in cats during this age period.[31]

Evidence from single cell electrophysiological experiments indicates that there are marked alterations during aging in several brain regions in a variety of species. Most of these changes reflect decreased function. Cerebellar Purkinje neurons in aged rats have slower discharge rates and show reduced excitability to afferent parallel fiber stimulation.[19,20] Spontaneous firing rates decrease in locus ceruleus and hippocampal neurons.[32-34] Spinal cord motorneurons in cats display conduction velocity decreases, membrane potential resistance increases, and alterations in monosynaptic inputs.[18] A recent study in aged rats indicates (similar to the present experiment) that there are decreases in spontaneous activity of Cd neurons.[35] In addition, decreases in the responsiveness of single cells in a number of areas in aged rats have been reported for the application of putative neurotransmitters.[36,37]

The changes in Cd neurophysiology and morphology may underlie some of the behavioral dysfunctions in aged cats. Behavioral data indicate that such animals have difficulty in processing information about the relevance of stimuli.[31] Cats over 10 years of age continue to react in situations in which cats of 1–3 years of age readily habituate. In addition, they do not appear to use information about previous reinforcement in the same way as young cats do because they can easily change previously reinforced preferences. Experimental lesions of the Cd produce behavioral disturbances that have some symptoms in common with the behavioral alterations exhibited by the aged cats.[38] There is a marked change in the ability of cats with Cd damage to habituate to repeated stimuli. Unlike aged animals, however, cats with Cd lesions perseverate in responding to previously reinforced stimuli.

Deficits in specific neurotransmitter systems occur in the basal ganglia during aging.[2] In the Cd, most of these deficits have been associated with changes in the dopaminergic neurotransmission that can occur even by mid-life periods.[2-4,39,40] It is possible that the electrophysiological alterations that we have observed in both 6–7- and 11–14-year-old cats reflect dysfunctions within the dopaminergic nigrostriatal system. For example, the largest and most consistent decrease in the excitatory response occurred when SN was stimulated. It is possible that reduced responsiveness of the dopaminergic system might also underlie some of the changes evoked by CX stimulation. It has generally been hypothesized that dopamine functions as a modulator of synaptic transmission and is capable of both facilitating and inhibiting Cd inputs from other sources.[41-43]

There are a number of problems that could have influenced the outcomes of these studies. First, because the aged cats are anesthetized during recording experiments, it is possible that increased sensitivity to the anesthetic or to the conditions of the experiment confounds the results. In a recent study, though, results similar to those obtained in the present experiment are demonstrated in unanesthetized cats, thus indicating that artifacts of anesthesia or surgical preparation in the aged animals are not major variables.[44] Second, the morphological and neurophysiological correlations obtained in these experiments depend upon the assumption that the majority of recordings are made from medium-sized Cd spiny neurons. If this assumption is incorrect, then different types of neurons may have been sampled in the physiological and morphological experiments. However, when intracellular recording is combined with intracellular labeling to identify recorded neurons, results from different laboratories and from different species indicate that over 95% of the Cd neurons sampled are medium-sized spiny neurons.[11,16,45] Third, experiential variables may have affected the outcome of these studies. There are considerable data on rodents showing that environmental conditions have an important role in determining the severity and nature of age-related morphological and electrophysiological alterations.[24-28] Although cats from different populations were used and similar results were obtained from each population, all animals were maintained under laboratory conditions. Therefore, the present results may not be easily generalizable to cats maintained under other conditions. However, because some of these findings have been partially replicated in rodents, it is highly probable that many of the changes were due to the aging process. Results from a recent analysis of the effects of experience upon aging that used the cerebellum as a model system suggest that normal aging involves both loss and growth and that the relative contribution of each of these may depend upon experience.[46]

Neurophysiological alterations occur in Cd neurons well before major losses in dendritic length are apparent. It would seem that the functional alterations precede major anatomical disturbances in connectivity (the loss of dendritic segments) and that more subtle morphological disturbances underlie the physiological changes. Because recordings were not performed in cats over 14 years of age, it is difficult to determine if the neurophysiological changes would become more severe in these older animals. However, in order to further understand the mechanisms responsible for these changes and to provide therapeutic strategies for restoring function, experimentation should be directed at the middle-aged groups of animals. It is during this time that functional, biochemical, and morphological alterations are interacting to produce many of the phenomena described in this research.

REFERENCES

1. BUGIANI, O., S. SALVARANI, F. PERDELLI, G. L. MANCARDI & A. LEONARDI. 1978. Eur. Neurol. **17:** 286–291.
2. FINCH, C. E., P. K. RANDALL & J. F. MARSHALL. 1981. Ann. Rev. Gerontol. Geriatr. **2:** 49–87.
3. GOVONI, S., P. LODDO, P. F. SPANO & M. TRABUCCHI. 1977. Brain Res. **138:** 565–570.
4. MCGEER, E. G., H. C. FIBIGER, P. L. MCGEER & V. WICKSON. 1971. Exp. Gerontol. **6:** 391–396.
5. LEVINE, M. S., A. M. ADINOLFI, R. S. FISHER, C. D. HULL, N. A. BUCHWALD & J. P. MCALLISTER. 1986. Neurobiol. Aging **7:** 277–286.
6. LEVINE, M. S., R. L. LLOYD, C. D. HULL, R. S. FISHER & N. A. BUCHWALD. 1987. Brain Res. **401:** 213–230.
7. DIFIGLIA M., P. PASIK & T. PASIK. 1976. Brain Res. **114:** 245–256.
8. KEMP, J. M. & T. P. S. POWELL. 1971. Philos. Trans. R. Soc. London Ser. **B262:** 383–401.
9. FISHER, R. S., M. S. LEVINE, C. D. HULL & N. A. BUCHWALD. 1982. Dev. Brain Res. **3:** 443–462.
10. LEVINE, M. S., R. S. FISHER, C. D. HULL & N. A. BUCHWALD. 1982. Dev. Brain Res. **3:** 429–441.
11. LEVINE, M. S., R. S. FISHER, C. D. HULL & N. A. BUCHWALD. 1986. Dev. Brain Res. **24:** 42–62.
12. WILLIAMS, R. S., R. J. FERRANTE & V. S. CAVINESS. 1978. J. Neuropathol. **37:** 13–33.
13. HULL, C. D., J. P. MCALLISTER, M. S. LEVINE & A. M. ADINOLFI. 1981. Dev. Brain Res. **1:** 309–332.
14. BUCHWALD, N. A., D. D. PRICE, L. VERNON & C. D. HULL. 1973. Exp. Neurol. **38:** 311–323.
15. HULL, C. D., G. BERNARDI, D. D. PRICE & N. A. BUCHWALD. 1973. Exp. Neurol. **38:** 324–336.
16. KITAI, S. T., J. D. KOCSIS, R. J. PRESTON & M. SUGIOMORI. 1976. Brain Res. **109:** 601–606.
17. LEVINE, M. S., A. M. ADINOLFI, R. S. FISHER, N. A. BUCHWALD & C. D. HULL. 1985. Proc. XII Int. Anat. Congr.: 403.
18. CHASE, M. H., F. R. MORALES, P. A. BOXER & S. J. FUNG. 1985. Exp. Neurol. **90:** 471–478.

19. ROGERS, J., M. A. SILVER, W. J. SHOEMAKER & F. E. BLOOM. 1980. Neurobiol. Aging **1:** 3–11.
20. ROGERS, J., S. F. ZORNETZER & F. E. BLOOM. 1981. Neurobiol. Aging **2:** 15–25.
21. CHERUBINI, E., G. NOVACK, C. D. HULL, N. A. BUCHWALD & M. S. LEVINE. 1979. Brain Res. **173:** 331–336.
22. SCHEIBEL, M. E., R. D. LINDSAY, U. TOMIYASU & A. B. SCHEIBEL. 1975. Exp. Neurol. **47:** 392–403.
23. SCHEIBEL, M. E., R. D. LINDSAY, U. TOMIYASU & A. B. SCHEIBEL. 1976. Exp. Neurol. **53:** 420–430.
24. CONNOR, J. R., JR., M. C. DIAMOND & R. E. JOHNSON. 1980. Exp. Neurol. **68:** 158–170.
25. HINDS, J. W. & N. A. MCNELLY. 1977. J. Comp. Neurol. **171:** 345–368.
26. HOLLINGSWORTH, T. & M. BERRY. 1975. Philos. Trans. R. Soc. London Ser. **B270:** 227–264.
27. RUTLEDGE, L. T., C. WRIGHT & J. DUNCAN. 1974. Exp. Neurol. **44:** 209–228.
28. SCHADE, J. P. & C. F. BAXTER. 1960. Exp. Neurol. **2:** 158–178.
29. BUELL, S. J. & P. D. COLEMAN. 1981. Brain Res. **214:** 23–41.
30. FLOOD, D. G., S. J. BUELL, C. H. DEFIORE, G. J. HOROWITZ & P. D. COLEMAN. 1985. Brain Res. **345:** 366–368.
31. LEVINE, M. S., R. L. LLOYD, R. S. FISHER, C. D. HULL & N. A. BUCHWALD. 1987. Neurobiol. Aging **8:** 253–263.
32. BARNES, C. A. 1979. J. Comp. Physiol. Psychol. **93:** 74–104.
33. BARNES, C. A. & B. L. MCNAUGHTON. 1979. Exp. Aging Res. **5:** 195–206.
34. OLPE, H. R. & M. W. STEINMANN. 1982. Brain Res. **251:** 174–176.
35. STERN, W. C., W. W. PUGH & P. J. MORGANE. 1985. Aging **6:** 245–248.
36. JONES, R. S. G. & H-R. OLPE. 1983. Neurobiol. Aging **4:** 97–99.
37. MARWAHA, J., B. J. HOFFER & R. FREEDMAN. 1981. Neurobiol. Aging **2:** 95–98.
38. VILLABLANCA, J. R. & C. E. OLMSTEAD. 1982. Acta Neurobiol. Exp. **42:** 225–297.
39. SEVERSON, J. A. & C. E. FINCH. 1980. Brain Res. **199:** 147–162.
40. SEVERSON, J. A. & C. E. FINCH. 1980. Fed. Proc. Fed. Am. Soc. Exp. Biol. **39:** 508.
41. ABERCROMBIE, E. D. & B. L. JACOBS. 1985. Brain Res. **358:** 27–33.
42. MERCURI, N., G. BERNARDI, P. CULABRISI, A. CUTUGNO, G. LEVI & P. STANZIONE. 1985. Brain Res. **358:** 110–121.
43. SCHNEIDER, J. S., M. S. LEVINE, C. D. HULL & N. A. BUCHWALD. 1984. J. Neurosci. **4:** 930–938.
44. LEVINE, M. S., J. S. SCHNEIDER, R. L. LLOYD, R. S. FISHER, C. D. HULL & N. A. BUCHWALD. 1987. Brain Res. **405:** 389–394.
45. VANDERMAELEN, C. P. & S. T. KITAI. 1981. Brain Res. Bull. **5:** 725–733.
46. GREENOUGH, W. T., J. W. MCDONALD, R. M. PARNISARI & J. E. CAMEL. 1986. Brain Res. **380:** 136–143.

DISCUSSION OF THE PAPER

D. MORGAN (*University of Southern California, Los Angeles, CA*): Is there any anatomical evidence for those axon collaterals? In your EM, it actually looked as if you had dendritic appositions. Did you find dendrite bundling?

M. S. LEVINE (*Mental Retardation Research Center, Los Angeles, CA*): No, not a lot of that. I do not know, but we have not yet looked at the axon collaterals in aged animals. That is one of the things that we intend to do and we will probably do it with immunohistochemistry to try to identify the neurotransmitter.

M. H. WOOLLACOTT (*University of Oregon, Eugene, OR*): Can you comment on any motor coordination differences between your 15- and 18-year-old cats and your younger cats?

LEVINE: All of the cats used in these experiments went through a series of behavioral tests that included a neurological examination. Now, I have good news and bad news depending upon how you feel about the caudate nucleus. If you feel that the caudate nucleus is a structure that has to be involved in pure motor function, I have bad news for you because none of the cats were neurologically deficient; their motor responses and their reflexes were perfectly normal. In fact, in many cases, their performance was better than some of the younger cats. However, there were deficits in cognitive ability that you pick up in these cats, but I think that is another subject. There were no marked differences between 15- and 18-year-old animals.

UNIDENTIFIED DISCUSSANT: What is the life span of the cat?

LEVINE: I do not know. Some people say cats live to 25 years of age, but the oldest animal in any of these experiments was 22 years of age. That animal was a delicate animal and we did not use it in a recording experiment because we did not think that it would survive a long-term experiment. On the other hand, all the other cats were very healthy animals.

UNIDENTIFIED: How homogeneous were these cats in terms of breeds?

LEVINE: It was a mongrel population and it was not a genetically pure one. Our initial set of animals was not by any stretch of the imagination homogeneous genetically.

UNIDENTIFIED: Therefore, depending upon their genetic makeup, could there have been aging at different rates?

LEVINE: Yes.

The Sympathoadrenal Medullary Functions in Aged Rats under Anesthesia[a]

MIEKO KUROSAWA, AKIO SATO, YUKO SATO,
AND HARUE SUZUKI

Department of Physiology
Tokyo Metropolitan Institute of Gerontology
35-2 Sakaecho, Itabashiku
Tokyo 173, Japan

The most important summary of aging research to date seems to have been written by N. W. Shock, whose fundamental work (1972) indicated that various physiological functions gradually decrease with age, but at different rates.[1] As it is obvious that the motor, autonomic, and endocrinological functions are interacting, it is important to know the individual age-related autonomic and endocrinological changes if one is to better understand the motor function.

In contrast to the general decline, it has been reported that catecholamines, especially noradrenaline, in systemic blood increase during aging;[2-6] however, adrenaline in systemic blood has been measured with inconsistent results.[4,7-9] Adrenaline and noradrenaline are important humoral factors in controlling glucose metabolism, the cardiovascular and respiratory systems, certain parts of the motor system, etc.

Adrenaline is secreted exclusively by the adrenal gland, while noradrenaline is secreted from both the adrenal gland and sympathetic postganglionic nerve terminals. The secretions of adrenaline and noradrenaline from the adrenal gland are regulated by a sympathetic preganglionic nerve. The present work focuses on changes in the sympathoadrenal medullary functions during aging in anesthetized rats. There have been numerous studies concerning the age-related changes in catecholamines in systemic blood.[2-9] However, many of these studies are not accurate reflections of adrenal medullary functions because of metabolic alterations in systemic blood circulation and because of large doses of noradrenaline secreted from the postganglionic nerve terminals of the general sympathetic system. Therefore, first of all, it seems to be important to directly measure the secretion rates of both adrenaline and noradrenaline from the adrenal gland and the adrenal sympathetic ongoing nerve activity during aging. We have just done this in our laboratory[10] and the results will be reviewed briefly.

It should be emphasized that all experiments using rats in our laboratory were performed under anesthesia. Additionally, respiration (using an artificial respirator), body temperature, etc., were strictly controlled.[11]

[a] This work was supported, in part, by Grant-in-Aid of the Japan Medical Association; Grant-in-Aid for Co-operation Research (A) No. 60304043 from the Ministry of Education, Science, and Culture; Research Grant for Cardiovascular Diseases (No. 61–5) from the Ministry of Health and Welfare; and a grant for aging from Shiseido Company.

SYMPATHOADRENAL MEDULLARY FUNCTIONS DURING AGING UNDER ANESTHETIZED AND RESTING CONDITIONS

Catecholamine Concentrations in Systemic Blood in Anesthetized Rats

At first, adrenaline and noradrenaline concentrations in the systemic blood plasma were measured under urethane-chloralose anesthesia and resting conditions in young adult male Wistar rats (of 81–229 days of age) and aged male Wistar rats (of 768–916 days of age). Both adrenaline and noradrenaline concentrations were significantly greater in the aged rats, as is shown in FIGURES 1A and 1B. A tendency to develop hypertension during aging is well known in humans; in rats, though, it is characteristic that the arterial blood pressure is not significantly increased in the aged (shown in FIGURE 1C).

Changes in Adrenal Catecholamine Secretion Rate during Aging

The secretion rates of both of the catecholamines from the adrenal gland were directly measured. A thin polyethylene tube was inserted into an adrenal vein and a small amount of adrenal blood was collected as described previously.[11] The adrenaline and noradrenaline in this adrenal venous blood plasma were separated by high performance liquid chromatography and they were then measured by an electrochemical detector. Concentrations of noradrenaline and adrenaline in the adrenal venous blood were almost 50 times (for noradrenaline) to 1000 times (for adrenaline) higher than those in systemic blood.

FIGURE 2 shows the secretion rates of adrenaline and noradrenaline for 69 male Wistar rats from 81 to 916 days of age. The average secretion rates of adrenaline and noradrenaline increased almost proportionally with age after 300 days up to 800 days,

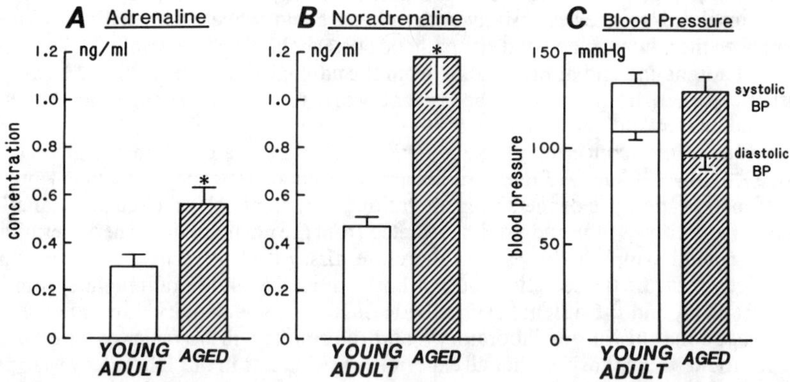

FIGURE 1. Concentrations of adrenaline (A) and noradrenaline (B) in systemic blood plasma, and systemic arterial blood pressure (C) in young adult (81–229 days old) and aged (768–916 days old) rats anesthetized with urethane-chloralose. The means ± SE for adrenaline in 9 young adult and 7 aged rats were 0.30 ± 0.05 and 0.56 ± 0.07 ng/mL, respectively, while those for noradrenaline in young adult and aged rats were 0.47 ± 0.04 and 1.18 ± 0.18 ng/mL, respectively. The means ± SE of systolic and diastolic blood pressure (BP) in 22 young adult rats were 135 ± 5 and 109 ± 4 mm Hg, respectively, while those in 19 aged rats were 130 ± 8 and 96 ± 7 mm Hg, respectively. *: $p < 0.01$ by Student's t test (from reference 12).

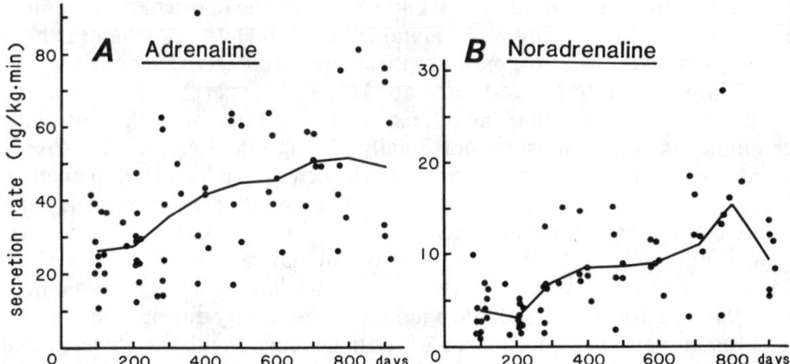

FIGURE 2. Secretion rates of adrenaline (A) and noradrenaline (B) from the adrenal gland in 69 urethane-chloralose–anesthetized rats of various ages (81–916 days old). Midlines drawn in (A) and (B) show the mean secretion rates for each age group (modified from reference 10).

although there was a great deal of variation. When the variations in the secretion rates of 24 young adult rats (81–217 days) and 18 aged rats (682–916 days) were compared, the young adult rat ranges were relatively narrow, while the aged rat ranges were widespread (as shown in FIGURE 2 and reference 12).

Changes in Adrenal Sympathetic Single Nerve Filament Activity during Aging

Single nerve filaments were dissected from the preganglionic sympathetic nerve innervating the adrenal gland and their ongoing activities were recorded in an anesthetized and resting state. Two typical examples in young adult and aged rats are shown in FIGURE 3A. In FIGURE 3B, the results from all 102 filaments dissected from 34 different rats (92–923 days old) are plotted. At ages of 100 to 300 days, the mean ongoing dis-

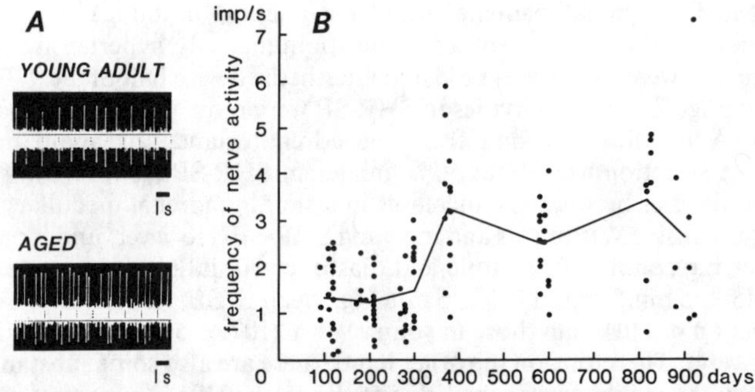

FIGURE 3. Spontaneous ongoing activity of 102 single adrenal sympathetic nerve filaments in 34 urethane-chloralose–anesthetized rats of different ages from 92 to 923 days—A: examples of single nerve filament activities of young adult (110-day-old) and aged (815-day-old) rats; B: dots represent the data from a single filament and the midline represents the mean values for nerve filament activities at different age groups (modified from reference 10).

charge rate was about 1.4 impulses/s. At 400 days, the mean discharge rate increased to 3.2 impulses/s. This increase was maintained up to 900 days. As before, the variations of the discharge rates also increased with age as did the secretion rates of catecholamines (as shown in FIGURE 3 and reference 12).

The present data show that the adrenal secretion rates of both adrenaline and noradrenaline increased almost proportionally with age and that these increased catecholamine secretion rates were accompanied by increased adrenal sympathetic nerve activities. Thus, these data suggest that an increase in adrenal sympathetic nerve activity with age is responsible for an increase in adrenal chromaffin cellular functions, which may ultimately result in an increase in adrenal catecholamine secretion.

This may be the first demonstration of increases in adrenal catecholamine secretion as well as in adrenal sympathetic ongoing nerve activity during aging in anesthetized and resting rats. These results are in good agreement with the previous findings of increased catecholamine contents[13,14] and catecholamine synthesizing enzyme activity[14,15] in the adrenal gland.

At present, the most important question is the mechanism by which aging produces such increases in adrenal sympathetic nerve activities. A decrease in baroreceptor sensitivity, a decrease in central inhibitory mechanisms, or an increase in central excitatory mechanisms might be causative factors. At this moment, though, we do not have any answers.

It is interesting to note that arterial blood pressure is not significantly increased despite the significant increase in the sympathoadrenal medullary functions in the aged rats. If it is possible to speculate that an age-related increase in other sympathetic nerve activities also exists in a similar way as the adrenal sympathetic nerve, then the maintenance of normal blood pressure in aged rats might be most likely explained by decreased responsiveness of the blood vessels[16] and cardiac muscles[17,18] to catecholamines.

Changes in Sympathoadrenal Medullary Functions in Stroke-prone Spontaneously Hypertensive Rats (SHR-SP)

With the above-mentioned question in mind, it is interesting to note that the sympathetic neuronal mechanisms of production and maintenance of hypertension in the genetically controlled spontaneously hypertensive rats (SHR) have been analyzed by other researchers.[19-23] Using the techniques employed in our aging studies, we have also investigated the sympathoadrenal medullary functions in young normotensive male Wistar Kyoto rats (WKY) and stroke-prone spontaneously hypertensive rats (SHR-SP); both groups were 15–20 weeks old and anesthetized with halothane.[24] The adrenal sympathetic ongoing nerve activities in SHR-SP were more than twice those in WKY (FIGURE 4). Adrenaline secretion from the adrenal gland was about double and noradrenaline secretion was about 50% greater in SHR-SP (FIGURE 5). Thus, there are some similarities between the increases in sympathoadrenal medullary functions in aged normotensive Wistar rats and in young SHR-SP. However, under our anesthetized and resting conditions, systolic and diastolic arterial blood pressures in young SHR-SP (215 ± 5 mm Hg and 156 ± 5 mm Hg, mean ± SE, respectively) were significantly higher ($p < 0.01$) than those in young WKY (107 ± 5 mm Hg and 73 ± 5 mm Hg, respectively). Therefore, on the other hand, there are also some substantial differences between the regulatory mechanisms of the arterial blood pressures in aged normotensive rats and in young SHR-SP.

Schramm and Chornoboy[22] have studied the effects of excitatory and inhibitory descending systems originating in the brain stem and projecting on spinal sympathetic neurons in SHR. Their finding was that adrenal sympathetic nerves in SHR exhibited

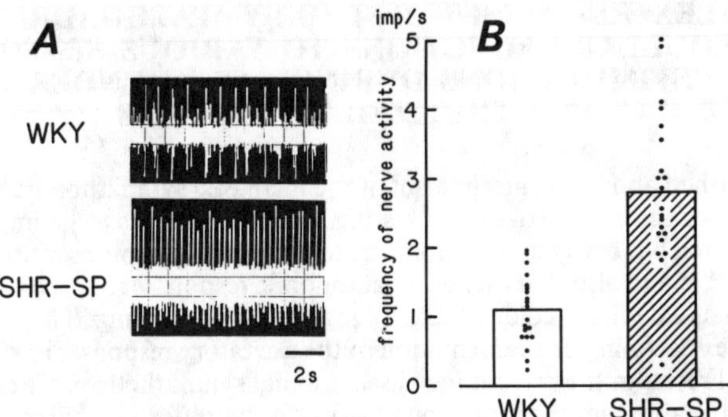

FIGURE 4. Spontaneous activity of single adrenal sympathetic nerve filaments in five normotensive (20 filaments) WKY and five SHR-SP (21 filaments) (15–20 weeks in age) anesthetized with halothane. WKY: Wistar Kyoto rats; SHR-SP: stroke-prone spontaneously hypertensive rats. (A) Examples of single nerve filament recordings; (B) dots represent the frequency of individual single nerve filament activities and columns show the mean frequencies of all fibers dissected in WKY and SHR-SP (from reference 24).

much larger responses than normal rats after stimulation of the descending sympathoexcitatory pathways. Takano *et al.*[23] found that the amount of substance P and the number of substance-P receptors in the region of the intermediolateral cell column at the spinal cord increased in SHR. They suggested that the activity of that excitatory descending pathway containing substance P would be increased in SHR. Fukuda *et al.*[20] reported an increased sensitivity of carotid chemoreceptor activity in SHR, while Nosaka and Wang[21] and Coote and Sato[19] emphasized a decreased sensitivity of baroreceptor activity in SHR. Such changes in the chemoreceptor and baroreceptor sensitivities seem to result in an increase in sympathetic nerve activity. Therefore, studies of the sympathoadrenal medullary functions of young SHR (or SHR-SP) may give us valuable insights into the sympathetic neural mechanisms involved in normotensive aged rats.

FIGURE 5. Spontaneous secretion rates of adrenaline (A) and noradrenaline (B) from the adrenal gland in five WKY and five SHR-SP (15–20 weeks in age) anesthetized with halothane. Dots represent the secretion rate of catecholamine of an individual animal and columns show the mean secretion rates of all animals (from reference 24).

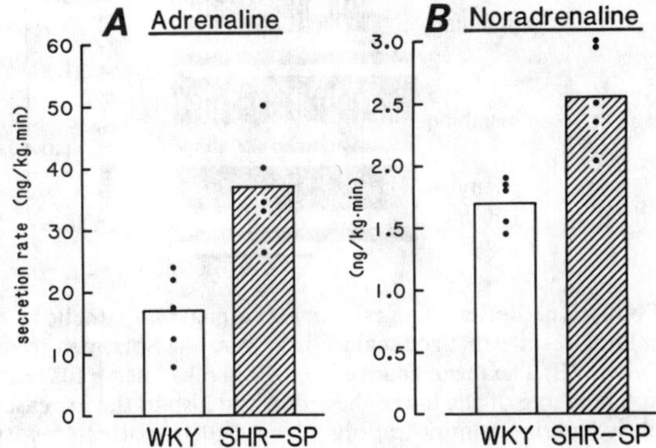

REFLEX RESPONSES OF THE SYMPATHOADRENAL MEDULLARY FUNCTIONS TO VARIOUS SENSORY STIMULATIONS DURING AGING UNDER ANESTHETIZED CONDITIONS

As mentioned above, the mechanism of the increased sympathoadrenal medullary functions under the anesthetized and resting conditions seems to be important to investigate. It often has been reported that baroreflex or baroreceptor sensitivity decreases during aging[25-29] and also that excitatory autonomic responses to some stressful stimulations (such as exercise,[30] cold,[31,32] etc.[33]) augment during aging. These may indicate that baroreflex declining or augmentation of the excitatory responses to various stimuli (or both) will result in the present increased adrenal sympathetic nerve activity. However, it is noticeable that most previous works on the reflex responses of autonomic functions during aging were performed on the effector organs. Therefore, it also becomes interesting to know whether or not the reflex ability of the adrenal sympathetic nerve itself would change during aging.

The purpose of the experiments to be reported on next will be to examine further the reflex responses of the adrenal sympathetic nerve to sensory stimulations of arterial baroreceptors and cutaneous mechanoreceptors during aging. First, though, our previous works on reflex responses of adrenal sympathetic nerve and catecholamine secretions evoked by these sensory stimulations in young adult rats will be introduced.[11,34,35]

Reflex Responses of the Sympathoadrenal Medullary Functions in Anesthetized Young Adult Rats

Single filaments of the adrenal sympathetic nerve were dissected and the effects of cutaneous noxious pinching, cutaneous innocuous brushing, and arterial baroreceptor stimulation were tested on each dissected filament. Single filaments showed spontaneous ongoing activity (FIGURE 6A, top) that was increased by pinching (FIGURE 6A,

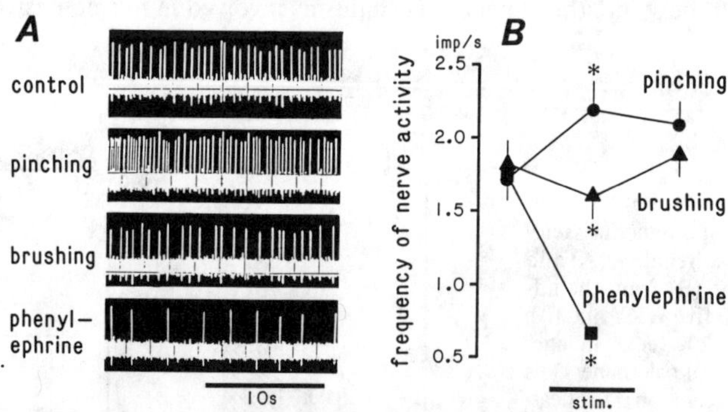

FIGURE 6. Reflex changes in single adrenal sympathetic nerve filament activity in 14 urethane-chloralose–anesthetized male Wistar rats. (A) Specimen recordings of single nerve filament activities. (B) The mean changes ($\pm$ SE) in all 46 nerve filament activities in response to pinching and brushing of the lower chest skin and also to the increased blood pressure after intravenous phenylephrine administration. *: $p < 0.01$ by paired t test (from reference 35).

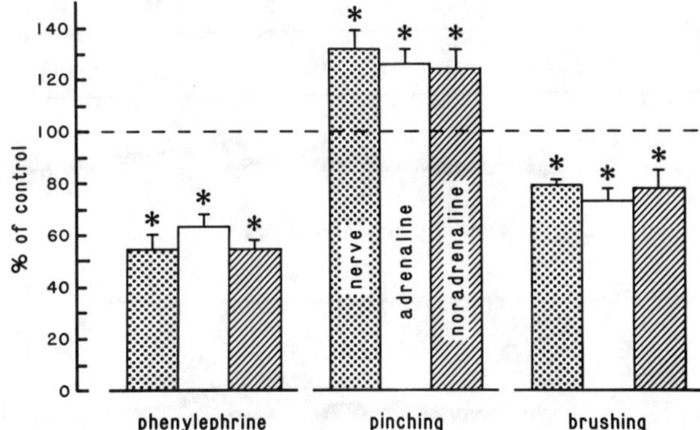

FIGURE 7. Reflex responses in adrenal sympathetic nerve mass discharge activities (stippled bar) and in adrenaline (open bar) and noradrenaline (hatched bar) secretion during baroreceptor stimulation by phenylephrine administration (left), pinching (middle), and brushing (right) in 39 urethane-chloralose–anesthetized rats. The magnitudes of the reflex responses are expressed as percentages of the prestimulus control levels. Each column represents the mean reflex response, and the vertical lines drawn in each column represent the standard error of the mean. *: $p <$ 0.01 by Student's t test or paired t test (modified from references 11 and 34).

second panel from top), decreased by brushing (FIGURE 6A, third panel from top), and decreased by arterial baroreceptor stimulation (FIGURE 6A, bottom). FIGURE 6B summarizes the data from all 46 filaments.

The responses of these single filaments to all three stimuli reasonably corresponded with the results of the mass discharges (which were recorded from a nerve not dissected to single filaments) in response to the same stimuli (as shown in FIGURE 7). Furthermore, the reflex responses of the adrenal nerve were generally proportional in magnitude to the reflex responses of adrenaline and noradrenaline secretions. Based on these facts, recordings of mass discharges from the adrenal sympathetic nerves were employed instead of single filament recordings in the following study of reflex responses during aging.

Reflex Responses of the Adrenal Sympathetic Nerve to Baroreceptor Stimulation during Aging

The experiments on reflex responses of the adrenal sympathetic nerve during aging were performed under halothane anesthesia of 1.0–1.2% depth.[36] Seven young adult rats (4 months old) and seven aged rats (26 months old) were employed. Artificial respiration was adjusted to maintain the end-tidal O_2 at about 18% for the young adult rats and at about 22% for the aged rats, respectively, in order to keep the level of arterial O_2 pressure at around 75–90 mm Hg (using the method as described previously[20]).

FIGURE 8 shows sample recordings of the reflex depression of the adrenal sympathetic nerve ongoing activity during increased arterial blood pressure evoked by an intravenous administration of phenylephrine in young adult (A,B) and aged (C,D) rats. The degree of the increase in arterial blood pressure after injections of the same doses of phenylephrine was less in aged animals than in the young ones ($p < 0.01$), as is

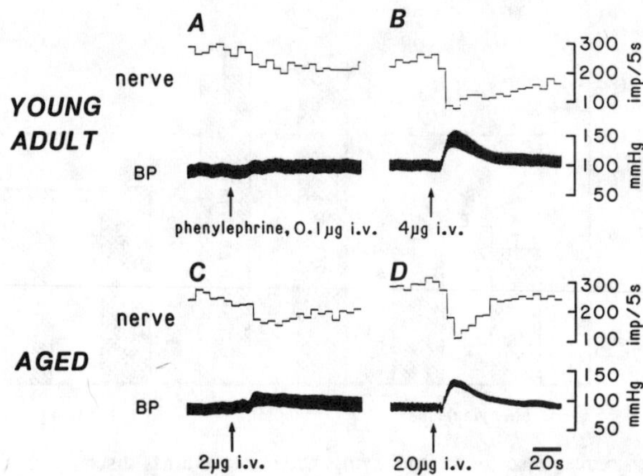

FIGURE 8. Reflex depression of the adrenal sympathetic nerve activity to baroreceptor stimulation by different doses of intravenous administration of phenylephrine in halothane-anesthetized young adult (4 months, A,B) and aged (26 months, C,D) male Wistar rats. Upper recordings: the mass nerve discharge activities are counted continuously every 5 s. Lower recordings: blood pressures. Note the difference in the dose of phenylephrine required to produce comparable increases in blood pressure for young adult and aged rats (modified from reference 36).

shown in FIGURE 9. This result is in good agreement with the previous work by Tuttle, who demonstrated a reduction of sensitivity to noradrenaline of aortic strips of aged rats.[16]

In the present experiment, we used different doses of phenylephrine in young adult and aged rats to produce comparable increases in blood pressure. For convenience, the increases in blood pressure were classified into four groups based on the degree of responses. In the first group, the increases in blood pressure ranged between 10 to 19 mm Hg; the second group, between 20 and 39 mm Hg; the third group, between

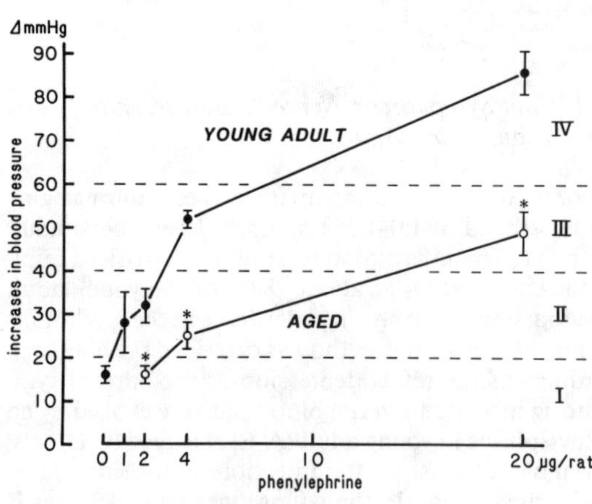

FIGURE 9. Effects of intravenous administration of different doses of phenylephrine on the blood pressure of young adult (4 months, closed circles) and aged (26 months, open circles) rats. Abscissa: doses of phenylephrine administered to each rat. Ordinate: increases in blood pressure. The increase in blood pressure was classified into four groups: the first (I) between 10 and 19 mm Hg; the second group (II) between 20 to 39 mm Hg; the third group (III) between 40 to 59 mm Hg; and the fourth group (IV) above 60 mm Hg. *: $p < 0.01$ by Student's t test (modified from reference 36).

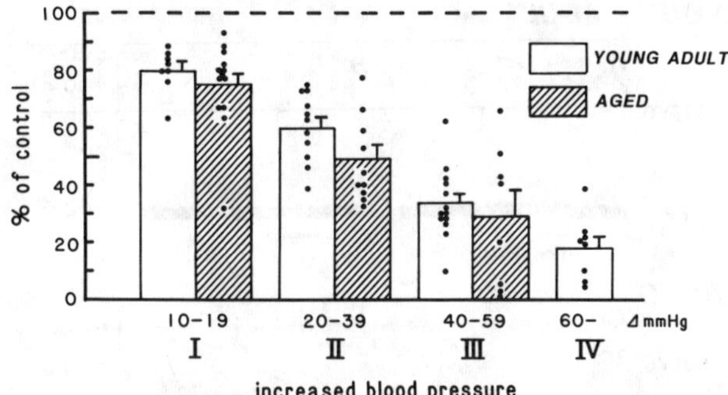

FIGURE 10. Reflex depression of adrenal sympathetic nerve activity to baroreceptor stimulation by intravenous phenylephrine administration in halothane-anesthetized rats. The magnitudes of reflex responses of the nerve activity during baroreceptor stimulations are expressed as percentages of the prestimulus control activity; that is, mean counts for 20 s following the maximum decrease response are compared with mean counts for 20 s before phenylephrine administration. Dots represent individual values ($\leq$2 values/rat) from seven young adult rats (4 months old) and seven aged rats (26 months old). Columns and vertical bars on the columns show the mean responses and SE of all data. Responses of the young adult rats are represented by open bars and those of the aged rats are shown by hatched bars. No significant differences between the young adult and aged rats were seen in the I–III classified groups when tested by Student's *t* test. There was no data for the aged rats in the IV group (modified from reference 36).

40 and 59 mm Hg; the fourth group, above 60 mm Hg. However, it was difficult to increase the blood pressure more than 60 mm Hg in the aged rats; thus, accordingly, we had no fourth group for the aged rats. The effects of increases in blood pressure of similar magnitudes on the adrenal sympathetic nerve activities were compared for young and aged groups. Increased blood pressures of 10–19 mm Hg, 20–39 mm Hg, 40–59 mm Hg, and above 60 mm Hg produced reflex decreases in adrenal sympathetic nerve activity in a pressure-dependent manner (as summarized in FIGURE 10). There were no significant differences between the reflex responses in the young adult and aged rats. From these results, it can therefore be concluded that baroreflex responses of the adrenal sympathetic nerve are quite well maintained in the aged rats.

In contrast to the present findings on the sympathetic baroreflex, the major discussions about baroreflex response in aged animals and human beings have centered on decreases in that response.[26-29] It should be kept in mind, though, that most previous experiments on the baroreflexes have been carried out by measuring heart rate and blood pressure, which are regulated not only by sympathetic nerves, but also by parasympathetic nerves and even by some hormones. The previous reports leave no doubt that the overall baroreflex response—including all responses at receptors, peripheral and central nervous systems, effectors, and neuroeffector transmission—decreases during aging. In fact, the present result demonstrating attenuation of increases in blood pressure during aging after the administration of phenylephrine strongly suggests that there are remarkable age-related decreases in the responsiveness of the blood vessel.[16] In spite of some age-related declines of the overall baroreflexes, the present findings on the adrenal sympathetic baroreflex support the well-maintained function of that reflex at the sympathetic preganglionic level in the aged provided that baroreceptors were sufficiently stimulated. In this respect, however, the present result does not intend to

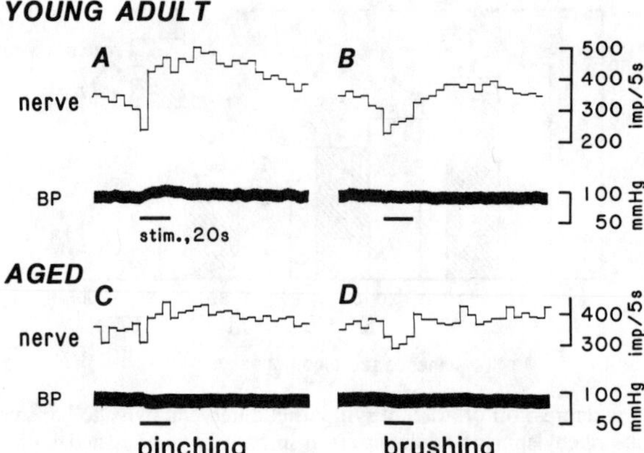

FIGURE 11. Sample recordings of adrenal sympathetic nerve reflex responses to pinching (left) and brushing (right) of lower chest skin for 20 s (indicated by horizontal bars) in halothane-anesthetized young adult (4 months, A,B) and aged (26 months, C,D) rats. Upper recordings: mass discharge nerve activities counted continuously every 5 s. Lower recordings: blood pressures (BP) (modified from reference 36).

show any age-related changes in sensitivity of the baroreceptor and baroreceptor afferents themselves. In any case, from this evidence of the well-maintained baroreflex responses in aged rats, it is not possible to explain the above-mentioned age-related increases in ongoing adrenal sympathetic nerve activity.

Reflex Responses of the Adrenal Sympathetic Nerve to Cutaneous Sensory Stimulations during Aging

FIGURE 11 shows sample recordings of excitatory and inhibitory reflex responses of the adrenal sympathetic nerve elicited by noxious pinching and innocuous brushing cutaneous stimulation in young adult (A,B) and aged (C,D) rats.

FIGURE 12 summarizes the results of these excitatory and inhibitory reflex responses during pinching and brushing in both young adult and aged rats. Both excitatory and inhibitory reflex responses produced by pinching and brushing of the skin were quite well maintained during aging. However, both the well-maintained inhibitory responses to the cutaneous brushing and the excitatory responses to cutaneous pinching within the control ranges during aging may not explain the age-related increases in adrenal sympathetic ongoing nerve activity.

CONCLUDING REMARKS

Spontaneous ongoing sympathetic nerve activity and catecholamine secretion rates from the adrenal gland were both increased during aging in anesthetized and resting rats. The increases in sympathoadrenal medullary functions during aging were reflected by the increased concentrations of catecholamines in systemic blood. In spite of those increases in the sympathoadrenal medullary functions in aged anesthetized rats, ar-

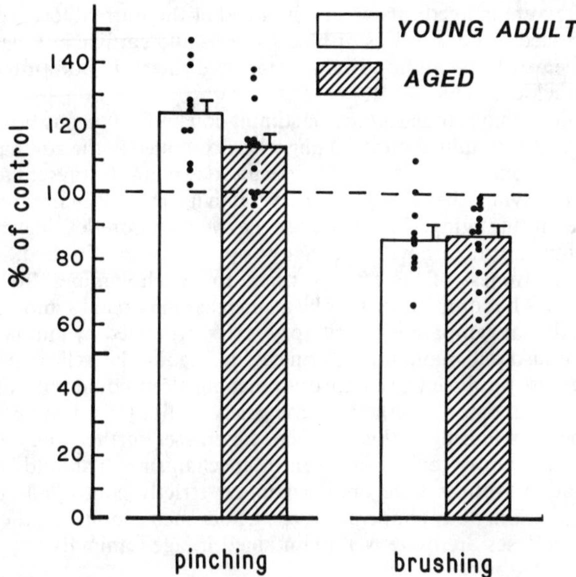

FIGURE 12. Summary of adrenal sympathetic nerve reflex responses to pinching (left) and brushing (right) of the lower chest skin for 20 s in seven young adult rats (4 months, open bar) and seven aged rats (26 months, hatched bar). The magnitudes of reflex responses of the nerve activity are expressed as percentages of the prestimulus control activity; that is, in the case of pinching, mean counts for 20 s starting 5 s after the onset of stimulation were compared with mean counts for 20 s before the stimulation, while in the case of brushing, mean counts for 20 s during the stimulation period were compared with mean counts for 20 s before the stimulation. Responses to pinching were 124 ± 4% (mean ± SE) and 114 ± 4%, while responses to brushing were 86 ± 4% and 87 ± 3% in young adult and aged rats, respectively. Dots represent the data (≤ 2 data/rat) from each animal. Columns and vertical bars show the mean responses and SE of all data (modified from reference 36).

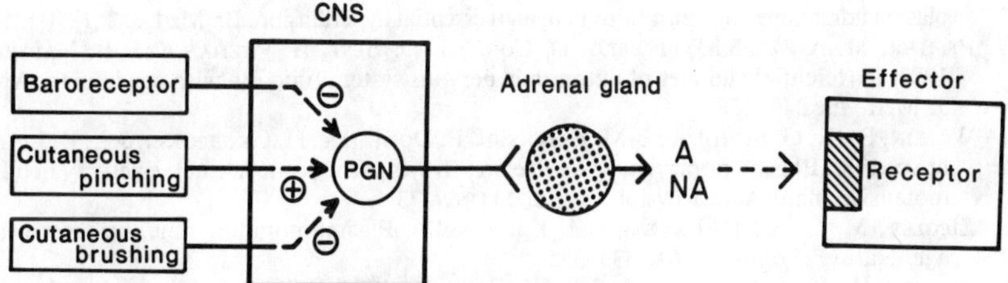

FIGURE 13. Diagram of an adrenal sympathetic preganglionic neuron (PGN) innervating adrenal chromaffin cells from which adrenaline (A) and noradrenaline (NA) are secreted. The reflex responses are influenced in excitatory and inhibitory manners by stimulations of baroreceptors and cutaneous mechanoreceptors. The secreted catecholamines affect the effector organs via their receptors. In the present study, the age-related increase in PGN activity was demonstrated under the anesthetized and resting conditions. The excitatory and inhibitory reflex effects on the PGN activity were well maintained during aging. CNS: central nervous system.

terial blood pressure in aged rats was maintained at the normal level of young adult rats. The decreased responsiveness of blood vessels and cardiac muscles to catecholamines also seemed to be an important age-related factor in addition to the above-noted present evidence (FIGURE 13).

The reflex depressions to baroreceptor stimulation and cutaneous brushing (FIGURE 13) were quite well maintained during aging when examined at the adrenal sympathetic preganglionic neuronal level. Thus, it is difficult to explain the present age-related increase in adrenal sympathetic ongoing nerve activity by well-maintained inhibitory reflex responses during aging. This is because the overall baroreflex, in general, suffered an overall decline in function with age that was probably conditioned, in part, by the decreased responsiveness of the effector organ to catecholamines. To a degree, this overall decline may be compensated for by an increase in adrenal sympathetic ongoing activity. The adrenal sympathetic excitatory reflex produced by cutaneous pinching (FIGURE 13) was also well maintained during aging. Again, the well-maintained excitatory reflex response produced by cutaneous pinching alone could not support the age-related increase in adrenal sympathetic ongoing nerve activity. Some other central mechanisms must be contributing to this age-related increase. Further study is under investigation in our laboratory to find such central mechanisms. It should be emphasized once more that the results were obtained under strictly controlled conditions for anesthesia, respiration, body temperature, etc. Under such conditions, the adrenal sympathetic nerve reflexes are quite well maintained in aged animals.

ACKNOWLEDGMENTS

The authors are grateful to T. Matsuzaki, A. Suzuki, and H. Hotta for their technical assistance.

REFERENCES

1. SHOCK, N. W. 1972. Energy metabolism, caloric intake and physical activity of the aging. *In* Nutrition in Old Age (Xth Symposium of the Swedish Nutrition Foundation). L. A. Carlson, Ed.: 12–23. Almqvist & Wiksells. Stockholm.
2. CHRISTENSEN, N. J. 1973. Plasma noradrenaline and adrenaline in patients with thyrotoxicosis and myxoedema. Clin. Sci. Mol. Med. **45:** 163–171.
3. FRANCO-MORSELLI, R., J. L. ELGHOSI, E. JOLY, S. DI GIUILIO & P. MEYER. 1977. Increased plasma adrenaline concentrations in benign essential hypertension. Br. Med. J. **2:** 1251–1254.
4. PFEIFER, M. A., C. R. WEINBERG, D. COOK, J. D. BEST, A. REENAN & J. B. HALTER. 1983. Differential changes of autonomic nervous system function with age in man. Am. J. Med. **75:** 249–258.
5. WALLIN, B. G., G. SUNDLÖF, B-M. ERIKKSON, P. DOMINIAK, H. GROBECKER & L. E. LINDBLAD. 1981. Plasma noradrenaline correlates to sympathetic muscle nerve activity in normotensive man. Acta Physiol. Scand. **111:** 69–73.
6. ZIEGLER, M. G., C. R. LAKE & I. J. KOPIN. 1976. Plasma noradrenaline increases with age. Nature (London) **261:** 333–335.
7. AVAKIAN, E. V., S. M. HORVATH & R. W. COLBURN. 1984. Influence of age and cold stress on plasma catecholamine levels in rats. J. Auton. Nerv. Syst. **10:** 127–133.
8. CHIUEH, C. C., S. M. NESPOR & S. L. RAPOPORT. 1980. Cardiovascular, sympathetic and adrenal cortical responsiveness of aged Fischer-344 rats to stress. Neurobiol. Aging **1:** 157–163.
9. MCCARTY, R. 1981. Aged rats: diminished sympathetic-adrenal medullary responses to acute stress. Behav. Neural Biol. **33:** 204–212.

10. Ito, K., A. Sato, Y. Sato & H. Suzuki. 1986. Increases in adrenal catecholamine secretion and adrenal sympathetic nerve unitary activities with aging in rats. Neurosci. Lett. **69:** 263–268.

11. Araki, T., K. Ito, M. Kurosawa & A. Sato. 1984. Responses of adrenal sympathetic nerve activity and catecholamine secretion to cutaneous stimulation in anesthetized rats. Neuroscience **12:** 289–299.

12. Sato, A., Y. Sato & H. Suzuki. 1987. Changes in sympatho-adrenal medullary functions during aging. *In* Organization of the Autonomic Nervous System: Central and Peripheral Mechanisms. C. Polosa & F. R. Calaresu, Eds.: 27–36. Alan R. Liss. New York.

13. Hökfelt, B. 1951. Noradrenaline and adrenaline in mammalian tissues. Acta Physiol. Scand. **25**(suppl. 92): 1–134.

14. Kvetňanský, R., E. Jahnová, T. Torda, V. Štrbák, V. Baláž & L. Macho. 1978. Changes of adrenal catecholamines and their synthesizing enzymes during ontogenesis and aging in rats. Mech. Ageing Dev. **7:** 209–216.

15. Reis, D. J., R. A. Ross & T. H. Joh. 1977. Changes in the activity and amounts of enzymes synthesizing catecholamines and acetylcholine in brain, adrenal medulla, and sympathetic ganglia of aged rat and mouse. Brain Res. **136:** 465–474.

16. Tuttle, R. S. 1966. Age-related changes in the sensitivity of rat aortic strips to norepinephrine and associated chemical and structural alterations. J. Gerontol. **21:** 510–516.

17. Lakatta, E. G. 1980. Age-related alterations in the cardiovascular response to adrenergic mediated stress. Fed. Proc. Fed. Am. Soc. Exp. Biol. **39:** 3173–3177.

18. O'Connor, S. W., P. J. Scarpace & I. B. Abrass. 1981. Age-associated decrease of adenylate cyclase activity in rat myocardium. Mech. Ageing Dev. **16:** 91–95.

19. Coote, J. H. & Y. Sato. 1977. Reflex regulation of sympathetic activity in the spontaneously hypertensive rat. Circ. Res. **40:** 571–577.

20. Fukuda, Y., A. Sato & A. Trzebski. 1987. Carotid chemoreceptor discharge responses to hypoxia and hypercapnia in the normotensive and spontaneously hypertensive rats. J. Auton. Nerv. Syst. **19:** 1–11.

21. Nosaka, S. & S. C. Wang. 1972. Carotid sinus baroreceptor functions in the spontaneously hypertensive rat. Am. J. Physiol. **222:** 1079–1084.

22. Schramm, L. P. & E. S. Chornoboy. 1982. Sympathetic activity in spontaneously hypertensive rats after spinal transection. Am. J. Physiol. **243:** R506–R511.

23. Takano, Y., W. B. Sawyer & A. D. Loewy. 1985. Substance P mechanisms of the spinal cord related to vasomotor tone in the spontaneously hypertensive rat. Brain Res. **334:** 105–116.

24. Sato, A., Y. Sato, K. Shimamura & H. Suzuki. 1986. An increase in the sympathoadrenal medullary function in stroke-prone spontaneously hypertensive rats under anesthetized and resting conditions. Neurosci. Lett. **72:** 309–314.

25. Andresen, M. C. 1984. Short- and long-term determinants of baroreceptor function in aged normotensive and spontaneously hypertensive rats. Circ. Res. **54:** 750–759.

26. Docherty, J. R., D. Fitzgerald & K. O'Malley. 1986. Age-related reduction of baroreflex tachycardia without loss of β-adrenoceptor-mediated tachycardia in Sprague-Dawley rats. J. Cardiovasc. Pharmacol. **8:** 376–380.

27. Gribbin, B., T. G. Pickering, P. Sleight & R. Peto. 1971. Effect of age and high blood pressure on baroreflex sensitivity in man. Circ. Res. **29:** 424–431.

28. Rothbaum, D. A., D. J. Shaw, C. S. Angell & N. W. Shock. 1974. Age differences in the baroreceptor response of rats. J. Gerontol. **29:** 488–492.

29. Shimada, K., T. Kitazumi, N. Sadakane, H. Ogura & T. Ozawa. 1985. Age-related changes of baroreflex function, plasma norepinephrine, and blood pressure. Hypertension **7:** 113–117.

30. Norris, A. H., N. W. Shock & M. J. Yiengst. 1953. Age changes in heart rate and blood pressure responses to tilting and standardized exercise. Circulation **8:** 521–526.

31. McCarty, R. 1986. Age-related alterations in sympathetic-adrenal medullary responses to stress. Gerontology **32:** 172–183.

32. Palmer, G. J., M. G. Ziegler & C. R. Lake. 1978. Response of norepinephrine and blood pressure to stress increases with age. J. Gerontol. **33:** 482–487.

33. ROWE, J. W. & B. R. TROEN. 1980. Sympathetic nervous system and aging in man. Endocr. Rev. **1:** 167–179.
34. ITO, K., A. SATO, K. SHIMAMURA & R. S. SWENSON. 1984. Reflex changes in sympatho-adrenal medullary functions in response to baroreceptor stimulation in anesthetized rats. J. Auton. Nerv. Syst. **10:** 295–303.
35. ITO, K., A. SATO, K. SHIMAMURA & R. S. SWENSON. 1984. Convergence of noxious and non-noxious cutaneous afferents and baroreceptor afferents onto single adrenal sympathetic neurons in anesthetized rats. Neurosci. Res. **1:** 105–116.
36. KUROSAWA, M., A. SATO, Y. SATO & H. SUZUKI. 1987. Undiminished reflex responses of adrenal sympathetic nerve activity to stimulation of baroreceptors and cutaneous mechanoreceptors in aged rats. Neurosci. Lett. **77:** 193–198.

DISCUSSION OF THE PAPER

G. S. ROTH (*NIA, Baltimore, MD*): I am curious about the relationship between blood pressure and spontaneous neuronal firing, especially in that first slide comparing the normal Wistar *kyoto* with the spontaneously hypertensive. The neuronal activity was higher, of course, in the hypertensive, but I noticed that there was one rat that was very low. What was the blood pressure of that particular animal?

A. SATO (*Tokyo Metropolitan Institute of Gerontology, Tokyo, Japan*): A very good question, but I do not remember.

UNIDENTIFIED DISCUSSANT: Are those mean blood pressures in your study?

SATO: I gave both systolic and diastolic blood pressures. The upper part was for systolic and the lower part was for diastolic.

C. CHIUEH (*National Institute of Mental Health, Bethesda, MD*): What kind of anesthetic agent did you use in your study?

SATO: Mostly, we used urethane-chloralose; however, for reflex studies and also for SHR studies, we used halothane anesthesia of 1.0–1.2%.

UNIDENTIFIED DISCUSSANT: The innervation of a number of effector tissues of the noradrenergic terminals in aged rats varies tremendously. For example, the kidney does not change its innervation pattern significantly between 3 and about 28 months of age. The spleen and the lymph nodes, though, are quite denervated to the point where they are less than 10% of what they had in a noradrenergic content and also in fibers. Therefore, I want to throw out a suggestion about why activity may change with aging. Hugo Bedadosky from the Swiss Research Institute has done some rather provocative studies in germ-free animals versus regular animals raised in a typical vivarium. During antigen stimulation, there is a marked suppression of norepinephrine release and turnover. If the animals are raised in germ-free conditions, the norepinephrine turnover and levels are considerably higher. In aging, though, one of the hallmarks of the immune dysfunction is a lack of responsiveness to antigen. Now, not only do you get the problem in the periphery, but it also happens in the central nervous system in key hypothalamic sites. This can even be mimicked by injecting supernatant from stimulated lymphocyte cultures. Therefore, this could be a compensatory change that is being put forth by the autonomic nervous system because of the lack of a factor from the immune system that tends to hold it in check during normal aging. This is a testable hypothesis and it is something that fits in with the known literature from the Swiss Research Institute.

Neostriatal Dopamine Uptake and Reversal of Age-related Movement Disorders with Dopamine-Uptake Inhibitors[a]

C. ANTHONY ALTAR[b] AND JOHN F. MARSHALL[c]

[b]Research Department
CIBA-GEIGY Pharmaceuticals Division
Summit, New Jersey 07901

[c]Department of Psychobiology
University of California
Irvine, California 92717

INTRODUCTION

The age-related degeneration of the nigrostriatal dopamine projection has been well characterized in rodents and primates including man. In rodents, the decline of striatal dopamine concentration occurs in senescence[1-4] and the decline of the D-2 class of dopamine receptors is evident by midage.[4-6] In the human caudate nucleus, the reductions of dopamine[7,8] and D-2 receptors [5,9] are progressive throughout adulthood and old age. Normal aging of the neostriatum is also associated with a decrement in dopamine biosynthetic capacities and a preservation — or even an enhancement — of dopamine catabolic processes (see references 10 and 11 for reviews). These alterations appear to play a major role in the etiology of some of the movement disorders of the aged because neurosurgical[12] or pharmacological[13,14] procedures that elevate dopamine concentrations or the density of D-2 sites in the striatum improve motor functions of old rodents.

Because the synaptic concentration of dopamine is regulated in large part via the uptake of the transmitter,[15] the viability of this uptake system could also substantially influence the appearance of movement disorders of old age. The high-affinity, sodium-dependent uptake of dopamine into dopaminergic nerve endings of striatal slices[16] or synaptosomes[17] has been reported to be unaffected in aging rats, although the affinity of this system is lower in the aged mouse striatum.[18] Interestingly, a preservation of dopamine-uptake capacities in the aged striatum could synergize with the declining pool of releasable dopamine to limit further the synaptic actions of dopamine. Such a role by the high-affinity uptake system would suggest that dopamine-uptake blockers may be efficacious in the treatment of dopamine-dependent motor decline of the elderly. To test these ideas, we have measured dopamine concentrations and the integrity of

[a] This research was supported by USPHS Grant Nos. AG 00538 and NS 20122 to J. F. Marshall. C. A. Altar was supported in part by USPHS Training Grant No. AG 00096.

the high-affinity dopamine-uptake system in the striatum and olfactory tubercle of the aged Fischer (F344) rat. Our studies demonstrate that striatal dopamine uptake is unaltered during the adult life span of the F344 rat despite significant losses of striatal dopamine. Additional experiments reveal that treatment with inhibitors of dopamine uptake markedly reverses the age-related decline in swim performance of these aged animals.

RELATIONSHIP BETWEEN THE CONCENTRATION AND UPTAKE OF DOPAMINE IN THE STRIATUM OF THE ADULT RAT

Several studies have indicated that the capacity of the high-affinity dopamine-uptake system reflects the density of dopamine innervation during, for example, ontogeny[19] or degeneration of the dopamine nerve fibers of the nigrostriatal pathway.[20-22] This degeneration, when induced by an infusion of 8 µg of the selective dopamine neurotoxin, 6-hydroxydopamine, into the region of nigrostriatal cell bodies, results in a parallel loss of dopamine, dopamine uptake, and the number of neuronal boutons containing small granular vesicles (FIGURE 1). The loss of these markers (which reflects the loss of dopamine nerve terminals) is complete within two days following the 6-hydroxydopamine infusion. These similar rates of loss indicate that the extent of high-

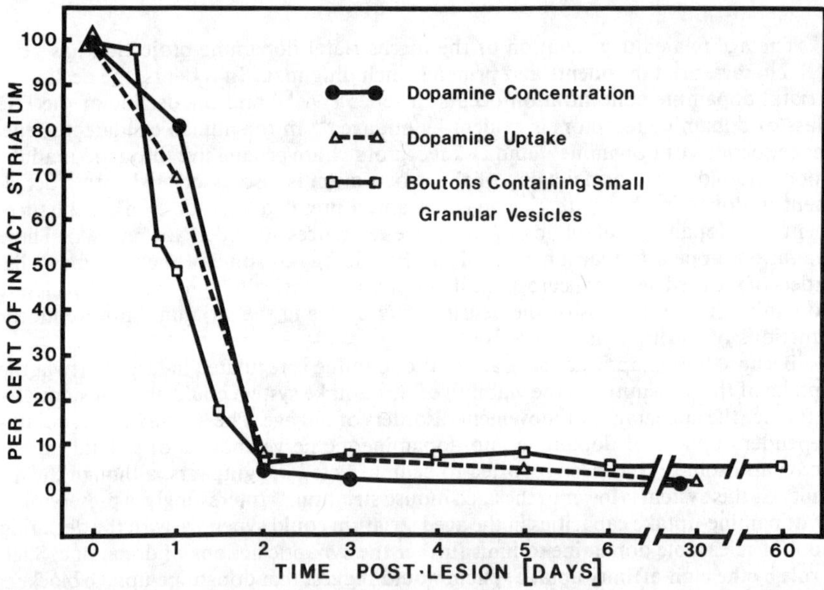

FIGURE 1. Time course of dopamine terminal degeneration in the neostriata of rats after 8-ng injections of 6-hydroxydopamine along the mesostriatal dopamine projection. Decreases in the dopamine concentration,[39] dopamine uptake,[21] and the number of boutons that contain small granular vesicles[40] are plotted during the postlesion interval as a function of the content in the lesioned (left) neostriatum versus that in the intact (right) neostriatum. Reprinted with permission from reference 21.

affinity dopamine uptake and the concentration of dopamine are proportional to each other following extensive lesions of the nigrostriatal pathway.

To determine whether this proportionality is maintained throughout a large range of less complete dopamine denervations, we measured the residual concentration of dopamine and the uptake of dopamine after three days following the intranigral infusion of 1, 2, or 4.5 μg of 6-hydroxydopamine.[22] Because the degeneration of nigrostriatal neurons is complete after two days following 6-hydroxydopamine infusions (FIGURE 1), it can be assumed that the measure of dopamine or its high-affinity uptake after three days following the lesion is derived exclusively from the population of surviving neurons. Indeed, the loss of dopamine correlated very highly ($r = 0.93$; $p < 0.01$) with the loss of high-affinity dopamine uptake (FIGURE 2). Based on the linear regression equation (FIGURE 2), the residual dopamine concentration approximates the residual amount of dopamine uptake when the losses of dopamine are less than about 90%. Thus, dopamine content reflects dopamine uptake over virtually the entire range of dopaminergic denervations of the adult rat striatum.

RELATIONSHIP BETWEEN STRIATAL DOPAMINE CONTENT AND UPTAKE IN THE AGED RAT

The parallel relationship between dopamine content and uptake in the young adult rat suggests that the well-characterized loss of striatal dopamine in the aged rat[1-4] may

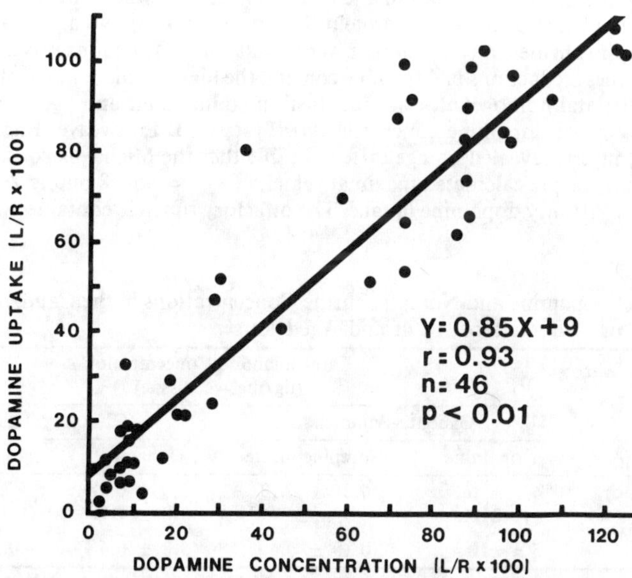

FIGURE 2. The loss of dopamine concentration is proportional and nearly equal to the loss of dopamine uptake in the striatum following partial nigrostriatal denervation. The dopamine concentration loss (x-axis) is expressed as the ratio of the dopamine concentrations in the left (lesioned) and right (intact) hemispheres. A similar ratio was calculated for the loss of dopamine uptake (y-axis) of a 5×10^{-7} M dopamine concentration.

parallel a loss of high-affinity dopamine uptake. To determine this directly, young adult (4–8-month-old) and aged (26–30-month-old) male Fischer 344 rats were obtained from the National Institute on Aging and housed individually in a colony (24 ± 1 °C, lights on from 0700 to 1900 h). Five adult and five aged rats were killed by decapitation, and the striatum and olfactory tubercle of both hemispheres were rapidly dissected from a 2.5-mm-thick coronal section of the forebrain. The left and right striata and olfactory tubercles were homogenized, and the catecholamine content and high-affinity [³H]dopamine uptake were measured. The pooled striata or olfactory tubercles of each rat were homogenized in 20 vol 0.32 M sucrose (maintained at 2–4 °C) using 10 strokes of a glass-Teflon homogenizer. Next, 250 µL of the homogenate was added to 750 µL of cold 0.1 N perchloric acid solution, and catecholamine concentrations were determined by an alumina extraction HPLC procedure.[23] The remainder of the sucrose homogenate was immmediately centrifuged (900 × g for 10 min, 2–4 °C), and 50-µL aliquots of the supernatant were used for protein determinations[24] or analysis of [³H]dopamine uptake. Uptake assays were conducted by mixing 50 µL of supernatant with 950 µL of Krebs-Henseleit HCO₃ buffer (pH 7.2–7.35).[25] Thirty-two parts of dopamine (Sigma Chemicals) to one part [³H]dopamine (Dupont-NEN, Boston, Massachusetts, 25–35 Ci/mmol) were mixed in each tube to achieve final dopamine concentrations of 5–1000 nM. The tubes were incubated at 37 °C for eight minutes (during which time uptake is linear) and the reaction was terminated at 2 °C. Alternate tubes contained 20 µM benztropine mesylate (Merck, Sharp and Dohme) to define specific dopamine uptake. At a dopamine concentration of 0.1 µM, dopamine uptake was inhibited by approximately 90%.

Relative to young adult rats, aged animals had significant reductions in the dopamine concentration of the striatum and olfactory tubercle whether expressed per mg tissue weight (TABLE 1) or per mg protein (results not shown). No age-related change in the norepinephrine concentration or wet weights of these regions was observed. In contrast to these reductions in dopamine content, the high-affinity uptake of [³H]dopamine into striatal homogenates was identical in young adult and aged rats over the 200-fold range of dopamine concentrations (FIGURE 3). Lineweaver-Burke analysis (FIGURE 3, insert) revealed no age difference in either the Michaelis constant (K_m = 0.11–0.12 µM) or the calculated maximal velocity (V_{max} = 96–98 pmoles/mg tissue/8 min) of high-affinity dopamine uptake. The olfactory tubercle contained insufficient

TABLE 1. Dopamine and Norepinephrine Concentrations in the Caudate-Putamen and Olfactory Tubercle of Adult and Aged Rats[a]

	Catecholamine Concentration (ng/mg wet tissue)			
	Caudate-Putamen		Olfactory Tubercle	
	Dopamine	Norepinephrine	Dopamine	Norepinephrine
Aged (30 mo)	4.7 ± 0.3[b] (−21%)	0.21 ± 0.13 n.c.	2.9 ± 0.3[c] (−24%)	0.34 ± 0.04 n.c.
Adult (8 mo)	5.9 ± 0.4	0.18 ± 0.4	3.8 ± 0.4	0.36 ± 0.07

[a] Values are mean ± SEM (N = 5 per group). Wet weights for tissues in mg were (mean ± SEM): 45.6 ± 1.0 (for adult striatum), 49 ± 3.3 (for aged striatum), 22 ± 2.3 (for adult olfactory tubercle), and 21 ± 3.3 (for aged olfactory tubercle); n.c. = not changed from the adult group.

[b] $p < 0.001$ compared with adult group by t tests.

[c] $p < 0.01$ compared with adult group by t tests.

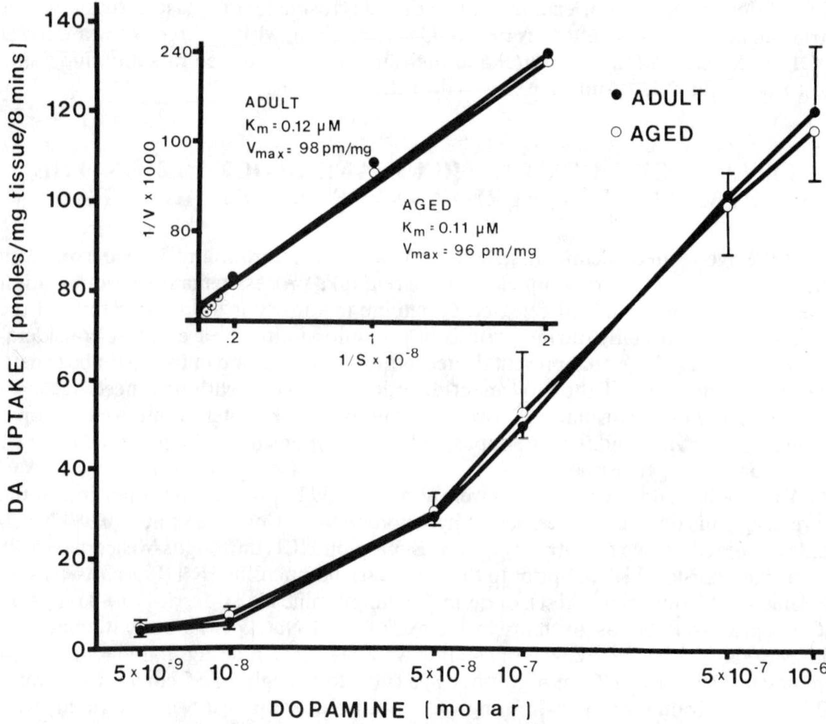

FIGURE 3. Equivalent affinity and capacity of dopamine (DA) uptake into homogenates of adult or aged rat striatum ($n = 5$ per group). The insert illustrates the results plotted by Lineweaver-Burke analysis. Reprinted with permission from reference 41.

tissue for a complete kinetic analysis in each animal. However, the uptake of striatal homogenates from 8-month-old animals at a [³H]dopamine concentration of 5×10^{-7} was 63 ± 7 pmol/mg tissue/8 min and did not differ significantly from the value of 56 ± 6 obtained with 30-month-old rats.

These neurochemical findings confirm the frequently reported decline in dopamine concentration that occurs in aged rodents.[1-4] However, the high-affinity transport system remained remarkably unchanged relative to young adult animals. Because the extent of high-affinity dopamine uptake reflects the density of catecholamine innervation during[20] (FIGURE 1) and after (FIGURE 2) neuronal degeneration, the present results with high-affinity dopamine uptake suggest that the dopaminergic innervation of the rat striatum or olfactory tubercle does not decline in senescence. If the dopamine nerve terminal density remains unchanged in senescent animals, then the observed decline in dopamine content in the striatum and olfactory tubercle most likely reflects a reduction in the amount of dopamine per neuron. In support of this possibility, McNeill *et al.*[26] reported age-related decreases in the catecholamine histofluorescence per cell body in the substantia nigra pars compacta and dorsal portion of the ventral tegmental area of mice. Declines in the size of the dopamine pool per neuron could result from the age-related retardation of synthesis and the accelerated degradation of dopamine.[10,11] For example, the reduced tyrosine hydroxylase activities in the striatum and olfactory tubercles of old F344 rats, along with the trends toward lower DOPAC concentrations in striatal and mesolimbic areas of aged rats and mice, suggest that dopamine turnover is lowered in these neurons.[1,2,27,28]

EFFECTS OF DOPAMINE REUPTAKE BLOCKADE ON THE IMPAIRED SWIM PERFORMANCE OF THE AGED RAT

If the age-related decline of striatal dopamine concentration reflects decreases in the pool of releasable dopamine and if the reuptake process remains at young adult levels, then the recapture of released dopamine might occur more efficiently in the aged striatum especially during periods of rapid dopamine release. These considerations suggest that drugs that prevent the recapture of released dopamine might be beneficial in treating some of the movement disorders associated with advanced age such as impaired swim performance.[14] Two compounds that are potent inhibitors of dopamine uptake *in vitro* and *in vivo*, bupropion and nomifensine,[29-33] were tested for their effects on swim performance.

Young adult and aged F344 rats were administered bupropion, nomifensine, or the norepinephrine uptake blocker, desmethylimipramine,[15] or just the vehicle (0.9% NaCl) and were tested for their swimming ability. Bupropion HCl (Burroughs-Wellcome, 25–75 mg/kg, administered 30 min prior to the swim test), nomifensine HCl (Hoechst-Roussel, 5–8 mg/kg, 15 min prior to test), or desmethylimipramine HCl (Merril-Dow, 15 mg/kg, 30 min prior to test) was given i.p. in 2–5 mL of 0.9% NaCl per kg body weight, with doses calculated as the free base. The rats were placed in a hexagonal glass tank (60 cm maximal width × 76 cm high) that was filled to a height of 55 cm with tap water (22–24 °C). Evaluation of swimming was conducted by an observer who rated swim performance during the test and by videotaping the sessions for later quantitative behavioral analysis. An observer experienced in rating swim performance evaluated the "vigor" and "success" of each animal at one-minute intervals for the duration of the test (12 minutes for bupropion, 15 minutes for nomifensine or desmethylimipramine). Rating scales were from zero (poorest performance) to three (best performance), using criteria previously established.[14] In general, the vigor scale reflects the strength and constancy with which each rat moves its limbs, while the success scale reflects the animal's ability to maintain its head above the water surface. The observer who rated the swim performances was uninformed as to the drug treatment of the animals. To minimize the distress of the animals, they were removed from the tank whenever they remained below the water surface for a period of 15 seconds. On those occasions in which animals were removed, they were assigned ratings of zero and were considered to have spent zero seconds with their noses above water for the remainder of the test. After the tests, the animals were towel-dried and placed in a warmed cage. At least 48 hours separated swim tests.

Another measure of swim performance was obtained by reviewing the videotapes of each swim session and recording the number of seconds out of each minute that the rat spent with its nose above or below the surface of the water.

The aged rats swam less well than did the young adult animals in both experiments (FIGURE 4; ANOVA p values < 0.02 for both vigor and success measures). However, bupropion and nomifensine each significantly improved the swimming of the aged rats (ANOVA p values < 0.006 for both vigor and success measures). The aged rats swam significantly better when given 25–50 mg/kg bupropion or 5–8 mg/kg nomifensine relative to their performance when given the vehicle. The highest dose of bupropion

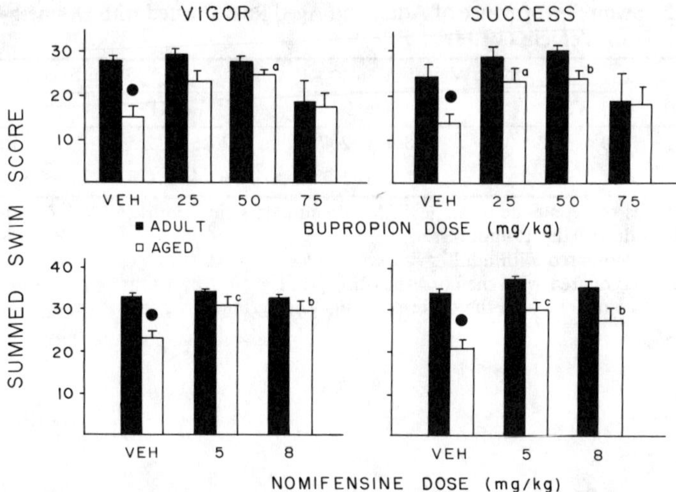

FIGURE 4. Improvement of swim vigor and success of aged rats given bupropion (top: n = 6–12 per group) or nomifensine (bottom: n = 10–15 per group). The swim scores were summed for the duration of the 12-min test (bupropion) or 15-min test (nomifensine). Symbols: ● = $p < 0.02$ versus adult given vehicle; a = $p < 0.05$, b = $p < 0.01$, c = $p < 0.001$ versus vehicle group by t tests. Reprinted with permission from reference 41.

(75 mg/kg) failed to facilitate the swimming of aged rats; perhaps this was because it induced conflicting or fatiguing behaviors during the swim test such as repetitive, stereotyped head movements that were observed in the home cage. Importantly, no significant effects on swim vigor or swim success following bupropion or nomifensine administration were observed in young adult animals. The norepinephrine uptake blocker, desmethylimipramine (15 mg/kg), had no effect on the swim performance of aged rats, but it did result in a small and significant impairment in the swimming of adult animals (TABLE 2).

Based on the quantitative review of the videotapes of the swim sessions, the aged rats spent less time with their heads above water as the swim test progressed ($p < 0.001$) (FIGURE 5). However, both the 50 mg/kg dose of bupropion ($p < 0.05$) and the 5 mg/kg dose of nomifensine ($p < 0.01$) significantly increased the time that the rats spent with their heads above water relative to vehicle treatment. For nomifensine, the interaction between drug and test duration was significant ($p < 0.001$).

PHARMACOLOGICAL INTERVENTION AND AGE-RELATED DECLINES IN MOTOR FUNCTION

In summary, the behavioral and neurochemical findings of this experiment suggest that the preservation of dopamine-uptake sites in the aged striatum may synergize with the declining pool of releasable dopamine to limit further this transmitter's synaptic actions. This conclusion suggests a novel pharmacological approach for reversing the well-documented impairments in sensorimotor functions occurring in senescence.

TABLE 2. Swim Performance of Adult and Aged Rats Treated with Desmethylimipramine (DMI) or Vehicle (VEH)[a]

	Swim Vigor		Swim Success	
	VEH	DMI	VEH	DMI
Aged	20.4 ± 2.5^b	18.0 ± 2.4^b	17.5 ± 2.5^b	16.8 ± 2.7^b
Adult	34.2 ± 0.5	31.2 ± 1.0^c	35.4 ± 0.9	31.4 ± 1.5^d

[a] The values represent the mean $\pm$ SEM of summed swim scores ($N = 7$ for aged, $N = 10$ for adult) during the 15-min test.
[b] $p < 0.01$ compared with adult swim scores by t tests.
[c] $p < 0.01$ compared with the corresponding VEH groups by t tests.
[d] $p < 0.02$ compared with the corresponding VEH groups by t tests.

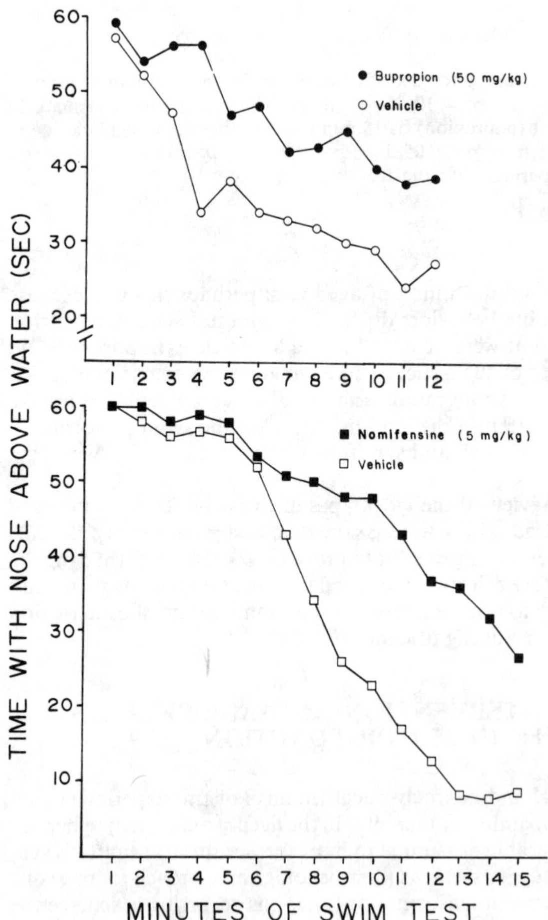

FIGURE 5. Mean number of seconds per minute that aged rats maintained their noses above the surface of the water after treatment with the saline vehicle or bupropion (top: 9 rats) or nomifensine (bottom: 15 rats). Reprinted with permission from reference 41.

Compared to existing pharmacological agents, dopamine-uptake inhibitors may represent a more selective means of treating movement disorders because their ability to increase dopamine in the synapse depends upon the ongoing rate of dopamine release. In contrast to precursors of dopamine biosynthesis such as L-dopa that can be converted to dopamine extraneuronally or directly acting dopamine agonists such as bromocriptine, the uptake inhibitors should elevate synaptic dopamine receptor stimulation to the greatest extent during periods of maximal dopamine release. By inhibiting the high-affinity transport of dopamine, these drugs elevate its concentration in the synapse after release. Therefore, unlike L-dopa or dopamine agonist treatments, which would uniformly elevate D_2 receptor activation, dopamine-uptake blockers should amplify synaptic dopamine levels and D_2 activation in proportion to dopamine neuron activity. Indeed, bupropion or nomifensine each greatly improved the swimming of aged animals. Although both compounds are also inhibitors of the high-affinity transport of norepinephrine in brain,[33,34] the preferential norepinephrine uptake blocker, desmethylimipramine, did not improve the swimming of aged rats and impaired the swimming of the adult animals. In view of previous work from several laboratories,[12–14] the improvement in motor performance seen after nomifensine or bupropion probably depends upon the ability of these drugs to elevate synaptic concentrations of dopamine. Thus, a more selective dopamine-uptake blocker may improve motor performance even more than did nomifensine or bupropion.

The use of dopamine-uptake inhibitors should also be effective in treating conditions in which striatal dopamine content is only moderately reduced (i.e., normal aging);[24] however, it will not be effective if extensive degeneration of dopamine neurons has already occurred (i.e., in late stages of parkinsonism).[35] In fact, many elderly individuals develop impairments of movement and posture that resemble the early stages of parkinsonism.[36] Both bupropion[37] and another dopamine-uptake inhibitor, mazindol,[38] have moderate antiparkinsonian properties. Accordingly, Delwaide and colleagues[38] have suggested that dopamine reuptake blockers, when used in Parkinson's disease, must be prescribed early in the course of the disorder, which is when appreciable numbers of properly functioning dopaminergic neurons are present.

REFERENCES

1. DEMAREST, J. T., G. D. REIGLE & K. E. MOORE. 1980. Characteristics of dopaminergic neurons in the aged male rat. Neuroendocrinology 31: 222–227.
2. OSTERBURG, H. H., H. G. DONAHUE, J. A. SEVERSON & C. E. FINCH. 1981. Catecholamine levels and turnover during aging in brain regions of male C57 BL/6J mice. Brain Res. 224: 337–352.
3. STRONG, R., T. SAMORAJSKI & Z. GOTTESFELD. 1982. Regional mapping of neostriatal neurotransmitter systems as a function of aging. J. Neurochem. 39: 831–836.
4. JOSEPH, J. A., R. E. BERGER, B. T. ENGEL & G. S. ROTH. 1978. Age-related changes in the nigrostriatum: A behavioral and biochemical analysis. J. Gerontol. 33: 643–649.
5. SEVERSON, J. A., & C. E. FINCH. 1980. Reduced dopaminergic binding during aging in the rodent striatum. Brain Res. 199: 147–162.
6. O'BOYLE, K. M. & J. L. WADDINGTON. 1984. Loss of rat striatal dopamine receptors with aging is selective for D-2 but not D-1 sites. Eur. J. Pharmacol. 105: 171–174.
7. CARLSSON, A. & B. WINBLAD. 1976. Influence of age and time interval between death and autopsy on dopamine and 3-methoxytyramine levels in human basal ganglia J. Neural Transm. 38: 171–176.
8. RIEDERER, P. & ST. WUKETICH. 1976. Time course of nigro-striatal degeneration in Parkinson's disease. J. Neural Transm. 38: 277–301.
9. SEVERSON, J. A., J. MARCUSSON, B. WINBLAD & C. E. FINCH. 1982. Age correlated loss of dopaminergic binding sites in human basal ganglia. J. Neurochem. 39: 1623–1631.

10. LYTLE, L. D. & C. A. ALTAR. 1979. Diet, central nervous system, and aging. Fed. Proc. Fed. Am. Soc. Exp. Biol. **38:** 2017–2022.

11. FINCH, C. E., P. K. RANDALL & J. F. MARSHALL. 1981. Aging and basal ganglia functions. *In* Annual Rev. Gerontol. Geriatr. Vol. 2. C. Eisdorfer, Ed.: 49–85.

12. GAGE, G. H., S. B. DUNNETT, U. STENEVI & A. BJÖRKLUND. 1983. Aged rats: Recovery of motor impairments by intrastriatal nigral grafts. Science **221:** 966–969.

13. JOSEPH, J. A., R. T. BARTUS, D. CLODY, D. MORGAN, C. FINCH, B. BEER & S. SESACK. 1983. Psychomotor performance in the senescent rodent: Reduction of deficits via striatal dopamine receptor up-regulation. Neurobiol. Aging **4:** 313–319.

14. MARSHALL, J. F. & N. BERRIOS. 1979. Movement disorders of aged rats: reversal by dopamine receptor stimulation. Science **206:** 477–479.

15. IVERSEN, L. L. 1974. Uptake mechanism for neurotransmitter amines. Biochem. Pharmacol. **23:** 1927–1935.

16. THOMPSON, J. M., J. R. WHITAKER & J. A. JOSEPH. 1981. [^{3}H]Dopamine accumulation and release from striatal slices in young, mature, and senescent rats. Brain Res. **224:** 436–440.

17. STRONG, R., T. SAMORAJSKI & Z. GOTTESFELD. 1984. High affinity uptake of neurotransmitters in rat neostriatum: effects of aging. J. Neurochem. **43:** 1766–1768.

18. JONEC, V. & C. E. FINCH. 1975. Aging and dopamine uptake by subcellular fractions of the C57BL/6J male mouse brain. Brain Res. **91:** 197–215.

19. TENNYSON, V. M., R. E. BARRETT, G. COHEN, L. COTÉ, R. HEIKKILA & C. MYTILINEOU. 1972. The developing neostriatum of the rabbit: correlation of fluorescence histochemistry, electron microscopy, endogenous dopamine levels, and [^{3}H]dopamine uptake. Brain Res. **46:** 251–285.

20. BELL, L. J., L. L. IVERSEN & N. J. URETSKY. 1970. Time course of the effects of 6-hydroxydopamine on catecholamine-containing neurons in rat hypothalamus and striatum. Br. J. Pharmacol. **40:** 790–799.

21. ALTAR, C. A., S. O'NEIL & J. F. MARSHALL. 1984. Sensorimotor impairment and elevated levels of dopamine metabolites in the neostriatum occur rapidly after intranigral injections of 6-hydroxydopamine or gamma-hydroxybutyrate in awake rats. Neuropharmacology **23:** 309–318.

22. ALTAR, C. A., M. R. MARIEN & J. F. MARSHALL. 1987. Time course of adaptation in dopamine synthesis, metabolism and release following nigrostriatal lesions: Implications for behavioral recovery from brain injury. J. Neurochem. **48:** 390–399.

23. REFSHAUGE, C., P. T. KISSINGER, R. DREILING, R. FREEMAN & R. N. ADAMS. 1974. New high performance liquid chromatographic analysis of brain catecholamines. Life Sci. **14:** 311–322.

24. BRADFORD, M. M. 1976. A rapid and sensitive model for the quantification of microgram quantities of protein utilizing the principle of protein-dye binding. Anal. Biochem. **72:** 248–254.

25. COYLE, J. T. & J. AXELROD. 1983. Development of the uptake and storage of L-[^{3}H]norepinephrine in the rat brain. J. Neurochem. **18:** 2061–2075.

26. MCNEILL, T. H., L. L. KOEK & J. W. HAYCOCK. 1984. Age-correlated changes in dopaminergic nigrostriatal perikarya of the C57 BL/6NNia mouse. Mech. Ageing Dev. **24:** 293–307.

27. MEMO, M., L. LUCCHI, P. F. SPANO & M. TRABUCCHI. 1980. Aging process affects a single class of dopamine receptors. Brain Res. **202:** 488–492.

28. REIS, D. J., R. A. ROSS & T. H. JOH. 1977. Changes in the activity and amounts of enzymes synthesizing catecholamines and acetylcholine in brain, adrenal medulla, and sympathetic ganglia of aged rat and mouse. Brain Res. **136:** 465–474.

29. COOPER, B. R., T. J. HESTER & R. A. MAXWELL. 1980. Behavioral and biochemical effects of the antidepressant bupropion (Wellbutrin): Evidence for selective blockade of dopamine uptake *in vivo*. J. Pharmacol. Exp. Ther. **215:** 127–134.

30. HUNT, P., M-H. KANNENGIESSER & J-P. RAYNAUD. 1974. Nomifensine: a new potent inhibitor of dopamine uptake into synaptosomes from rat brain corpus striatum. J. Pharm. Pharmacol. **26:** 370–371.

31. ROSS, S. B. 1979. The central stimulatory action of inhibitors of the dopamine uptake. Life Sci. **24:** 159–168.

32. SAMANIN, R., S. BERNASCONI & S. GARATTINI. 1975. The effect of nomifensine on the depletion of brain serotonin and catecholamines induced respectively by fenfluramine and 6-hydroxydopamine in rats. Eur. J. Pharmacol. **34:** 377–380.

33. SOROKO, F. E., N. B. MEHTA, R. A. MAXWELL, R. M. FERRIS & D. H. SCHROEDER. 1977. Bupropion hydrochloride [(±)α-t-butylamino-3-chloropropiophenone HCl]: a novel antidepressant agent. J. Pharm. Pharmacol. **29:** 767–770.

34. SCHACHT, U. & W. HEPTNER. 1974. Effect of nomifensine (HOE 984), a new antidepressant, on uptake of noradrenaline and serotonin and on release of noradrenaline in rat brain synaptosomes. Biochem. Pharmacol. **23:** 3413–3422.

35. BERNHEIMER, H., W. BIRKMAYER, O. HORNYKIEWICZ, K. JELLINGER & F. SEITILBERGER. Brain dopamine and the syndromes of Parkinsonism and Huntington: Clinical, morphological, and neurochemical correlations. J. Neurol. Sci. **20:** 415–455.

36. MORTIMER, J. A. & D. D. WEBSTER. 1982. Comparison of extrapyramidal motor function in normal aging and Parkinson's disease. *In* The Aging Motor System. J. A. Mortimer, F. J. Pirozzola & G. J. Masetta, Eds.: 217–241. Praeger. New York.

37. GOETZ, C. G., C. M. TANNER & H. L. KLAWANS. 1984. Bupropion in Parkinson's disease. Neurology **34:** 1092–1094.

38. DELWAIDE, P. J., P. MARTINELLI & J. SCHOENEN. 1983. Mazindol in the treatment of Parkinson's disease. Arch. Neurol. **40:** 788–790.

39. NEVE, K. A., M. R. KOZLOWSKI & J. F. MARSHALL. 1982. Plasticity of neostriatal dopamine receptors after nigro-striatal injury: Relationship to recovery of sensorimotor functions and behavioral supersensitivity. Brain Res. **244:** 33–44.

40. HÖKFELT, T. & U. UNGERSTEDT. 1973. Specificity of 6-hydroxydopamine-induced degeneration of central monoamine neurones: An electron and fluorescence microscopic study with special reference to intracerebral injection of the nigro-striatal dopamine system. Brain Res. **60:** 269–297.

41. MARSHALL, J. F. & C. A. ALTAR. 1986. Striatal dopamine uptake and swim performance of the aged rat. Brain Res. **379:** 112–117.

DISCUSSION OF THE PAPER

P. LeWITT (*Lafayette Clinic, Detroit, MI*): If nomifensine has been tried in combination with levodopa and as a solo agent without effect, do you think that this could just be a consequence of there not being enough dopamine there for the reuptake blockade to be significant? Or do you think there are other problems in that situation?

A. ALTAR (*CIBA–GEIGY Corporation, Summit, NJ*): That is a very interesting point. You do not need the uptake of L-dopa into a dopamine neuron for the conversion to dopamine to occur. In that case, the concomitant use of the dopamine uptake inhibitor may not be that efficacious because you are flooding the system with dopamine, which is not dependent upon production by L-dopa uptake into the nerve terminal. In addition, this suggests that one reason why a selective dopamine uptake inhibitor may be more useful than a direct acting agonist or an indirect acting agonist (such as L-dopa) is that the uptake inhibition may best restore dopamine concentrations in the synapse during periods of maximal depolarization of those neurons. Therefore, what you are getting is not a sustained increase from a low level of dopamine that is present in the injured striatum; instead, what you may get is a marked increase. Furthermore, this increase is modulated by the extent of ongoing demands, so when demands are made, patients can mobilize these neurons during emergency situations. It may be that you are going to get an increase that is parallel with the firing rate of these residual dopamine neurons. Then, in that context, you would not expect much effect by dopamine-uptake inhibitors when you have no neurons left because there would be no substrate on which the inhibitors could act.

LeWITT: Now that is important whether the surviving terminals have a regulatory role or if their role is to just dump dopamine. However, did you assess the order of magnitude of the effects of levodopa or dopamine itself in improving swimming performance as has been done in the past?

ALTAR: We have not. However, in a 1979 paper by Berrios and Marshall, they looked at apomorphine and L-dopa and each of these drugs was able to reverse the swimming impairments.

LeWITT: Was it of the order of magnitude as the improvements you saw?

ALTAR: It was certainly no greater. It was approximately the same magnitude and I am sure that it was no greater because the aged animals never exceeded the young adults in swim performance.

D. INGRAM (*NIA, Baltimore, MD*): Were the rats naive performers or were they well practiced in swimming performance?

ALTAR: These animals were naive at the beginning of the study. All swim tasks and drug administrations, though, were made in a completely counterbalanced order so these animals were quite practiced by the end. Thus, the experiment was not confounded by a learning effect because of the counterbalanced nature of the design.

INGRAM: What would happen if you gave animals an anxiolytic? Swim performances are often used in animal models of depression. Floating, in fact, is alleviated by anxiolytics, and floating would be a performance within this task that would weigh the performance on the aging animals downward.

ALTAR: Floating? We never observed floating in these studies.

Upregulation of Striatal Dopamine Receptors and Improvement of Motor Performance in Senescence

J. A. JOSEPH[a] AND G. S. ROTH[b]

[a]Division of Behavioral Sciences
Armed Forces Radiobiology Research Institute
Bethesda, Maryland 20814-5415

[b]Gerontology Research Center
Francis Scott Key Medical Center
Baltimore, Maryland 21044

INTRODUCTION

The authors of several previous chapters in this volume have presented a great deal of data showing that decrements in motor control are an important consequence of aging. Their systematic evaluations, as well as those of others (e.g., references 1–3), have indicated that deficits in motor performance vary directly with the level of difficulty of the task, with the most demanding task exhibiting the greatest debilitating effects of age. Behavioral tasks such as those involving simple reaction speed in humans[4] or accurate paw placement in rodents[2] show no change with age. However, in tests that require the organism to exhibit balance, strength, coordination, and/or sensory-motor integration (such as those that assess postural stability[5–8] or complex reaction time[4]), consistent age-related declines are observed. The deficits observed in these examinations can be translated to losses of independence for the elderly because they appear as components of such everyday tasks as walking or driving an automobile. It is known, for example, that the likelihood of automobile accidents[9] as well as the occurrence of life-threatening accidental falls increase in the elderly.[10]

Importantly, striking interspecies similarities can be found between the rodent and human in these declines. Thus, the rodent may serve as a useful model for delineating the basic mechanisms of motor control (especially central motor control) and examining how these mechanisms change with age. With this understanding, methods might be developed that could retard these age-related changes or enhance performance in individuals where the changes have already occurred.

One central system that has received a great deal of attention is that of the nigrostriatal system. Systematic research has demonstrated a primary involvement of this system in the mediation of motor behavior and has indicated its significant role in the decline of motor performance in senescence. The purposes of the present review are to elaborate upon this relationship and to show how manipulations designed to modulate nigrostriatal functioning can have a profound effect on motor performance.

ALTERED STRIATAL DOPAMINERGIC FUNCTION AND PSYCHOMOTOR PERFORMANCE

The evidence implicating the nigrostriatal DA system in the decline of motor behavioral function in senescence is derived primarily from three sources. The first is provided from experiments in which striatal dopaminergic function was pharmacologically or surgically altered in young animals. It has been known for a long time that interference with the striatal dopaminergic system in young animals by such compounds as reserpine[11,12] or α-methyl-p-tyrosine[13] will compromise postural tone and decrease locomotor activity. L-Dopa can reverse reserpine's effects on spontaneous locomotor activity and it also affects locomotor activity when given alone.[14] When various dopamine-receptor antagonists are given in sufficient doses, both man and lower animals exhibit catalepsy and akinesia in numerous experiments. In fact, these organisms tend to resist being moved out of static equilibrium and exhibit exaggerated bracing in response to having their positions changed. In addition, doses of neuroleptics that do not produce catalepsy still induce decrements in the righting reflex, as well as in balance and coordination. In one study, for example, 22% of the animals (cats) given as little as 0.25 mg/kg of chlorpromazine showed decrements in performance on many of the tasks described above.[15]

When striatal dopaminergic function was altered in rats via bilateral injections of 6-hydroxydopamine (6-OHDA) into the nigrostriatal fiber bundles, the animals showed signs of sensorimotor impairment—namely, akinesia, limb dysfunction, rigidity, and impairments in orientation to sensory stimuli.[16,17] Recovery was highly correlated with the extent of development of striatal DA receptor denervation supersensitivity and with the amount of DA remaining in the lesioned striatum.[17]

The second source of evidence that suggests a link between the striatal dopaminergic system and motor behavior can be derived from the clinical data of patients suffering from Parkinson's disease, tardive dyskinesia, or akathisia.[18] In the case of Parkinson's disease, there appears to be reduced dopaminergic receptor binding in the putamen,[19,20] lowered dopamine levels in the basal ganglia,[21] and cell loss in the substantia nigra.[21] Similarly, persons who have intravenously self-administered meperidine contaminated with N-methyl-4-phenyl-1,2,3,6-tetrahydropyridine (MPTP) will develop severe parkinsonian-like movement aberrations.[22] MPTP is known to be a neurotoxin that selectively destroys cells in the substantia nigra.[23,24] In both Parkinson's disease and MPTP poisoning, some alleviation of symptoms can be achieved by enhancing striatal DA levels with L-dopa.

Finally, a third source of evidence of striatal DA involvement in age-related declines in movement can be provided from studies that have examined these changes in the senescent organism. McGeer and McGeer[25] have reported that out of 400,000 nigral cells present at birth in the human, less than 200,000 survive to age 75. If their regression line is extrapolated, the projected number of cells surviving at age 100 would be 140,000. These numbers may be compared to the 60,000 to 120,000 range reported for Parkinson patients.[26] These changes appear to occur in concert with alterations in nigrostriatal morphology, such as axonal dilations in the nigrostriatal pathways, accumulations of lipofuscin granules, and markedly reduced DA histofluorescence in the pars compacta of the substantia nigra.[27]

In the caudate, many of the indices of DA functioning appear to be much more variable between the human and rodent. For example, while age-related declines in striatal DA levels are seen with some regularity in the aged human,[28] DA loss is more intrastriatally regionally selective[29] or not observed[30] in the aged rodent. Moreover, recent evidence indicates that there are no age-related declines in KCl-induced release[31] or reuptake[31] of DA from superfused striatal tissue slices in the rat. If other aspects of synaptic functioning are considered, interspecies variations become even more salient. This is seen in two important DA synthetic enzymes, tyrosine hydroxylase (TH) and dopa decarboxylase (DDC), that show no consistent changes as a function of age. Tyrosine hydroxylase activity in the human shows either no decrease in the activity[32] or primary decreases before 20 years of age.[21] In the rodent, the findings range from those that report significant decreases in TH activity after 10 months of age in rat[21] to those that show no significant age-related declines with senescence in the mouse[33,34] or rat.[35] Findings with respect to DDC range from those that show a 66% decline in human[36] to those that show a 0% decline in rat[35] and mouse.[33] Because motor behavioral changes are similar in the aged rat and human, these interspecies inconsistencies in striatal DA synaptic functioning suggest that other indices should be considered to account for decreased performance.

One synaptic index that has shown remarkably consistent age-related changes in rodent and human is the decrease in striatal receptor binding. Our first report indicated a 35% decline in haloperidol binding with no loss of binding affinity in the aged rat.[37] This observation has been repeated numerous times under a variety of experimental conditions using various experimental models, including human,[38] rat,[39] mouse,[40] and rabbit.[41] (These findings are discussed in detail elsewhere in this volume, so only a brief overview will be presented here.) The actual percentage of decline as a function of age depends upon the particular dopamine-sensitive ligand that is utilized. Findings from studies using 3H-spiroperidol, for example, which may be selective for the D2 receptor subtype, indicate consistent decreases in D2 receptor concentrations of about 36–66% that occur over the life span of the animal.[37,40] More recent studies using dopamine agonists such as 3H-2-amino-6,7-dihydroxy-1,2,3,4-tetrahydronaphthalene (3H-ADTN) or 3H-N-propylnorapomorphine (3H-PNA) (which bind to the high affinity component of the D2[41] in the absence of guanine nucleotides) indicate decreases in the proportion of high to low affinity D2 sites that occur in concert with the decrease of D2 sites in mice from 3 to 12 months of age[42] (see also Severson, this volume).

Under certain assay conditions, 3H-ADTN also binds to the high affinity form of the striatal D1 receptor.[43] In fact, it has been shown that the age-related loss in density of this form of the receptor may be greater than 50%.[44] If the low affinity form of the D1 receptor (cyclase-linked[45]) is assessed, the results from at least one laboratory show parallel losses between D1 receptor (assessed with 3H-piflutixol) and DA-stimulated adenylate cyclase activity that are greatest between 3 and 12 months of age in the rat.[46] However, results from other laboratories using Sprague-Dawley rats[42] or C57BL6 mice[47] indicate no change in striatal D1 receptor levels throughout the life span. Examination of postmortem human material indicates an actual increase in D1 receptors with age.[48]

Therefore, these findings suggest that there are increases in the striatal D1/D2 receptor ratio in senescence, which is a finding that has been confirmed in humans (see Wong, this volume). In addition, there are some indications that the biosynthetic rates of both D1[49] and D2 receptor[49,50] subtypes show declines in animals beginning at about 12 months of age.[50] However, even in the face of alterations in striatal DA receptor number, D1/D2 ratio, high to low agonist binding components, and synthetic rate, it is interesting to note in this regard that the dopamine receptors that remain in senescent animals appear to function in a manner similar to those of young animals. Recent experiments in which the function of striatal DA autoreceptors was assessed by examining the effects of haloperidol application to superfused striatal slices from 6- and 24-month-old animals indicated no age-related decrements in the ability of this antagonist to block the DA autoreceptor and enhance KCl-induced DA release from these slices (e.g., 500 µM haloperidol + 30 mM KCl pmoles DA/mg protein released = 140 + 10, 6 mo; 130 + 8, 24 mo).[51]

FUNCTIONAL CONSEQUENCES OF EXPERIMENTAL MANIPULATIONS OF STRIATAL DA RECEPTOR DENSITY

In our initial observations, we found that if old and young rats were unilaterally lesioned in the left substantia nigra and if rotational behavior[52] was examined following graded doses of amphetamine (AMPH), then the old group showed less rotational behavior than the young group.[37] The interesting finding, though, was that when these same animals were given apomorphine (a DA agonist), there was no difference in rotational behavior between the young and old groups. It had been shown previously[52] that the denervated striatal DA receptors would proliferate after lesioning and that agonists, such as apomorphine, would have a greater effect on the lesioned, "upregulated" striatum, thereby resulting in increased contralateral (to the lesion) turning. However, because no age-related differences in contralateral turning were seen, these findings suggested that increases in striatal DA receptor density could still occur in the striata from the old animals and that these striata had retained their "plastic" capabilities.

This hypothesis was supported by a subsequent experiment in which unilaterally lesioned (6-OHDA) young and old rats were tested initially with AMPH and then later with lergotril, a potent DA agonist. Age-related deficits in rotation were seen with respect to the former of these compounds, but not with the latter. Results from the biochemical analyses indicated that both 3H-spiroperidol binding and DA-stimulated adenylate cyclase activity were higher in the lesioned striata than in the nonlesioned striata irrespective of age or sex.[53]

In addition to rotational behavior, other tasks requiring coordinated control of motor and reflexive responses (such as suspension time on a horizontal wire[2] or on an inclined wire-mesh screen,[54-56] as well as the length of time that it takes for a rodent to traverse a wooden rod or plank[56]) showed significant declines with age. In an effort to further explore the generality of the "upregulation effect" to these types of tasks, performance was examined in young, middle-aged and old mice following chronic haloperidol administration and withdrawal. This neuroleptic is a potent DA receptor antagonist. It induces striatal DA receptor upregulation by producing a functional denervation of these receptors. The results indicated that haloperidol-treated animals of all age groups showed better performance than those that were given chronic vehicle treatment.[56]

These findings were replicated in a later experiment[57] in which chronic prolactin (150 ng/h/7 days; Alzet minipumps) was administered to senescent animals. These animals improved on tests such as the inclined-screen and rod-walking tasks beginning 4–6 days after the pumps were implanted, and behavior declined within two weeks after the pumps were withdrawn. The induction of the behavioral improvements coincided with the increases in 3H-spiroperidol binding that had been reported previously.[58] Tests in other groups of animals also showed enhanced rotational behavior to intrastriatal DA following chronic prolactin treatment.[59] Although there have been some previous reports in which prolactin was administered directly[60] or in which prolactin was indirectly stimulated via domperidone[61] or stimulated through the implantation of prolactin-secreting pituitary tumors,[62] which have not shown increases in striatal 3H-spiperone binding, these studies only examined prolactin effects in young animals. We, however, have shown that the prolactin effect was even greater in old animals (37% increase in 3H-spiperone binding) than in young ones (15-20%).[58] It could be that some of these changes were missed in studies where old animals were not examined. It is also possible that if there was an overstimulation of prolactin production, such as might be expected following the implantation of a prolactin-secreting tumor, then the effect would be reversed. At the dose of prolactin that we employed, increased blood levels of prolactin were undetectable.

In addition to including increases in receptor density to enhance motor performance, we have employed one rather interesting method to retard the loss of striatal DA receptors and alter the age-related progressive deterioration of these behaviors. This method involves the use of dietary restriction. It has been known for a long time that if rats receive food only on alternate days (EOD) from the time that they are weaned, then life span is extended by 40% (see reference 63). Recent evidence indicates that striatal DA receptor concentrations as measured by both 3H-ADTN and specific 3H-spiroperidol binding are maintained at young levels well into middle age before declining and that 24-month-old EOD animals have striatal DA receptor complements that are equivalent to that of a 12-month-old ad-lib fed animal.[64] When rotational behavior was examined in these 24-month-old EOD animals, it was found to be comparable to that of young animals.[65]

Taken together, the data from all of these techniques that induce striatal DA receptor upregulation suggest a critical role for these receptors in the mediation of motor function in senescence. Furthermore, from these findings and those above, it might be postulated that there is a critical concentration range for striatal DA receptors. If the receptor number is lowered via age, then it could lead to a "cascade" of intrastriatal effects that might initially change the reciprocal inhibitory control between acetylcholine (ACh) and DA [e.g., loss of efficacy of DA agonists such as apomorphine to inhibit KCl-induced release of ACh,[66] and loss of efficacy of muscarinic agents such as carbachol to inhibit DA-stimulated cyclase activity (Joseph *et al.*, unpublished)]. This ultimately would result in decreased motor performance.

Conversely, increasing the concentration of DA receptors seems to reverse this "cascade" and, thus, motor performance is improved on a variety of tasks. In fact, it appears that the "striatal dopaminergic receptor-motor behavioral link may be stronger in old animals than it is in young." In a recent experiment,[67] both old and young animals were treated with the irreversible DA receptor antagonist, N-ethoxycarbonyl-2-ethoxy-1,2-dihydroquinoline (EEDQ), and tested at various times on the inclined screen. The results indicated that although young animals had returned to pre-EEDQ levels of performance at 48 hours post-EEDQ, their striatal DA receptor concentrations were only at 40% of control for both the D1 and D2 receptor subtypes. Old animals did not reach pre-EEDQ levels of inclined-screen performance even when tested at 192 hours post-EEDQ (45% of control), despite the fact that their striatal DA receptor concentrations were closer to pre-EEDQ levels than those in young animals (90% and 60% of control for the D1 and D2 receptor subtypes, respectively). Hence, in young animals, the return to pre-EEDQ levels of performance is, to some extent, independent of the recovery of pre-EEDQ concentrations of striatal DA receptors; subsequent attempts to compromise inclined performance in young animals by treating them at 48 hours post-EEDQ with spiroperidol (2 mg/kg) have been unsuccessful. These findings suggest that when striatal function is compromised in young animals, they are able to utilize other control mechanisms, possibly extrastriatal, in their behavioral recovery that are unavailable to old animals. One of these areas may be the cerebellum. It has been shown in a number of studies that cerebellar function is morphologically altered and physiologically compromised in senescence (see chapters by Hoffer and Rogers, this volume). Therefore, the old animal is probably less able to utilize cerebellar mediation in its post-EEDQ recovery than is the young animal. Consequently, the old animal must rely more heavily on the return of pre-EEDQ levels of striatal DA functioning for its recovery.

Unfortunately, because of the nonspecific nature of some of these upregulation and downregulation procedures used to alter striatal DA function, it is difficult, at this point, to specify which DA-receptor subtype may be most critical in the regulation of these types of motor tasks. However, evidence from three sources suggests that it might be the D2 receptor subtype: (a) there is a more progressive age-related change in the concentration of this striatal DA receptor subtype than in that of the D1, cyclase-linked receptors; (b) historically, there is a well-established link between D2 receptor function and motor performance;[68] and (c) in ongoing experiments from this laboratory, only D2 receptor blockade via 2 mg/kg spiperone has been found to be effective in disrupting inclined screen performance. Doses of the D1 antagonist SCH 23390 as high as 3 mg/kg were found to be ineffective in disrupting performance. In this regard, though, there are some recent reports that have shown that the D1 receptors have a role in the mediation of rotational behaviors.[69] Therefore, the exact specification of the role of each of these receptor subtypes in mediating age changes in motor function awaits further research. However, clinically, it is clear that the development and utilization of techniques that take advantage of these "plastic capabilities" could result ultimately in improved motor performance in the elderly.

REFERENCES

1. BARTUS, R. T. 1979. *In* Aging, Vol. 10: Sensory Systems and Communications in the Elderly. J. M. Ordy, Ed.: 35–73. Raven Press. New York.
2. WALLACE, J. E., E. KRAUTER & B. A. CAMPBELL. 1980. J. Gerontol. **35:** 364–370.
3. WELFORD, A. T. 1982. *In* The Aging Motor System. J. A. Mortimer, F. J. Pirozzolo & G. J. Maletta, Eds.: 159–188. Praeger. New York.
4. WELFORD, A. T. 1977. *In* Handbook of the Psychology of Aging. J. E. Birren & K. W. Schaie, Eds.: 450–497. Van Nostrand–Reinhold. Princeton, New Jersey.
5. HASSELKUS, B. R. & G. M. SHAMBES. 1975. J. Gerontol. **30:** 661–667.
6. SHELDON, J. H. 1963. Gerontol. Clin. **5:** 129–138.
7. WOOLLACOTT, M. H., A. SHUMWAY-COOK & L. NASHNER. 1982. Same source as reference 3.
8. MURRAY, M. P., R. C. KORY & B. T. CLARKSON. 1969. J. Gerontol. **24:** 169–178.
9. McFARLAND, R. A., G. S. TUNE & A. T. WELFORD. 1964. J. Gerontol. **19:** 190–197.
10. RIFFLE, K. 1982. Geriatr. Nurs. **May-June:** 165–169.
11. BLASCHKO, H. & T. L. CHRUSCIEL. 1960. J. Physiol. **151:** 272–284.
12. CARLSSON, A., M. LINDQUIST & T. MAGNUSSON. 1957. Nature **180:** 1200.
13. RECH, R. H., H. K. BORYS & K. E. MOORE. 1966. Exp. Ther. **153:** 412–419.
14. SMITH, C. B. & P. B. DEWS. 1962. Psychopharmacologia **3:** 55–59.
15. CARP, J. S. & R. J. ANDERSON. 1979. Pharmacol. Biochem. Behav. **10:** 513–520.
16. MARSHALL, J. F. 1979. Brain Res. **17:** 311–324.
17. KOZLOWSKI, M. R. & J. F. MARSHALL. 1981. Exp. Neurol. **74:** 318–323.
18. BERNHEIMER, H. W., O. BIRKMAYER, K. HORNYKIEWICZ, K. JELLINGER & F. J. SEITELBERGER. 1973. J. Neurol. Sci. **20:** 415–455.
19. REISINE, T. D., J. Z. FIELDS & H. I. YAMAMURA. 1977. Life Sci. **21:** 335–345.
20. LEE, T., P. SEEMAN, A. RAJPUT & I. J. FARLEY. 1978. Nature **273:** 59–61.
21. McGEER, P. L. & E. G. McGEER. 1978. *In* Parkinson's Disease II. Aging and Neuroendocrine Relationships. C. E. Finch, D. E. Potter & A. D. Kenny, Eds.: 41–57. Plenum. New York.
22. LANGSTON, J. W., P. BALLARD, J. W. TETRUD & I. IRWIN. 1983. Science **219:** 979–980.
23. HEIKKILA, R. E., A. HESS & R. C. DUVOISIN. 1984. Science **224:** 1451–1453.
24. HALLMAN, H., J. LANGE, L. OLSON, I. SHOMBER & G. JANSON. 1985. J. Neurochem. **44:** 117–127.
25. McGEER, P. L., E. G. McGEER & J. S. SUZUKI. 1977. Arch. Neurol. **34:** 33–35.

26. MORTIMER, J. A. & D. D. WEBSTER. 1982. Same source as reference 3.
27. McNEILL, T. H., L. I. KOEK & J. W. HAYCOCK. 1984. Mech. Aging Dev. **24:** 293–307.
28. CARLSSON, A. & B. WINBLAD. 1976. J. Neural Transm. **38:** 271–276.
29. STRONG, R., T. SAMORAJSKI & Z. GOTTESFELD. 1982. J. Neurochem. **39:** 831–836.
30. PAPAVASILIOU, P. S., S. T. MILLER, L. J. THAL, L. J. NERDER, G. HOULIHAN, S. N. RAO & J. M. STEVENS. 1981. Life Sci. **28:** 2947–2952.
31. THOMPSON, J. M., J. WHITAKER & J. A. JOSEPH. 1981. Brain Res. **224:** 436–440.
32. ROBINSON, D. S., R. L. SOURKES, A. NIES, L. S. HARRIS, S. SPECTOR, D. L. BARTLET & I. S. KAYE. 1977. Arch. Gen. Psychiatry **34:** 89–92.
33. REIS, D. J., R. A. ROSS & T. H. JOH. 1977. Brain Res. **136:** 465–474.
34. WALLER, S. B., D. K. INGRAM, M. A. REYNOLDS & E. D. LONDON. 1981. Age **4:** 143.
35. JOSEPH, J. A., C. FILBURN, L. P. TZANKOFF, J. M. THOMPSON & B. T. ENGEL. 1980. Neurobiol. Aging **1:** 119–125.
36. McGEER, P. L. & E. G. McGEER. 1976. J. Neurochem. **26:** 65–76.
37. JOSEPH, J. A., R. E. BERGER, B. T. ENGEL & G. S. ROTH. 1978. J. Gerontol. **33:** 643–649.
38. SEVERSON, J. A., J. MARCUSSON, B. WINBLAD & C. E. FINCH. 1982. J. Neurochem. **39:** 1623–1631.
39. SEVERSON, J. A. & C. E. FINCH. 1980. Fed. Proc. Fed. Am. Soc. Exp. Biol. **39:** 508.
40. SEVERSON, J. A. & C. E. FINCH. 1980. Brain Res. **192:** 147–162.
41. HAMBLIN, M. W., S. E. LEFF & I. CREESE. 1984. Biochem. Pharmacol. **33:** 877–887.
42. SEVERSON, J. A. & P. K. RANDALL. 1985. J. Pharmacol. Exp. Ther. **233:** 361–369.
43. HAMBLIN, M. W. & I. CREESE. 1982. Life Sci. **30:** 1587–1595.
44. THAL, L. J., S. G. HOROWITZ, B. DVORKIN & M. H. MAKMAN. 1980. Brain Res. **192:** 185–194.
45. KEBABIAN, J. W. & D. CALNE. 1979. Nature **277:** 93–96.
46. HENRY, J. M., C. R. FILBURN, J. A. JOSEPH & G. S. ROTH. 1986. Neurobiol. Aging **7:** 357–361.
47. O'BOYLE, K. M. & J. L. WADDINGTON. 1984. Eur. J. Pharmacol. **105:** 171–174.
48. MORGAN, D. G., J. O. MARCUSSON, B. WINBLAD & C. E. FINCH. 1984. Soc. Neurosci. Abstr. **10:** 445.
49. HENRY, J. M. & G. S. ROTH. 1984. Life Sci. **35:** 899–904.
50. LEFF, S. E., R. GARIANO & I. CREESE. 1984. Proc. Natl. Acad. Sci. USA **81:** 3910–3914.
51. JOSEPH, J. A., T. DALTON & W. HUNT. 1986. Soc. Neurosci. Abstr. **12:** 1468.
52. UNGERSTEDT, U. 1971. Acta Physiol. Scand. Suppl. **367:** 69–93.
53. JOSEPH, J. A., C. R. FILBURN & G. S. ROTH. 1981. Life Sci. **29:** 575–584.
54. DEAN, R. L., J. SCOZZAFAVA, J. A. GOAS, B. REGAN, B. BEER & R. T. BARTUS. 1981. Exp. Aging Res. **35:** 427–451.
55. BARTUS, R. T. 1979. *In* Aging, Vol. 10: Sensory Systems and Communications in the Elderly. J. M. Ordy, Ed.: 35–73. Raven Press. New York.
56. JOSEPH, J. A., R. T. BARTUS, D. CLODY, D. MORGAN, C. FINCH, B. BEER & S. SESACK. 1983. Neurobiol. Aging **4:** 313–319.
57. JOSEPH, J. A. & A. S. LIPPA. 1986. Neurobiol. Aging **7:** 37–40.
58. LEVIN, P., M. HAJII, J. A. JOSEPH & G. S. ROTH. 1983. Life Sci. **32:** 1743–1749.
59. JOSEPH, J. A., G. S. ROTH & A. S. LIPPA. 1986. Neurobiol. Aging **7:** 31–35.
60. MORGAN, D. G., C. V. MOBBS, C. P. ANDERSON, Y. N. SINHA & C. FINCH. Eur. J. Pharmacol. In press.
61. MORGAN, D. G., Y. N. SINHA & C. E. FINCH. 1984. Neuroendocrinology **38:** 407–410.
62. CRONIN, M. J., A. RECHES, R. M. MacLEOD & I. S. LOGIN. 1983. Eur. J. Pharmacol. **91:** 229–234.
63. BURROWS, C. H. & G. C. KOKKONEN. 1977. *In* Advances in Nutrition. Vol. 1. H. H. Draper, Ed.: 253–298. Plenum. New York.
64. ROTH, G. S., D. K. INGRAM & J. A. JOSEPH. 1984. Brain Res. **300:** 27–29.
65. JOSEPH, J. A., J. WHITAKER, G. S. ROTH & D. K. INGRAM. 1983. Neurobiol. Aging **4:** 191–197.
66. THOMPSON, J. M., C. L. MAKINO, J. R. WHITAKER & J. A. JOSEPH. 1984. Brain Res. **299:** 169–173.
67. HENRY, J. M., J. A. JOSEPH & G. S. ROTH. Brain Res. In press.
68. CREESE, I. 1982. Trends Neurosci. Res. **Feb:** 40–43.
69. BARONE, P., T. DAVIS, A. R. BROWN & T. N. CHASE. 1986. Eur. J. Pharmacol. **123:** 109–114.

DISCUSSION OF THE PAPER

B. HOFFER (*University of Colorado Health Sciences Center, Denver, CO*): Have you given some thought to making measurements that are more linked to what we consider D2 function to be, that is, inhibitory coupling to the cyclase doing GTPase assay, and to things that might relate more to the molecular function of D2 striatal receptors? Do you have any data in this regard?

J. A. JOSEPH (*Armed Forces Radiobiology Research Institute, Bethesda, MD*): There is a very nice paper by Rabin in *Neurobiology of Aging* where he averaged some of these parameters. No changes were seen in the catalytic subunits.

D. MORGAN (*University of Southern California, Los Angeles, CA*): There is a great deal of variability in the prolactin effects among the various investigators. I think that the differences may be the result of using different strains of species. However, if there are no prolactin receptors in the striatum or nigra and if there is no prolactin there, how is it possibly doing anything?

JOSEPH: I do not know. However, if you take all of the papers concerned with this issue where no upregulation of striatal DA receptor stimulation is seen, you will see that the studies utilized intense prolactin stimulation to try to obtain an effect. When people have seen something, they tend to use very low doses. Therefore, it may be some kind of a compensatory response to very low stimulation. When we looked for changes in plasma prolactin levels in these animals, we could not see any differences between treated animals and controls.

J. SEVERSON (*Amersham Corporation, Arlington Heights, IL*): Do you see any slowed responses or slowed recovery of the D1 receptor after EEDQ administration? If so, is it similar to the slowed response of the D2 receptor?

JOSEPH: Yes.

SEVERSON: Is there a slowed recovery of D1 also?

JOSEPH: Yes, they are both slower in the old animal.

Exercise Effects on Aged Motor Function[a]

WANEEN W. SPIRDUSO,[b] HOLDEN H. MacRAE,[c]
PRISCILLA G. MacRAE,[c] JACQUIN PREWITT,[d] AND
LANCE OSBORNE[d]

[b]Department of Physical and Health Education
Institute for Neurological Science Research
University of Texas–Austin
Austin, Texas 78712

[c]Department of Sports Medicine
Pepperdine University
Malibu, California 90265

[d]University of Texas
Health Science Center at Dallas
Dallas, Texas 75235

Aging degrades speeded performance in time-constrained tasks primarily by changes in the central nervous system. Motor responses such as simple, discrimination, and choice reaction time might therefore be viewed as behavioral "windows" into the central nervous system.[1] Age differences in performance on some of these tasks may be reduced substantially by selecting subjects for speed[2] or by exposing them to extraordinary practice sessions.[3,4] Nevertheless, one of the most consistent observations of behavioral change related to aging remains the insidious and pervasive slowing in almost all types of speeded performance.[5]

Why do these types of performance slow with age? This question has led to a search for task components that might be disproportionately vulnerable to aging. Very early, Weiss[6] discovered that the major slowing in a choice reaction response occurred primarily centrally rather than peripherally. An unresolved issue is whether these central changes represent a generalized slowing of CNS function or differential age effects upon specific stages of information processing.

Birren[1] suggested that a "general primary mechanism within the nervous system" ages, thereby affecting most psychomotor speeded performance. He described his mechanism as representing the general integrity of the central nervous system. Arenberg[7] suggested that this general primary mechanism represents an overall structural deterioration; this is in opposition to flawed control processes at various stages of processing such as encoding, filtering, or memory. Analyses of age effects on specific stages of processing have generally indicated that all stages are slowed by aging. Several investigators[7–9] found encoding deficits, and Salthouse and Somberg,[5] using Sternberg's[10]

[a] This work was supported in part by Grant No. NS20827.

363

memory scanning procedure, found deficits in memory scanning, stimulus encoding, and response preparation and execution. Baylor and Spirduso[11] also found age effects on response selection and response programming. Salthouse and Somberg[5] concluded that because age differences could not be easily localized to a specific information processing stage, there must be a generalized speed reduction in all central nervous system activity.

Hick's[12] law states that choice reaction time (CRT) can be predicted by the equation, $CRT = a + b[\log_2(N)]$, where a = the structural or basic speed of the sensory and motor apparatus, b = the rate of processing additional information, and N = the number of stimulus-response alternatives. The component a is viewed as simple reaction time because, theoretically, no uncertainty exists about what to do; the only uncertainty is about when to do it. Therefore, age effects on structural and functional integrity of the central nervous system would affect primarily the a component (Rabbitt;[4] Rabbitt & Vyas[13]), whereas age effects on efficiency of processing information in one or more stages would influence the slope, which is the b component of the equation.[14-16] Although Salthouse and Somberg[17] defined the slope component of the "rate of extracting information" somewhat differently than is used in paradigms using multiple stimuli displays, they nevertheless found that the slope was not affected by age.

The locus of age-related degradation of speeded performance is an important question to answer because it addresses the issue of plasticity of behavioral function. How inevitable and irreversible is age-related deterioration of speeded psychomotor performance? If psychomotor slowing is the result of structural deterioration of the central nervous system, then the decline may be more difficult to modify or postpone. On the other hand, plasticity of function might be prolonged only by health or nutrition-related changes in physiological function, not by practice or usage. However, if the behavioral slowing is primarily in control mechanisms that have been hypothesized as stages of information processing, the interventions such as practice and learned strategy changes might defer an age-related decline.

One intervention, suggested as early as 1968 by Botwinick and Thompson,[18] that has been purported to postpone age-related decline of psychomotor function is that of chronic exercise. Investigators who sample unusual populations of highly physically fit elderly individuals report that they are significantly faster in reactivity. At least six investigators and their colleagues who studied these types of samples have reported a relationship between systematic exercise and simple, discrimination, or choice reaction time[11,19] (see Spirduso[20] for review). Results from all of these studies were dependent upon the assumption that the exercised subjects were highly physically fit, inasmuch as subjects were categorized on the basis of their self-report of daily physical activity. However, recent researchers who addressed this issue by directly measuring physical fitness levels in a pre- and post-exercise design have also reported faster reactivity in physically fit individuals. Although a few reports have failed to find this relationship, the preponderance of evidence supports a relationship between physical fitness levels and psychomotor speeded performance (see Spirduso[20] for a discussion of this issue).

If physical fitness produced by chronic physical activity is related to psychomotor speed in the aged, what types of performance are affected? What components of these tasks are influenced? What are the mechanisms by which systematic physical activity might enhance psychomotor performance? One approach to these questions is to compare individuals differing in age and physical fitness level on several psychomotor tasks in which successful performance depends heavily on different stages of information processing. If physically fit individuals differ only in simple reaction time (a measure of basic sensory and motor apparatus speed) and not on trailmaking (a measure of scanning and stimulus identification), then physical fitness may influence a general central nervous system speed-reduction factor, but not specific stages of information processing.

The present study was conducted to determine which performances of several tasks were related to physical fitness level as inferred from the self-reports of the subjects of their chronic physical activity. Tasks were selected because success on each was thought to rely on different components of psychomotor performance.

METHODS

Subjects

The subjects were women categorized according to age and physical activity level as follows: 20–29 years, active (A, $N = 10$); 20–29 years, nonactive (NA, $N = 20$); 50–59 years (A, $N = 18$; NA, $N = 14$); 60–69 years (A, $N = 16$; NA, $N = 14$); and 70–79 years (A, $N = 10$; NA, $N = 9$). Subjects for all groups were screened to exclude those with abnormal body weight, medication, smoking, disease, and poor vision, and those who were not licensed automobile drivers. Subjects were accepted into active age groups if they reported that they walked/jogged/ran a minimum of three miles per day, three days per week, and had been maintaining this schedule for at least five years.

Tests

Simple Reaction Time (SRT)

The task was selected to measure structural integrity or basic speed of the sensory motor apparatus. Subjects were seated in a dental chair with their right foot on a microswitch that simulated the accelerator of an automobile. When a red light was illuminated, the subject lifted the right foot from the "accelerator" and placed it as quickly as possible on a microswitch that simulated an automobile brake. A warning bell preceded the presentation of the stimulus light by a randomly assigned interval of from two to four seconds. The foot switches were mounted adjacently at 40° angles to the subject; the wood block containing the brake microswitch was 18 cm to the left and slightly above the accelerator switch. SRT was the latency in milliseconds from the stimulus light onset to the activation of the accelerator microswitch. Subjects received one block of 15 trials. The score was the mean of the second block, with latencies above or below two standard deviations deleted.

Discrimination Reaction Time (DRT)

Performance on this task relies heavily on stimulus identification and comparison in order to make a discrimination. The task was similar to the SRT task above except that the display panel contained two lights, red and green. If the red light was illuminated, as in the SRT task, the subject lifted the right foot quickly from the accelerator to the brake. If the green light was illuminated, however, the subject did not respond. The probability of illumination for each light was 50%. Therefore, the task required stimulus discrimination prior to a decision to move. The simulated automobile apparatus was designed to increase the ecological validity of these measures, thereby minimizing novelty of the task. Novelty is known to be an age-related contaminant in experiments of reactivity. Subjects received one block of 28 trials; 8 of these were the green stimulus light, or the "no-go" condition. The score was the mean of those responses to the red light that were within two standard deviations of the subject's mean.

Stationary Tapping (S-Tap)

Performance on this task appears to rely on structural integrity of the central and peripheral motor system and central response programming. The subject, holding an 18-cm-long electronic stylus in the preferred hand, tapped it in place against a 2.5 × 12.7 cm steel plate as many times as possible in 10 s. The plate was large enough so that accuracy of tapping was not a factor. The score for each trial was the total number of taps in 10 s. The subject's score for the test was the average of three trials.

Between Target Tapping (T-Tap)

Performance on this task, by involving visual and proprioceptive serial comparisons of limb and target locations, relies on processing movement-generated error information and in error corrections. The subject, holding the electronic stylus in the preferred hand, tapped between two copper targets, each 2.5 × 12.7 cm, spaced 17.8 cm apart. The score for each trial was the total number of contacts made on the two targets within a 10-s time period. The score for the test was the average of three trials.

Trailmaking (TM)

Performance on this task requires scanning and stimulus identification. The subject, when ready, turned over a paper that contained 25 small circles (1 cm diameter), each numbered consecutively from 1 to 25. The subject placed the pencil on circle number 1, then drew a line from it to circle number 2, then to circle 3, and continued in this fashion until circle 25 was connected. The score for the trial was the number of seconds necessary to move the pencil from circle number 1 to circle number 25. The average of three trials constituted the subject's score.

Digit Symbol Substitution (DSS)

Performance on this task relies on stimulus identification, encoding, and short-term memory. The subject was presented with several rows of randomly ordered numbers, 1–9. Each number was associated with a symbol and the subject drew the appropriate matched symbol underneath each presentation of the numbers 1–9 as quickly as possible. The score was the average number of symbols matched within a 60-s time period over three trials.

Test Administration

Subjects were scheduled in a counterbalanced design three at a time and were assigned to one of three laboratory testing stations: reaction time, tapping, or trailmaking and digit symbol substitution. At the conclusion of each testing period, subjects rotated to the next station until tests were completed. Each test was conducted by an experienced, well-trained experimenter. Each subject was tested three consecutive days at the same time of day, but the order of test presentation was different on each day.

Experimental Design and Analysis

The experimental design was a three-way between-within factorial ANOVA. The between factors were activity level (active/nonactive) and age (20–29/50–59/60–69/70–79 years), and the within-subject factor was the days of testing (1–3). Dependent variables were SRT, DRT, discrimination time (DRT − SRT), stationary tapping, between target tapping, trailmaking, and digit symbol substitution for the separate ANOVAs. SRT and DRT trial latencies that were above or below two SDs were deleted from the analysis, and the means of the subjects were calculated with these trials excluded. Discrimination time was calculated by subtracting SRT from DRT for each subject.

RESULTS

TABLE 1 is a summary of all the ANOVAs. Performance on four of the seven tasks was related to activity level, as shown by either a significant main effect (SRT, DRT, and DT) or by an interaction with age (S-Tap). As expected, the main effect for age was significant on all variables, and the main effect of practice (days) was also significant on all variables where it was measured. The only two-way interaction that proved to be significant was the age × days interaction on trailmaking; here, the 70-year-old subjects made dramatically greater gains from day 1 to day 3 than the other three groups. On all other tests, all age groups improved in a similar pattern.

Reaction Time

The simple reaction time of physically active women was significantly faster than that of the sedentary women in the 20–29 (10%) and 50–59 (8%) year groups only

TABLE 1. Summary of Probability Levels for Analyses of Variance Attributable to Activity Level, Age, and Test Sessions (Days) for All Variables[a]

Variable	Activity Level	Age	Days	Act X Age	Act X Days	Age X Days	Activity X Age X Days
SRT	0.02	<0.001	<0.001	0.06			0.10
DRT	0.002	<0.001	<0.001				
DT	0.04	0.03	N/A		N/A	N/A	N/A
S-Tap		<0.001	<0.001	0.05	0.09		
TM		<0.001	<0.001			0.03	
T-Tap		<0.001	<0.001			0.07	
DSS		<0.001	<0.001				

[a] SRT = simple reaction time. DRT = discrimination reaction time. DT = discrimination time (DRT − SRT). S-Tap = stationary tapping. TM = trailmaking. DSS = digit symbol substitution. N/A = not applicable. Discrimination time was calculated on the third day only.

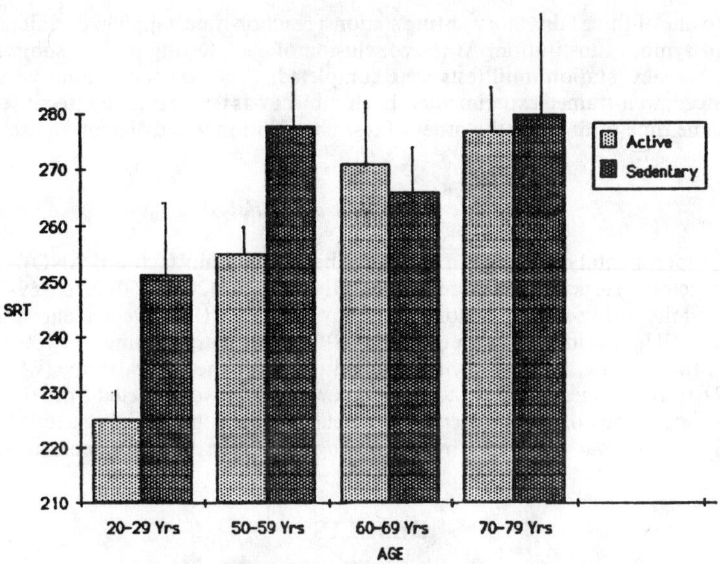

FIGURE 1. Simple reaction times (SRT) of subjects categorized as active or nonactive at each of four decades. Error bars are standard errors of the mean. SRT = latency in ms from the onset of a stimulus light to the release of a foot microswitch.

($F_{1,97}$ = 5.5, p = 0.02). However, on the discrimination reaction variable, the physically active women at all ages tested were significantly faster than the sedentary women ($F_{1,97}$ = 9.76, p = 0.002). The differences between the physically active and sedentary women on DRT at each age were 12%, 12%, 8%, and 4% from the 20–29

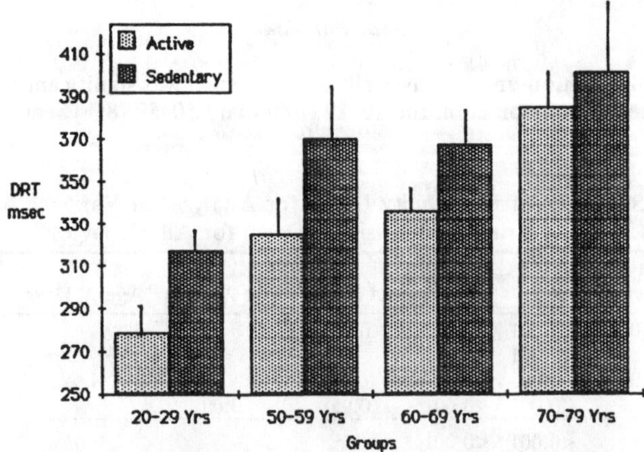

FIGURE 2. Discrimination reaction times (DRT) of subjects categorized as active or nonactive at each of four decades. Error bars are standard errors of the mean. DRT = latency in ms from the onset of the designated stimulus light, which is when a nondesignated light may or may not be activated.

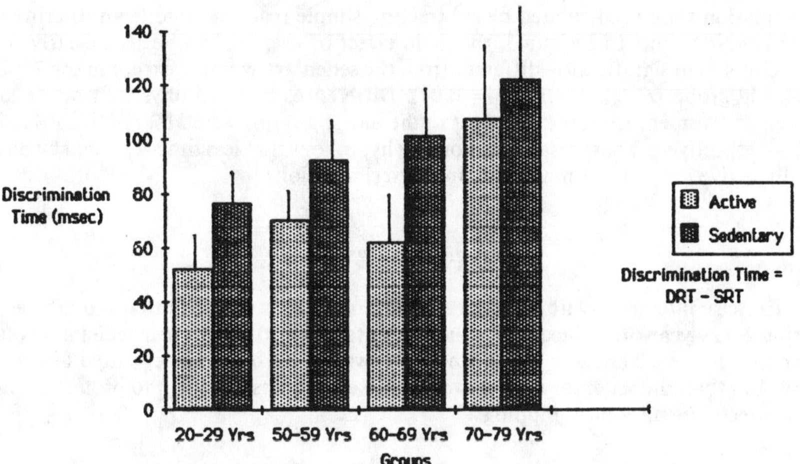

FIGURE 3. Discrimination times (DT) of subjects categorized as active or nonactive at each of four decades. Error bars are standard errors of the mean. DT = DRT (FIGURE 2) − SRT (FIGURE 1).

to the 70–79 year groups, respectively. Overall, exercise was associated with faster reaction time (see FIGURES 1 and 2).

Discrimination Time

DT is thought to be a measure of the actual time taken to make the decision. It is dissociated from the general speed of the sensory and motor apparatus. Hence, dis-

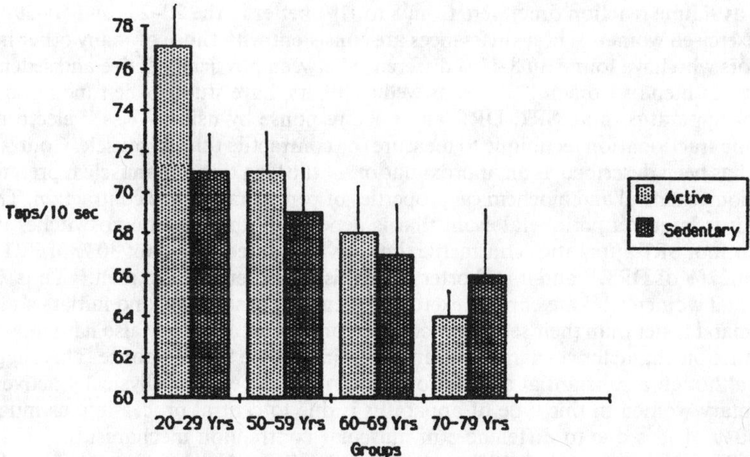

FIGURE 4. Stationary tapping (S-Tap) of subjects categorized as active or nonactive at each of four decades. Error bars are standard errors of the mean. The ordinate is the total number of contacts made in 10 s.

crimination time is calculated by subtracting simple reaction time from discrimination reaction time. In FIGURE 3, the main effect of exercise can be seen clearly. The exercisers were significantly different from the sedentary women, except in the 70–79-year-old group ($F_{1,102} = 4.38$, $p = 0.04$). Differences between physically active and sedentary women, from the youngest to the oldest groups, were 31%, 24%, 39%, and 12%, respectively. These results support the hypothesis that less time is needed by physically active subjects to make a simple discrimination.

Stationary Tapping

Exercise interacted with age (as can be seen in FIGURE 4) such that only the exercising 20–29-year-old subjects generated more taps per 10 s than their sedentary counterparts ($F_{3,97} = 2.66$, $p = 0.05$). The 20–29-year-old exercisers generated 8% more taps/10 s than the sedentary young women. Exercise does not seem to protect against age effects on stationary tapping.

Conclusion

The tasks selected for study in the above investigations were indeed measuring different parameters because intercorrelations among them ranged from $r = 0.0$ to 0.69. Most of the intercorrelations were below 0.45.

DISCUSSION

Enhanced physical fitness, as might be inferred from a lifestyle of chronic exercise, appears to be related to psychomotor performance reflecting primarily the basic speed of the sensory and motor apparatus as it conducts simple discriminations and choices. Performances depending upon the structural integrity of the central nervous system, such as simple reaction time, were from 8 to 11% better in the 20–29- and 50–59-year-old exercised women. These differences are consistent with those of many other investigators who have found an 8–11% difference between physically active and sedentary groups of men or women.[19-21] We, as well as others, have studied the function of the motor apparatus in an SRT, DRT, and CRT response by using Weiss's[6] electromyographic fractionation technique to measure the contractile time of muscle. Contractile time has been described as an approximation of the "lag time" in muscle representing the biomechanical and biochemical properties of peripheral muscle contraction. Therefore, it is largely a peripheral event that is dependent upon the microswitches used. In our foot SRT apparatus, contractile time has accounted for about 30% of SRT and about 27% of DRT,[11] and it is shorter in exercised women[11,22] and men.[23] Thus, both men and women who are chronic exercisers identify the stimulus and initiate a motor command faster than their sedentary counterparts. Moreover, they also have muscular contraction characteristics that consume less time in the SRT response. This suggests that although a substantial amount of the difference between physically active and sedentary women in this type of apparatus is due to central processing, as much as 28–30% of it is due to differences in muscular contraction mechanisms.

DRT, which was from 9–12% faster in physically active women, relies heavily on basic sensory and motor programming speed, but also requires a single discrimination between two stimuli. The motor response is identical to that used in the simple reaction time task; the only difference between DRT and SRT, as assumed by the subtraction method, is a stimulus discrimination stage. When the latency necessary for a simple reaction (SRT) and the contractile time are subtracted from the discrimination time (DRT − SRT), the resulting time attributed to making the discrimination is observed to be significantly shorter in the chronic exercisers. In our study, that amount of time ranged from 52 ms in the young runners (15% of DRT) to 122 ms in the old sedentary group (30% of DRT). The older and more sedentary women took longer to make the discrimination. These results are similar to earlier results showing that the performance of both male and female older exercisers in relatively uncomplicated choice reaction time paradigms having only one or two alternatives is approximately 11% faster than that of sedentary older individuals.[19,20]

Stationary tapping, which was significantly faster only in the young runners, is a measure of motor outflow or motor programming. Performance on this task is relatively stable, especially within each day where subjects vary little from trial to trial. The average amount of improvement from the first to the third day was 3–4% and the greatest amount of improvement for one group was 6%. In comparison, simple and discrimination responses improved 5–10% over the three-day testing session. Unlike the task demands of simple and discrimination reaction times, the motor programming necessary in stationary tapping requires the programming of a neuromotor integration of muscles that were not used predominantly in fast walking or running (the exercise activity). Therefore, stationary tapping is probably a clearer representation of the physical training effects on central motor programming that are dissociated from exercise effects on the peripheral motor apparatus (as might be expressed by contractile time). This suggests that physical activity may be related less to open-loop central motor programming in the aged and more to reactivity attributes.

The observation that SRT and stationary tapping (both purported to be measures of structural integrity of the central nervous system) were not significantly faster in the two oldest running groups (60–69; 70–79 years) may have at least two explanations. The first and most probable is that the subjects in the two oldest groups did not maintain as high a physical fitness level as those in the 20–29- and 50–59-year-old groups. Although all subjects declared that they walked or ran at better than a 10-min-mile pace at least 3–5 miles/day, 5 days/week, it is possible that the oldest women maintained a pace much closer to the minimum in terms of both time and distance than did the younger groups. Botwinick and Storandt,[24] two of the few researchers to find no relationship between exercise and reactivity in older subjects, did however report such a relationship in their younger subjects. The physical activity level of their active group was relatively low and could have accounted for the failure to find a relationship. In studies that rely upon the self-reports of activity levels of the subjects, only estimates of physical fitness status are available, and age-related differential fitness levels always remain as an alternative interpretation. The second explanation is that high levels, in an absolute sense, of cardiovascular and aerobic capacity may be necessary to express the highest functioning of the central nervous system and no amount of physical training in older individuals can produce those required levels.

Psychomotor performances that depend more on scanning, stimulus identification, encoding, processing movement-generated error information, and short-term memory were not related to exercise status at any age. These more complex psychomotor tasks certainly tax information processing capacities, as was shown in the dramatic inverse relationship between age and performance. However, exercised women were not significantly better; in fact, the means of physically active and sedentary groups at all ages were almost identical on trailmaking, digit symbol substitution, and target tapping. The contribution of basic sensory and motor speed and the simple discriminations of choices of response selection to these more complex tasks may be a contribution so small that enhancements of these basic mechanisms are undetectable from an observation of the task performance.

A NEUROCHEMICAL MECHANISM OF EXERCISE EFFECTS ON CENTRAL NERVOUS SYSTEM FUNCTION

Our results and those of others suggest that chronic exercise may exert a protective effect on those central nervous systems mediating sensorimotor processing. These findings are consistent with studies in animals that indicate that exercise changes the levels of neurotransmitters and their metabolites in these same brain regions. In order to determine the possible subcellular mechanisms within the central nervous system that might be responsible for the protective effects of exercise on psychomotor performance, we have, in parallel to our studies in humans, explored neurochemical correlates of exercise in the rat. Our focus has been on dopamine because it is well known that adequate functioning of the dopaminergic neurotransmitter system in the basal ganglia is necessary for normal motor responses. Parkinson's diseased individuals, known to have delayed reaction times, have lost virtually all of their dopaminergic nigrostriatal neurons.[25] Even in normal aging, as evidenced by animal research, the nigrostriatal dopamine system deteriorates selectively with aging.[26,27] Although some have questioned the importance of this system in reaction-type responses,[25] we have reported several experiments using a rodent model that provide evidence for tight linkage between rapid movement initiation and an intact nigrostriatal dopamine system.[28-31]

The trophic effects of chronic physical activity on brain neurotransmitter function are far from clear, but preliminary evidence suggests that chronic adaptations of neurotransmitter systems in the physiological response to systematic exercise bouts may be considerable. Brown[32] reported that resting levels of norepinephrine in cerebrum and serotonin in midbrain were higher in rats that experienced daily treadmill running for 8 weeks. Chronic exercise[33,34] also has been shown to alter cholinergic blocking drugs. Under the leadership of R. E. Wilcox, we have studied more specifically the issue of exercise effects upon one of the neurotransmitter systems (dopamine) that has been linked by us and others to speeded movement initiation. D_2 dopamine receptor binding in striatum was significantly higher in young rats that had experienced 12 weeks of treadmill running, one hour/day,[35] which is a finding that has been corroborated recently by de Castro and Duncan.[36] Similarly, we found D_2 dopamine binding to be higher in 21-month-old presenescent rats that had experienced the same exercise protocol as the young rats. Dopamine receptor density, as expressed by B_{max}, was also significantly higher in old runners than in old controls.[37] Finally, the ratio of D_2 dopamine binding to a dopamine metabolite, DOPAC (suggesting the "coupling" between transmitter and receptor), was higher in treadmill-trained young rats.[38]

Because DA parameters cannot be measured prior to treadmill running in the same animals that are assessed following the exercise program, it is only appropriate to conclude that exercise seems related to the characteristics of D_2DA receptor binding (receptor density) and the relationship between binding and dopamine metabolites. If the relationship is causal, then chronic exercise may have the capacity to defer age-related declines in the dopaminergic system, which is a system thought to be highly related to speeded movement initiation. Thus, either an optimum level of aerobic capacity or repetitive physical activity may decelerate age-related degradation of nigrostriatal dopamine neurons and striatal D_2 dopamine receptors.

A multitude of physiological adaptations occur in response to chronic and intense physical exercise, only one of which may be a change in brain neurotransmitters. The leap from an apparent relationship between exercise and one neurotransmitter in rodents — albeit one that is important in the initiation of movement — is a great one. Nevertheless, the results from these preliminary studies of exercise effects on neurotransmitters, and from studies of apparent exercise effects on human reactive psychomotor performance, suggest that exercise may in fact postpone age-related degradation of psychomotor reactivity and that it may do this, at least in part, by preserving the nigro-striatal dopaminergic system.

REFERENCES

1. BIRREN, J. E., A. M. WOODS & M. V. WILLIAMS. 1980. Behavioral slowing with age: causes, organization, and consequences. *In* Aging in the 1980s: Psychological Issues. L. W. Poon, Ed. Amer. Psychol. Assoc. Washington, D.C.
2. GOTTSDANKER, R. 1982. Age and simple reaction time. J. Gerontol. **37:** 342–348.
3. MURRELL, F. H. 1970. The effect of extensive practice on age differences in reaction time. J. Gerontol. **25:** 268–274.
4. RABBITT, P. M. A. 1980. A fresh look at the changes in reaction time in old age. *In* The Psychobiology of Aging. D. G. Stein, Ed. Elsevier/North-Holland. New York/Amsterdam.
5. SALTHOUSE, T. A. & B. L. SOMBERG. 1982. Isolating the age deficit in speeded performance. J. Gerontol. **37:** 59–63.
6. WEISS, A. D. 1965. The locus of reaction time change with set, motivation, and age. J. Gerontol. **20:** 60–64.
7. ARENBERG, D. 1980. Comments on processes that account for memory decline with age. *In* New Directions in Memory and Aging. L. W. Poon, J. L. Fozard, L. S. Cermak, D. Arenberg & L. W. Thompson, Eds. Erlbaum. Hillsdale, New Jersey.
8. SIMON, J. R. 1968. Signal processing time as a function of aging. J. Exp. Psychol. **78:** 76–80.
9. SIMON, J. R. & A. R. POURAGHABAGHER. 1978. The effect of aging on the stages of processing in choice reaction tasks. J. Gerontol. **33:** 553–561.
10. STERNBERG, S. 1969. The discovery of processing stages: extensions of Donder's method. *In* Attention and Performance, Vol. II. W. G. Koster, Ed. North-Holland. Amsterdam.
11. BAYLOR, A. M. & W. W. SPIRDUSO. Effects of systematic exercise on components of reaction time in older women. J. Gerontol. Submitted.
12. HICK, W. E. 1952. On the rate of gain of information. Q. J. Exp. Psychol. **4:** 11–26.
13. RABBITT, P. M. A. & S. M. VYAS. 1970. An elementary preliminary taxonomy for some errors in laboratory choice reaction time tasks. Acta Psychol. **33:** 56–76.
14. SUCI, G. J., M. D. DAVIDOFF & W. W. SURWILLO. 1960. Reaction time as a function of stimulus information and age. J. Exp. Psychol. **60:** 242–244.
15. ANDERS, T. R. & J. L. FOZARD. 1973. Effects of age upon retrieval from primary and secondary memory. Dev. Psychol. **9:** 411–415.
16. ANDERS, T. R., J. L. FOZARD & T. D. LILLYQUIST. 1972. Effects of age upon retrieval from short memory. Dev. Psychol. **6:** 214–217.
17. SALTHOUSE, T. A. & B. L. SOMBERG. 1982b. Time-accuracy relationships in young and old adults. J. Gerontol. **37:** 349–353.
18. BOTWINICK, J. & L. W. THOMPSON. 1968. Age differences in reaction time: An artifact? Gerontologist **8:** 25–28.
19. RICKLI, R. & B. SHARMAN. 1986. Motor performance of women as a function of age and physical activity level. J. Gerontol. **41:** 645–649.
20. SPIRDUSO, W. W. 1982. Physical fitness in relation to motor aging. *In* The Aging Motor System. J. A. Mortimer, F. J. Pirozzolo & G. J. Maletta, Eds. Praeger. New York.
21. DUSTMAN, R. E., R. O. RUHLING, E. M. RUSSELL, D. E. SHEARER, H. W. BONEKAT, J. W. SHIGEOKA, J. S. WOOD & C. BRADFORD. 1984. Aerobic exercise training and improved neuropsychological function of older adults. Neurobiol. Aging **5:** 35–42.
22. HART, B. 1981. The effect of age and habitual activity on the fractionated components of resisted and unresisted response time. Med. Sci. Sports Exercise **13:** 78.

23. CLARKSON, P. M. 1978. The effect of age and activity level in simple and choice fractionated response time. Eur. J. Appl. Physiol. **40:** 17–25.
24. BOTWINICK, J. & M. STORANDT. 1974. Cardiovascular status depressive effect and other factors in reaction time. J. Gerontol. **29:** 543–548.
25. MARSDEN, C. D. 1982. The mysterious motor function of the basal ganglia: The Robert Wartenberg lecture. Neurology **32:** 514–539.
26. RANDALL, P. K. 1980. Functional aging of the nigrostriatal system. Peptides **1**(suppl. 1): 177–184.
27. WILCOX, R. E. 1984. Changes in biogenic amines and their metabolites with aging and alcoholism. *In* Alcoholism in the Elderly. J. T. Hartford & T. Samorajski, Eds.: 85–115. Raven Press. New York.
28. SPIRDUSO, W. W., L. D. ABRAHAM & M. D. WOLF. 1981. Effects of chlorpromazine on escape and avoidance responses: a closer look. Pharmacol. Biochem. Behav. **14:** 433–438.
29. SPIRDUSO, W. W., P. E. GILLIAM & R. E. WILCOX. 1984. Speed of movement initiation predicts differences in 3H-spiroperidol receptor binding in rats. Psychopharmacologia **83:** 205–209.
30. SPIRDUSO, W. W., P. E. GILLIAM, T. J. SCHALLERT, M. UPCHURCH, D. M. VAUGHN & R. E. WILCOX. 1985. Reactive capacity: a sensitive behavioral marker of movement initiation and nigrostriatal dopamine function. Brain Res. **325:** 49–55.
31. MACRAE, P. G., W. W. SPIRDUSO & R. E. WILCOX. Movement initiation and nigrostriatal dopamine function: the effects of age and practice. Brain Res. In press.
32. BROWN, B. S., T. PAYNE, C. KIM, G. MOORE, P. KREBS & W. MARTIN. 1979. Chronic response of rat brain norepinephrine and serotonin levels of endurance training. J. Appl. Physiol. Respir. Environ. Exercise Physiol. **46:** 19–23.
33. MCMASTER, S. N. & J. M. CARNEY. 1985. Exercise-induced changes in scheduled controlled behavior. Physiol. Behav. **35:** 337–341.
34. MCMASTER, S. B. & J. M. CARNEY. 1985. Changes in drug sensitivity following acute and chronic exercise. Pharmacol. Biochem. Behav. **23:** 191–194.
35. GILLIAM, P. E., W. W. SPIRDUSO, T. P. MARTIN, T. J. WALTERS, R. E. WILCOX & R. P. FARRAR. 1984. The effects of exercise training on 3H-spiperone binding in rat striatum. Pharmacol. Biochem. Behav. **20:** 863–867.
36. DECASTRO, J. M. & G. DUNCAN. 1985. Operantly conditioned running: effects on brain catecholamine concentrations and receptor densities in the rat. Pharmacol. Biochem. Behav. **23:** 495–500.
37. MACRAE, P. G., W. W. SPIRDUSO, G. D. CARTEE, R. P. FARRAR & R. E. WILCOX. 1987. Endurance training effects on striatal D2 dopamine receptor binding and striatal dopamine metabolites in presenescent older rats. Psychopharmacologia **92:** 236–240.
38. MACRAE, P. G., W. W. SPIRDUSO, G. D. CARTEE, R. P. FARRAR & R. E. WILCOX. Endurance training effects on striatal D2 dopamine receptor binding, striatal dopamine metabolite levels, and the initiation of movement. Neurosci. Lett. In press.

DISCUSSION OF THE PAPER

A. ALTAR (*CIBA-GEIBY Corporation, Summit, NJ*): You state that if you had only as little as a 15% decrease in the dopamine concentration of the striatum, you could observe impairments of reaction time. Is this in the old or young animal?

W. SPIRDUSO (*University of Texas, Austin, TX*): No, these were in young animals that were dopamine depleted.

ALTAR: How about in the older animal?

SPIRDUSO: We did not do that particular lesioning in the older animal.

ALTAR: It would be very interesting to see if you could get an even smaller amount of depletion to show a significant impairment in those animals. However, my other question concerns the treadmill experience. Over six months, you notice considerable change in the dopamine system both in terms of D_2 receptors and dopamine metabolites. How soon after the last treadmill experiment or after the last treadmill experience were these animals killed?

Spirduso: Forty-eight hours.

Altar: That is a fairly good period of time. Did you ever take young control animals after just a single treadmill experience and kill them 48 hours later to show that there was not these kinds of changes?

Spirduso: No, we did not do that in young rats.

Altar: It seems like a long period of time, so one may not see the change; however, it may be worth doing.

Spirduso: We were interested in resting levels and changes in resting levels. We tried to avoid the acute effects that might occur as a result of the running.

D. Morgan (*University of Southern California, Los Angeles, CA*): We obtained some brains from animals that were exercised for six weeks and then not allowed to exercise for three weeks. When we looked at the striatal DA receptors, we did not see anything. Have you looked at times longer than 48 hours after there was exercise to see if this effect dissipates with time?

Spirduso: No, we have been fairly rigorous with the 48-hour time.

Neuropharmacological Intervention with Motor System Aging

PETER A. LeWITT

Lafayette Clinic
Department of Neurology
Wayne State University School of Medicine
Detroit, Michigan 48207

With increasing age, there is no obvious biologically programmed schedule for decline in motor capabilities nor any compelling "theme" that currently directs attempts at therapeutic intervention. These realities need to be confessed at the start in order to dispel any undue expectations by readers that they will learn at what point "aging" begins or what can be done about it. While neuropharmacology has become extremely sophisticated and capable in symptomatic control of a variety of CNS disorders such as epilepsy, depression, parkinsonism, and psychosis, there has been little advance in understanding and treating those deficits appearing with normal aging. Many of the effective pharmacological approaches with CNS illness have been guided by knowledge of the disease state against which antagonism, enhancement, or other modes of drug intervention could restore previous function. In the case of normal aging, however, it is unclear which of the many neurochemical changes with age are in of themselves "pathological" (in the sense of being an equivalent of a disease state), nonessential alterations, "useful" compensations, or secondary consequences of loss in cellular elements such as neurotransmitter-bearing neurons.[1] Unfortunately, the identity of aging mechanisms in the CNS motor system cannot be read from the imprint of CNS neurodegenerative disorders such as Alzheimer's disease. Although it can have associated parkinsonism, along with the emergence of regressive motor reflexes, even severely demented Alzheimer's disease subjects are generally without deficits of motor control; this is true despite the extensive neuronal and neurochemical losses in cortical and subcortical systems of the CNS. Several spontaneously developing movement disorders appearing with advancing age (such as essential tremor, orofacial dyskinesia, torticollis, and restless leg syndrome) do not reveal in their features or symptomatic therapeutics (TABLE 1) obvious targets for relieving deficits of normal aging. Even parkinsonism, which superficially resembles an exaggeration of some age-related motor changes, is limited as a model for reasons to be discussed. The pharmacological rationales for several of the medications in TABLE 1, as well as the pathophysiology of these disorders, await further understanding.

At some point past maturity, every individual experiences elements of a uniform array of motor deficits. These may become evident in situations of specialized clinical testing as in settings of everyday life.[2-6] By the seventh decade, the neurological examination in healthy subjects has typically changed to reveal a number of deficits due to peripheral and central changes in the nervous system. These changes include subdued muscle-stretch reflexes, decreased muscular strength and work rate,[7] impaired upward gaze, release of certain involuntary reflexes (snout, palmomental sign, etc.), less acute perception of touch and vibration, and mildly decreased abilities of fine

TABLE 1. Medication Treatment of Movement Disorders

Parkinsonism: levodopa, bromocriptine, anticholinergics, amantadine,
  other synergistic therapies (e.g., deprenyl)
Essential tremor: beta-blockers, primidone, ethanol
Dyskinesia: tetrabenazine, reserpine, neuroleptics, cholinergic agents,
  bromocriptine (low-dose), clonazepam, α-methyl-para-tyrosine, sedatives
Dystonia: anticholinergics, levodopa, bromocriptine, clonazepam,
  baclofen, carbamazepine, lithium, neuroleptics, botulinum injection
Myoclonus: 5-hydroxytryptophan, clonazepam, valproate, lisuride,
  piracetam
Tics: clonidine, neuroleptics, tetrabenazine, clonazepam
Restlessness & Akathisia: benzodiazepines, beta-blockers,
  anticholinergics, clonidine
Ataxia: thyrotropin-releasing hormone (?)
Muscular weakness: anabolic steroids

coordination and rapid alternating movements of the hands.[5,8] While most of these deficits are innocuous and not necessarily pathological, the functional disturbances of gait fluidity, straight posture, base of stepping, and surety of balance together constitute a syndrome that disables many individuals that are otherwise neurologically healthy.[9,10] Although the causes of gait disturbance can be multifactorial, the contributions of aging-derived CNS pathophysiology to these problems have not yet been clarified.

Comparative changes over the postmaturity years in other motor activities have been measured using semiquantitative techniques developed by Potvin and colleagues.[10] In a cross-sectional study of normals ranging from 27–75 years of age, certain abilities such as the manipulation of a safety pin or tying a bowknot showed little decline. More substantial deficits with age accompanied tests of buttoning, cutting food, handwriting speed, and arising from a chair. Even though the balancing and coordination test of "tandem gait" was generally intact, the ability to balance on one leg with eyes closed tended to be markedly impaired. This deficit was evident in physically conditioned 80-year-old subjects active at jogging.[11] However, the evidence to link age-related disabilities such as imbalance to discrete anatomical or neurochemical systems of the brain and spinal cord has been extremely limited and circumstantial. For example, despite the substantial loss of cortical and subcortical neurons with normal aging,[12] there is relatively little dropout of neurons or other pathological change in cerebellar nuclei or brain-stem systems mediating balance control.[13] Although certain regions of the cerebral cortex can be identified as sites at which lesions would impair walking, the specificity of aging-derived changes in cortical motor neurons for the disturbance of gait is a difficult association to make, particularly with the relatively good preservation of other motor skills.

As in the elderly, impaired gait, balance, and posture control are prominent features in Parkinson's disease, and they can be the least likely to improve with dopaminergic and other forms of medication therapy. Furthermore, slowness and decreased dexterity of movement in parkinsonism resemble, in some ways, other deficits with advancing age. It should be noted, though, that Parkinson's disease commonly has the early presentation of several findings — resting tremor, rigidity, micrographia, masked facies — that are generally not prominent in the neurological exam of the normal elderly. Because Parkinson's disease is so often a disorder of advanced age, it is difficult in most patients to know which components of their deficits are contributed by their aging process in the face of the major impairments caused by the degenerative disease. With the advent of a selective neurotoxin, 1-methyl-4-phenyl-1,2,3,6-tetrahydropyridine (MPTP), that can duplicate clinical and biochemical features of idiopathic Parkinson's disease in man, the ability to study parkinsonian changes of motor control in isolation from aging has been possible.[14,15] The neurochemical changes produced by MPTP have been limited to the nigrostriatal dopaminergic pathways in animal studies, and MPTP-parkinsonian subjects recover symptomatically from their permanent motor deficits during levodopa or other dopaminergic therapy. The specificity of bradykinesia, imbalance, postural disturbance, and rigidity to this selective dopamine-deficiency state (lacking the decreases in noradrenergic, serotonergic, and other neurotransmitter/neuromodulator substances additionally found in aging and in idiopathic Parkinson's disease) emphasizes that parkinsonian symptom complex can be regarded as solely that of decreased nigrostriatal dopaminergic neurotransmission.

The analogy of Parkinson's disease to normal aging has proven to be a fruitful model for studying several patterns of deficit in motor control.[16] Decline in striatal content of dopamine and its synthetic enzyme, tyrosine hydroxylase, is found with increasing human age.[17,18] However, the most substantial decline in tyrosine hydroxylase is in the first three decades of life, and little change occurs thereafter.[18] One concept derived from earlier studies of Parkinson's disease[19] (and now the human model of MPTP-induced parkinsonism[14]) is that approximately 80% of striatal dopamine needs to be lost before clinical features of parkinsonism emerge. Cell counts of substantia nigra neurons (by regression line analysis) show significant declines with normal aging, but counts in the range of parkinsonians would not be found until approximately 100 years of age by this analysis.[18] Moreover, the remaining neurons appear to be capable of increasing their output of dopamine.[19] If the nigrostriatal system has a significant reserve of dopaminergic function, then age-related decline might not reach the threshold needed to unmask parkinsonian motor deficits during a normal life span. Could some of the features of motor impairment with normal aging be derived from "subparkinsonian" deficits in dopaminergic neurotransmission?

This question was addressed by a study of 10 normal subjects, aged 59–72 years, who participated in a double-blind crossover study of placebo versus levodopa.[20] Receiving the drug (as Sinemet) in the dose range of 400–800 mg/day for six weeks, these subjects were given a regimen generally therapeutic for most parkinsonian patients. No subject had significant neurological abnormalities at enrollment, and a 5-element clinical rating scale showed no parkinsonian signs (except for one or two equivocal features in a few patients). As compared to the placebo phase, levodopa-treated subjects developed no changes in their clinical ratings nor subjective experience of improved dexterity, gait, or other motor functioning. Assessment of simple reaction time and hand speed of movement showed a slight (but statistically insignificant) improvement during the levodopa phase, and there was no change in resting and action tremor amplitude. Neuropsychological evaluations of these subjects[21] revealed a significant improvement of effort-demanding cognitive operations (but not more "automatic" tasks) with levodopa treatment. The latter findings, along with observations of enhanced electroretinogram b wave amplitude,[20] indicate central dopamine effects from medication in this study. It is of interest that untreated subjects of similar age with idiopathic Parkinson's disease, when tested with the same neuropsychological battery,[21] had deficits of more effortful cognitive operations in a pattern opposite to the improvements that came about in the age-matched normals treated with levodopa. Levodopa and the dopaminergic ergot agonist, bromocriptine, have been investigated for therapeutic effect in senile dementia. While levodopa may bring about improvement in memory and other neuropsychological features,[22,23] no change in the motor exam was reported in patients affected just with senile dementia. Other studies have failed to find any benefits for cognition from levodopa or another monoamine neurotransmitter enhancement in Alzheimer's dementia.

In Alzheimer's disease, large-scale losses can be found in a number of neurotransmitter and neuropeptide systems. Although the extensive dropout in cortical and subcortical neurons could be the major explanation for these observations, it is also possible that some components of the biochemical pathology could be more primary deficiency states in preserved neuronal systems. Due to the optimism along these lines, most attempts to enhance geriatric brain function have been directed at lessening the impaired mental performance as found in dementia.[24-26] For the most part, motor functioning has not been evaluated, and medication trials have not been carried out with normal elderly controls. A variety of pharmacological approaches have been investigated for improving cognition. These have included drugs with regulatory effects on CNS circulation (based on unproven assumptions that decrease in brain blood flow with aging contributes to cognitive impairment). Cyclandelate, papaverine, and isoxsuprine as vasodilators have been claimed to bring about improvements in EEG and various cognitive operations in patients with cerebrovascular "insufficiency". With pyrithioxine and naftidrofuryl, augmentation of glucose utilization by the aged brain has also been reported;[27] however, the lack of an established mode of therapeutic effect or critical assessment of clinical results likely accounts for the obscurity of these "remedies". Hydergine, a mixture of ergot alkaloids widely used for treatment of impaired mental abilities with aging, has several actions on cerebral metabolism. Though extensively studied in animal and human models of aging and dementia, little is known of its pharmacological actions in improving cognitive performance.[28] Piracetam, a compound with a number of CNS effects, including enhanced metabolism and improved recovery from experimental anoxic insult, also has been claimed to improve human cognitive functioning[29] and parkinsonism[30] through unestablished mechanisms.

The extensive literature that exists for the effects of indirect sympathomimetics such as dextroamphetamine, methylphenidate, and pemoline fails to support a role for this class of drug in improving motor disorders of the aged.[31] That involuntary movements, ataxic gait, and enhanced physiological tremor can sometimes be side effects of these drugs might suggest that drugs acting against the "hyperadrenergic" state found with increasing age[32] might be a reasonable theme for improving age-related decline in motor performance. A study currently under way by the author will assess the effects of chronic clonidine therapy in normal elders and may shed some light on this question.

The search for effective pharmacotherapy of aging-related motor impairment needs to look beyond the model of parkinsonism for other disorders with clues to reversible deficits. For example, the cerebellar system undergoes significant morphological and neurochemical change with age and could account for some components of impaired gait and coordination. Interventions enhancing cholinergic outflow[33] and cerebellar thyrotropin-releasing hormone metabolism[34] in ataxic individuals have been reported to bring about symptomatic improvements, and tremor from structural damage to deep cerebellar nuclei can respond to primidone.[35] Perhaps trials with these medications in the normal elderly might enhance cerebellar functioning that was lost with age. Other mechanisms of the CNS that lose vitality with age, such as the speed of information processing or comprehension of complex information, could also be behind functional losses in the initiation, accuracy, or synergy of movement. Hence, pharmacological approaches for improving motor control may have to be targeted beyond primary pathways mediating movement.

REFERENCES

1. LeWitt, P. A. & D. B. Calne. 1982. Neurochemistry and pharmacology of the aging motor system. *In* The Aging Motor System. J. A. Mortimer, F. J. Pirozzolo & G. J. Maletta, Eds.: 36–59. Praeger. New York.

2. Critchley, M. 1956. Neurological changes in the aged. *In* The Neurologic and Psychiatric Aspects of the Disorders of Aging. Vol. 35. J. E. Moore, H. H. Merritt & R. J. Masselink, Eds.: 198–223. Williams & Wilkins. Baltimore.

3. Smith, B. H. & P. K. Sethi. 1975. Aging and the nervous system. Geriatrics **30:** 109–115.

4. Kokmen, E., R. W. Bossemeyer, J. Barney & W. J. Williams. 1977. Neurological manifestations of aging. J. Gerontol. **32:** 411–419.

5. Albert, M. L., Ed. 1984. Clinical Neurology of Aging. Oxford University Press. New York/London.

6. Skre, H. 1972. Neurological signs in a normal population. Acta Neurol. Scand. **48:** 575–606.

7. Shock, N. W. & A. H. Norris. 1970. Neuromuscular coordination as a factor in age changes in muscular exercise. *In* Physical Activity and Aging. D. Brunner & E. Jokl, Eds.: 92–105. University Park Press. Baltimore.

8. Sudarsky, L. & M. Ronthal. 1983. Gait disorders among elderly patients: a study of fifty patients. Arch. Neurol. **40:** 740–743.

9. Sabin, T. D. 1982. Biologic aspects of falls and mobility limitations in the elderly. J. Am. Geriatr. Soc. **30:** 51–58.

10. Potvin, A. R., K. Syndulko, W. W. Tourtellotte, J. A. Lemmon & J. H. Potvin. 1980. Human neurologic function and the aging process. J. Am. Geriatr. Soc. **28:** 1–9.

11. Katzman, R. & R. Terry. 1983. Normal aging of the nervous system. *In* The Neurology of Aging. R. Katzman & Terry, Eds.: 15–50. Davis. Philadelphia.

12. Kemper, T. 1984. Neuroanatomical and neuropathological changes in normal aging and in dementia. *In* Clinical Neurology of Aging. M. L. Albert, Ed.: 9–52. Oxford University Press. New York/London.

13. Hanley, T. 1974. Neuronal fallout in the aging brain: a critical review of the quantitative data. Age Aging **3:** 133–151.

14. Burns, R. S., P. A. LeWitt, M. H. Ebert, H. Pakkenberg & I. J. Kopin. 1985. The clinical syndrome of striatal dopamine deficiency: parkinsonism induced by 1-methyl-4-phenyl-1,2,3,6-tetrahydropyridine (MPTP). N. Engl. J. Med. **312:** 1418–1421.

15. Ballard, P., J. W. Tetrud & J. W. Langston. 1985. Permanent human parkinsonism due to 1-methyl-4-phenyl-1,2,3,6-tetrahydropyridine (MPTP): seven cases. Neurology **35:** 949–956.

16. Terävainen, H. & D. B. Calne. 1983. *In* The Neurology of Aging. R. Katzman & R. Terry, Eds.: 85–109. Davis. Philadelphia.

17. Carlsson, A. & B. Winblad. 1976. Influence of age and time interval between death and autopsy on dopamine and 3-methoxytyramine levels in human basal ganglia. J. Neural Transm. **38:** 271–276.

18. McGeer, E. G. 1978. Aging and neurotransmitter metabolism in human brain. *In* Alzheimer's Disease: Senile Dementia and Related Disorders. R. Katzman, R. D. Terry & K. L. Bick, Eds.: 427–440. Raven Press. New York.

19. Hornykiewicz, O. 1983. Dopamine changes in the aging human brain: functional considerations. *In* Aging Brain and Ergot Alkaloids. A. Agnoli, G. Crepaldi, P. F. Spano & M. Trabucchi, Eds.: 9–14. Raven Press. New York.

20. Newman, R. P., P. A. LeWitt, M. Jaffe, D. B. Calne & T. A. Larsen. 1985. Motor function in the normal aging population: treatment with levodopa. Neurology **35:** 571–572.

21. Newman, R. P., H. Weingartner, S. A. Smallberg & D. B. Calne. 1984. Effortful and automatic memory: effects of dopamine. Neurology **34:** 805–807.

22. Weingartner, H., S. Burns, R. Diebel & P. A. LeWitt. 1984. Cognitive impairments in Parkinson's disease: distinguishing between effort-demanding and automatic cognitive processes. Psychiatr. Res. **11:** 223–235.

23. Van Woert, M. H., G. Heninger, V. Rathey & M. B. Bowers. 1970. L-DOPA in senile dementia. Lancet **i:** 573–574.

24. Drachman, D. A. & S. Stahl. 1975. Extrapyramidal dementia and levodopa. Lancet **i:** 809.

25. REISBERG, B., S. H. FERRIS & S. GERSHON. 1979. Psychopharmacologic aspects of cognitive research in the elderly: some current perspectives. Interdiscip. Top. Gerontol. **15**: 132–152.

26. GREENWALD, B. S. & K. L. DAVIS. 1983. Experimental pharmacology of Alzheimer's disease. Adv. Neurol. **38**: 87–102.

27. GOODNICK, P. J. & S. GERSHON. 1983. Chemotherapy of cognitive disorders. *In* Aging of the Brain. D. Samuel, S. Gershon, V. E. Grimm & G. Toffano, Eds.: 349–361. Raven Press. New York.

28. LEHMANN, H. E. 1979. Psychopharmacotherapy in psychogeriatric disorders. *In* Brain Function and Old Age, p. 456–479. Springer-Verlag. Berlin/New York.

29. HOROWSKI, R. & R. J. MCDONALD. 1983. Experimental and clinical aspects of ergot derivatives used in the treatment of age-related disorders. *In* Aging Brain and Ergot Alkaloids. A. Agnoli, G. Crepaldi, P. F. Spano & M. Trabucchi, Eds.: 283–303. Raven Press. New York.

30. ABUZZAHAB, F. S., G. E. MERWIN, R. L. ZIMMERMAN & M. C. SHERMAN. 1977. A double-blind investigation of Piracetam (Nootropil) versus placebo in geriatric memory. Pharmakopsychiatrie **10**: 49–56.

31. IIZUKA, J. 1978. Piracetam in der modernen pharmakotherapie des Parkinsons-syndroms. Med. Welt **29**: 1381–1388.

32. PRIEN, R. F. 1983. Psychostimulants in the treatment of senile dementia. *In* Alzheimer's Disease: The Standard Reference. B. Reisberg, Ed.: 381–386. Free Press. New York.

33. ROWE, J. W. & B. R. TROEN. 1980. Sympathetic nervous system and aging in man. Endocr. Rev. **1**: 167–179.

34. KARK, R. A. P. 1981. Double-blind triple-crossover trial of low-doses of oral physostigmine in inherited ataxias. Neurology **31**: 288–292.

35. CAMPANELLA, G., A. FILLA, G. DE MICHELE, A. MAGGIO, A. MENGANO, L. IORIO & P. CARTONI. 1986. A double-blind trial with TRH-T in inherited ataxias. Ann. Neurol. **20**: 151.

36. LEWITT, P. A., K. MAURITZ & J. N. SANES. 1984. Cerebellar kinetic tremor (KT) responsive to primidone and to visual suppression. Neurology **34**(suppl. 1): 265.

DISCUSSION OF THE PAPER

A. ALTAR (*CIBA–GEIGY Corporation, Summit, NJ*): What was the name of the one dopamine uptake inhibitor that you tried with modest success?

P. LEWITT (*Lafayette Clinic, Detroit, MI*): We looked at pemoline, the brand name for which is Cylert.

ALTAR: Perhaps you might not abandon all hope yet with dopamine uptake blockade. For example, there are these other drugs that have met with modest success in the clinic and that also have given some of the data that we presented with the swimming test where dramatic exercise was required. It might be of interest to look at these kinds of drugs combined with, say, an exercise program for these patients. Have you ever looked at the combination of these drugs with these situations where motoric demands are heightened?

LEWITT: We have not. However, we currently have a study about to begin looking at pemoline again in parkinsonian patients and also in depressed individuals. Perhaps, then, we could incorporate indices of their activity to the data that we will be collecting, but this is something that we are just about to begin doing.

J. SEVERSON (*Amersham Corporation, Arlington Heights, IL*): Is there any reason to believe that a drug like Parnate might be effective in this situation?

LEWITT: Because Parnate is a monoamine oxidase inhibitor, it would increase endogenous monoamine metabolism. However, this seems an indirect way. A lot of depressed individuals have been treated with it and the data might be out there. If a precursor does not work, though, then this more indirect way of enhancing neurofunction might not either.

J. SLADEK (*University of Rochester Medical School, Rochester, NY*): As long as we are on the topic of MAO inhibitors, would you like to comment on antioxidative strategies using such substances as deprenyl or tocopherol?

LEWITT: There are a number of possibilities for the causation of Parkinson's disease. One of the current popular ones is that there is a self-destruction by oxidative or oxidation-generated products such as superoxide free radicals that could damage neurons. Some thought has been given to strategies that either quench these free radicals or block their production with drugs such as the monoamine oxidase B inhibitor, deprenyl. In fact, if these cumulative damages to the neuron could be lessened, then perhaps the progression of Parkinson's disease might be slowed down too. This has been made much more exciting by the observation that a monoamine oxidase B inhibitor such as deprenyl can block the toxicity of MPTP. There seems to be a step of activation needed and, based on this, there is the thought that if there are other exogenous toxins similar to it that might be causing the loss of neurons in Parkinson's disease, then that could be one way to slow the disease. There is a study plan to evaluate this in California and a larger prospective study in the United States. Unfortunately, there is not a shred of evidence to say that there is such a toxin; it is just an enticing hypothesis at this point.

D. MORGAN (*University of Southern California, Los Angeles, CA*): I want to comment on that last point. I believe that amphetamine treatment in monkeys has been shown to produce 6-hydroxydopamine; thus, there may be some evidence that boosted release can actually result in some hydroxylated toxins that may themselves help to autodestroy the terminals. In fact, that was a strategy we approached using pergolide treatment, so there may be a number of approaches to looking at protected strategies. One of them is simply trying to block the formation of hydroxylated derivatives like that.

LEWITT: That is a good point. In fact, with the increased stresses that are placed on the dopaminergic neuron by the 80%-plus losses of those neurons in Parkinson's disease, it is conceivable that this could be a mechanism for the progression of the disease. Getting to that 80% point might be via normal aging attrition, and D. B. Calne gave a slide suggesting that there might be mechanisms of acceleration, which is a good possibility. Certainly, the generation of catecholamines (the productivity per neuron) is such that the free radicals that are part of the normal process of the metabolism of the dopamine could well produce enough damage over a lifetime. Moreover, it might be the efficacy of the protective mechanisms, the quenching of these free radicals, or their deposition as neuromelanin that could be the process that prevents the disease from occurring in everyone of us.

Intracerebral Neuronal Grafting in Experimental Animal Models of Age-related Motor Dysfunction[a]

F. H. GAGE,[b] P. BRUNDIN,[c] R. STRECKER,[c]
S. B. DUNNETT,[c] O. ISACSON,[c] AND
A. BJORKLUND[c]

[b]Department of Neurosciences
University of California, San Diego
La Jolla, California 92093

[c]Department of Histology
University of Lund
Lund, Sweden

INTRODUCTION

Age-related motor decline is not a unitary process and it is important to dissociate motor decline from motivational decline, sensory inattention, and cognitive disorientation. In addition, deficits in balance and coordination of central nervous system origin must be dissociated from motor deficits of peripheral origin such as muscle atrophy. The problem is compounded when looking at the aging organism because all of these changes can be occurring to a small degree simultaneously, thereby giving the picture of a major deficit. Enough is known about the underlying anatomy of these different systems to believe that each system acts with some independence. However, less is known about how each of these systems interacts with each other, especially in relation to age-related decline.

It is clear from both clinical and experimental literature that the extrapyramidal system plays a pivotal role in motor function. This is particularly evident in Parkinson's disease and Huntington's chorea. In addition, within the extrapyramidal system, the dopaminergic innervation from the ventral mesencephalon plays a prominent role in modulating many aspects of motor behavior. Specifically, decline of dopamine (DA) function with age is associated with a general decline in motor function.

The ascending dopamine systems are associated with motor function. Of particular importance is the close proximity of the A10 or ventral tegmental area to the A8 and A9, the nigrostriatal system. Though the two cell populations are adjacent to each other, there is much less overlap of their target areas. Therefore, A8 projects primarily to the striatum (albeit in a topographical organization), while the A10 has a more diffuse projection system to areas including the prefrontal cortex, accumbens, lateral

[a] This work was supported by grants from the American Parkinson Disease Association, NIA (No. AGO6088), the Office of Naval Research, and the Margaret and Herbert Hoover Jr. Foundation.

383

septum, and amygdala. Because of the clear reproducible deficits that can be modeled with lesions of these systems selectively, they have been the target of many experiments that have attempted to establish structure-function relationships. Intracerebral neuronal grafting has been used extensively and successfully with these models and has provided the framework for clinical studies presently under way. Our focus has been on the use of neuronal grafting as a basic tool for the neurobiologist to understand basic brain mechanisms.

This review will summarize first the basic methods used and the principal anatomical and biochemical results. Subsequently, the functional studies will be summarized from three separate systems: (a) the nigrostriatal system, (b) the mesolimbic system, and (c) the aged neostriatum. In the final section, some suggestions about the mechanism of action will be presented.

GRAFTS OF FETAL MESENCEPHALON TO THE NEOSTRIATUM

Two principal techniques have been used to graft fetal CNS tissue to the previously denervated striatal regions. The first one involves the transplantation of solid pieces of tissue to a surgically prepared transplantation cavity in which the graft is placed in direct contact with the denervated striatum. In this procedure, good graft survival is ensured by preparing the cavity in such a way that the graft can be placed on a richly vascularized surface (e.g., the pia in the choroidal fissure) that can serve as a "culturing bed" for the grafts.[1] This cavity is in direct communication with the lateral ventricle, which may allow the CSF to circulate through the graft cavity and thus probably help the graft to survive, particularly during the early postoperative period. In the case of the striatum, we have adopted a two-stage surgical procedure.[2-3] First, a cavity is made in the dorsal parietal cortex to expose the dorsal surface of the head of the caudate-putamen. After a few weeks, when a new vessel-rich pia has grown over the surfaces of the cavity, the cavity is reopened and a graft is placed onto the exposed striatal surface.

The second technique that we have used involves injection of dissociated cell suspensions into the depth of the brain.[4-5] In this technique, pieces of fetal CNS tissue are trypsinized and mechanically dissociated into a milky cell suspension. Small volumes of the suspension can then be stereotaxically injected into the desired site using a microsyringe. A major advantage of this technique is that it allows precise and multiple placements of the cells. The technique also makes possible accurate monitoring of the number of cells injected by counting the density of cells in the suspension.[6] For the remainder of this section, the first technique will be referred to as the "solid graft" technique and the second technique will be referred to as the "cell suspension" technique.

Anatomy

Grafts of mesencephalic DA-rich tissue to the denervated striatum in hydroxydopamine (6-OHDA) lesioned rats have been studied by catecholamine fluorescence histochemistry and by tyrosine hydroxylase (TH) immunohistochemistry.[3,7,8]

With the delayed transplantation procedure, the survival rate of solid nigral grafts is greater than 95% and, on the average, they show a 1.5–3-fold increase in volume.[2,3] Solid nigral grafts positioned in a dorsal cortical cavity reinnervate the dorsal third of the denervated caudate putamen. Fluorescent DA cells are frequently seen to cluster with dendritic arborization perpendicular to the layer of aggregated DA cells in an arrangement reminiscent of the normal pars compacta–pars reticulata organization of the intact substantia nigra. Bundles of axons are seen to course through the graft and to ramify into a dense terminal plexus in the gray matter of the host neostriatum. Occasionally, ingrowth is seen into cortical areas that are medial, rostral, and lateral to the graft, but the preferential direction of growth of the ingrowing DA axons is into the proximal portions of the striatum, where they reinnervate from one-tenth to a maximum of one-half of the nucleus's volume at the longest survival times (six months or longer). A similar pattern of graft survival and growth is seen when solid grafts are placed into a lateral cortical cavity, which results in an equivalent rich ingrowth into proximal (ventrolateral) regions of the striatum.[9]

The survival and growth of DA-rich suspension grafts have been studied in different brain sites.[10] The implanted DA neurons survive in clusters or aggregates at the injection site. Although the DA neurons survive quite well in several different brain sites, their fiber outgrowth into the surrounding host tissue varies markedly from one area to another.[10] Thus, rich fiber outgrowth is seen only into areas that are normally richly innervated by DA fibers (such as the caudate putamen and nucleus accumbens), whereas DA cells implanted into normally poorly innervated areas (such as parietal cortex, globus pallidus, lateral hypothalamus, and substantia nigra) demonstrate very little fiber growth into the surrounding host tissue. In the striatum, the DA fibers radiate out in a halo with a radius of about 1.5–2 mm around the implant. Each DA cell deposit reaches only subportions of the striatum, and extensive reinnervation of the striatum will require several implants in different sites. On the other hand, though, the regionally restricted fiber outgrowth from each implant will allow observations of regionally confined effects on behavior (this feature will be dealt with later in this section).

Reinnervation of the denervated target is only efficient if the DA neurons are placed into or immediately adjacent to the target. DA implants placed along the course of the nigrostriatal pathway (i.e., into the lateral hypothalamus, internal capsule, or globus pallidus) have not been seen to grow any axons into the striatum.[10] However, this does not necessarily mean that grafted mesencephalic DA neurons are unable to extend their axons over longer distances. In fact, Aguayo *et al.*[11] have recently shown that DA axons growing from solid nigral grafts, placed over the tectum, can reach the caudate putamen along a piece of sciatic nerve placed as a bridge (running over the parietal cortex) between the nigral graft and the denervated striatum, which is a distance of about 2 cm. In addition, Gage *et al.*[12] have shown that these combined graft-bridges are functional.

At the electron microscopic level, Freund *et al.*[8] used tyrosine hydroxylase (TH) immunocytochemistry to trace DA synapses in the neostriatum reinnervated by solid nigral grafts. They identified abundant graft-derived TH-positive synapses on neuronal elements in the host neostriatum. As in normal animals,[13] the principal target was the dendrites of the spiny neurons, the majority of which are likely to be the striatal projection neurons.

Biochemistry

For grafted DA neurons as well, measurements of DA turnover and synthesis rates *in vivo* indicate that the implanted DA neurons are capable of restoring DA neurotransmission in the initially denervated target.[14,15]

With solid nigral grafts placed on the dorsal striatal surface, as described above, the DA concentrations were restored from less than 0.5% in the 6-OHDA-lesioned neostriatum to a mean of 13.6% (maximum = 36%) in the reinnervated neostriatum. Moreover, measurements of the rate of DOPA accumulation after DOPA decarboxylase inhibition and measurements of the DA metabolite, DOPAC, indicated a restitution of normal (or even above normal) DA synthesis and release rates in the new "nigrostriatal" connections established by the grafted DA neurons.

Nigral suspension implants restored neostriatal DA levels to an average of 13–18%, with the highest individual values reaching about 50% of control. DOPAC was restored from about 5% of control (in the 6-OHDA denervated rats) to an average of about 20% of normal in the animals with grafts. The DOPAC:DA ratio and the DOPA accumulation rates indicated that the DA turnover and synthesis in the grafted neurons were, on the average, some 50–100% higher than in the intrinsic nigrostriatal pathway.

MODEL CATECHOLAMINE MOTOR DEFICITS

Nigrostriatal

Bilateral 6-OHDA lesions of ascending dopamine pathways produce a syndrome of behavioral impairments—similar to bilateral electrolytic lesions of the lateral hypothalamus—in which rats are profoundly aphagic, adipsic, akinetic, and negligent of stimuli on both sides of the body.[16] Because animals with such lesions require intensive and sustained postoperative care to be kept alive, the bilateral lesion model has not proved convenient for the routine assessment of DA graft function. By contrast, unilateral 6-OHDA lesions of the ascending mesotelencephalic DA fibers leave one side of the brain intact for the animal to maintain basic regulatory functions, yet induce motor and sensorimotor asymmetries that are readily quantified.

The simplest and most widely used test of motor asymmetry in both unilateral 6-OHDA-lesioned and dopamine-grafted rats has been the rotational model of Ungerstedt.[16,17] Unilateral lesioned rats show postural bias and spontaneous ipsilateral turning (i.e., towards the side of the lesion) for a few days or weeks following surgery. Although spontaneous turning recovers thereafter, ipsilateral rotation can be readily reinstated by activating the animal, for example, by pinching the tail, placing it in a novel environment, or by injections of the stimulant drug, amphetamine. Conversely, the DA-receptor agonist, apomorphine, induces contralateral rotation, which is thought to be attributable to the development of receptor supersensitivity on the lesioned side.

Transplanted DA neurons reinnervating the neostriatum have been found to be effective in reversing apomorphine- and amphetamine-induced rotation in unilaterally lesioned animals. This is true for all three major procedures described above, namely, intraventricular graft placement,[18,19] solid grafts into a dorsal parietal cavity,[3] and suspension grafts injected directly into the caudate putamen.[8] Interestingly, whereas in each case the dopamine-rich grafts have been seen to provide a complete or even overcompensation of amphetamine-induced rotation, the apomorphine response is reduced by 30–70% but never completely abolished. This is probably attributable both to the observation that the apomorphine response is more variable and is critically dependent upon the extent of the lesion and that striatal segments distal to the graft remain deafferented so that supersensitivity is never fully abolished. In addition to drug-induced rotation, spontaneous and tail pinch-induced turnings have also been seen to be significantly ameliorated following dorsal parietal graft placement.[20]

As more extensive studies of rats with unilateral 6-OHDA lesions and DA grafts have been conducted on a variety of functional tests,[2,9,20,21] it has become apparent that graft-derived recovery is dependent upon graft placement in parallel with the known topographic organization of striatal function.[22–24] Therefore, to summarize a range of observations, reinnervation of dorsal caudate putamen is a requirement for amelioration of both spontaneous and drug-induced rotation,[2,20,21] and reinnervation of ventral and lateral caudate putamen is a requirement for reinstatement of sensorimotor attention and responsiveness on the contralateral side of the body.[9,21]

Mesolimbic

Injections of the specific catecholamine neurotoxin, 6-OHDA, into the mesotelencephalic DA bundle produce a profound akinesia in addition to the regulatory and sensorimotor effects of the lesion.[25-27] Some animals are not only spontaneously akinetic, but they also fail to show a normal locomotor activation following injection of moderate doses of the presynaptic dopaminergic stimulant, amphetamine.[28,29] However, the precise neuroanatomical substrate for this effect remains unclear.

The mesolimbocortical DA neurons — which originate in the ventral tegmental area (VTA, A10 of Dahlstrom and Fuxe)[30] and project rostrally to innervate the nucleus accumbens, olfactory tubercle, prefrontal cortex, anteromedial striatum, and septum among others[31,32] — appear to provide one essential substrate for the regulation of locomotor activity. Injections of DA directly into the nucleus accumbens induced and increased locomotor activity,[33-35] and haloperidol injected into the nucleus accumbens inhibited peripherally injected amphetamine-induced locomotor activity.[36] Lesion studies support a similar conclusion: 6-OHDA lesions of the nucleus accumbens block amphetamine-induced locomotor activity[37-39] and thus result in a locomotor hyperactivity following an injection of a low dose of the DA receptor agonist, apomorphine.[37,38]

The designs of the studies of locomotor activity differ from the other functional measures, which have all been conducted on rats with extensive unilateral DA deafferentation. By contrast, locomotor activity is only mildly affected by unilateral lesions, although a "supersensitive" apomorphine response can still be elicited from rats in which one side remains intact.[39] Rather, in order to study the effect in animals with bilateral lesions without inducing debilitating aphagia and adipsia, 6-OHDA injections have been restricted to the midline VTA.[40-41] This destroys the mesolimbocortical DA projecting to the nucleus accumbens and frontal cortex[16,32] (which is believed to be involved principally in the akinesia and other locomotor impairments induced by full bilateral lesions[38]), but leaves the more lateral DA systems originating in the substantia nigra relatively intact. VTA lesions alone block the stimulant effects of amphetamine, whereas injections of the DA receptor agonist, apomorphine, induce a marked locomotor activation at low doses that has no effect on normal animals, presumably by action on supersensitive denervated receptors. Following transplantation of mesencephalic grafts into the nucleus accumbens or prefrontal cortex, a rapid recovery of the stimulant effect of amphetamine is seen by four weeks. In contrast, a reduction in apomorphine-supersensitive activation only becomes apparent from about 12 weeks after grafting, which may reflect the dynamic nature of receptor sensitivity dependent on both the extent and physiological activity of graft-derived reinnervation.

Of the range of impairments following either unilateral or bilateral 6-OHDA lesions, only the adipsia (and perhaps also the aphagia) in bilaterally lesioned animals has remained unresponsive to DA-rich grafts.[20,21]

Grafting in Brains of Aged Rats

Graft Survival and Fiber Outgrowth

The first stage in our study of neural implants in the aged rat brain was to demonstrate that such transplants could survive well in the aged brain and that they were able to provide appropriate reinnervation of the host.[42] To this end, neuronal cell suspensions prepared from the ventral mesencephalon of rat embryos were implanted into the depth of the intact neostriatum of 21- to 23-month-old female rats of the same strain. Graft survival assessed 3–4 months after grafting was comparable to that seen in our previous studies of young adult recipients. Fiber outgrowth into the host brain was evaluated in animals that were subjected to lesions of the intrinsic nigrostriatal system 6–10 days before killing. Dense dopaminergic fiber outgrowth was seen within a zone of up to about 1 mm radius around the nigral implants. The overall magnitude of fiber outgrowth was less than that generally seen in previously denervated targets in young adult recipients. However, the outgrowth seen in the aged rats with intact afferent inputs appeared to be as extensive as in young recipients when the grafts were placed in nondenervated targets.[43] The distribution of the fibers from the implants in the host suggested that the pattern found in the nondenervated targets of the aged recipients was more diffuse and partly different from the normal pattern. Therefore, it is an interesting possibility that synapse loss in intrinsic connections[44,45] may influence the patterning of the graft-derived innervation and, in fact, improve the ability of implants to terminate in the otherwise intact target of the aged host brain.

Motor Coordination Skills

Motor performance was assessed on four measures adapted from the battery described by Campbell *et al.*:[46] (a) the ability to maintain balance on and to successfully reach a safety platform at either end of a narrow bridge of square cross section; (b) the ability to maintain balance on a similar bridge of round cross section; (c) the period of time that the animal could sustain its own weight clinging suspended from a taut wire; and (d) the ability to descend in a coordinated manner on a vertical pole covered with wire mesh. Prior to transplantation, the aged rats were significantly impaired on the four measures as compared to the young control animals. On the square and round bridges, young rats had no difficulty walking and exploring along the rod, and they generally reached the platform within 30–60 seconds. By contrast, before transplantation, the aged rats had greater difficulty maintaining balance. Most animals fell off the bridges or they alternatively lay on the bridges without attempting to walk (they clung tightly with all four paws or they clung with the forepaws while the hind paws hung freely). Twelve weeks after transplantation, the aged rats with nigral grafts — but not the aged controls or the rats with septal grafts — showed marked and significant improvement in their balance and limb coordination on both the square and round bridges.[47] Typically, they could walk along the bridge without falling, they displayed gait posture similar to that of the young rats, and they fell less frequently than did the other aged rats. On the wire-mesh-covered pole, the aged rats descended more rapidly before transplantation than did the young controls, with frequent falling, slipping, or sliding down backwards. Although the aged rats with nigral transplants had a tendency to descend in a more controlled and coordinated manner (with the head-down orientation that was seen in the young controls), the differences from the other aged rats did not reach significance on this measure. The aged rats showed no difference between groups in either body weight or in latency to fall from the taut wire; this suggests that enhanced motor coordination in the aged rats with nigral grafts was not attributable to nonspecific differences in weight or strength of these animals.

SUMMARY

The combined morphological, biochemical, electrophysiological, and behavioral data summarized above show that implanted embryonic nerve cells in some cases can substitute quite well for a lost intrinsic neuronal system in mammals. The intracerebral implants probably exert their effects in several ways. The functional effects seen with grafts placed into one of the cerebral ventricles (such as those described in the studies of Perlow *et al.*,[16] Freed *et al.*,[19] and Gash *et al.*[48]) are thus probably explained on the basis of a diffuse release of an active amine or peptide into the host CSF and adjacent brain tissue. In other instances, as in animals with DA-rich grafts reinnervating the neostriatum, we believe that the available data provide quite substantial evidence that the behavioral recovery is caused by the ability of the grafted neurons to reinnervate relevant parts of the host brain. This is illustrated by the studies mentioned above that show that the degree of functional recovery in 6-OHDA-lesioned rats with nigral transplants is directly correlated with the extent of striatal DA reinnervation and that the "profile" of functional recovery is dependent on that area of the striatal complex that is reinnervated by the graft. This point is particularly well illustrated in a further study[49] in which rats with electrodes implanted into the center of intracortical nigral grafts were allowed to "self-stimulate" via the graft. The results show that the graft can indeed sustain self-stimulation behavior and that the rate of lever-pressing is related to the proximity between the electrode tip and the DA-containing neurons in the graft. This strongly supports the notion that the implanted DA neurons can transmit behaviorally meaningful and temporally organized information to the host brain via their efferent connections.

To what extent the intracerebral implants can be functionally integrated with the host brain is still poorly known, though, and it therefore remains an interesting question for further investigation. The chances for extensive integration may be greatest for neuronal suspension grafts implanted as deposits directly into the depth of the brain, but even solid grafts inserted as whole pieces into the brain have, in several cases, been seen to become reinnervated from the host brain in adult and developing recipients. Nevertheless, a recent HRP study[8] failed to detect any host afferents to intracortical solid nigral grafts, despite the fact that these grafts had themselves formed extensive DA connections in the host striatum and had produced behavioral recovery. This suggests that implanted neurons can also function well in the absence of some — or perhaps even all — of their normal afferent inputs.

Available data indicate that implanted embryonic central neurons can substitute to some degree for a lost set of afferents to a denervated brain region in adult rats and can replace a lost intrinsic neuronal system in normalizing the rat's behavior. This indicates a remarkable plasticity of the mature rat CNS in incorporating new neuronal elements into its already established circuitries.

Neuronal replacement by neural implants is a striking further example of how the brain can allow new elements to be inserted and linked into its own functional subsystems. Obviously, there must be definite limitations as to which types of neurons or functional subsystems can successfully be manipulated in this way. Neural implants would seem most likely to have behaviorally meaningful functional effects with types of neurons that normally do not convey, or link, specific or patterned messages (e.g., in sensory or motor input and output systems). Indeed, functional or behavioral recovery in the neuronal replacement paradigm has so far been demonstrated primarily for neurons of the types that normally appear to act as tonic regulatory level-setting systems.

Mesencephalic DA neurons are commonly conceived of as modulatory or level-setting systems that tonically regulate the activity of the neostriatal and hippocampal neuronal machineries.[50,51] Removal of the dopaminergic control mechanisms results in severe inhibition or impairment of neostriatal functions, respectively. Functional recovery seen after reinstatement of dopaminergic transmission by drugs or by neural implants can thus be interpreted as a reactivation of an inhibited, but otherwise intact, neuronal machinery.

The nigral DA neurons are normally proposed to act by regulating, or gating, the response of the striatal output neurons to the excitatory (probably glutaminergic) cortical input. This could be achieved as a result of an interaction of the dopaminergic and cortical inputs on the same dendrites or dendritic spines (as suggested, for example, by Schwarcz *et al.*,[52] Brown and Arbuthnott,[53] and Godukhin *et al.*[54]). Removal of the nigrostriatal DA input, as in the "DA-lesioned" animal, results in an inhibition of neostriatal function and in an increase in the threshold for initiation of motor acts from the cortex. The grafted DA neurons act by reducing or normalizing the threshold for behavioral response to cortical (or other) inputs.

An interesting implication of this model is that it may be sufficient for the nigral grafts to reinstate dopaminergic transmission in the reinnervated target in a tonic and relatively nonspecific manner in order to compensate for at least some of the lesion-induced or age-related behavioral impairments. Because temporally or spatially patterned inputs to the grafted neurons may not be necessary for the maintenance of such tonic activity, this mode of action would allow for behavioral recovery to occur even in the absence of afferent connections from the host. Indeed, our biochemical studies on nigral grafts reinnervating the neostriatum indicate that the grafted DA neurons can maintain a sufficiently high spontaneous activity even in the absence of any major afferents from the host brain. This recently has been confirmed and extended by Zetterstrom *et al.*[55] using dialysis measurements of tonic catecholamine release. The reason for this tonic control by the grafts may be that local regulation, even in the intact situation, at the terminal level (e.g., through local transmitter interactions or presynaptic autoreceptors) may play an important role in the maintenance of tonic, baseline transmission in the aminergic systems.

ACKNOWLEDGMENT

We thank Sheryl Christenson for her skill in typing.

REFERENCES

1. STENEVI, U., A. BJORKLUND & N-AA. SVENDGAARD. 1976. Transplantation of central and peripheral monoamine neurons to the adult rat brain: Techniques and conditions for survival. Brain Res. **114:** 1–20.
2. BJORKLUND, A., S. B. DUNNETT, U. STENEVI, M. E. LEWIS & S. D. IVERSEN. 1980. Reinnervation of the denervated striatum by substantia nigra transplants: Functional consequences as revealed by pharmacological and sensorimotor testing. Brain Res. **199:** 307–333.
3. BJORKLUND, A. & U. STENEVI. 1979. Reconstruction of the nigrostriatal dopamine pathway by intracerebral nigral transplants. Brain Res. **177:** 555–560.
4. BJORKLUND, A., R. H. SCHMIDT & U. STENEVI. 1980. Functional reinnervation of the neostriatum in the adult rat by use of intraparenchymal grafting of dissociated cell suspensions from the substantia nigra. Cell Tissue Res. **212:** 39–45.
5. BJORKLUND, A., U. STENEVI, R. H. SCHMIDT, S. B. DUNNETT & F. H. GAGE. 1983. In-

tracerebral grafting of neuronal cell suspensions. I. Introduction and general methods of preparation. Acta Physiol. Scand. Suppl. **522:** 1–10.

6. BRUNDIN, P., O. ISACSON & A. BJORKLUND. 1985. Monitoring of cell viability in suspensions of embryonic CNS tissue and its criterion for intracerebral graft survival. Brain Res. **331:** 251–259.

7. FREED, W. J., J. M. MORISHISA, E. SPOOR, B. J. HOFFER, L. OLSON, A. SEIGER & R. J. WYATT. 1981. Transplanted adrenal chromaffin cells in the rat brain reduce lesion-induced rotational behavior. Nature **292:** 351–352.

8. FREUND, T., P. BOLAM, A. BJORKLUND, U. STENEVI, S. B. DUNNETT & A. D. SMITH. 1985. Synaptic connections of nigral transplants reinnervating the host neostriatum: A TH-immunocytochemical study. J. Neurosci. **5:** 603–616.

9. DUNNETT, S. B., A. BJORKLUND, U. STENEVI & S. D. IVERSEN. 1981. Grafts of embryonic substantia nigra reinnervating the ventrolateral striatum ameliorate sensorimotor impairments and akinesia rats with 6-OHDA lesions of the nigrostriatal pathway. Brain Res. **229:** 209–217.

10. BJORKLUND, A., U. STENEVI, R. H. SCHMIDT, S. B. DUNNETT & F. H. GAGE. 1983. Intracerebral grafting of neuronal cell suspensions. II. Survival and growth of nigral cells implanted in different brain sites. Acta Physiol. Scand. Suppl. **522:** 11–22.

11. AGUAYO, A. J., BJORKLUND A., U. STENEVI & T. CARLSTEDT. 1984. Fetal mesencephalic neurons survive and extend long axons across peripheral nervous system grafts inserted into the adult rat striatum. Neurosci. Lett. **45:** 53–58.

12. GAGE, F. H., U. STENEVI, T. CARLSTEDT, G. FOSTER, A. BJORKLUND & A. J. AGUAYO. 1985. Anatomical and functional consequences of grafting mesencephalic neurons into a peripheral nerve "bridge" connected to the denervated striatum. Exp. Brain Res. **60:** 584–589.

13. FREUND, T. F., J. F. POWELL & A. D. SMITH. 1984. Tyrosine hydroxylase-immunoreactive synaptic boutons in contact with identified striatonigral neurons with particular reference to dendritic spines. Neuroscience **13:** 1189–1215.

14. SCHMIDT, R. H., A. BJORKLUND, U. STENEVI, S. B. DUNNETT & F. H. GAGE. 1983. Intracerebral grafting of neuronal cell suspension. III. Activity of intrastriatal nigral suspension implants as assessed by measurements of dopamine synthesis and metabolism. Acta Physiol. Scand. Suppl. **522:** 23–32.

15. SCHMIDT, R. H., M. INGVAR, O. LINDVALL, U. STENEVI & A. BJORKLUND. 1982. Functional activity of substantia nigra grafts reinnervating the striatum: Neurotransmitter metabolism and (14C)-2-deoxy-D-glucose autoradiography. J. Neurochem. **38:** 737–748.

16. UNGERSTEDT, U., T. LJUNGBERG & C. RANJE. 1977. Dopamine neurotransmission and the control of behaviour. *In* Psychobiology of the Striatum. A. R. Cools, A. H. M. Lohman & J. H. L. van den Bercken, Eds.: 85–97. Pergamon. Elmsford, New York.

17. UNGERSTEDT, U. & G. W. ARBUTHNOTT. 1970. Quantitative recording of rotational behavior in rats after 6-hydroxydopamine lesions of the nigrostriatal dopamine system. Brain Res. **24:** 485–493.

18. PERLOW, M. J., W. J. FREED, B. J. HOFFER, A. SEIGER, L. OLSON & R. J. WYATT. 1979. Brain grafts reduce motor abnormalities produced by destruction of nigrostriatal dopamine system. Science **204:** 643–647.

19. FREED, W. J., M. J. PERLOW, F. KAROUM, A. SEIGER, L. OLSON, B. J. HOFFER & R. J. WYATT. 1980. Restoration of dopaminergic function by grafting of fetal rat substantia nigra to the caudate nucleus: Long-term behavioural, biochemical and histochemical studies. Ann. Neurol. **8:** 510–519.

20. DUNNETT, S. B., A. BJORKLUND, U. STENEVI & S. D. IVERSEN. 1981. Behavioural recovery following transplantation of substantia nigra in rats subjected to 6-OHDA lesions of the nigrostriatal pathway. I. Unilateral lesions. Brain Res. **215:** 147–161.

21. DUNNETT, S. B., A. BJORKLUND, R. H. SCHMIDT, U. STENEVI & S. D. IVERSEN. 1983. Intracerebral grafting of neuronal cell suspensions. IV. Behavioral recovery in rats with unilateral 6-OHDA lesions following implantation of nigral cell suspensions in different brain sites. Acta Physiol. Scand. Suppl. **522:** 29–37.

22. KELLY, P. H., P. W. SEVIOUR & S. D. IVERSEN. 1975. Amphetamine and apomorphine responses in the rat following 6-OHDA lesions of the nucleus accumbens septi and corpus

striatum. Brain Res. **94:** 507–522.

23. KELLEY, A. E., V. B. DOMESICK & W. J. H. NAUTA. 1982. The amygdalostriatal projection in the rat — an anatomical study of anterograde and retrograde tracing methods. Neuroscience **7:** 615–630.

24. DUNNETT, S. B. & S. D. IVERSEN. 1982. Sensorimotor impairments following localized kainic acid and 6-hydroxydopamine lesions of the neostriatum. Brain Res. **248:** 121–127.

25. FINK, J. S. & G. P. SMITH. 1979. Decreased locomotor and investigatory exploration after denervation of catecholamine terminal fields in the forebrain of rats. J. Comp. Physiol. Psychol. **93:** 34–65.

26. MARSHALL, J. F., J. S. RICHARDSON & P. TEITELBAUM. 1974. Nigrostriatal bundle damage and the lateral hypothalamic syndrome. J. Comp. Physiol. Psychol. **87:** 808–880.

27. WILLIS, G. L., G. C. SMITH & B. P. McGRATH. Deficits in locomotor behavioral and motor performance after central 6-hydroxydopamine or peripheral L-DOPA. Brain Res. **226:** 279–286.

28. FIBIGER, H. C., H. P. FIBIGER & A. P. ZIS. 1973. Attenuation of amphetamine-induced motor stimulation and stereotypy by 6-hydroxydopamine in the rat. Br. J. Pharmacol. **47:** 683–692.

29. FINK, J. S. & G. P. SMITH. 1980. Relationship between selective denervation of dopamine terminal fields in the anterior forebrain and behavioral responses to amphetamine and apomorphine. Brain Res. **201:** 107–127.

30. DAHLSTROM, A. & K. FUXE. 1964. Evidence for the existence of monoamine-containing neurons in the central nervous system. Acta Physiol. Scand. Suppl. **232:** 1–55.

31. ALBANESE, A. & D. MINCIACCHI. 1983. Organization of the ascending projections from the ventral tegmental areas: a multiple fluorescent retrograde tracer study in the rat. J. Comp. Neurol. **216:** 406–420.

32. LINDVALL, O. & A. BJORKLUND. 1978. Organization of catecholamine neurons in the rat central nervous system. *In* Handbook of Psychopharmacology, Vol. 8. L. L. Iversen, S. D. Iversen & S. H. Snyder, Eds.: 139–231. Plenum. New York.

33. COSTALL, B. & R. J. NAYLOR. 1975. The behavioral effects of dopamine applied intracerebrally to areas of the mesolimbic system. Eur. J. Pharmacol. **32:** 87–92.

34. DILL, R. E., D. L. JONES, J. C. GILLIN & G. MURPHY. 1979. Comparison of behavioral effects of systemic L-DOPA and intracranial dopamine in mesolimbic forebrain of non-human primates. Pharmacol. Biochem. Behav. **10:** 711–716.

35. PIJNENBERG, A. J. J. & J. M. VAN ROSSUM. 1973. Stimulation of locomotor activity following injection of dopamine into nucleus accumbens. J. Pharm. Pharmacol. **25:** 1003–1005.

36. PIJNENBERG, A. J. J., W. M. M. HONIG & J. M. VAN ROSSUM. 1975. Inhibition of D-amphetamine-induced locomotor activity by injection of haloperidol into the nucleus accumbens of the rat. Psychopharmacology **41:** 87–95.

37. JOYCE, E. M. & G. F. KOOB. 1981. Amphetamine-, scopolamine- and caffeine-induced locomotor activity following 6-hydroxydopamine lesions of the mesolimbic dopamine system. Psychopharmacology **73:** 311–313.

38. KELLY, P. H., P. W. SEVIOUR & S. D. IVERSEN. 1975. Amphetamine and apomorphine responses in the rat following 6-OHDA lesions of the nucleus accumbens septi and corpus striatum. Brain Res. **94:** 507–522.

39. ROBBINS, T. W., D. C. S. ROBERTS & G. F. KOOB. 1983. The effect of D-amphetamine and apomorphine upon operant behavior and schedule-induced licking in rats with 6-hydroxydopamine-induced lesions of the nucleus accumbens. J. Pharmacol. Exp. Ther. **224:** 662–673.

40. DUNNETT, S. B., F. H. GAGE, A. BJORKLUND, U. STENEVI, W. C. LOW & S. D. IVERSEN. 1982. Hippocampal deafferentation: transplant-derived reinnervation and functional recover. Scand. J. Psychol. Suppl. **I:** 104–111.

41. NADAUD, D., J. P. HERMAN, H. SIMON & M. LeMOAL. 1984. Functional recovery following transplantation of ventral mesencephalic cells in rats subjected to 6-OHDA lesions of the mesolimbic dopaminergic neurons. Brain Res. **304:** 137–141.

42. GAGE, F. H., A. BJORKLUND, U. STENEVI & S. B. DUNNETT. 1983. Intracerebral grafting of neuronal cell suspensions. VIII. Cell survival and axonal outgrowth of dopaminergic

and cholinergic cells in the aged brain. Acta Physiol. Scand. Suppl. **522:** 67–75.

43. GAGE, F. H. & A. BJORKLUND. 1985. Enchanced graft survival in the hippocampus following selective denervation. Neuroscience 17(1): 89–98.
44. GEINISMAN, Y., W. BONDAREFF & J. T. DODGE. 1977. Partial deafferentation of neurons in the dentate gyrus of the senescent rat. Brain Res. **134:** 541–545.
45. HOFF, S. F., S. W. SCHEFF, L. S. BERNARDO & C. W. COTMAN. 1982. Lesion-induced synaptogenesis in the dentate gyrus of aged rats: I. Loss and reacquisition of normal synaptic density. J. Comp. Neurol. **205:** 246–252.
46. CAMPBELL, B. A., E. E. KRAUTER & J. E. WALLACE. 1980. Animal Models of Aging: Problems and Perspectives. D. G. Stein, Ed.: 201–226. Elsevier/North-Holland. Amsterdam/New York.
47. GAGE, F. H., S. B. DUNNETT, A. BJORKLUND & U. STENEVI. 1983. Aged rats: recovery of motor coordination impairments by intrastriatal nigral grafts. Science **221:** 966–969.
48. GASH, D., J. R. SLADEK & C. D. SLADEK. 1980. Functional development of grafted vasopressin neurons. Science **210:** 1367–1369.
49. FRAY, P. J., S. B. DUNNETT, S. D. IVERSEN, A. BJORKLUND & U. STENEVI. 1983. Nigral transplants reinnervating the dopamine-depleted neostriatum can sustain intracranial self-stimulation. Science **219:** 416–419.
50. KRNJEVIC, K. & N. ROPERT. 1982. Electrophysiological and pharmacological characteristics of facilitation of hippocampal population spikes by stimulation of the medial septum. Neuroscience **7:** 2165–2183.
51. STRICKER, E. M. & M. J. ZIGMOND. 1976. Recovery of function after damage to central catecholamine-containing neurons: a neurochemical model for the lateral hypothalamic syndrome. *In* Progress in Physiological Psychology and Psychobiology. J. M. Sprague & A. E. Epstein, Eds.: 121–188. Academic Press. New York.
52. SCHWARCZ, R., J. CREESE, J. T. COYLE & S. H. SNYDER. 1978. Dopamine receptors localized on cerebral cortical afferents to rat corpus striatum. Nature **271:** 766–768.
53. BROWN, J. R. & G. W. ARBUTHNOTT. 1983. The electrophysiology of dopamine (D2) receptors. A study of the actions of dopamine on corticostriatal transmission. Neuroscience **10:** 349–355.
54. GODUKHIN, O. V., A. D. ZHARIKOVA & A. YU. BUDANTSEV. 1984. Role of presynaptic dopamine receptors in regulation of the glutamatergic neurotransmission in rat neostriatum. Neuroscience **12:** 377–383.
55. ZETTERSTROM, T., P. BRUNDIN, F. H. GAGE, T. SHARP, O. ISACSON, S. B. DUNNETT, U. UNGERSTEDT & A. BJORKLUND. 1986. *In vivo* measurement of spontaneous release and metabolism of dopamine from intrastriatal nigral grafts using intracerebral dialysis. Brain Res. **362:** 344–349.

DISCUSSION OF THE PAPER

J. SLADEK (*University of Rochester Medical School, Rochester, NY*): Can you address the specificity of the type of nerve cell in reversing functions or improving functions? If you put VTA neurons into the caudate for motor deficits, will that reverse the deficits?

F. GAGE (*University of California, San Diego, CA*): We have not been separating our fetal tissue into VTA and substantia nigra. Those of you who have tried to do fetal grafting at E11 or E10 in the rat recognize that the separation of A10 and A8 would be difficult.

UNIDENTIFIED DISCUSSANT: Can you elaborate on your medial frontal cortex work? Are there any postlesion behavioral deficits or postgrafting behavioral changes that you could pin on the VTA medial frontal cortex system rather than on things like the accumbens?

GAGE: We saw an increase in the response to amphetamine in the prefrontal group as well as in terms of locomotor activity. There was an increase with just grafts into the prefrontal cortex and there was no way that those axons projected to the accumbens, so it is associated with the motor response as well. Presently, with these VTA animals, we have an extensive study that has injections into the prefrontal cortex and the accumbens and septal area. We then look at the animals in water-maze performance in terms of some of the cognitive deficits that appear with the VTA lesions and find that the animals are severely impaired on these tests as well. The problem is for an experiment to dissociate whether or not these are really cognitive impairments or whether or not they are part of the motor problems. By selectively grafting one area or another, we are beginning to see improvement in the animals on one dimension or another. In fact, it does look like grafts to the prefrontal cortex help the animals in some of the spatial localization problems.

UNIDENTIFIED DISCUSSANT: I was interested in the comment that your grafts did not work quite as well in the animals that were more severely impaired. In the data we presented earlier, we divided our animals into an impaired and unimpaired group and then looked at the dendritic structure in terms of the neurons that were regressed and the neurons that were not. We set up an experiment where we hoped to show a linear relationship between declining motor function and declining dendritic structure, but it did not happen that way. You can have a very significant loss of motor function in terms of rotorod and balance beam testing, but dendritic structure remains stable until you get to the very end. In the very severely handicapped animal, the dendritic structure falls off so that you have regression. Therefore, maybe what is happening in that severe group is that the postsynaptic cell that the graft is looking for is not there.

GAGE: Yes.

T. McNEILL (*University of Rochester, Rochester, NY*): Furthermore, in that intermediate group, even though they are showing motor impairment, the dendritic structure still exists. Maybe, if you would produce a cortical striate lesion and try your graft, then it would mimic that same thing.

GAGE: That is a very good idea. I also think of it in terms of the underlying problem that exists between cerebellum and caudate in regard to explaining motor deficits. We may be observing dopaminergic deficits in the early stages that can be restored by dopaminergic grafts or dopaminergic function.

Paralleling this is a threshold effect on cerebellum; once the two reach their vortex, the dopamine grafts alone are not going to have any effect because another system is affected as well. One is going to have to work with both systems at that severe state, so I do not think that it is going to be one system or another. Obviously, there are multiple systems involved.

C. COTMAN (*University of California, Irvine, CA*): In the old animals, do the dopamine neurons grow over longer distances? Secondly, it seems like cholinergic neurons may be able to grow over longer distances too. Can you comment on that?

GAGE: If dopamine neurons are grafted in the spinal cord, they can grow up to a centimeter in six months. However, that is a target area for dopamine neurons. It depends on the target area that you are putting the cells in because they will not grow well in substantia nigra. Cholinergic neurons also will not grow if they are not in an appropriate target area. I think that is a phenomenon that is true for any cell—you have to match the cells with the appropriate target area.

Ganglioside Treatment in the Recovery of the DA Nigrostriatal System in Different Experimental Conditions

A. CONSOLAZIONE AND G. TOFFANO

Fidia Research Laboratories
35031 Abano Terme, Italy

Cognitive, sensory, and motor deficits are still today often dramatic consequences of brain damage. In fact, although great improvements have occurred in the last decades in diagnosing and localizing brain injury, effective treatments for reducing lesion-induced malfunction and for facilitating repair processes are still lacking. Yet, during the last few years, basic neurobiological studies have supplied increasing evidence that opportunities may exist provided the variables are understood. Neurons of the central nervous system (CNS) and, in particular, synapses are now known to be potentially able "to modify their function, to be replaced, and to increase or decrease in number when required".[1] This phenomenon, known as neuronal plasticity, is very complex and has been suggested to underlie the possibility for the occurrence of not only functional, but also morphofunctional compensatory processes following brain damage. Hopefully, comprehension of this phenomenon will, in the near future, provide novel pharmacological strategies effective in minimizing the consequences of brain injury. In this regard, the involvements of neuronotrophic factors (NTFs) and gangliosides — in particular, monosialoganglioside GM_1 (nomenclature according to Svennerholm[2]) — are now being analyzed with increasing attention.

BRAIN INJURY AND NEURONOTROPHIC FACTORS

CNS injury, whether it be acute or chronic, is associated not only with primary, but also secondary neuronal cell damage and death. Pharmacological treatments aimed at minimizing or preventing neuronal cell death may be expected to greatly ameliorate prognosis.

NTFs, known for many years to be essential for the regulation of neuronal cell survival and fiber outgrowth during development, have recently been suggested to be involved in the maintenance of cell survival and proper functional connectivity of neuronal cells throughout adulthood.[3] As such, a decrease in the availability or an increase in the requirement of NTFs (or both) following trauma, stroke, and perhaps neurodegenerative diseases may well underlie the secondary neuronal cell death and inability of the neurons to compensate for the loss of function.[3,4]

Recent support for this hypothesis derives from evidence indicating that the intracerebral administration of NTFs, in particular, nerve growth factor (NGF), is effective in both reducing neuronal cell death and in ameliorating behavioral outcome following injury of some neuronal cell types in the adult brain.[5-7] This indicates that improved neuronal cell survival and, hence, better conditions for facilitating functional repair can be achieved by at least two, not mutually exclusive, therapeutical strategies; that is, by increasing either the availability of NTFs (e.g., substitutive therapy) or the biological potency of the endogenously occurring NTF molecules (corrective therapy), or both. Whereas the former approach is still today at a very initial experimental stage, evidence is available that indicates that the latter approach is indeed feasible. In fact, NTFs are known to occur in the adult mammalian brain, and even though NTF activity has been reported to increase following CNS injury, this increase presumably occurs at a time subsequent to most neuronal cell death.[8,9] In addition, agents such as GM_1, known to increase neuronal cellular response to trophic signals at least *in vitro*,[10-13] have been demonstrated to positively affect CNS repair processes *in vivo*.

In line with the above-mentioned ideas, we will now briefly summarize the currently available *in vitro* and *in vivo* evidence with regard to the capability of GM_1 to facilitate neuronal repair processes in adult mammals following brain damage.

GM_1 AND NEURONOTROPHIC INTERACTIONS *IN VITRO*

The endogenously occurring GM_1 on the neuronal cell surface[14] is probably involved in the regulation of neurite outgrowth and regeneration not only during development, but also in the adult state (for review, see reference 15). Furthermore, exogenous GM_1 addition to culture medium has been reported to facilitate neurite outgrowth of a variety of clonal and primary neuronal cells *in vitro*.[16-21] When analyzed, this effect has been associated with enhanced neuronal cell development and survival. Interestingly, in most cases, the attainment of these GM_1 effects *in vitro* has been shown to be strictly dependent on the presence of adequate NTFs and to be associated with enhanced neuronal cell responsiveness to the NTF molecule.[10-13] The latter aspect is well exemplified in experiments utilizing fetal chick (E_8) dorsal root ganglion (DRG)[11] and pheochromocytoma (PC12)[10-13] cells *in vitro*. Both of these cell types are known to require NGF for neuritic outgrowth and expression of characteristic neuronal phenotypic traits. In both cases, the GM_1-induced facilitation of neuritic outgrowth was shown to necessitate the presence of NGF. GM_1 alone was totally ineffective. In addition, analogous results were obtained in primary neuronal cell culture model systems (e.g., ciliary ganglia and CNS mesencephalic neurons) known to necessitate trophic support other than NGF.[20,21] This has been interpreted as indicating that GM_1 can positively affect the efficacy of different NTF molecules acting on specific neuronal cell types.

Even though the molecular mechanisms underlying the exogenous GM_1 effects *in vitro* are still obscure, it has been postulated that they most likely occur via modifications of cell surface properties consequent to stable insertion of the GM_1 molecule into the neuronal plasma membrane.[22] However, NGF association with the PC12 cells has been reported to be apparently unaffected by GM_1. Alternative explanations may involve a modulation of cell surface transduction mechanisms or an enhancement of specific posttranslational events triggered by the NTF(s).

GM_1 EFFECTS FOLLOWING CNS INJURY

Parenteral GM_1 administration has been shown to be effective in ameliorating cognitive,[23,24] sensory,[25] and motor[26] deficits following different specific lesion paradigms.

We will summarize below our results concerning GM_1 effects following unilateral partial hemitransection of the dopamine (DA) nigrostriatal pathway in young adult rats. In addition, some experimental variables underlying GM_1 effects in this lesion paradigm will be examined.

Effect of GM₁ Treatment on Recovery of DA Nigrostriatal Parameters after Unilateral Partial Deafferentation in Young Adult Rats

Following unilateral partial hemitransection of the DA nigrostriatal pathway in young adult rats, animals show a decrease of tyrosine hydroxylase (TH) activity (about 50%), a decrease of TH immunopositive nerve terminals, and a decrease of homovanillic acid (HVA) content in the lesioned striatum with respect to the unlesioned contralateral striatum. In contrast, treatment with GM_1 induces a significant increase of TH activity in the lesioned striatum in a time- and dose-dependent manner. This effect is apparent already after two weeks of treatment (TABLE 1) and is associated with an increased number of TH immunofluorescent terminals in the partially denervated striatum;[27] in addition, it is associated with an increased number of TH immunopositive cell bodies in the substantia nigra ipsilateral to the lesion.[28]

Moreover, experiments utilizing retrograde transport of wheat-germ agglutinin conjugated to horseradish peroxidase (WGA-HRP) indicate that all the TH immunoreactive nigral cells in the GM_1-treated animals possess an intact connectivity to the striatum.[29]

The biochemical and immunohistochemical improvements elicited by GM_1 treatment are also of functional relevance. Apomorphine-induced rotational behavior, considered as an index of striatal DA denervation,[30] is significantly reduced in GM_1-treated animals with respect to the saline-treated ones (FIGURE 1).

The above findings indicate that parenteral administration of GM_1 is effective in facilitating the functional recovery of the nigrostriatal pathway following partial deafferentation. It must be recalled that this effect is closely correlated with maintenance in the number of TH positive cell bodies in the substantia nigra. Whether it is also associated with sprouting of TH positive fibers in the striatum, though, remains to be established.

TABLE 1. Effect of GM_1 Treatment on Striatal TH Activity after Partial Unilateral Hemitransection of the Nigrostriatal System[a]

	V_{max} as % of Control		
	Days after Hemitransection		
Treatment	8	14	56
Saline	45 ± 3.5	50 ± 3.0	53 ± 6.1
GM_1 (5 mg/kg)	50 ± 3.0	65 ± 5.0^b	80 ± 2.9^c
GM_1 (30 mg/kg)	48 ± 3.0	85 ± 4.8^c	89 ± 6.5^c

[a] The intraperitoneal treatment, either with saline or GM_1, was started on the second day after surgery and ended 24 hours before sacrifice. Data represent the V_{max} mean values of TH and are expressed as the percent of the respective unlesioned side. All means are from 6–8 determinations. The V_{max} of TH determined in the unlesioned side of the saline-treated group (19.7 ± 1.01 nmol $CO_2 \times h^{-1} \times mg^{-1}$ protein) was not significantly different from that of the GM_1-treated group at any time.

[b] $p < 0.05$.

[c] $p < 0.01$ versus the respective group treated with saline (Student's t test).

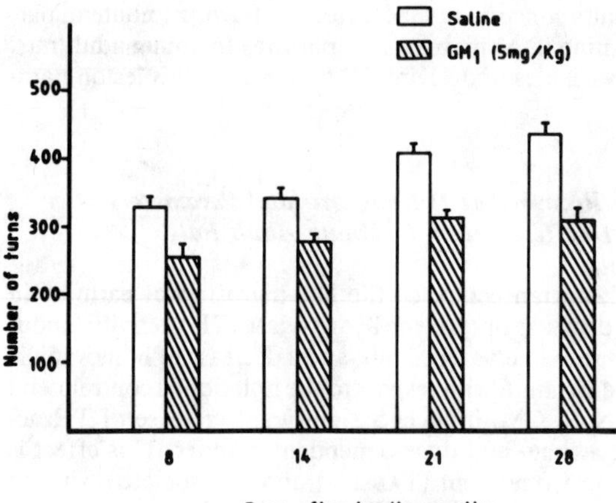

FIGURE 1. Effect of GM_1 after partial lesion of the nigrostriatal system on apomorphine-induced behavior. Turning behavior was analyzed in a rotometer by recording the number of full turns in both directions after injecting 1 mg/kg subcutaneously apomorphine over a period of 45 minutes. Fifteen animals were used in each determination. All values of GM_1-treated animals were statistically different ($p <$ 0.01) from those of the saline-treated group.

Effect of GM₁ Treatment on Striatal TH Activity in Different Experimental Conditions

In an attempt to have some further insight with regard to GM_1 effects following injury of the nigrostriatal pathway, we tested GM_1 effects in various experimental conditions.

In particular, in order to analyze whether the effect of GM_1 in facilitating the recovery of striatal dopaminergic parameters depends on the response of the remaining intact fibers of the ipsilateral side, we induced an almost total hemitransection that resulted in a 95% loss of striatal TH activity. In contrast to what is observed in the case of a less extensive mechanical lesion, GM_1 in our case is unable to facilitate recovery of striatal TH activity. This result suggests that the GM_1 effect is dependent on the extent of the lesion, thereby supporting the hypothesis that an essential prerequisite for triggering the repair process is the survival of an adequate number of the ipsilateral neurons.[31] As variations in the extent of the lesion can be expected to result in variations in trophic need, the occurrence of adequate NTF activity and GM_1 effects may be causally related.

In addition, we explored the role of the contralateral hemisphere in the repair process and found that the integrity of the interhemispheric nigrostriatal neuronal loop is another condition essential for the occurrence of the GM_1 effects.[32] This is not surprising because the reciprocal influence of the two nigrostriatal systems through intrathalamic connections is well documented.[33-35] These anatomical connections have been reported to increase following unilateral lesion of the substantia nigra.[36] Therefore, the effect of GM_1 is also related to the presence of regulatory signals derived from areas that can be located distant from the site of the primary damage. Interestingly, following partial unilateral hemitransection in young adult rats, we observed induction of NTF activity not only in the substantia nigra and striatum of the lesioned side, but in the unlesioned contralateral side as well.[37]

The fact that neuronal activity of both the substantia nigra and the caudate nucleus is altered by stimulation of visual or motor cortices[38] prompted us to perform an experiment in which the GM_1 effect was studied in partially hemitransected rats kept in darkness. These animals showed a lower striatal TH activity when compared to that of lesioned animals kept at a normal 12-hour light-dark cycle. In addition,

TABLE 2. Effect of Light and Darkness on GM_1-Induced Recovery of Striatal TH Activity after Partial Unilateral Hemitransection of the Nigrostriatal System[a]

| | V_{max} as % of Control | |
Treatment	Light	Darkness
Saline	45 ± 3.0	16 ± 3.5[b]
GM_1	93 ± 6.5[c]	13 ± 2.5[b]

[a] Intraperitoneal treatment, either with saline or GM_1 (30 mg/kg), was given for 30 days. Data represent the V_{max} mean values of TH and are expressed as the percent of the respective unlesioned side. Light means that animals were allowed to have a normal 12-hour light-dark cycle. Darkness means that the animals were kept in darkness for the whole period of the experiment.

[b] $p < 0.01$ versus light.

[c] $p < 0.01$ versus saline (Student's t test).

these animals did not show any recovery of striatal TH activity following GM_1 treatment (TABLE 2). Hence, an adequate sensory perception plays a relevant role in GM_1-induced brain repair and, more generally, in sensory-motor rehabilitation. Normal visual perception is known to contribute extensively to hormonal circadian rhythms, and hormones (such as triiodothyronine) are known to possess trophic activity *in vitro*.[39]

Another condition influencing the effect of GM_1 on the recovery of striatal TH activity following partial unilateral hemitransection is the age of the rats. Although GM_1 is capable of enhancing CNS repair in rats of all ages, we have observed that the treatment time necessary to obtain comparatively beneficial effects in hemitransected rats is dependent on the age of the animals. In fact, with increasing age, there

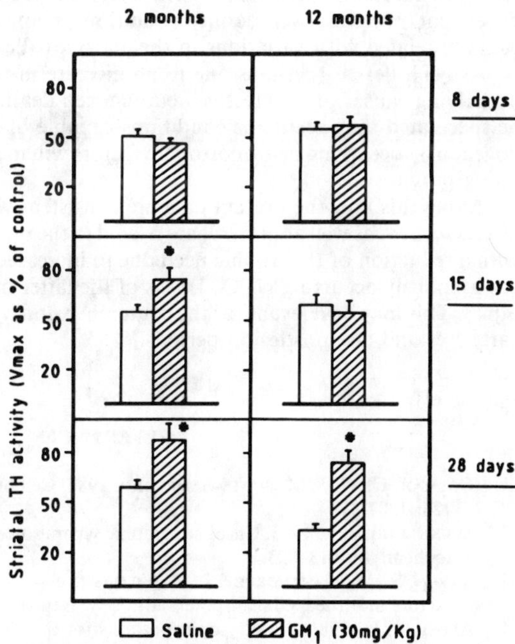

FIGURE 2. Treatment with GM_1 (30 mg/kg i.p.) was started on the second day after surgery. Data represent the V_{max} mean values of TH and are expressed as the percent of the respective unlesioned side. The V_{max} of TH determined in the striatum of the unlesioned side of the saline-treated group (18.9 ± 1.01 nmol $CO_2 \times h^{-1} \times mg^{-1}$ protein) was not significantly different from that of the GM_1-treated group at any time or age considered. GM_1 treatment had no effect on striatal TH activity of the unlesioned rats of both ages. The asterisk stands for $p < 0.01$ versus the respective saline-treated group.

occurs an increasing latency in the appearance of the GM_1 facilitatory effect on striatal TH activity (FIGURE 2). This observation therefore suggests that although lesion-induced neuronal plasticity can be manifested in aged mammals, it nonetheless occurs with increasing age at a much slower rate. Also noteworthy is the fact that lesion-induced increases of NTF activity have been reported to be delayed in aged rats with respect to young adult rats.[9]

Furthermore, we evaluated whether GM_1 could promote recovery of DA nigrostriatal parameters after destruction of the DA neurons with the specific neurotoxin, 6-hydroxydopamine (6-OHDA). For this purpose, 6-OHDA was unilaterally injected into either the medial forebrain bundle or into the substantia nigra. In both of these conditions, treatment with GM_1 failed to improve recovery.[31,40] However, although the underlying cause for this lack of GM_1 effect is currently unknown, we have observed, in contrast to the mechanical injury, that no induction of NTF activity occurs in the substantia nigra of the 6-OHDA lesioned rats.[37] This suggests that the trophic response may vary depending on the nature of the injury and that adequate titers of NTF(s) are perhaps needed for GM_1 facilitation of functional repair.

CONCLUSIONS

Several lines of evidence are available today that support the possibility that GM_1 can favorably modulate neuronal cell responsiveness to NTFs *in vitro*. Furthermore, the systemic administration of GM_1 has been shown to ameliorate the biochemical and behavioral outcome following brain damage to adult mammals. In many cases, these effects have been associated with enhanced neuronal cell survival. Interestingly, the intracerebral administration of NTF(s) has been reported to produce a similar effect.[6,7] In addition, although the GM_1 effects *in vivo* are, as exemplified in this report, dependent on certain well-defined conditions, many of these conditions appear to be causally related with variations in the entity of the trophic deficit.

As NTF deficit (perhaps due to an increase in trophic need) may be one of the underlying causes of progressive neuronal cell death following brain injury,[3,4] it can be speculated that agents or conditions capable of potentiating the efficacy of endogenously occurring neuronotrophic factors will most probably be useful in ameliorating prognosis.

Along this line, the present data are consistent with the possibility that the GM_1 effects *in vivo*, as well as *in vitro*, are related to the presence of NTFs and are associated with a reduction of the trophic need due to increased neuronal cell responsiveness to endogenously occurring NTFs. Levels of the latter may be inadequate soon after the injury. This may be relevant for the comprehension of GM_1 facilitatory effects at both early[41,42] and late postlesion periods.[24,43–45]

REFERENCES

1. COTMAN, C. W. & M. NIETO-SAMPEDRO. 1984. Cell biology of synaptic plasticity. Science **225:** 1287–1294.
2. SVENNERHOLM, L. 1963. Chromatographic separation of human brain gangliosides. J. Neurochem. **10:** 613–623.
3. VARON, S., M. MANTHORPE & L. R. WILLIAMS. 1984. Neuronotrophic and neurite-promoting factors and their clinical potentials. Dev. Neurosci. **6:** 73–100.
4. APPEL, S. H. 1981. A unifying hypothesis for the cause of amyotrophic lateral sclerosis, parkinsonism and Alzheimer's disease. Ann. Neurol. **10:** 499–505.

5. STEIN, D. G. 1981. Functional recovery from brain damage following treatment with nerve growth factor. *In* Functional Recovery from Brain Damage. M. W. van Hof & G. Mohn, Eds.: 423–443. Elsevier. Amsterdam/New York.

6. HEFTI, F. 1986. Nerve growth factor (NGF) promotes survival of septal cholinergic neurons after fimbrial transections. J. Neurosci. **6:** 2155–2162.

7. VARON, S., L. R. WILLIAMS & F. H. GAGE. 1987. Exogenous administration of neuronotrophic factors *in vivo* protects CNS neuron against axotomy-induced degeneration. Prog. Brain Res. **71:** 191–201.

8. NIETO-SAMPEDRO, M., E. R. LEWIS, C. W. COTMAN, M. MANTHORPE, S. D. SKAPER, G. BARBIN, F. M. LONGO & S. VARON. 1982. Brain injury causes a time dependent increase in neuronotrophic activity at the lesion site. Science **217:** 860–861.

9. WHITTEMORE, S. R., M. NIETO-SAMPEDRO, D. L. NEEDELS & C. W. COTMAN. 1985. Neuronotrophic factors for mammalian brain neurons: injury induction in neonatal, adult and aged rat brain. Dev. Brain Res. **20:** 169–178.

10. FERRARI, G., M. FABRIS & A. GORIO. 1983. Gangliosides enhance neurite outgrowth in PC12 cells. Dev. Brain Res. **8:** 215–221.

11. LEON, A., D. BENVEGNÙ, R. DAL TOSO, D. PRESTI, L. FACCI, O. GIORGI & G. TOFFANO. 1984. Dorsal root ganglia and nerve growth factor: a model for understanding the mechanism of GM1 effects of neuronal repair. J. Neurosci. Res. **12:** 277–287.

12. DOHERTY, P., J. G. DICKSON, T. P. FLANIGAN & F. S. WALSH. 1985. Ganglioside GM1 does not initiate but enhances neurite regeneration of nerve growth factor-dependent sensory neurones. J. Neurochem. **44:** 1259–1265.

13. KATOH-SEMBA, R., S. D. SKAPER & S. VARON. 1984. Interaction of GM1 ganglioside with PC12 pheochromocytoma cells: serum and NGF-dependent effects on neuritic growth (and proliferation). J. Neurosci. Res. **12:** 299–310.

14. YAMAKAWA, Y. & Y. NAGAI. 1978. Glycolipids at the cell surface and their biological functions. Trends Biochem. Sci. **3:** 128–131.

15. LEDEEN, R. W., R. K. YU, M. M. RAPPORT & K. SUZUKI. 1984. Ganglioside Structure, Function and Biomedical Potential. Plenum. New York.

16. DREYFUS, H., J. C. LUIS, S. HARTH & P. MANDEL. 1980. Gangliosides in culture neurons. Neuroscience **5:** 1647–1655.

17. ROISEN, F. J., H. BARTFELD, R. MAGELLE & G. YORKE. 1981. Ganglioside stimulation of axonal sprouting *in vitro*. Science **214:** 577–578.

18. BYRNE, M. C., R. W. LEDEEN, F. J. ROISEN, G. YORKE & J. R. SCLAFANI. 1983. Ganglioside-induced neuritogenesis: verification that gangliosides are the active agents and comparison of molecular species. J. Neurochem. **41:** 1214–1222.

19. SPOERRI, P. E. 1983. Effects of gangliosides on the *in vitro* development of neuroblastoma cells: an ultrastructural study. Int. J. Dev. Neurosci. **1:** 383–391.

20. DAL TOSO, R., A. LEON, D. PRESTI, D. BENVEGNÙ, L. FACCI, O. GIORGI & G. TOFFANO. 1984. Effect of monosialoganglioside on expression of dopaminergic characteristics of embryonic mesencephalic cells in cultures. Cellular and Pathological Aspects of Glycoconjugate Metabolism. Inserm **126:** 297–308.

21. SKAPER, S. D. & S. VARON. 1985. Ganglioside GM1 overcomes serum inhibition of neuritic outgrowth. Int. J. Dev. Neurosci. **3:** 187–198.

22. FACCI, L., A. LEON, G. TOFFANO, S. SONNINO, R. GHIDONI & G. TETTAMANTI. 1984. Promotion of neuritogenesis in mouse neuroblastoma cells by exogenous gangliosides. Relationship between the effect and the cell association of ganglioside GM1. J. Neurochem. **42:** 299–305.

23. SABEL, B. A., G. L. DUNBAR & D. G. STEIN. 1984. Gangliosides minimize behavioral deficits and enhance structural repair after brain injury. J. Neurosci. Res. **12:** 429–443.

24. CASAMENTI, F., L. BRACCO, L. BARTOLINI & G. PEPEU. 1985. Effects of ganglioside treatment in rats with a lesion of the cholinergic forebrain nuclei. Brain Res. **338:** 45–52.

25. CARMIGNOTO, G., R. CANELLA & S. BISTI. 1984. Can functional reorganization of area 17 following monocular deprivation be modified by GM_1 internal ester treatment? J. Neurosci. Res. **12:** 477–483.

26. SABEL, B. A., G. L. DUNBAR, W. M. BUTLER & D. G. STEIN. 1985. GM_1 gangliosides stimulate neuronal reorganization and reduce rotational asymmetry after hemitransections of the nigrostriatal pathway. Exp. Brain Res. **60:** 27–37.

27. TOFFANO, G., G. SAVOINI, F. MORONI, M. G. LOMBARDI, L. CALZÀ & L. F. AGNATI. 1983. GM1 ganglioside stimulates the regeneration of dopaminergic neurons in the central nervous system. Brain Res. **261:** 163–166.

28. AGNATI, L. F., K. FUXE, L. CALZÀ, F. BENFENATI, L. CAVICCHIOLI, G. TOFFANO & M. GOLDSTEIN. 1983. Ganglioside increase the survival of lesioned nigral dopamine neurons and favour the recovery of dopaminergic synaptic function in striatum of rats by collateral sprouting. Acta Physiol. Scand. **119:** 347–363.

29. CONSOLAZIONE, A., C. ALDINIO, L. CAVICCHIOLI, A. LEON & G. TOFFANO. 1987. Gangliosides as a tool for studying the repair of adult mammalian brain after injury. *In* Model System of Development and Aging of the Nervous System. A. Vernadakis, Ed.: 443–452. Nijhoff. The Hague.

30. UNGERSTEDT, U. 1978. 6-Hydroxydopamine-induced degeneration of central monoamine neurons. Eur. J. Pharmacol. **5:** 107–110.

31. TOFFANO, G., G. SAVOINI, F. APORTI, S. CALZOLARI, A. CONSOLAZIONE, G. MAURA, M. MARCHI, M. RAITERI & L. F. AGNATI. 1984. The functional recovery of damaged brain: the effect of GM1 monosialoganglioside. J. Neurosci. Res. **12:** 397–408.

32. TOFFANO, G., L. F. AGNATI, K. FUXE, C. ALDINIO, A. CONSOLAZIONE, G. VALENTI & G. SAVOINI. 1984. Effect of GM1 ganglioside treatment on the recovery of dopaminergic nigro-striatal neurons after different types of lesion. Acta Physiol. Scand. **122:** 313–321.

33. RUFFIEUX, A. & W. SCHULTZ. 1980. Dopaminergic activation of reticulate neurones in the substantia nigra. Nature **295:** 240–241.

34. CHERAMY, A., V. LEVIEL, F. DAUDET, B. GUIBERT, M. F. CHESSELET & J. GLOWINSKI. 1981. Involvement of the thalamus in the reciprocal regulation of the two nigrostriatal dopaminergic pathways. Neuroscience **6:** 2657–2668.

35. COLLINRIDGE, G. L. 1982. Electrophysiological evidence for the existence of crossed nigro-striatal fibers. Experientia **38:** 812–814.

36. PRITZEL, M., J. P. HOUSTON & M. SARTER. 1983. Behavioural and neuronal reorganization after unilateral substantia nigra lesions: evidence for increased interhemispheric nigro-striatal projections. Neuroscience **9:** 879–888.

37. CONSOLAZIONE, A., C. ALDINIO, D. PRESTI, R. DAL TOSO, A. LEON & G. TOFFANO. 1985. Correlation between long-term GM1 ganglioside effects on CNS repair and neuronotrophic activity. Soc. Neurosci. Abstr. no. 279.13.

38. NIEOULLON, A., A. CHERAMY & J. GLOWINSKI. 1978. Release of dopamine evoked by electrical stimulation of the motor and visual areas of the cerebral cortex in both caudate nuclei and in the substantia nigra in the cat. Brain Res. **145:** 69–83.

39. PUYMIRAT, J., A. BARRET, R. PICART, A. VIGNY, C. LOUDES, A. FAIVRE-BAUMAN & A. TIXIER-VIDAL. 1983. Triiodothyronine enhances the morphological maturation of dopaminergic neurons from fetal mouse hypothalamus cultured in serum-free medium. Neuroscience **10:** 801–810.

40. TOFFANO, G., G. SAVOINI, C. ALDINIO, M. VALENTI, M. G. LOMBARDI, F. MORONI, L. F. AGNATI & K. FUXE. 1984. A role for exogenous gangliosides in the functional recovery of adult lesioned nervous system. *In* Catecholamines: Neuropharmacology and Central Nervous System—Therapeutic Aspects. E. Usdin *et al.*, Eds.: 219–227. Alan R. Liss. New York.

41. BORZEIX, M. G. 1984. Drugs effect in an experimental stroke resulting from a transient cerebral oligaemia. Drugs Dis. **1:** 44–53.

42. KARPIAK, S. E. & S. P. MAHADIK. 1984. Reduction of cerebral edema with GM1 ganglioside. J. Neurosci. Res. **12:** 485–492.

43. ODERFELD-NOWAK, B., M. SKUP, J. ULAS, M. JEZIERSKA, M. GRADKOWSKA & M. ZAREMBA. 1984. Effect of GM1 ganglioside treatment on postlesion responses of cholinergic enzymes in rat hippocampus after various partial deafferentations. J. Neurosci. Res. **12:** 409–420.

44. SABEL, B. A., M. D. SLAVIN & D. G. STEIN. 1984. GM1 ganglioside treatment facilitates behavioral recovery from bilateral brain damage. Science **225:** 340–342.

45. KOJIMA, H., A. GORIO & G. JONSSON. 1985. GM1 ganglioside has a regrowth stimulatory effect on neurotoxin-induced lesion of noradrenaline nerve terminals in rat cerebral cortex. Neuroscience **13:** 1011–1022.

Effect of AL 721, a Novel Membrane Fluidizer, on the Binding Parameters of Brain Dopamine Receptors

LIDA ANTONIAN AND ARNOLD S. LIPPA

Matrix Research Laboratories
North Academic Complex
City College of New York
New York, New York

INTRODUCTION

Our studies have been directed towards understanding the molecular mechanism of D2 receptor function. Purification of the D2 receptor from its natural membrane environment is the first step in the biochemical characterization of the receptor. Our alternative approach in characterization of the receptor has been through modulation of receptor function by altering the lipid milieu of the plasma membrane. As a first step, the D2 receptor in canine striatum was purified 300–400-fold by affinity chromatography.[1] Reconstitution of the affinity-purified receptor with phospholipids has been shown to be essential for stabilization of the activity of the purified receptor.[2] Because it has been shown that an optimal lipid composition is essential for the retention of active purified D2 receptors, we have manipulated striatal membrane fluidity in order to determine its effect on membrane-bound D2 receptor activity. We have investigated the fluidization effects of a natural lipid mixture, AL 721, on the membrane-bound D2 receptors. Fluidization of the striatal membranes with this pharmacologically active lipid did not alter the capacity of the striatal dopamine receptors in either young or old rats. However, it restored the decreased affinity of the D2 receptor in the aged rats to the basal level found in the younger rats. These results suggest that removal of the natural lipids during purification diminishes the binding ability of the D2 receptor and that direct *in vitro* modulation of rat striatal membrane fluidity is effective in restoring the affinity of dopamine receptors, which have diminished upon aging.

METHODS

Purification of Dopamine D2 Receptors with Affinity Chromatography

Haloperidol hemisuccinate was synthesized as reported previously[1] and was used as a ligand for affinity chromatography. The hydrophilic affinity matrix, Sepharose amine-succinyl-amine haloperidol hemisuccinate (ASA-HHS), was used for the purification of canine striatal dopamine (D2) receptors.[1] P_2-P_3 pellets were prepared from canine striata in 50 mM TEAN buffer (50 mM tris base, 5 mM Na_2EDTA, 0.01% ascorbic acid, and 10 μM nialamide) and were solubilized in the presence of a 1% solution of digitonin containing 0.01% sodium azide. Sixteen mL of digitonin-solubilized preparation was applied to the affinity column, which was previously washed with TEAN buffer containing 0.01% digitonin, 0.01% sodium azide, and 1.0 M KCl. The digitonin-solubilized preparation was recycled through the column at 3.0 mL/h for 14–15 hours. After the unbound soluble preparation was eluted, the column was washed with a TEAN buffer containing 0.01% NaN_3, 0.1% digitonin, and 50 μM DTT until all measurable protein had eluted. Then, elution was continued with the same buffer with the addition of 20 μM haloperidol. One mL of each collected fraction was treated with 10 mg of charcoal for 15 min and was centrifuged at 9000 × g for 5 min. The supernatant was subjected to a ³H-spiroperidol binding assay. Nonspecific binding was measured in the presence of 1 μM (+)-butaclamol. One-dimensional electrophoresis was performed on column eluates that showed specific binding with ³H-spiroperidol. Two-dimensional IEF-PAGE analysis was performed on a column eluate that showed binding activity.

Incorporation of AL 721 into Striatal Membranes

A sonicated solution of AL 721 in 15 mM TEAN buffer (15 mM tris base, 5 mM Na_2EDTA, 0.02% ascorbic acid, and 10 μM nialamide) was prepared with a probe sonicator at a power setting of 20–30 watts for 15 minutes; the sonicated solution is stable for several days at 4 °C. Rat striata were dissected and stored at −70 °C until used. Membrane homogenates were prepared according to a previously reported procedure.[3] Equal volumes of the striatal homogenate and the AL 721 solution (1 mg/mL) were incubated at 25 °C with agitation for four hours. The incubation was terminated by centrifugation of the sample at 40,000 × g for 15 minutes. The pellet was rinsed with buffer to remove any adhering AL 721 and was then resuspended in the buffer at the original volume of the homogenate. The AL 721–treated tissue was then subjected to binding and fluidization studies.

Binding Studies of Striatal D2 Receptors

Saturation isotherms of ³H-spiroperidol (0.025–2.0 nM) binding to the D2 receptor in rat striatal homogenates were determined in a total volume of 1.2 mL. Ketanserin, at 100 nM, was included in order to mask serotonin S_2 receptors in the striata. Nonspecific binding was defined in the presence of 100 μM (−)-sulpiride. Agonist displacement of ³H-spiroperidol (∼250 pM) binding was performed at a concentration range of 10 nM to 10 μM.

Measurements of Lipid Fluidity

Membrane lipid microviscosity (η) was determined by fluorescence polarization (P) of a lipid probe, 1,6-diphenyl-1,3,5-hexatriene (DPH). A stock solution of 2.0 mM DPH in tetrahydrofuran was diluted to 2.0 μM with 15 mM TEAN buffer (pH = 7.4). A 0.5-mL sample of a membrane homogenate (containing about 40 μg of protein) was incubated with 4.5 mL of 2 μM DPH for 30 min at 25 °C. Steady-state polarization measurements were made at 25 °C on an SLM Model 4800 spectrofluorometer. The outputs, $I_\perp$ and $I_\parallel$, from the photomultiplier tubes were measured directly. $I_\perp$ and $I_\parallel$ are the fluorescence intensities polarized perpendicular and parallel to the polarization of the excitation beam, respectively. Use of appropriate membrane blanks and a cutoff filter above 470 nm eliminated light scattering and signal-to-noise effects during the polarization measurements. The excitation and emission wavelengths were 360 and 427 nm, respectively. The lipid microviscosity (the reciprocal of fluidity) was determined by the approximate empirical relation, $\eta = 2P/(0.46 - P)$.[4]

RESULTS

Purification of the dopamine receptor was performed in order to determine the essential biochemical factors for the retention of its bioactivity and in order to determine whether the receptor affinity states are a manifestation of the receptor interaction with other components of the membrane system. A derivative of haloperidol, haloperidol hemisuccinate (HHS), was used in an affinity chromatography matrix for the purification of digitonin-solubilized dopamine receptors from canine striatal homogenates. The affinity matrix, gel ASA-HHS, was prepared by coupling a hydrophilic spacer arm in a stepwise manner to CNBr-activated Sepharose 4B. Maximum absorption of receptors by ASA-HHS ranged from 81–100% of ^{3}H-spiroperidol binding sites in the solubilized preparation. A 50 mM TEAN buffer containing 0.01% NaN_3, 0.01% digitonin, 50 μM dithiothreitol, and 20 μM haloperidol was used for elution of receptors adsorbed to a column of ASA-HHS. Recovery of active receptors from the affinity column proved to be variable in multiple trials. In 30% of the trials, when receptors were adsorbed to the gel, the haloperidol wash eluted two well-separated active fractions (fractions 1 and 2) that represented 22% and 27% recovery of specific ^{3}H-spiroperidol binding in the solubilized preparation, respectively. In those experiments where specific binding of ^{3}H-spiroperidol was observed in the haloperidol eluates, approximately 350–460-fold purification was obtained (TABLE 1).

Fractions 1 and 2 showed similar protein profiles in SDS-PAGE analysis. Several protein bands were visible. A protein band of $M_r = 43,000$ was composed of at least four different components when separated by 2-D gel analysis, which included β and γ actin. In addition, α and β tubulins were identified at M_r values of 53,000 and 57,000. The 2-D gel analysis also revealed a number of protein spots at M_r values of 66,000 and 92,500. The coelution of receptor activity and cytoskeletal proteins in 30% of the affinity chromatography runs suggested that actin and tubulin had been solubilized with the dopamine receptor in the presence of the detergent digitonin. The variable successful recovery of active purified receptors suggested that the digitonin-receptor micellar particles did not contain the appropriate membrane-lipid composition. This may have consequently perturbed the receptor microenvironment that is crucial for receptor binding activity. Another report[2] on the affinity chromatography of the D2

TABLE 1. Purification of the Digitonin-solubilized Dopamine Receptor[a]

Sample	Receptor (cpm/300 μL)	Receptor (fmol/300 μL)	Total Volume (mL)	Protein (mg/mL)	Specific Activity (fmol/mg)
Solubilized preparation	1043	38.3	19	2.0	1.0
Fraction 1	234	8.58	2	0.011	379
Fraction 2	285	10.46	2	0.011	462

[a] Fractions 1 and 2 were eluted with haloperidol buffer. Low protein concentrations were measured by fluorescamine detection procedure. The ^{3}H-spiroperidol binding was performed at 4 °C. Nonspecific binding was measured in the presence of 1 μM (+)-butaclamol.

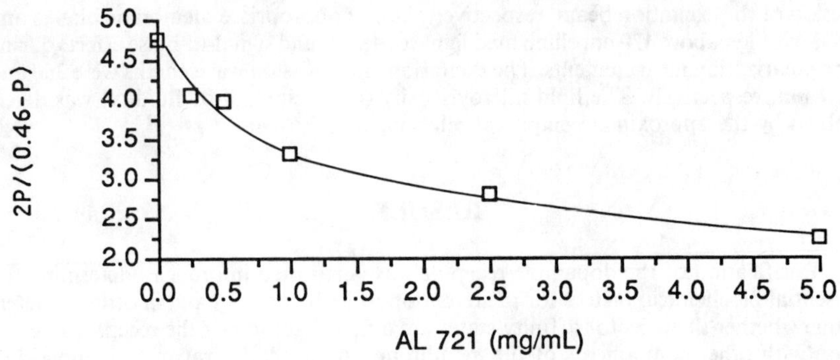

FIGURE 1. Effect of AL 721 on the microviscosity of rat striatal membranes.

receptor confirmed the diminished ability of the affinity-purified receptor to bind ^{3}H-spiroperidol. Reconstitution of the affinity-purified receptor with phosphatidylcholine was necessary for the binding activity to be observed.[2] Thus, it seems that an appropriate receptor conformation is necessary for retention of its binding activity in the purified state.

Optimal lipid fluidity and composition about the receptor is essential for physiologically functioning receptors.[5] The administration of ethanol has been reported to affect a variety of receptors through membrane fluidization.[5] The efficacy of AL 721 as a membrane fluidizer has been demonstrated in several receptor and cell systems.[6–8] AL 721 is a novel lipid mixture composed of neutral triglycerides, phosphatidylcholine, and phosphatidylethanolamine in a 7:2:1 ratio.[6,9] When dispersed in aqueous media, AL 721 forms chylomicron-like assemblies. For this reason, membrane fluidization *in vitro* with AL 721 occurs more efficiently than with pure phosphatidylcholine.[6] AL 721 appears to fluidize cellular membranes primarily through the extraction of membrane cholesterol, thereby enriching the phospholipid-to-cholesterol ratio of the membrane.[6]

AL 721 was shown to be a potent fluidizer of striatal membrane homogenates (FIGURE 1). The half-maximal effect of fluidization occurred between 500–1000 µg/mL of AL 721. Fluidity measurements on striatal membranes of young and old rats (7.39 and 7.29 poise, respectively) indicated no difference in their microviscosity. The viscosity of the striatal homogenate could be reduced upon AL 721 fluidization to 5.39 ± 0.47 (n = 2) and 4.20 ± 0.82 (n = 2) poise in young and old rats, respectively. Consequently, the effect of membrane fluidization on the binding characteristics of the membrane D2 receptor was investigated by measuring the binding properties of the dopamine receptor in the striata of young and old Wistar female rats. The old rats used in this study had a similar performance to the young animals in the inclined screen test. The ^{3}H-spiroperidol binding indicated a similarity in the number of the binding sites in both young and old animals (TABLE 2). However, the affinity of spiroperidol for the D2 receptor was three times greater (45.5 pM) for the younger animals as compared to the old (124 pM) (TABLE 2). Fluidization of the striatal homogenates with AL 721, though, restored the affinity in the older animals to the same level as the young rats, as shown in TABLE 2. The reduced number of binding sites in AL 721–treated young rats may have been due to the solubilization of the membrane receptors.

TABLE 2. Effect of AL 721 on the Binding Parameters of ^{3}H-Spiroperidol[a]

| | K_D (pM) | | B_{max} (fmoles/mg protein) | |
	Control	AL 721	Control	AL 721
Young	45.5 ± 6.3[b]	60.3 ± 8.8	354.5 ± 24.2[c]	227.5 ± 25.8[c]
	($n = 4$)	($n = 4$)	($n = 4$)	($n = 4$)
Old	124.3 ± 27.0[b]	71.6 ± 14.5	331.3 ± 33.5	264.6 ± 33.4
	($n = 4$)	($n = 5$)	($n = 4$)	($n = 5$)

[a] Values given are means $\pm$ SEM for the number of animals in parentheses. All animals were Wistar female rats. The young animals were 6 months of age. The old animals were over 20 months of age.
[b] $p < 0.05$ in a two-tailed t test.
[c] $p < 0.02$ in a two-tailed t test.

Agonist displacement of ^{3}H-spiroperidol binding was also investigated in striata of untreated young and old animals and in those treated with AL 721. The IC50 of apomorphine in old striata was greater than that in younger tissue (TABLE 3). *In vitro* fluidization with AL 721 effectively restored the affinity of the receptor for apomorphine in the older animals to levels found in younger ones. No significant variations in the affinity of ADTN were observed between young and old striata in either the absence or presence of membrane fluidization.

A preliminary test of the *in vivo* effect of AL 721 in old rats was performed (J. A. Joseph, personal communication). The injection of AL 721 (50 and 150 mg/injection) for eight days indicated an improved performance on the inclined screen as compared to the vehicle-injected animals. More thorough studies on the *in vivo* effects of AL 721 are under way.

DISCUSSION

Our results suggest that the pharmacological and biochemical functioning of the striatal D2 receptor is highly dependent on the composition of the lipids that surround the receptor protein. The affinity-purified striatal D2 receptor has shown variable recovery of binding activity. Therefore, elution of spiroperidol binding sites from the affinity column was successfully achieved in 30% of the trials. The binding ability of the affinity-purified pituitary D2 receptor was recovered by enriching the micellar

TABLE 3. Effect of AL 721 on the Binding of Dopamine Agonists[a]

| | Control | | AL 721 | |
	ADTN	APO	ADTN	APO
Young	3059 ± 262 (3)	578 ± 100 (3)[b]	2219 ± 420 (4)	801 ± 40 (3)
Old	2169 ± 399 (4)	904 ± 45 (4)[b,c]	1651 ± 144 (3)	631 ± 94 (3)[c]

[a] Values given are the IC50 means $\pm$ SEM for the number of animals in parentheses. All animals were Wistar female rats. The young rats were 6 months old. The old animals were over 20 months of age.
[b] $p < 0.05$ in a two-tailed t test between young and old.
[c] $p < 0.05$ in a two-tailed t test between control and AL 721–treated tissue.

detergent with a natural phospholipid.[2] Reconstitution of the purified receptor into an optimal lipid environment may restore activity by promoting the natural conformation of the receptor.

Various investigators have manipulated membrane fluidity with ethanol, lecithin, or cholesterol hemisuccinate and, as a result, they have observed changes in the capacity of the several types of membrane receptors. Age-related changes in the responsiveness of striatal D2 receptors have, in fact, been indicated.[10] For example, the rate of synthesis of striatal dopamine receptors is reduced by 25–35% in senescent rats when compared to mature rats.[11] Studies of the striatal β-adrenergic receptors have revealed a population of cryptic receptors that are stored in the membrane and that are inaccessible to neurotransmitters and drugs; however, they may be unmasked upon fluidization of the membranes by phospholipid methylation.[12] Our present results indicate that striatal membrane fluidization with AL 721 does not result in the appearance of a cryptic population of receptors. These findings are in agreement with those of Henry et al.,[13] who used ethanol and cholesterol hemisuccinate, respectively, for the fluidization and rigidification of striatal membranes. Our findings also indicate that the D2 receptor in the aged rat has a lower affinity for apomorphine and spiroperidol when compared with the young counterparts. Fluidization of striatal membranes with the pharmacologically active lipid, AL 721, can restore the diminished affinity of the receptor for its ligands. Alteration of the chemical composition of the striatal membrane was reflected in the degree of membrane fluidity, which was measured by fluorescence polarization. In contrast to our findings, Henry et al. reported a diminished affinity of the D2 receptor for spiroperidol binding when striatal tissue was rigidified with cholesterol hemisuccinate. In addition, changes in membrane fluidity have been affected by temperature variations. Fluidization of rat striatal membranes by elevation of temperature from 1 °C to 37 °C has been shown to increase the affinity of the D2 receptor for ^{3}H-spiroperidol by tenfold (from 510 to 53 pM).[14]

AL 721 fluidization of various types of cell membranes points to a common mode of action. For example, AL 721 provides a rapid and effective means of achieving membrane fluidization in human peripheral blood lymphocytes.[6] The effect of AL 721 on rodent serotonin and opiate receptors has also been reported.[7,15] AL 721, when administered to alcohol- or morphine-dependent animals, reversed tolerance-dependent membrane rigidification and markedly reduced withdrawal symptoms.[16,17]

Furthermore, AL 721 has demonstrated antiviral effects against envelope viruses such as HTLV-III/LAV [18] and Herpes simplex viruses I and II (R. Whitley, personal communication). Approximately 50% of the HTLV-III/LAV membrane is composed of lipids with cholesterol and phospholipids present in a molar ratio of 0.6. It is thought that changes in the HTLV-III/LAV envelope microviscosity as a result of exposure to AL 721 resulted in orientational changes in envelope glycoproteins and thereby decreased the ability of the virus to bind or fuse (or both) with T4 lymphocytes.[18]

In physiological membranes, cholesterol acts as a primary lipid rigidifier that increases viscosity in the membrane lipid bilayer.[19,20] Decreasing the cholesterol-to-phospholipid (C/PL) ratio increases membrane fluidity. The optimal AL 721 concentration that produced membrane fluidity in brain striatal and cortical tissue was determined to be 0.5–1.0 mg/mL. The mechanism by which this fluidization may be accomplished is believed to be primarily through extraction of cholesterol from the plasma membrane. Incubation of mouse thymic lymphocytes with AL 721 resulted in a maximum membrane cholesterol extraction of 47%.[21] The mechanism of fluidization of striatal membranes with AL 721 is believed to result from the same mechanism.

REFERENCES

1. ANTONIAN, L., E. ANTONIAN, R. B. MURPHY & D. I. SCHUSTER. 1986. Studies on the use of a novel affinity matrix, sepharose amine-succinyl-amine haloperidol hemisuccinate, ASA-HHS, for purification of canine dopamine (D2) receptor. Life Sci. **38:** 1847–1858.
2. SENOGLES, S. E., N. AMLIAKY, A. L. JOHNSON & M. G. CARON. 1986. Affinity chromatography of the anterior pituitary D2-dopamine receptor. Biochemistry **25:** 749–753.
3. ANTONIAN, L., J. A. JOSEPH, L. R. MEYERSON, J. COUPET, D. I. SCHUSTER, H. E. KATERINOPOULOS, A. P. S. NARULA & C. E. RAUH. 1986. Striatally-mediated response of some structurally rigid analogues of dopamine. Pharmacol. Biochem. Behav. **24:** 253–258.
4. SHINITZKY, M. & Y. BARENHOLZ. 1978. Fluidity parameters of lipid regions determined by fluorescence polarization. Biochim. Biophys. Acta **525:** 367–394.
5. HUNT, W. A. 1985. Alcohol and Biological Membranes. Chapter 2. Guilford Press. New York.
6. LYTE, M. & M. SHINITZKY. 1985. A special lipid mixture for membrane fluidization. Biochim. Biophys. Acta **812:** 133–138.
7. HERON, D. S., M. ISRAELI, M. HERSHKOWITZ, D. SAMUEL & M. SHINITZKY. 1981. Lipid-induced modulation of opiate receptors in mouse brain membranes. Eur. J. Pharmacol. **72:** 361–364.
8. HERON, D., M. SHINITZKY, N. ZAMIR & D. SAMUEL. 1982. Adaptive modulations of brain membrane lipid fluidity in drug addiction and denervation supersensitivity. Biochem. Pharmacol. **31:** 2435–2438.
9. SHINITZKY, M. 1984. Membrane fluidity and cellular function. *In* Physiology of Membrane Fluidity. Vol. 1. M. Shinitzky, Ed.: 1–51. CRC Press. Boca Raton, Florida.
10. JOSEPH, J. A., G. S. ROTH & J. R. WHITAKER. 1983. Importance of striatal dopamine receptor changes in senescence. *In* Intervation in the Aging Process. Part B: Basic Research and Preclinical Screening, p. 187–202. Alan R. Liss. New York.
11. LEFF, S. E., R. GARIANO & I. CREESE. 1984. Dopamine receptor turnover rates in rat striatum are age dependent. Proc. Natl. Acad. Sci. USA **81:** 3910–3914.
12. CIMINO, M., G. VANTINI, S. ALGERI, G. CURATOLA, C. PEZZOLI & G. STRAMENTINOLI. 1984. Life Sci. **34:** 2029–2039.
13. HENRY, J. M. & G. S. ROTH. 1986. Modulation of rat striatal membrane fluidity: effects on age-related differences in dopamine receptor concentrations. Life Sci. **39:** 1223–1229.
14. ZAHNISER, N. R. & P. B. MOLINOFF. 1983. Thermodynamic differences between agonist and antagonist interactions with binding sites for ^{3}H-spiroperidol in rat striatum. Mol. Pharmacol. **23:** 303–309.
15. HERON, D. S., M. SHINITZKY, M. HERSHKOWITZ & D. SAMUEL. 1980. Lipid fluidity markedly modulates the binding of serotonin to mouse brain membranes. Proc. Natl. Acad. Sci. USA **77:** 7463–7467.
16. PACE, U. 1983. The role of membrane fluidity in alcohol addiction. Dissertation. Weizmann Institute of Science. Israel.
17. HERON, D., M. SHINITZKY & D. SAMUEL. 1983. Alleviation of drug withdrawal symptoms by treatment with a potent mixture of natural lipids. Eur. J. Pharmacol. **83:** 253–261.
18. SARIN, P. S., R. C. GALLO, D. I. SCHEER, F. CREWS & A. S. LIPPA. 1985. Effects of a novel compound (AL 721) on HTLV-III infectivity *in vitro*. N. Engl. J. Med. **313:** 1289–1290.
19. SCHROEDER, F. 1985. Fluorescence probes unravel asymmetric structure of membranes. *In* Subcellular Biochemistry. Vol. 11. D. B. Roodyn, Ed.: 51–101. Plenum. New York.
20. WOOD, W. G., R. STRONG, L. S. WILLIAMSON & R. W. WISE. 1984. Changes in lipid composition of cortical synaptosomes from different age groups of mice. Life Sci. **35:** 1947–1952.
21. SHINITZKY, M. 1984. Possible reversal of tissue aging by a lipid diet. Abstract. *In* Alzheimer Disease: Advances in Basic Research and Therapies. Zurich.

DISCUSSION OF THE PAPER

D. MORGAN (*University of Southern California, Los Angeles, CA*): I am very concerned about what you observed in your binding data. First of all, no one has really observed a consistent change in the affinity of these receptors with age. Your change is relatively small—that is, you are talking about a threefold change when you have really got a two log-order magnitude of responsivity. Therefore, when you analyzed those data, were you using the actual data in terms of nanomoles or did you convert them into the log-scale affinity? Secondly, why do you think that you did not see any change in B_{max}?

L. ANTONIAN (*Matrix Research Laboratories, New York, NY*): With regard to changes in the affinity, these are significant changes and they have been reported in the literature. In fact, studies on the rate of turnover of the dopamine receptor in young and old animals have noted significant changes that are, again, approximately the same fold in the affinity of the receptor for spiroperidol binding. There is also thermodynamic evidence that shows that as you increase the fluidity of the membrane by increasing the temperature of the membrane from 1 °C to 37 °C, you can lower the affinity of the D2 receptor for spiroperidol binding by tenfold (this was done in the early 80s by Molinoff and his collaborators). Hence, there is evidence in the literature that there are affinity changes in the young and old regarding the dopamine receptor.

As far as B_{max} is concerned, these animals did not have any motor deficits when they were tested on the inclined screen test. Thus, as a result, they did not have any drop in the number of receptors.

MORGAN: Receptors and behaviors, though, do not always correspond. Perhaps, it is really the coupling between the receptor and some receptor mechanism that is really mediating these effects that you have.

ANTONIAN: We are hoping by manipulation of the lipid composition to see if the coupling has been affected in the dopamine receptor as reported by others.

Neurodegenerative Disorders and Aging

Alzheimer's Disease and Parkinson's Disease — Common Ground[a]

R. W. HAMILL, E. CAINE, T. ESKIN, L. LAPHAM,
I. SHOULSON, AND T. H. McNEILL

Department of Neurology and Brain Research
University of Rochester School of Medicine and Dentistry
Rochester, New York 14603

The two most common neurodegenerative disorders of the elderly are Alzheimer's disease (AD) and Parkinson's disease (PD). Over the age of 65, these disorders may afflict 5% and 1% of the population, respectively,[1,2] and the incidence of both disorders appears to be age dependent to some degree.[1,2] Over the last six years, a number of studies have begun to address the potential overlap of these two disease states, and two broad clinical subgroups may be distilled from these observations: AD with and without "extrapyramidal signs", and PD with and without dementia. Because the frequency of "extrapyramidal signs" (EPS) in AD and the frequency of dementia in PD are both quite substantial, consideration has been given to viewing these two illnesses as part of a continuum. Thus, a collective view of these disorders would include the following spectrum: classical AD, AD with EPS, AD + PD, PD with dementia, and classical PD. Inherent in such a scheme would be that specific clinical-including neuropsychological, pathological, or neuroscientific markers would identify such subgroups and perhaps provide information regarding the specific substrates that underlie clinical expression of disease states. Additionally, such observations might possibly permit new understandings of why certain neuronal populations fail, either in isolation or collectively. Data are accruing, but further clinical-neuropathological and neuroscientific studies are needed.

This brief report will review selective literature that addresses these aforementioned issues and present preliminary data from the Rochester Alzheimer Disease Project that address, in part, the relationship between AD and the presence of EPS. The term, EPS, will be used throughout this report—largely because it tends to be entrenched in the clinical literature—but a more pathophysiologically based term would be striatal motor dysfunction because we are referring to disturbances within midbrain dopaminergic and striatal neuronal systems.

CLINICAL STUDIES

The presence of striatal motor dysfunction (extrapyramidal signs—EPS) in AD has been reported to vary from 28% to 92% (TABLE 1). If either paratonia or

[a] These efforts were supported by the Rochester Alzheimer Disease Program Project supported by NIA Grant No. 1 PO1 AG03644.

TABLE 1. Extrapyramidal Signs in Alzheimer's Disease

Series	Patient Number	Age of Onset	Duration	Neuroleptics	EPS	%
Chui *et al.* (1985)	146	68 ± 9.8	4.6 ± 3.5	22	43/124	35%
Mayeux *et al.* (1985)	121	65 ± 9.9	3.5 ± 2.3	12	34/121	28%
Molsa *et al.* (1984)	143	71 ± 1.0	3.7 ± 0.1	—	131/143	92%
Sulkava (1982)	36	60 ± 4	6.0 ± 3.8	—	22/36	61%
Sulkava (1982)	35	74 ± 7	3.9 ± 2	—	22/35	65%

bradykinesia alone is considered to be representative of EPS, then its prevalence may reach 100%. In most series, rigidity (which occurs in approximately 60% of AD patients) appears to be the major clinical feature used to identify EPS, although flexion posture (50%), dyskinesias (15–20%), and tremor (5–10%) may all exist.[3,4] Because aging may normally be associated with such changes in motor function as altered posture, increased resistance to passive stretch (including some degree of paratonia), slowness of movement, and essential tremor, slight alterations in striatal motor function in AD patients must be viewed as possibly being a normal variant. The presence of EPS appears to influence the course of patients with AD. Compared to AD patients without EPS, patients experiencing striatal motor disturbances appear to have an increased incidence of myoclonus, hallucinations, and psychotic symptoms; moreover, they appear to have increased and more progressive mental impairment.[5,6] Although the reported cases to date suggest that age, family history, and duration of illness are not clearly related to the presence of EPS, additional prospective longitudinal studies will be needed to clarify these issues.

TABLE 2. Studies Providing Evidence on the Prevalence of Dementia in Parkinson's Disease[a]

Survey	No. of Patients	% with Dementia	Method of Assessment
Patrick & Levy (1922)	146	0	?
Lewy (1923)	70	64	?
Jones (1949)	194	40	interview + MSE[b]
Pollack & Hornabrook (1966)	131	20	interview + MSE
Mindham (1970)	89	35	retrospective
Sacks *et al.* (1972)	72	21	"clinical picture"
Celesia & Wanamaker (1972)	153	40	MSE
Martin *et al.* (1973)	100	81	interview MSE
Rajput & Rodzilsky (1975)	125	28	MSE
Marttila & Rinne (1976)	444	29	MSE
Sweet *et al.* (1976)	100	56	MSE retrospective
Mindham *et al.* (1976)	40	28	MSE
Liberman *et al.* (1979)	520	32	interview + MSE
Sroka *et al.* (1981)	93	28	MSE
Mindham *et al.* (1982)	40	28	MSE
De Smet *et al.* (1982)	75	36	retrospective
Rajput *et al.* (1984)	138	31	retrospective
Total	2530	35–1%	

[a] Adapted from reference 12.
[b] MSE = mental state examination.

The presence of dementia in Parkinson's disease was originally doubted because James Parkinson reported that the shaking palsy was not associated with intellectual deterioration. Initial studies in the mid-1960s[7] and early 1970s, though, clearly established that intellectual impairment was present in Parkinson's syndrome.[8,9] These initial studies indicated that perhaps 20–25% of patients with PD would have cognitive impairment. A subsequent study in 1973 suggested that up to 70–80% of patients would have at least mild dementia.[10] A more recent pathologically based study indicated that mental status changes in 55% of patients.[11]

In an attempt to define just how commonly patients with PD experience dementia, Brown and Marsden[12] reviewed the clinical data from 17 studies.[12] Although sampling methods and patient populations varied in the 2,530 patients studied, the clinical profiles described dementia in from 0–20% to approximately 80% of patients (TABLE 2). These authors, as have others, point out that the inclusion of various patient groups with "pseudo-Parkinsonism" may have inflated some of these numbers and that the actual prevalence of dementia in PD may be closer to 25%. Although prospective clinical-neuropathological studies are indicated to specifically define this issue, it seems clear that a substantial group of patients with PD will experience dementia. Whether this dementia is actually coexistent AD or not, though, is unclear.

NEUROPATHOLOGICAL STUDIES

Traditionally, AD and PD are viewed to have quite specific neuropathological changes. AD is associated with neuronal loss in specific brain areas, neurofibrillary tangles, senile plaques, and granulovacuolar change. Because these histological alterations may occur in normal aging (especially within limbic structures and, in particular, the hippocampus), the neuropathological diagnosis rests on the amount and geographical distribution of AD change. Therefore, the changes are not qualitative, but quantitative.[13–15] Neuropathologically, PD is associated with neuronal loss, free melanin pigment, Lewy bodies, and reactive cellular elements (e.g., gliosis, macrophages) in the substantia nigra. Similar changes will also occur in the locus ceruleus and, to some degree, in the dorsal motor nucleus of the vagus.

Clinical pathological correlations between AD patients with and without EPS are essentially lacking. However, there are a number of studies that indicate that the substantia nigra may be altered in patients with AD. Depigmentation of the nigra, reactive cellular elements, and Lewy bodies have all been described in the substantia nigra of patients with AD.[16,17] These observations, though, must be viewed with care because some changes (Lewy bodies) within the nigra may be age related.[17] Thus, if the presence of Lewy bodies is utilized to indicate the presence of PD-like changes in patients with AD, then the present data do not strongly support a clear overlap of PD in patients with AD. At the other end of the spectrum, PD patients appear to exhibit a higher incidence of AD change and, in some series, these changes are significantly greater than the alterations observed in age-matched controls. In one series, senile plaques, neurofibrillary tangles, and granulovacuolar change are described in 85–90% of patients with PD, whereas age-matched control patients exhibit such changes in only 15–20% of the cases.[18] Another report indicates that the histological changes of AD are present in approximately 33% of PD patients, which is a prevalence six times that found in age-matched controls.[11] However, not all reports support these observations, and other studies raise the question that age-related changes may be sufficient to suggest the coexistence of the two pathologies.

Recently, studies of the cellular pathology of neurodegenerative disorders have focused on specific changes in cell morphology and morphometry, as well as on cytoskeletal pathology in specific neuronal populations.[13,14] Neuron numbers are decreased in AD in specific regions of the brain with deficits in the hippocampus approaching 50%, especially in the CA1 area.[19] Similarly, neurons in the nucleus basalis may exhibit a 45–50% reduction in number and locus ceruleus neurons decline by 65–70%.[14] In contrast, cell numbers in the substantia nigra appear to be reduced by only 10%.[13] In addition to these alterations, abnormalities in the dendritic arbor of neurons occur in AD. In normal aging, a proliferation of dendritic surface appears to occur, possibly in relation to the expectant loss of adjacent neurons, and this response may be viewed as a possible compensatory response.[20] In patients with AD, an increase in dendritic extent fails to occur.[20,21] Similar studies of dendritic response in other neurodegenerative disorders have not been performed.

NEUROCHEMICAL STUDIES

Neurochemical deficits in both AD and PD reflect alterations in subcortical and brain stem neuronal populations. Recent reviews address the spectrum of neurochemical deficits in AD[1,2,22] and PD.[2,23–25] Initially, PD was generally viewed as a specific deficit in the dopaminergic neurons of the substantia nigra that project to the striatum. More recently, the spectrum of chemical pathology has increased: noradrenergic, serotoninergic, cholinergic, and peptidergic systems may all be involved. The exact relationship of these multiple transmitter deficits to the clinical presentation is not entirely clear. A similar broad spectrum of chemical pathology also exists in AD: cholinergic, noradrenergic, serotoninergic, peptidergic, and possibly dopaminergic systems fail. Initial observations suggested that a specific cholinergic deficit may exist in AD, but evidence for a multineuronal disorder accumulated quite rapidly. There is now clear support that neurochemical deficits in AD may be influenced by the age of onset of the disease: older patients may have a relatively pure cholinergic disorder of the hippocampus and temporal lobe, whereas younger patients exhibit a multineuronal disorder.[26,27]

Although cholinergic deficits in AD and dopaminergic deficits in PD appear to underlie the major clinical dysfunctions of these disorders, substantial alterations exist in a number of neurotransmitter systems in both disorders and these deficits overlap. For instance, it is not entirely clear what neurochemical deficits underlie the clinical differences between patients with classical AD and patients with AD plus EPS. In contrast, there is some suggestion that patients with PD plus dementia may have cholinergic deficits in the temporal lobe and substantia innominata. Furthermore, the neocortical alterations appear to correlate with the degree of intellectual impairment.[24] Although some studies show substantial alterations in the nucleus basalis in PD,[28,29] the morphological correlates of these biochemical changes are not entirely clear because other reports suggest that these alterations may not correlate with dementia.[30]

In summary, it is apparent that many critical clinical, pathological, and neurochemical features of AD and PD overlap and that a substantial amount of common ground exists between these most common neurodegenerative disorders of the elderly. Our own investigations of these disorders are just beginning.

CURRENT RESEARCH

The Rochester Alzheimer Disease Project, which initiated its research efforts approximately two years ago, is designed as a clinical, neuropsychological, neuropathological, and neuroscientific correlative study. The fundamental design was based on the hypothesis that AD is a multineuronal disorder and that specific clinical subtypes might exist that would reflect relatively specific changes in brain pathology, morphology, and chemistry. These preliminary observations, which relate to the aforementioned topic of the common ground of AP and PD, will focus on identifying morphological alterations in AD patients with and without EPS and in patients with PD.

METHODS AND MATERIALS

Tissues containing the basal ganglia and substantia nigra were collected at the time of autopsy from deceased patients diagnosed as having either Alzheimer's or Parkinson's disease. Control tissues were taken from cases without neurological or neuropsychiatric disorders. The time between death and tissue collection varied between four and six hours. Tissues used for light immunocytochemistry were immerse-fixed in 10% formalin, while fresh tissue used for Golgi staining was prepared by the Golgi Cox method according to the procedure of Van der Loos.[31] Tissues used for immunocytochemical staining were cut at 30 μm in the frontal plane on a Vibratome and were stained immunocytochemically for tyrosine hydroxylase following the procedure of Sternberger.[32] Tissue sections containing the striatum used for Golgi staining were cut in a coronal plane at 200 microns, and slides were coded so that it would be unknown during data gathering which slide came from which brain. A sample of 20 striatal neurons (based on a predetermined 95% confidence interval) was randomly chosen from each brain from among all well-impregnated cells. We examined only cells whose somas were in the center one-third of the section and whose dendrites were unobscured by overlying glia, blood vessels, other neurons, or nonspecific deposits of stain. Based on previous observations, terminal dendritic segments were required to be tapered at their tips and to lack spines, thus indicating the complete impregnation of the dendrite. For our study, medium spiny (medium spiny I) neurons were analyzed. Profiles of the cell soma and dendrites were traced using a 40× objective lens and a camera lucida drawing tube. Cells were entered into an IBM microcomputer system using a digitizing tablet and DAN software.[33] Analysis of dendritic parameters of medium spiny I neurons included total and terminal segment lengths, as well as the number of dendritic segments per neuron.

RESULTS

Qualitative examination of the striatum showed that medium spiny (MS) I neurons were characterized by a round or ovoid cell body and that they represented the majority of all impregnated neurons in the putamen and caudate nuclei. MS neurons had four to eight primary dendrites that emerged from the cell soma, with subsequent branches radiating in all directions. MS neurons had smooth primary dendrites with increasing spin density on secondary and distal segments. Although the density of cellular impregnation varied from case to case, more impregnated neurons appeared in control than in the PD group. Medium spiny neurons were always the most prevalent cell type in the striatum and were distributed equally between the putamen and caudate nucleus. Many dendrites and most axon segments had irregular contours with focal swellings.

For both control and Parkinson's disease brain, we identified five populations of

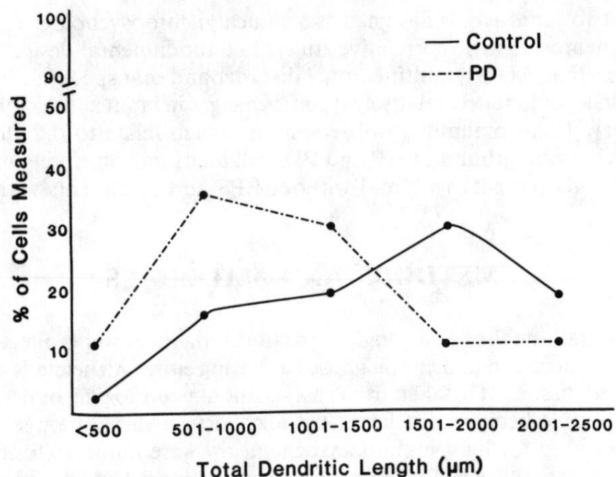

FIGURE 1. Distribution of medium spiny neurons in the striatum of control and Parkinson's diseased brain. There is a significant increase in neurons with small dendritic arbors in Parkinson's disease.

MS neurons based on their total and terminal lengths. The smallest population was a group of cells with short dendrites; the total dendritic length was less than 500 μm. The largest population in control brains had robust dendritic arbors between 1500–2000 μm (FIGURE 1). In general, our quantitative data showed the MS neurons in the putamen of normally aged individuals had longer and more branching dendrites than those with Parkinson's disease (FIGURE 2). Medium spiny neurons in parkinsonian brain were atrophic with severely degenerated dendritic arbors and few dendritic spines. In addition, Parkinson's disease cells were characterized by an overall loss of total and terminal dendritic length, as well as an increase in the number of small, shrunken

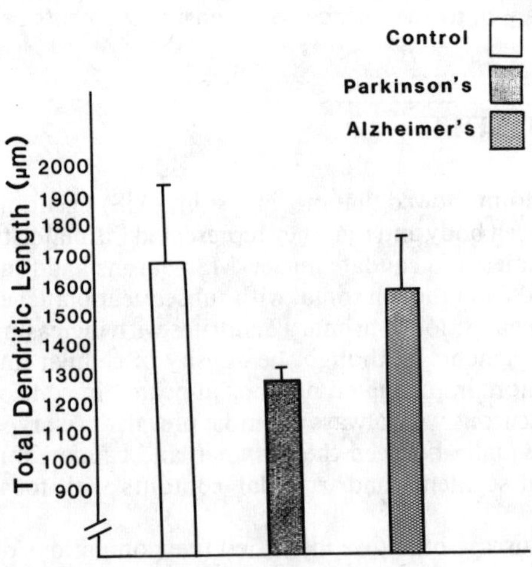

FIGURE 2. Total dendritic length of MS neurons in control, Parkinson's diseased brain, and Alzheimer's diseased brain. There is a significant decrease in total dendritic length in Parkinson's disease, but not in Alzheimer's disease.

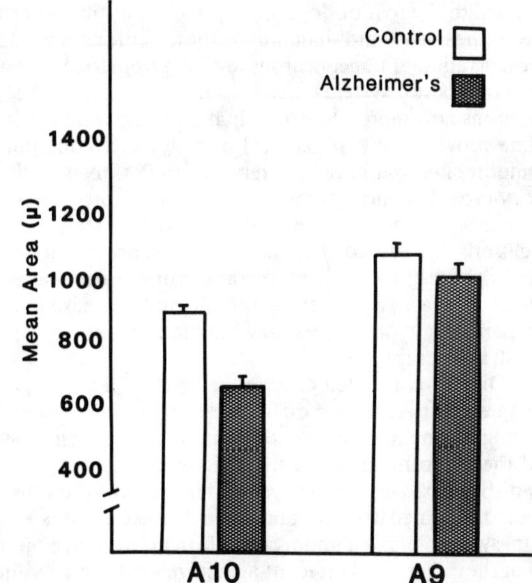

FIGURE 3. Mean cross-sectional area of A9 and A10 neurons taken from control and Alzheimer's diseased brain. Mean ± SEM.

atrophic cells (FIGURES 1 and 2). In Alzheimer's brain, there was also a trend towards a decrease in the total dendritic length of MS neurons of the striatum; however, this was not significantly different from controls (FIGURE 2).

Brown reaction product localizing the antiserum against tyrosine hydroxylase was found both in perikarya and processes of medium-sized neurons of the pars compacta of the substantia nigra and in small-sized neurons of the ventral tegmental area of Tsai. These neuron populations correspond respectively to the A9 and A10 cell groups described by Dahlstrom and Fuxe[34] in the rodent. Immunoreactive fibers of the nigro-striatal and mesolimbic dopamine systems course dorsomedially from these nuclei towards the midline and they ascend as part of the medial forebrain bundle to the striatum or cortex (or both). Qualitative examination shows that while the staining intensity of A9 and A10 neurons is not significantly different between control and Alzheimer's diseased brain, there is a significant difference in the size of A10 neurons. As shown in FIGURE 3, there is a significant decline in the mean cross-sectional area of A10 neurons, while the mean cross-sectional area of A9 neurons remains unchanged. If Alzheimer's patients are divided into cases without EPS and cases with EPS, the mean cross-sectional areas of A9 cells are significantly different. Similarly, A10 neurons from Alzheimer's cases with EPS showed the most significant reduction in mean cross-sectional area. The observations, though, are quite preliminary because the number of patients studied is limited. Nevertheless, these observations support the concept that specific neural substrates may underlie disease heterogeneity.

DISCUSSION

These data show that there is a significant regression of dendritic arbors of medium spiny neurons in Parkinson's disease. Whether this apparent failure of growth is directly related to the loss of dopaminergic afferent fibers or other projection neuron systems from the cortex and thalamus to these neurons is not known. However, transneuronal degeneration of target neurons resulting from lesions of afferent inputs has been reported in a number of systems. In addition, because it has been shown that the medium spiny neurons now represent a principal target population for dopaminergic afferents,[35] our data provide a morphological basis for the reduction of dopaminergic postsynaptic binding sites that have been reported in Parkinson's disease.[36] In addition, our findings may provide a morphological basis for the progressive nature of Parkinson's disease, as well as for the ultimate failure of L-dopa therapy. It may be suggested that surviving cells are still able to alter their dendritic arbor during the initial stages of the disease and thus respond to drug therapy. Furthermore, as the disease progresses, neuronal death increases and there is a significant decrease in the number of neurons to which dopaminergic precursors may interact. This, of course, results in the ultimate failure of drug therapy.

Disease-correlated changes in the A10 but not A9 neurons in Alzheimer's disease suggest that AD has a differential effect on selected cell populations of dopamine-containing neurons of the midbrain that have been shown to project to different regions of the striatum and cortex. Previous studies using retrograde transport of the horse-radish peroxidase have shown that neurons of the substantia nigra project topographically to the neostriatum and cortex.[37] Because it is known that mesolimbic nigrostriatal systems play an important role in motor and cognitive functioning, it is suggested that the differential effect of age-correlated changes and subsets of dopamine neurons of the midbrain may, in part, underlie the wide range of motor functions and cognitive deficits that have been associated with Alzheimer's disease. In addition, if our preliminary observations hold, a change in the A9 neurons in Alzheimer's disease cases with EPS will indicate that specific neural substrates may define disease heterogeneity.

REFERENCES

1. KATZMAN, R. 1986. Alzheimer's disease. N. Engl. J. Med. **315**(15): 964–973.
2. QUINN, N. P., M. N. ROSSOR & C. D. MARSDEN. 1986. Dementia and Parkinson's disease — pathological and neurochemical considerations. Br. Med. Bull. **42**: 86–90.
3. SULKAVA, R. 1982. Alzheimer's disease and senile dementia of Alzheimer type. Acta Neurol. Scand. **65**: 636–650.
4. MÖLSA, P. K., R. J. MARTTILA & U. K. RINNE. 1984. Extrapyramidal signs in Alzheimer's disease. Neurology **34**(7): 1114–1116.
5. MAYEUX, R., Y. STERN & S. SPANTON. 1985. Heterogeneity in dementia of the Alzheimer type: evidence of subgroups. Neurology **35**: 453–461.
6. CHUI, H. C., E. L. TENG, V. W. HENDERSON & A. C. MOY. 1985. Clinical subtypes of dementia of the Alzheimer type. Neurology **35**(11): 1544–1550.
7. POLLOCK, M. & R. W. HORNABROOK. 1966. The prevalence, natural history and dementia of Parkinson's disease. Brain **89**: 429–448.
8. LORANGER, A. W., H. GOODELL, F. H. McDOWELL *et al.* 1972. Intellectual impairment in Parkinson's syndrome. Brain **95**: 405–412.
9. CELESIA, G. G. & W. WANAMAKER. 1972. Psychiatric disturbances in Parkinson's disease. Dis. Nerv. Syst. **33**: 577–583.
10. MARTIN, W. E., R. B. LOEWENSON, J. A. RESCH & A. B. BAKER. 1973. Parkinson's disease. A clinical analysis of 100 patients. Neurology **23**: 783–790.
11. BOLLER, F., T. MIZUTANI, U. ROESSMAN & P. GAMBETTI. 1980. Parkinson disease, dementia, and Alzheimer's disease: clinicopathological correlations. Ann. Neurol. **7**: 329–335.
12. BROWN, R. G. & C. D. MARSDEN. 1984. How common is dementia in Parkinson's disease? Lancet **2**: 1262–1265.

13. MANN, D. M. A. 1986. The neuropathology of Alzheimer's disease: a review with pathogenetic, aetiological, and therapeutic considerations. Mech. Ageing Dev. **31:** 213–255.
14. PRICE, D. L., P. J. WHITEHOUSE & R. G. STRUBLE. 1986 (January). Cellular pathology in Alzheimer's and Parkinson's diseases. Trends in Neuroscience.
15. PRICE, D. L. 1986. New perspectives on Alzheimer's disease. Annu. Rev. Neurosci. **9:** 489–512.
16. FORNO, L. S. 1981. Pathology of Parkinson's disease. *In* Butterworths International Medical Reviews, Neurology 2. Movement Disorders. C. D. Marsden & S. Fahn, Eds. Butterworths. London.
17. JELLINGER, K. & W. GRISWOLD. 1982. Cerebral atrophy in Parkinson syndrome. Exp. Brain Res. (suppl. 5): 26–35.
18. HAKIM, A. M. & G. MATHIESON. 1979. Dementia in Parkinson's disease. A neuropathologic study. Neurology **29:** 1209–1214.
19. BALL, M. J. 1977. Neuronal loss, neurofibrillary tangles and granulovacuolar degeneration in hippocampal cortex of ageing and demented patients. Acta Neuropathol. **42:** 73–80.
20. BUELL, S. J. & P. D. COLEMAN. 1981. Quantitative evidence for selective dendritic growth in normal human aging but not in senile dementia. Brain Res. **214:** 23–41.
21. BUELL, S. J. & P. D. COLEMAN. 1979. Dendritic growth in the aged human brain and failure of growth in senile dementia. Science **206:** 854–856.
22. TERRY, R. D. & P. DAVIES. 1980. Dementia of the Alzheimer type. Annu. Rev. Neurosci. **3:** 77–95.
23. HORNYKIEWICZ, O. 1981. Brain neurotransmitter changes in Parkinson's disease. *In* Butterworths International Medical Reviews, Neurology 2. C. D. Marsden & S. Fahn, Eds.: 41–58. Butterworths. London.
24. DUBOIS, B., M. RUBERG, F. JAVOY-AGID, A. PLOSKA & Y. AGID. 1983. A subcortico-cortical cholinergic system is affected in Parkinson's disease. Brain Res. **288:** 213–218.
25. SCATTON, V., F. JAVOY-AGID, L. ROQUIER, B. DUBOIS & Y. AGID. 1983. Reduction of cortical dopamine, noradrenaline, serotonin and their metabolites in Parkinson's disease. Brain Res. **275:** 321–328.
26. ROSSOR, M. N., L. L. IVERSEN, G. P. REYNOLDS, C. Q. MOUNTJOY & M. ROTH. 1984. Neurochemical characteristics of early and late onset types of Alzheimer's disease. Br. Med. J. **288:** 961–964.
27. FRANCIS, P. T., A. M. PALMER, N. R. SIMS, D. M. BOWEN, A. N. DAVISON, M. M. ESIRI, D. NEARY, J. S. SNOWDEN & G. K. WILCOCK. 1985. Neurochemical studies of early-onset Alzheimer's disease. N. Engl. J. Med. **313**(1): 7–11.
28. WHITEHOUSE, P. J., J. C. HEDREEN, C. L. WHITE III & D. L. PRICE. 1983. Basal forebrain neurons in the dementia of Parkinson disease. Ann. Neurol. **13**(3): 243–248.
29. ROGERS, J. D., D. BROGAN & S. S. MIRRA. 1985. The nucleus basalis of Meynert in neurological disease: a quantitative morphological study. Ann. Neurol. **17**(2): 163–170.
30. NAKANO, I. & A. HIRANO. 1984. Parkinson's disease: neuron loss in the nucleus basalis without concomitant Alzheimer's disease. Ann. Neurol. **15:** 415–418.
31. VAN DER LOOS, H. 1956. Une combinaison de deux vieilles methodes histologiques pour le systeme nerveux centra. Monatsschr. Psychiatr. Neurol. **132:** 330–334.
32. STERNBERGER, L. A. 1974. Immunocytochemistry. Prentice–Hall. Englewood Cliffs, New Jersey.
33. MOYER, A., V. MOYER & P. D. COLEMAN. 1985. An inexpensive PC based system for quantification of neuronal processes. Soc. Neurosci. **11:** 261.18.
34. DAHLSTROM, A. & K. FUXE. 1964. Evidence for the existence of monamine-containing neurons in the central nervous system. I. Demonstration of monamines in the cell bodies of brain stem neurons. Acta Physiol. Scand. **62:** 1–55.
35. FREUND, T. F., J. F. POWELL & A. D. SMITH. 1984. Tyrosine hydroxylase-immunoreactive boutons in synaptic contrast with identified striatonigral neurons with particular reference to dendritic spines. Neuroscience **13**(4): 1189–1215.
36. SEVERSON, J. A., J. MAECUSSON, B. WINBLAD & C. E. FINCH. 1982. Age-correlated loss of dopaminergic binding sites in human basal ganglia. J. Neurochem. **39:** 1623–1631.
37. MOORE, R. Y. & F. E. BLOOM. 1978. Central catecholamine neuron systems: anatomy and physiology of the dopamine systems. *In* Annual Review of Neuroscience, Vol. 1. W. M. Cowan, Z. W. Hall & E. R. Handel, Eds.: 126–169. Annual Reviews. Palo Alto, California.

DISCUSSION OF THE PAPER

D. MORGAN (*University of Southern California, Los Angeles, CA*): We have recently analyzed 180 samples of caudate putamen from Alzheimer's disease and in control patients and basically support everything you said — that is, the change in the dopamine system both postsynaptically and presynaptically is extremely small and probably not statistically significant in Alzheimer's disease.

R. HAMILL (*University of Rochester School of Medicine and Dentistry, Rochester, NY*): If you look in the literature, there are reports of dopamine receptors being altered in the striatum in Alzheimer's disease; however, a lot of times the patient population for that study is not entirely clear. On the other hand, in many other studies, there is not much of a change reported at all.

MORGAN: We see absolutely no change of D2 or D1 receptors in Alzheimer's disease. As I said, we have 180 samples from five different sources, so there is probably a 20% loss in dopamine and a 50% loss in serotonin in that area, but there is nothing that would account for any major motor side effect.

Aged Mice Show More Severe Motor Deficits and Morphological Changes following MPTP Treatment than Their Younger Counterparts[a]

M. GUPTA[b] AND B. K. GUPTA

Department of Neurobiology and Anatomy
University of Rochester School of Medicine
Rochester, New York 14642

Aging is associated with decreased dopamine levels in the striatum.[1] This decrease is markedly enhanced in patients with Parkinson's disease,[2] which is a neurodegenerative disorder of elderly humans characterized by degeneration of the nigrostriatal dopaminergic and other monoaminergic systems. McGeer *et al.*[3] reported that substantia nigra neurons diminish in number with age, thereby leading to diminished levels and synthesis of dopamine in terminal fields. MPTP is known to cause destruction of the nigrostriatal dopamine system in humans, in nonhuman primates, and in rodents.[4-10] The present study was undertaken to investigate whether MPTP treatment in aged mice, when superimposed upon the normal age-related alterations in some monoamine systems, results in more severe damage to the nigrostriatal system and other dopaminergic systems. Male C57BL/6 mice at 2 and 21 months of age were injected intraperitoneally with serial doses of MPTP at 15 mg/kg body weight. Mice were sacrificed by decapitation. The brains were removed and processed for fluorescence histochemistry using the sucrose–potassium phosphate–glyoxylic acid (SPG) method.[11]

Aged mice treated with MPTP showed marked motor dysfunction characterized by a striking paucity of movements, a stiffness of hind limbs, and an initial resting tremor of the whole body. Such symptoms were either less evident or not present in the young adults treated with MPTP. Neuroanatomical studies revealed a decreased number of fluorescent cell bodies in the substantia nigra pars compacta in both the young adult and aged mice (FIGURES 1a–d). In addition, there was a marked reduction in the number and intensity of fluorescent dopaminergic cell bodies in the ventral tegmental area in treated aged mice, whereas this region remained unaltered in the treated young mice (FIGURES 2a–d). These studies suggest that aged mice are more sensitive to MPTP treatment than the young adult counterparts and show more severe motor deficits and neuroanatomical changes following MPTP treatment.

[a] This work was supported by USPHS Grant Nos. RO3-MH41435 and R23-NS24291.

[b] Current address: Department of Psychiatry, Louisiana State University School of Medicine, Shreveport, Louisiana 71130.

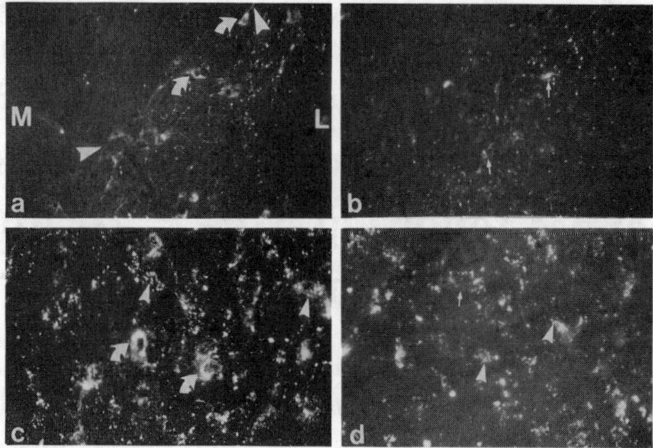

FIGURE 1. Sections through the substantia nigra from (a) control young adult mouse, (b) MPTP-treated young adult, (c) 21-month-old normal control, and (d) MPTP-treated 21-month-old mouse. All were processed for fluorescence histochemistry using the SPG method. Large arrows in FIGURES 1a and 1c point to fluorescent perikarya in the dopaminergic neurons of the substantia nigra pars compacta. Also, note the presence of fluorescent processes (large arrowheads). The number and intensity of fluorescence in the treated animals (FIGURES 1b and 1d) appear to be reduced (small arrows). In addition, the 21-month-old animals show a large amount of granular lipofuscin pigment (small arrowheads). M = Medial and L = Lateral, which point to the orientation for all the photomicrographs. FIGURES 1a and 1b are magnified ×106, while FIGURES 1c and 1d are magnified ×212. (The whole figure, though, is reduced to 55%.)

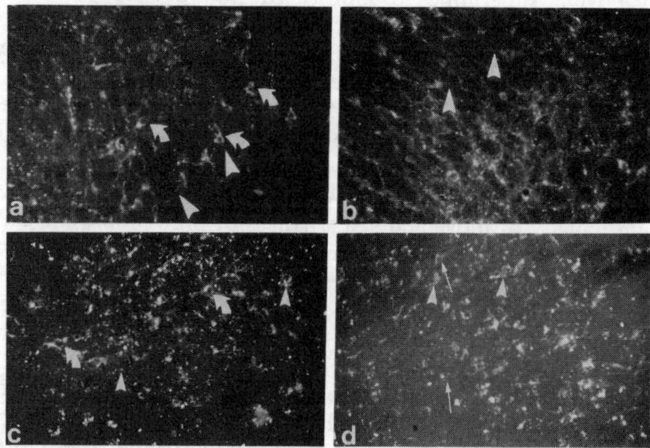

FIGURE 2. Sections through the ventral tegmental area from (a) control young adult mouse, (b) MPTP-treated young adult, (c) 21-month-old normal control, and (d) MPTP-treated 21-month-old mouse. Note the presence of a large number of fluorescent profiles (large arrows) and processes (large arrowheads) in the young adult control (FIGURE 1a) and in the MPTP-treated group (FIGURE 1b). The 21-month-old group shows a large amount of lipofuscin pigment (small arrowheads) in both the control and treated group. The 21-month-old treated animals also show reduced intensity and number of fluorescent cell bodies (small arrows) compared to the control aged animals (×106). (The whole figure, though, is reduced to 55%.)

REFERENCES

1. CARLSSON, A. & B. WINBLAD. 1976. J. Neurol. Transm. **38:** 271–276.
2. HORNYKIEWICZ, O. 1982. *In* Movement Disorders. C. D. Marsden & S. Fahn, Eds.: 41–58. Butterworths. London.
3. MCGEER, P. L., E. G. MCGEER & J. S. SUZUKI. 1977. Arch. Neurol. **34:** 33–35.
4. DAVIS, G. C., A. C. WILLIAMS, S. P. MARKEY, M. H. EBERT, E. D. CAINE, C. M. REICHERT & I. J. KOPIN. 1979. Psychiatry Res. **1:** 249–254.
5. LANGSTON, J. W., P. BALLARD, J. W. TETRUD & I. IRWIN. 1983. Science **219:** 979–980.
6. BURNS, R. S., C. C. CHIUEH, S. P. MARKEY, M. H. EBERT, D. M. JACOBOWITZ & I. J. KOPIN. 1983. Proc. Natl. Acad. Sci. USA **80:** 4546–4550.
7. BURNS, R. S., S. P. MARKEY, J. M. PHILLIPS & C. C. CHIUEH. 1984. Can. J. Neurol. Sci. **11:** 166–168.
8. HEIKKILA, R. E., A. HESS & R. C. DUVOISIN. 1984. Science **224:** 1451–1453.
9. GUPTA, M., D. L. FELTEN & D. M. GASH. 1984. Brain Res. Bull. **13:** 737–742.
10. GUPTA, M., D. L. FELTEN & S. Y. FELTEN. 1985. *In* MPTP—A Neurotoxin Producing a Parkinsonian Syndrome. S. P. Markey, N. Castagnoli, Jr., A. J. Trevor & I. J. Kopin, Eds.: 399–402. Academic Press. New York.
11. DE LA TORRE, J. C. 1980. Neurosci. Lett. **17:** 339–340.

Tendon Reflexes in the Aged

GARY KAMEN AND DAVID M. KOCEJA

Motor Control Laboratory
Indiana University
Bloomington, Indiana 47405

Previous reports of neurological examinations in older adults indicated that these patients usually exhibited a less vigorous tendon reflex than younger individuals.[1,2] However, deVries *et al.*[3] measured the Achilles tendon reflex and obtained no significant difference between the young and old groups. This report presents the first of a series of experiments designed to determine the quality of segmental reflex function in older adults.

Subjects consisted of nine aged (mean age = 72.5 years) and ten college-age (mean age = 25.4 years) subjects. Patellar tendon reflexes were tested while the subject was seated, blindfolded, and listening to music through headphones. The tendon tap stimulus was delivered using a rubber-tipped solenoid capable of delivering a blow that was supramaximal for the reflex response. Consistent force taps were assured by monitoring the output of a piezoelectric force transducer mounted in series with the solenoid. Reflex force was measured by strain gauges mounted on a plate placed in front of the ankle. In addition to the assessment of the right leg patellar tendon reflexes, a conditioning stimulus was applied to the left patellar tendon using an identical solenoid apparatus, which was followed by a test reflex stimulus applied to the right patellar tendon at intertap intervals of 0, 25, 50, 75, 150, and 300 ms. Peak force and contraction time (CT), which is the interval between reflex force onset and maximal reflex force, were recorded on a pen recorder.

Tendon reflex force was 57% higher in the old than in the young subjects ($p < 0.05$). CT was also longer in the old (79.0 ms) than in the young (74.6 ms) subjects ($p < 0.05$). Therefore, the aged subjects produced a greater force over a longer period of time.

The conditioning reflex stimulus applied to the contralateral patellar tendon affected the right tendon reflex at both short and long intertap intervals. At short latencies (about 25 ms), there was a depression of the tendon reflex. At longer latencies (75 and 150 ms), an enhancement of the tendon reflex was observed. This enhancement was especially great in the old subjects at 150 ms following the conditioning stimulus.

There are two important observations that can be made from these data. First, aged individuals with no clinical neurological deficit manifest greater patellar tendon reflexes than young subjects; and, second, long latency responses to a contralateral conditioning stimulus are different in the two subject groups. At present, we have not determined whether the differences in the control tendon reflex can be attributed to age-related neuromuscular or connective tissue changes, or whether the long latency response is of spinal or supraspinal origin. However, these findings show that the conditioned tendon reflex protocol, in concert with other experimental strategies, may be useful in examining reflex function in aged individuals.

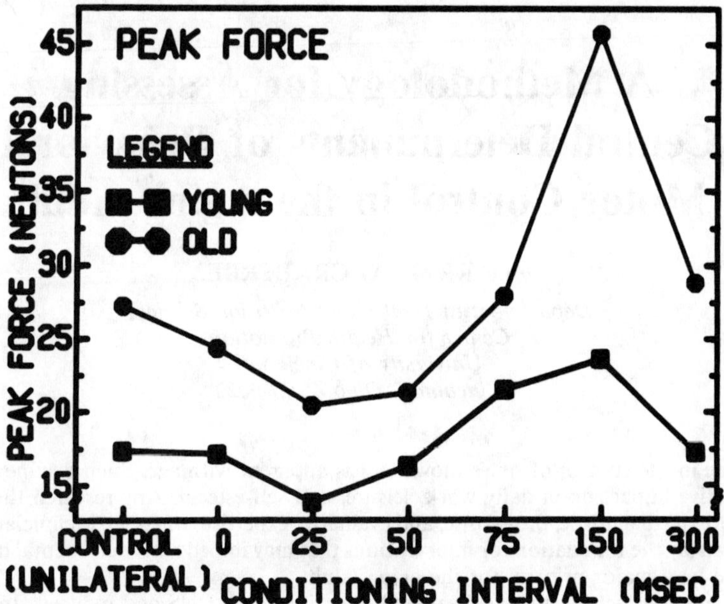

FIGURE 1. Peak reflex force during the control (right tendon reflex only) trials and during the trials in which a tendon tap stimulus was applied to the contralateral leg prior to a test stimulus in the right leg. Note that the reflex force was always greater in the old than in the young subjects.

REFERENCES

1. BHATIA, S. P. & R. E. IRVINE. 1973. Electrical recording of the ankle jerk in old age. Gerontol. Clin. **15:** 357–360.
2. MILNE, J. S. & J. WILLIAMSON. 1972. The ankle jerk in older people. Gerontol. Clin. **14:** 86–88.
3. DEVRIES, H. A., R. A. WISWELL, G. T. ROMERO & E. HECKATHORNE. 1985. Changes with age in monosynaptic reflexes elicited by mechanical and electrical stimulation. Am. J. Phys. Med. **64:** 71–81.

A Methodology for Assessing Central Determinants of Behavioral Motor Control in the Aging Adult

DARRYL A. CRABTREE

Department of Health and Nutrition Services
Center for Health Promotion
University of Cincinnati
Cincinnati, Ohio 45221-0022

Decline in the control of one's movement is apparent with age. Such decline exerts a negative impact upon daily work, leisure, and self-esteem. Any research that can improve the diagnostic, prognostic, and evaluative expertises of geriatric clinicians and that can lay the foundation for interventions that may impede this detrimental decline should be a major priority for the aging adult.

Peripheral factors such as decreased integrity of the PNS and reduced strength, flexibility, and endurance play integral roles in such decline. Overt motor disorders often implicate specific motor areas of the CNS, such as the motor cortex, premotor cortex, basal ganglia, red nucleus, cerebellum, and pyramidal and extrapyramidal tracts. However, motor decline also may be the result of generalized aging of the CNS.

Therefore, an apparent need exists for the development of a safe, noninvasive methodology for assessing what may be termed as "behavioral motor control". Operationally, this construct may be thought of as the percursive influence of psychological information-processing mechanisms on motor output. The ability to measure behavioral motor control could have a positive impact on the understanding of "normalcy" in aging. If so, a criteria then would exist that could enhance the expertises of geriatric clinicians in their diagnostic, prognostic, and evaluative work with "abnormal aging" and dementia.

The development of such an innovative assessment methodology is a major priority at the University of Cincinnati Center for Health Promotion. The Battery of Behavioral Motor Control is being designed to assess the central determinants of behavioral motor control in the elderly. The battery uses motor response data from 20 test items to assess neurobehavioral mechanisms that are precursive to motor output. The battery is comprehensive in that it tests numerous information-processing mechanisms. The battery is balanced in that each information mechanism is assessed separately with regard to its temporal and spatial parameters. The battery is discriminative in that it separates central from peripheral control and maximizes the among-subject variance.

A long-range research agenda has been initiated. All protocols and instrumentation have been completed, validation research is under way, and the establishment of standardized norms are to begin soon. The assessment methodology will help to provide behavioral markers of normal aging, which will, in turn, facilitate improved (1) diagnoses of abnormal aging, (2) "staging" and prognoses of the diseases of abnormal aging, and (3) criteria for evaluation of biomedical and behavioral interventions. Clinical data from cross-sectional and longitudinal studies (made possible with the use of validated protocols, instrumentation, and normative measures) will provide a discriminant analysis data base invaluable to the geriatric clinician. Furthermore, the instruments and protocols of this battery will be studied with the elderly as possible means of rehabilitation, remediation, and maintenance of the functional status of these precursive central determinants of motor control.

Index of Contributors